国际经典内科学教科书

第10版
Cecil Essentials of Medicine
希氏内科学精要
中英双语版

原　著　**Edward J. Wing, MD, FACP, FIDSA**
Former Dean of Medicine and Biological Sciences
Professor of Medicine
Warren Alpert Medical School of Brown University, Providence, Rhode Island

Fred J. Schiffman, MD, MACP
Sigal Family Professor of Humanistic Medicine
Vice Chair, Department of Medicine
Warren Alpert Medical School of Brown University, Providence, Rhode Island

中英双语版　编辑委员会　主任委员　王　辰

第 4 分册
胃肠疾病·肝脏与胆道系统疾病

主　译　房静远　杨爱明　贾继东

北京大学医学出版社

XISHI NEIKEXUE JINGYAO（DI 10 BAN） DI 4 FENCE　WEICHANG JIBING・GANZANG YU DANDAO XITONG JIBING（ZHONGYING SHUANGYU BAN）

图书在版编目（CIP）数据

希氏内科学精要：第 10 版．第 4 分册，胃肠疾病・肝脏与胆道系统疾病：汉、英／（美）爱德华・温（Edward J. Wing），（美）弗雷德・谢夫曼（Fred J. Schiffman）原著；房静远，杨爱明，贾继东主译．-- 北京：北京大学医学出版社，2024. 11. -- ISBN 978-7-5659-3263-2

Ⅰ. R5

中国国家版本馆 CIP 数据核字第 2024FS8085 号

北京市版权局著作权合同登记号：图字：01-2024-4518

Elsevier (Singapore) Pte Ltd.
3 Killiney Road, #08-01 Winsland House I, Singapore 239519
Tel: (65) 6349-0200; Fax: (65) 6733-1817

Cecil Essentials of Medicine, Tenth Edition
Copyright © 2022 by Elsevier, Inc. All rights are reserved, including those for text and data mining, AI training, and similar technologies.
Publisher's note: Elsevier takes a neutral position with respect to territorial disputes or jurisdictional claims in its published content, including in maps and institutional affiliations.
Previous editions copyrighted 2016, 2010, 2007, 2004, 2001, 1997, 1993, 1990, and 1986.
ISBN-13: 978-0-323-72271-1

This translation of Cecil Essentials of Medicine, Tenth Edition by Edward J. Wing and Fred J. Schiffman was undertaken by Peking University Medical Press and is published by arrangement with Elsevier (Singapore) Pte Ltd.
Cecil Essentials of Medicine, Tenth Edition by Edward J. Wing and Fred J. Schiffman 由北京大学医学出版社进行翻译，并根据北京大学医学出版社与爱思唯尔（新加坡）私人有限公司的协议约定出版。
《希氏内科学精要（第 10 版）第 4 分册　胃肠疾病・肝脏与胆道系统疾病（中英双语版）》（房静远　杨爱明　贾继东　主译）
ISBN: 978-7-5659-3263-2
Copyright © 2024 by Elsevier (Singapore) Pte Ltd. and Peking University Medical Press.
All rights reserved. No part of this publication may be reproduced or transmitted in any form or by any means, electronic or mechanical, including photocopying, recording, or any information storage and retrieval system, without permission in writing from Elsevier (Singapore) Pte Ltd. and Peking University Medical Press.

注　意

本译本由北京大学医学出版社独立完成。相关从业及研究人员必须凭借其自身经验和知识对文中描述的信息数据、方法策略、搭配组合、实验操作进行评估和使用。由于医学科学发展迅速，临床诊断和给药剂量尤其需要经过独立验证。在法律允许的最大范围内，爱思唯尔、译文的原文作者、原文编辑及原文内容提供者均不对译文或因产品责任、疏忽或其他操作造成的人身及（或）财产伤害及（或）损失承担责任，亦不对由于使用文中提到的方法、产品、说明或思想而导致的人身及（或）财产伤害及（或）损失承担责任。

Published in China by Peking University Medical Press under special arrangement with Elsevier (Singapore) Pte Ltd. This edition is authorized for sale in the People's Republic of China only, excluding Hong Kong SAR, Macau SAR and Taiwan. Unauthorized export of this edition is a violation of the contract.

希氏内科学精要（第 10 版）　第 4 分册　胃肠疾病・肝脏与胆道系统疾病（中英双语版）

主　　译：房静远　杨爱明　贾继东
出版发行：北京大学医学出版社
地　　址：（100191）北京市海淀区学院路 38 号　北京大学医学部院内
电　　话：发行部 010-82802230；图书邮购 010-82802495
网　　址：http://www.pumpress.com.cn
E - m a i l：booksale@bjmu.edu.cn
印　　刷：北京信彩瑞禾印刷厂
经　　销：新华书店
策划编辑：高　瑾
责任编辑：梁　洁　　责任校对：靳新强　　责任印制：李　啸
开　　本：889 mm×1194 mm　1/16　印张：17　字数：630 千字
版　　次：2024 年 11 月第 1 版　2024 年 11 月第 1 次印刷
书　　号：ISBN 978-7-5659-3263-2
定　　价：120.00 元
版权所有，违者必究
（凡属质量问题请与本社发行部联系退换）

中英双语版 编辑委员会

主任委员

王　辰

委　员（按姓氏笔画排序）

王　洁	王伊龙	王建祥	巴　一	代华平	宁　光	宁晓红	朱　兰
任景怡	刘海鹰	李小鹰	李梦涛	李雪梅	杨爱明	张福杰	郑金刚
房静远	赵　晶	赵明辉	郝　伟	姜　辉	栗占国	贾继东	夏维波
黄　慧	黄晓军	曹　彬	彭　斌	潘　慧

第 1 分册　内科学概论・呼吸与危重症医学・术前和术后照护
　　　　　　主译　王　辰　代华平　赵　晶　黄　慧

第 2 分册　心血管疾病
　　　　　　主译　郑金刚　任景怡

第 3 分册　肾脏疾病
　　　　　　主译　李雪梅　赵明辉

第 4 分册　胃肠疾病・肝脏与胆道系统疾病
　　　　　　主译　房静远　杨爱明　贾继东

第 5 分册　血液疾病
　　　　　　主译　黄晓军　王建祥

第 6 分册　肿瘤疾病
　　　　　　主译　王　洁　巴　一

第 7 分册　内分泌疾病与代谢疾病・女性健康・男性健康・骨与骨矿物质代谢疾病
　　　　　　主译　宁　光　朱　兰　姜　辉　夏维波　潘　慧

第 8 分册　肌肉骨骼与结缔组织疾病
　　　　　　主译　栗占国　李梦涛

第 9 分册　感染性疾病
　　　　　　主译　刘海鹰　张福杰　曹　彬

第 10 分册　神经疾病・老年医学・缓和医疗・酒精和物质使用
　　　　　　主译　彭　斌　王伊龙　李小鹰　宁晓红　郝　伟

医学名词审定指导

任慧玲　李晓瑛　冀玉静　张燕舞　李军莲

中英双语版 序言

让我国医学生与国际医学生站在同一起跑线上的首要之事，是为其提供具有世界先进水平的标准教材。我们应争取使每一位医学生都能接触到内容经典、充分代表现代医学水平的国际权威原文教材并力求准确翻译，提供原文与中文双语对照版本，使医学生和医生在学习中形成双语医学词语、概念、概念间逻辑及由此构成的医学知识体系。在这样的思想驱动下，国际经典内科学教科书《希氏内科学精要（第10版）》中英双语版应运而生。

《希氏内科学》原著以其论述严谨准确、系统全面，被誉为"标准的内科学参考书"。自1927年首次出版以来，在内科学领域渐享世界级声誉，成为全球众多优秀医学院校，包括哈佛医学院、斯坦福大学医学院、约翰斯·霍普金斯大学医学院、牛津大学医学部、剑桥大学医学院、墨尔本大学医学院、新加坡国立大学医学院及多伦多大学医学院等普遍采用的内科学参考书。首版《希氏内科学精要》则诞生于1986年，旨在凝炼其全本的精华和要点，以最为简洁明确的方式向以医学生为主体的医学界精辟传达《希氏内科学》的核心信息，包括书中所体现出的人文精神。此后，每版精要本都力求凝炼地反映当时最新医学成果和医疗实践指南，愈来愈成为各国医学生、住院医师、专培医师及教师学习和传授内科学的主要教本，在世界医学教材体系中居引领地位。《希氏内科学》和《希氏内科学精要》两个版本不仅在英语国家被广泛使用，更被翻译为葡萄牙语、西班牙语、希腊语、意大利语、日语、简体中文版，为全球医学界广泛采用。

中国的医学生、住院医师、专培医师需要培养国际专业信息获取能力。将精要本原文引进并准确翻译，以中英文对照的形式呈现，便于读者进行双语对照阅读和学习，使之在学习理解国际标准医学内容的同时，学习好中英文医学词语，为国际医学交流打好基础。相信此举对于提高我国的医学教育水平，培养国际型医学人才至为有益。

《希氏内科学精要》精练地涵盖了内科学的所有主要领域，包括心血管疾病、呼吸疾病与危重症、消化疾病、肾脏疾病、内分泌和代谢疾病、风湿疾病、血液疾病、肿瘤、感染性疾病、神经与老年疾病等，构建了较为系统的知识体系。在翻译引进过程中，我们遵循将相关内容集中的原则，将原书按系统器官拆分为十个分册，使其更具有专科阅读的对应性，以更加灵活轻便的形式为读者提供多样化的阅读选择。

为确保译文质量，我们在译者遴选上采取了严谨的标准。从《希氏内科学（第26版）》翻译团队中择优选取责任心强、译文优质的译者，同时吸纳了临床医学专业"101"计划核心教材的编者团队。每个分册均由主译专家带领各自译者团队完成翻译、审校、交叉互审、通审四级审校工作。这些译者具备扎实的英语与专业能力，他们在翻译过程中，深入理解原文，准确阐述作者思想，并多角度审视译文的准确性、流畅性与风格一致性，确保译文的忠实性、规范性与可读性，在不同的语言和文化间架起坚实的桥梁。尤其值得称赞的是，对原著中疏漏或不够完善之处，译文中以"译者注"的形式加以适当解释和说明，使译文内容在忠实于原著的基础上更为准确。

本书读者定位于具有一定学习能力和基础的高等医学院校医学专业8年制、5年制学生以及相关医学专业人员，可作为医务人员的内科学参考书、住院医师规范化培训和专科医师规范化培训辅导教材、研究生入学考试辅导教材、内科学教师参考书、内科学各专科医师复习回顾其他专科知识的重要读本。

呼吸与危重症医学教授
中国医学科学院院长
北京协和医学院校长
2024年11月

对学习者教科书重要。

对学医者内科学重要。

世界上的内科学教科书，

首推《希氏内科学精要》。

中文是中国医生主要执业用语。

英文是国际医学交流的主要文字。

学习医学，当以双语对应阅读为好。

如此，可获纵横国际之效。

本书力求有助于此。

In Memoriam

Thomas E. Andreoli, MD

Dr. Thomas Andreoli, along with Drs. Lloyd Hollingsworth (Holly) Smith, Jr., Fred Plum, and Charles C.J. Carpenter, was one of the four founding editors of *Cecil Essentials of Medicine*. He served as editor for editions one through eight before he passed away on April 14, 2009. Dr. Andreoli was born in the Bronx, New York, in 1935, attended Catholic primary and high schools, and graduated from St. Vincent College and the Georgetown School of Medicine. He trained as a resident at Duke University under legendary Chair of Medicine Dr. Eugene Stead, who recognized him as a brilliant physician and scientist and encouraged his research career. Dr. Andreoli received his research training at the NIH and then in the laboratory of Dr. Tosteson at Duke. His research focused on the biochemical and biophysical properties of renal tubular cell membranes and their role in water and electrolyte transport. He made fundamental discoveries on the normal renal physiology, illuminating the way to subsequent work by many others on renal health and disease. His research was recognized with numerous awards and election to honorific societies both in the United States and in Europe. Dr. Andreoli also served as editor of *The American Journal of Physiology: Renal Physiology* and Editor in Chief of *Kidney International*.

Tom's national prominence and leadership qualities were recognized early in his career when he became head of Nephrology at the University of Alabama in Birmingham. There he helped faculty and trainees develop outstanding research, organized clinical services, and created a hemodialysis program to build one of the outstanding Divisions of Nephrology in the country. In 1979, Dr. Andreoli was appointed Chair of the Department of Internal Medicine at the University of Texas, Houston, where he assembled an outstanding faculty focused on research, clinical care, and teaching. In 1988, he accepted the position as Chairman of Internal Medicine at the University of Arkansas School of Medicine, a position he held until his death. There he again assembled a distinguished faculty who were outstanding researchers but also dedicated to outstanding clinical care and teaching. Morning report and clinical rounds with Dr. Andreoli were rigorous and riveting, focusing on the individual patient, not only their diagnoses and treatment but also on each patient's personal concerns and well-being. Dr. Andreoli was revered by medical students, his house staff, faculty, and colleagues, and I (EJW) personally can attest to what he regarded as his most cherished role—the mentorship and education of the next generation of physicians.

One of Dr. Andreoli's great interests was *Cecil Essentials of Medicine*, for which he was the editor/chief editor for eight of its ten editions, an interest that reflected his commitment to the education of students, house staff, and other physicians in the "essentials" of Internal Medicine.

Dr. Andreoli was devoted to his family. He was married to Elizabeth Berglund Andreoli from 1987 until his death. He was previously married to Dr. Kathleen Gainor Andreoli, mother of his three children and their ten grandchildren. Being of Italian ancestry and from Bronx, New York, it is not surprising that Dr. Andreoli was a passionate fan of the New York Yankees, Italian opera, which he could sing in Italian, and Frank Sinatra.

Dr. Andreoli's legacy lives on in his numerous previous students, house staff, colleagues, and in this book.

缅 怀

托马斯·安德里奥利博士

托马斯·安德里奥利（Thomas E. Andreoli）博士携手李奥德·霍灵斯沃斯·史密斯［Lloyd Hollingsworth（Holly）Smith］博士、弗雷德·普拉姆（Fred Plum）博士和查尔斯·卡彭特（Charles C.J. Carpenter）博士同为《希氏内科学精要》的创始编者。他在2009年4月14日去世前，曾担任该书第1至第8版的编者。安德里奥利博士于1935年出生于美国纽约布朗克斯区，就读于天主教小学和中学，后毕业于圣文森特学院和乔治城大学医学院。他在杜克大学医学院接受住院医师培训期间师从著名内科主任尤金·斯特德（Eugene Stead）博士，后者将其视为杰出的医生和科学家，并鼓励他投身科研事业。安德里奥利博士在美国国立卫生研究院接受科研训练后，前往杜克大学托斯特森（Tosteson）博士的实验室继续深造。他重点研究肾小管细胞膜的生化和生物物理特性及其在水和电解质转运中所发挥的作用。他在正常肾脏生理学方面的重要发现为后续关于肾脏健康和疾病的研究铺平了道路。安德里奥利博士的研究工作荣获多个学术奖项，并入选美国和欧洲的多个荣誉学会。他还担任《美国生理学杂志：肾脏生理学篇》（*The American Journal of Physiology*：*Renal Physiology*）的编辑以及《国际肾脏杂志》（*Kidney International*）的主编。

安德里奥利博士担任阿拉巴马大学伯明翰分校肾脏病学系主任后不久，即因其杰出领导力而赢得全美业内声誉。他帮助本校师生们取得科研突破，负责临床业务的组织实施，并因开创血液透析业务而使该科跻身全美顶级肾脏内科之列。1979年，安德里奥利博士被任命为得克萨斯大学休斯敦分校内科学系主任，他在该系组建了一支科研、临床诊疗和教学并重的优秀教职团队。自1988年起，他担任阿肯色大学医学院内科学系主任，直至辞世。在这里他再次组建了一支卓越的教职团队，他们不仅科研工作出色，临床诊疗和教学工作也出类拔萃。安德里奥利博士带领的晨会报告和查房非常严谨而引人入胜，不仅尽心竭力于每位患者的诊断和治疗，还关注到他们每个人的个体情况和福祉。安德里奥利博士深受医学生、住院医师、教职人员和同事的崇敬，我（EJW）可以证明，他最珍视的角色当属培养和教育下一代医生。

安德里奥利博士对《希氏内科学精要》倾注了满腔热忱，先后担任了该书10版中8版的编者/主编，践行他为医学生、住院医师和其他各科医生们传授内科学"精要"的承诺。

安德里奥利博士高度重视家庭。他与第二任妻子伊丽莎白·伯格兰德·安德里奥利（Elizabeth Berglund Andreoli）的婚姻从1987年延续到辞世。他与第一任妻子凯瑟琳·盖娜·安德里奥利（Kathleen Gainor Andreoli）博士育有三个子女和十个孙辈。作为意大利裔和纽约布朗克斯人，安德里奥利博士是纽约洋基队、意大利歌剧（他能用意大利语演唱）和美国著名歌手、演员、主持人弗兰克·辛纳屈（Frank Sinatra）的忠实拥趸。安德里奥利博士将永远被他的众多学生、住院医师和同事怀念，并因本书而流芳百世。

In Memoriam

Charles C.J. Carpenter, MD

Dr. Charles C.J. Carpenter joined Drs. Thomas Andreoli, Lloyd Hollingsworth Smith, Jr., and Fred Plum as a founder of *Cecil Essentials of Medicine*. He served as editor for seven editions and was followed in that role by Dr. Ivor Benjamin and then Dr. Edward Wing. Sadly, Chuck passed away on March 19, 2020, surrounded by his wife and children. He was Professor Emeritus of Medicine at The Warren Alpert Medical School of Brown University and Physician-in-Chief Emeritus at The Miriam Hospital.

Chuck was born in Savannah, Georgia, on January 5, 1931. He attended college at Princeton and medical school at Johns Hopkins where he also did his house staff training, including chief residency, and then joined the Johns Hopkins faculty. With his young family, he travelled to Calcutta, India, where he carried out landmark studies for the treatment of cholera.

Before coming to Brown in 1986, he was Chair of Medicine at Baltimore City Hospital and Case Western Reserve University.

His contributions to medical science and clinical care were many. While in Calcutta, using basic scientific evidence coupled with practical approaches, Dr. Carpenter developed "oral rehydration therapy" to address the cholera epidemic there. This treatment has saved millions of lives. While at Case, one of his innovations was to develop the nation's first Division of Geographic Medicine because of his strong belief that all physicians should be medical citizens of the world. In 1987, as he became deeply involved in the clinical management of persons living with HIV, he initiated a unique program in which Brown University faculty and trainees assumed responsibility for all HIV care in the Rhode Island State prison system.

Dr. Carpenter served as Chairman of the American Board of Internal Medicine and President of the Association of American Physicians. He has been a member of the NIH AIDS Executive Committee, the National Advisory Allergy and Infectious Diseases Council, and the USPHS AIDS Task Force. He was Chair of the Antiretroviral Treatment Panel of the International AIDS Society-USA and authored their recommendations on antiretroviral treatment. He also served as Chair of the Treatment Committee to evaluate the President's Emergency Plan for HIV/AIDS Relief. He became the director of the Brown University International Health Institute and the director of the Lifespan/Brown Center for AIDS Research with several Boston hospitals.

Throughout his career, Dr. Carpenter was the recipient of many international, national, and regional awards, accepting each with characteristic humility. With both small and large groups of learners, Chuck made certain that every member of his team was well educated, and each felt that they contributed to the well-being of their patients. His ability to sit calmly at the bedside, hold the patient's hand, comfort them, and listen in a genuinely focused way, influenced so many physicians. He was truly grateful for the opportunity to care for those less fortunate than he, and the feeling of being privileged to do so was clearly transmitted to all. Dr. Carpenter was a wonderful blend of profound compassion combined with the adherence to scholarship and teaching. Sir William Osler wrote that physicians should "Do the kind thing and do it first." Chuck lived by this precept. Vigor and insight characterized his approach to clinical and ethical challenges, always with younger colleagues at his side. In a recent tribute to him, many emphasized that Dr. Carpenter dedicated his life to his patients, many of whom were the most vulnerable members of society. We hope that we will have some of his strength and use his example as our compass as we are challenged to reduce suffering and improve the health of all for whom we are responsible.

He is survived by his wife of 61 years, Sally; three sons, Charles, Murray, and Andrew; and seven grandchildren.

缅 怀

查尔斯·卡彭特博士

查尔斯·卡彭特（Charles C.J. Carpenter）博士与托马斯·安德里奥利（Thomas E. Andreoli）博士、李奥德·霍灵斯沃斯·史密斯（Lloyd Hollingsworth Smith）博士和弗雷德·普拉姆（Fred Plum）博士共同开创了《希氏内科学精要》。他共担任了7版的编者，嗣后由艾弗·本杰明（Ivor Benjamin）博士和爱德华·温（Edward Wing）博士接任。查尔斯·卡彭特博士于2020年3月19日在妻子和子女们的陪伴下辞世。他曾担任布朗大学沃伦·阿尔珀特医学院的内科学系名誉教授和米里亚姆医院的名誉主任医师。

查尔斯·卡彭特博士于1931年1月5日出生于美国佐治亚州萨凡纳市。他在普林斯顿大学获得学士学位后进入约翰斯·霍普金斯大学医学院，并完成了包括住院总医师在内的住院医师培训，随后加入了约翰斯·霍普金斯大学的教职团队。他曾携妻子和年幼的孩子前往印度加尔各答，在当地对霍乱的治疗进行了具有里程碑意义的研究工作。

在1986年入职布朗大学之前，他曾担任巴尔的摩市医院和凯斯西储大学医学院的内科学主任。

他在医学科学研究和临床诊疗领域建树颇多。在加尔各答期间，基于基础科学证据及临床实践，查尔斯·卡彭特博士开创了"口服补液疗法"以遏制当地的霍乱疫情。这一疗法拯救了数百万人的生命。秉承医生无国界的世界公民理念，他在凯斯西储大学做了一项开创性工作，建立了美国首个地缘医学部（研究地理环境因素对人体健康和疾病影响的学科）。1987年，他深度参与人类免疫缺陷病毒（HIV）携带者的临床管理，并发起了一个独特的项目——由布朗大学教职团队和医学生们承担罗德岛州监狱系统内所有艾滋病相关诊疗工作。

查尔斯·卡彭特博士曾担任美国内科医师委员会主席和美国医师协会主席。他曾是美国国立卫生研究院艾滋病行政委员会、美国国家过敏与传染病咨询委员会以及公共卫生服务部艾滋病工作组的成员。他还曾担任国际艾滋病学会-美国分会抗逆转录病毒治疗组主席，并撰写了抗逆转录病毒治疗建议。他还担任过艾滋病治疗委员会主席，该委员会负责评估美国总统防治艾滋病紧急救援计划；曾担任布朗大学国际健康研究所所长，以及大学与多家波士顿当地医院合办的生命周期/布朗大学艾滋病研究中心主任。

查尔斯·卡彭特博士在职业生涯中获得过诸多国际性、全美和地区性奖项，同时展现其谦逊品格。无论学员人数多寡，查尔斯·卡彭特博士都会确保人人都能受到良好教育，并让他们感到自己也对患者的健康做出了贡献。他能够安静地坐在病床边，握住患者的手，安慰他们，并全神贯注地听取患者倾诉，这一举动深深地感染了许多医生。他十分珍视诊治不幸染病者的机会，并且能够将这种殊荣感传递给所有人。查尔斯·卡彭特博士完美地融汇了对患者的宅心仁厚与对学术和教学的坚守。威廉·奥斯勒（William Osler）爵士曾写道，医生应该"行善事，为人先"，而这正是查尔斯·卡彭特博士一生奉行的信条。他在面对临床和伦理挑战时充满活力和洞察力，始终重视提携年轻同事。许多人的悼词中都重点指出，查尔斯·卡彭特博士将毕生致力于患者福祉，其中许多人属于社会上最弱势群体。我们希望，在我们面临减少患者痛苦及改善其健康状况的挑战时，能够拥有他的力量，并以他为榜样获得指引。

查尔斯·卡彭特博士与妻子萨丽（Sally）共度了61年的婚姻时光，育有查尔斯（Charles）、穆雷（Murray）和安德鲁（Andrew）三子以及七个孙辈。

ABOUT THE EDITORS

Dr. Edward J. Wing was an editor of *Cecil Essentials of Medicine,* editions 8 and 9, and is the lead editor of edition 10. He graduated from Williams College in 1967 and from the Harvard Medical School in 1971. He was a resident in Internal Medicine at the Peter Bent Brigham and completed an Infectious Diseases Fellowship at Stanford University. Joining the faculty at the University of Pittsburgh in 1975, he focused his NIH-funded research on mechanisms of cell-mediated immunity as well as various clinical aspects of Infectious Diseases. From 1990 to 1998, the University and UPMC appointed him as Physician-in-Chief at Montefiore Hospital, then Chief of Infectious Diseases, and finally Interim Chair of Medicine.

In 1998, Dr. Wing became Chair of Medicine at Brown University (1998–2008) where he consolidated the department across hospitals, practice plans, and training programs. As Dean of Medicine and Biological Sciences at Brown University (2008–2013) he strengthened ties with affiliated hospitals (Lifespan and Care New England), increased research, and oversaw the construction of a new medical school building. International exchange programs with medical schools in Kenya, the Dominican Republic, and Haiti were established during his years as chairman and dean. Dr. Wing has cared for patients with HIV since the beginning of the epidemic in outpatient clinics. He continues to be active in research, clinical care, and teaching.

Dr. Fred J. Schiffman, who along with Dr. Edward Wing is editor of *Cecil Essentials of Medicine,* 10th edition, attended Wagner College and then the New York University School of Medicine, from which he graduated in 1973. He performed his early house staff training at Yale-New Haven Hospital and then spent two years at the National Cancer Institute. He returned to Yale as Chief Medical Resident followed by a hematology fellowship. He became Medical Director of Yale's Primary Care Center before coming to Brown University in 1983, where he has been a leader in the medical residency program as well as Associate Physician-in-Chief at The Miriam Hospital.

Dr. Schiffman holds The Sigal Family Professorship in Humanistic Medicine at The Warren Alpert Medical School of Brown University. His scholarly interests include the structure and function of the human spleen and the intersection of the arts and medical care. He has directed or championed many projects and programs, including those that encourage and reinforce wellness and resilience in patients, families, and caregivers. He began a novel program that places medical students and physicians with other nonmedical professionals as they share in the viewing of works of art in the Museum of the Rhode Island School of Design. Dr. Schiffman recently led a Brown University edX course entitled, "Artful Medicine: Art's Power to Enrich Patient Care," with worldwide participation. Dr. Schiffman has also edited texts on hematologic pathophysiology, consultative hematology, and the anemias.

原著主编

爱德华·温（Edward J. Wing）博士是《希氏内科学精要》第8版和第9版的编者，以及第10版的主编。他先后于1967年和1971年毕业于威廉姆斯学院和哈佛医学院。他曾在彼得·本特·布里格姆医院任内科住院医师，后在斯坦福大学完成了传染病学的专科医师（Fellowship）课程。自1975年加入匹兹堡大学医学院以来，他通过美国国立卫生研究院资助的研究项目，探索细胞介导免疫的机制以及传染病学各领域的临床诊疗工作。1990—1998年期间，他先后被匹兹堡大学及其医学中心任命为蒙特菲奥里医院的主任医师、传染病科主任，后担任内科临聘主任。

1998年起，温博士担任布朗大学医学院的内科主任（1998—2008年）。在此期间，他在不同医院、实践计划和培训项目间对内科进行整合。在担任布朗大学医学与生物科学院院长（2008—2013年）期间，他加强了与各附属医院（Lifespan医院和Care New England医院）间的联系，提升了科研工作的水准，并为医学院建成了一座新楼。在担任主任和院长期间，他还建立了与肯尼亚、多米尼加共和国和海地的医学院的国际交流项目。温博士自艾滋病流行初期便在门诊诊治艾滋病患者，并始终工作在科研、临床和教学一线。

弗雷德·谢夫曼（Fred J. Schiffman）博士与爱德华·温（Edward Wing）博士共同担任《希氏内科学精要》第10版的主编。他就读于瓦格纳学院，随后进入纽约大学医学院，并于1973年毕业。他在耶鲁大学附属纽黑文医院接受早期住院医师培训，随后在美国国家癌症研究所工作了两年。回到耶鲁大学后，他担任住院总医师，然后完成了血液学专科医师课程，随后成为耶鲁初级保健中心医学主任。他于1983年入职布朗大学，领导医学住院医师项目并担任米里亚姆医院的副主任医师。

谢夫曼博士担任布朗大学沃伦·阿尔珀特医学院人文医学系的西格尔家庭医学教授。他的学术兴趣涵盖人体脾脏的结构和功能，以及艺术与医疗的交叉融合。他主持或参与了许多项目和计划，其中包括许多旨在鼓励和加强患者、家人和医护人员的福祉与康复能力的项目。他所创办的一个新项目可以让医学生和医生与其他非医学专业人士一起，共同欣赏罗德岛设计学院博物馆的艺术作品。谢夫曼博士近期还主持了布朗大学名为"艺术与医学：艺术赋能患者照护"的edX课程，此课程的参与者来自全球多个国家。谢夫曼博士还出版了有关血液病理生理学、血液科会诊和贫血的著作。

原著者名单

Jinnette Dawn Abbott, MD
Rajiv Agarwal, MD
Marwa Al-Badri, MD
Hyeon-Ju Ryoo Ali, MD
Jason M. Aliotta, MD
Khaldoun Almhanna, MD, MPH
Mohanad T. Al-Qaisi, MD
Zuhal Arzomand, MD
Akwi W. Asombang, MD, MPH
Su N. Aung, MD, MPH
Christopher G. Azzoli, MD
Christina Bandera, MD
Debasree Banerjee, MD
Mashal Batheja, MD
Jeffrey J. Bazarian, MD, MPH
Selim R. Benbadis, MD
Ivor J. Benjamin, MD, FAHA, FACC
Eric Benoit, MD
Marcie G. Berger, MD
Clemens Bergwitz, MD
Nancy Berliner, MD
Jeffrey S. Berns, MD
Pooja Bhadbhade, DO
Ratna Bhavaraju-Sanka, MD
Tanmayee Bichile, MD
Ariel E. Birnbaum, MD
Charles M. Bliss, Jr., MD
Andrew S. Blum, MD, PhD
Bryan J. Bonder, MD
Russell Bratman, MD
Glenn D. Braunstein, MD
Alma M. Guerrero Bready, MD
Richard Bungiro, PhD
Anna Marie Burgner, MD, MEHP
Jonathan Cahill, MD
Andrew Canakis, DO
Benedito A. Carneiro, MD, MS
Brian Casserly, MD
Abdullah Chahin, MD, MA, MSc
Philip A. Chan, MD
Kimberle Chapin, MD
William P. Cheshire, Jr., MD
Waihong Chung, MD, PhD
Emma Ciafaloni, MD

Joaquin E. Cigarroa, MD
Michael P. Cinquegrani, MD
Andreea Coca, MD, MPH
Harvey Jay Cohen, MD
Scott Cohen, MD, MPH
Beatrice P. Concepcion, MD, MS
Nathan T. Connell, MD, MPH
Maria Constantinou, MD
Roberto Cortez, MD
Timothy J. Counihan, MD, FRCPI
Anne Haney Cross, MD
Cheston B. Cunha, MD, FACP
Joanne S. Cunha, MD
Susan Cu-Uvin, MD
Noura M. Dabbouseh, MD
Kwame Dapaah-Afriyie, MD, MBA
Erin M. Denney-Koelsch, MD
Andre De Souza, MD
An S. De Vriese, MD, PhD
Neal D. Dharmadhikari, MD
Leah Dickstein, MD
Don Dizon, MD, FACP, FASCO
Robyn T. Domsic, MD, MPH
Kim A. Eagle, MD
Michael G. Earing, MD
Pamela Egan, MD
Wafik S. El-Deiry, MD, PhD, FACP
Mitchell S. V. Elkind, MD, MS
Tarra B. Evans, MD
Michael B. Fallon, MD
Dimitrios Farmakiotis, MD
Francis A. Farraye, MD
Ronan Farrell, MD
Panayotis Fasseas, MD, FACC
Mary Anne Fenton, MD
Fernando C. Fervenza, MD, PhD
Sean Fine, MD
Arkadiy Finn, MD
Timothy Flanigan, MD
Brisas M. Flores, MD
Andrew E. Foderaro, MD
Theodore C. Friedman, MD, PhD
Joseph Metmowlee Garland, MD, AAHIVM

Eric J. Gartman, MD
Abdallah Geara, MD
Raul Macias Gil, MD
Timothy Gilligan, MD, FASCO
Michael Raymond Goggins, MB BCh BAO, MRCPI
Geetha Gopalakrishnan, MD
Vidya Gopinath, MD
Susan L. Greenspan, MD, FACP
Osama Hamdy, MD, PhD
Johanna Hamel, MD
Sajeev Handa, MD, SFHM
Mitchell T. Heflin, MD, MHS
Robert G. Holloway, MD, MPH
Christopher S. Huang, MD
Zilla Hussain, MD
T. Alp Ikizler, MD
Iris Isufi, MD
Carlayne E. Jackson, MD
Paul G. Jacob, MD, MPH
Matthew D. Jankowich, MD
Niels V. Johnsen, MD, MPH
Jessica E. Johnson, MD
Rayford R. June, MD
Tareq Kheirbek, MD, ScM, FACS
Alok A. Khorana, MD, FACP, FASCO
Sena Kilic, MD
David Kim, MD
James Kleczka, MD
James R. Klinger, MD
Patrick Koo, MD, ScM
Pooja Koolwal, MD
Mary P. Kotlarczyk, PhD
Nicole M. Kuderer, MD
Awewura Kwara, MD
Jennifer M. Kwon, MD, MPH
Richard A. Lange, MD, MBA
Jerome Larkin, MD
Alfred I. Lee, MD, PhD
Daniel J. Levine, MD
David E. Lewandowski, MD
Kelly V. Liang, MD, MS
Kimberly P. Liang, MD, MS
David R. Lichtenstein, MD

扫描二维码了解更多信息

Douglas W. Lienesch, MD
Geoffrey S.F. Ling, MD, PhD
Ester Little, MD, FACP
Yi Liu, MD
Nicole L. Lohr, MD, PhD
John R. Lonks, MD, FACP, FIDSA, FSHEA
Gary H. Lyman, MD, MPH
Jeffrey M. Lyness, MD
Shane Lyons, MD, MRCPI, MRCP(UK)
Diana Maas, MD
Talha A. Malik, MD, MSPH
Sonia Manocha, MD
Susan Manzi, MD, MPH
Frederick J. Marshall, MD
F. Dennis McCool, MD
Russell J. McCulloh, MD
Kelly McGarry, MD, FACP
Eavan Mc Govern, MD, PhD
Robin L. McKinney, MD
Anthony Mega, MD
Shivang Mehta, MD
Douglas F. Milam, MD
Maria D. Mileno, MD
Abhinav Kumar Misra, MBBS, MD
Orson W. Moe, MD
Niveditha Mohan, MBBS
Larry W. Moreland, MD
Alan R. Morrison, MD, PhD
Steven F. Moss, MD
Christopher J. Mullin, MD, MHS
Sinéad M. Murphy, MB, BCh, MD, FRCPI
Sagarika Nallu, MD, FAAP, FAAN, FAASM
Javier A. Neyra, MD, MSCS
Ghaith Noaiseh, MD
Thomas A. Ollila, MD
Steven M. Opal, MD
Biff F. Palmer, MD
Jen Jung Pan, MD, PhD
Anna Papazoglou, MD
Aric Parnes, MD
Nayan M. Patel, DO, MPH
Ari Pelcovits, MD
Mark A. Perazella, MD
Michael F. Picco, MD, PhD
Kate E. Powers, DO
Laura A. Previll, MD, MPH
Nilum Rajora, MD
Adolfo Ramirez-Zamora, MD
John Reagan, MD
Rebecca Reece, MD
Harlan Rich, MD, AGAF, FACP
Jennifer H. Richman, MD
Lisa R. Rogers, DO
Ralph Rogers, MD
Michal G. Rose, MD
James A. Roth, MD
Sharon Rounds, MD
Jason C. Rubenstein, MD
Abbas Rupawala, MD
Jenna Sarvaideo, DO
Ramesh Saxena, MD, PhD
Fred J. Schiffman, MD, MACP
Ruth B. Schneider, MD
Kristin A. Seaborg, MD
Anil Seetharam, MD
Stuart Seropian, MD
Jigme Michael Sethi, MD
Sanjeev Sethi, MD, PhD
Elizabeth Shane, MD
Esseim Sharma, MD
Shani Shastri, MD, MPH
Barry S. Shea, MD
Lauren Shevell, MD, MPH
Joseph A. Smith, Jr., MD
Robert J. Smith, MD
Davendra P.S. Sohal, MD, MPH
Christopher Song, MD, FACC
Thomas Sperry, MD
Jeffrey M. Statland, MD
Emily M. Stein, MD
Jennifer L. Strande, MD, PhD
Rochelle Strenger, MD
Thomas R. Talbot, MD, MPH
Christopher G. Tarolli, MD, MSEd
Yael Tarshish, MD
Pushpak Taunk, MD
Philip Tsoukas, MD
Allan R. Tunkel, MD, PhD
Jeffrey M. Turner, MD
Zoe G.S. Vazquez, MD
Stacie A. F. Vela, MD
Paul M. Vespa, MD, FCCM, FAAN, FANA, FNCS
Wanpen Vongpatanasin, MD
Marcella D. Walker, MD
Eunice S. Wang, MD
Sharmeel K. Wasan, MD
Thomas J. Weber, MD
Brandon J. Wilcoxson, MD
Edward J. Wing, MD, FACP, FIDSA
Ellice Wong, MD
John J. Wysolmerski, MD
Rayan Yousefzai, MD
Thomas R. Ziegler, MD
Rebecca Zon, MD

ACKNOWLEDGMENTS

Dr. Schiffman and I wish to thank first of all, the authors of the 128 chapters that make up the tenth edition of *Cecil Essentials of Medicine*. They have worked diligently to compose the material for each chapter and apply their mastery as they added the newest information, in clear language, to the text. Their efforts are apparent in the excellence of the book, and we are immensely grateful for their work. We wish to also thank Marybeth Thiel, Jennifer Ehlers, and Dan Fitzgerald from Elsevier who guided and supported our work as editors and whose expertise has made this volume possible. Finally, we are always thankful to our wives, Dr. Rena Wing and Ms. Gerri Schiffman, without whose love, support, and especially humor, this book would not have happened.

致　谢

　　谢夫曼博士和我首先要致谢《希氏内科学精要》第10版全书128章的各位作者。感谢他们精益求精地撰写每一章节，并运用其专业知识，以简明的语言将前沿资讯呈现在书中。正是他们的辛勤努力确保了本书的卓越地位，对他们唯有由衷的感激。我们还要感谢爱思唯尔出版集团的玛丽贝丝·蒂尔（Marybeth Thiel）、詹妮弗·埃勒斯（Jennifer Ehlers）和丹·菲茨杰拉德（Dan Fitzgerald），他们对本书的编辑工作给予了指导和支持，其专业水准保障了本书的完稿。最后，要特别感谢我们的妻子——蕾娜·温（Rena Wing）博士和盖瑞·谢夫曼（Gerri Schiffman）女士，对她们的爱和支持，特别是积极乐观的心态始终心存感激，她们为本书的圆满完成发挥了不可或缺的作用。

总目录

第 1 分册

第 1 篇　内科学概论　Introduction to Medicine
第 2 篇　呼吸与危重症医学　Pulmonary and Critical Care Medicine
第 3 篇　术前和术后照护　Preoperative and Postoperative Care

第 2 分册

心血管疾病　Cardiovascular Disease

第 3 分册

肾脏疾病　Renal Disease

第 4 分册

第 1 篇　胃肠疾病　Gastrointestinal Disease
第 2 篇　肝脏与胆道系统疾病　Diseases of the Liver and Biliary System

第 5 分册

血液疾病　Hematologic Disease

第 6 分册

肿瘤疾病　Oncologic Disease

第 7 分册

第 1 篇　内分泌疾病与代谢疾病　Endocrine Disease and Metabolic Disease
第 2 篇　女性健康　Women's Health
第 3 篇　男性健康　Men's Health
第 4 篇　骨与骨矿物质代谢疾病　Diseases of Bone and Bone Mineral Metabolism

第 8 分册

肌肉骨骼与结缔组织疾病　Musculoskeletal and Connective Tissue Disease

第 9 分册

感染性疾病　Infectious Disease

第 10 分册

第 1 篇　神经疾病　Neurologic Disease
第 2 篇　老年医学　Geriatrics
第 3 篇　缓和医疗　Palliative Care
第 4 篇　酒精和物质使用　Alcohol and Substance Use

第4分册
胃肠疾病·肝脏与胆道系统疾病

第 4 分册译者名单

主　译

房静远　杨爱明　贾继东

译　者（按姓氏笔画排序）

马　红　首都医科大学附属北京友谊医院	吴颜延　中国医学科学院北京协和医院
王　宇　首都医科大学附属北京友谊医院	张冠华　首都医科大学附属北京友谊医院
王　艳　首都医科大学附属北京友谊医院	陈　倩　华中科技大学同济医学院附属同济医院
王吉林　上海交通大学医学院附属仁济医院	陈萦晅　上海交通大学医学院附属仁济医院
王冰琼　首都医科大学附属北京友谊医院	陈慧敏　上海交通大学医学院附属仁济医院
王晓明　首都医科大学附属北京友谊医院	武丽娜　首都医科大学附属北京友谊医院
王倩怡　首都医科大学附属北京友谊医院	单　姗　首都医科大学附属北京友谊医院
尤　红　首都医科大学附属北京友谊医院	房静远　上海交通大学医学院附属仁济医院
左秀丽　山东大学齐鲁医院	赵新颜　首都医科大学附属北京友谊医院
冯云路　中国医学科学院北京协和医院	段维佳　首都医科大学附属北京友谊医院
刘　苓　四川大学华西医院	费贵军　中国医学科学院北京协和医院
孙亚朦　首都医科大学附属北京友谊医院	贾继东　首都医科大学附属北京友谊医院
苏文雨　上海交通大学医学院附属仁济医院	郭　涛　中国医学科学院北京协和医院
李佳宁　中国医学科学院北京协和医院	黄志寅　四川大学华西医院
李晓青　中国医学科学院北京协和医院	蒋青伟　中国医学科学院北京协和医院
李淑香　首都医科大学附属北京友谊医院	谢　思　清华大学附属北京清华长庚医院
杨爱明　中国医学科学院北京协和医院	谢元鸿　上海交通大学医学院附属仁济医院
肖英莲　中山大学第一附属医院	谭　蓓　中国医学科学院北京协和医院
吴　晰　中国医学科学院北京协和医院	魏　来　清华大学附属北京清华长庚医院

第4分册目录

第1篇　胃肠疾病　Gastrointestinal Disease

1. Common Clinical Manifestations of Gastrointestinal Disease: Abdominal Pain, 4
   胃肠疾病常见临床表现：腹痛，5

2. Common Clinical Manifestations of Gastrointestinal Disease: Gastrointestinal Hemorrhage, 12
   胃肠疾病常见临床表现：消化道出血，13

3. Common Clinical Manifestations of Gastrointestinal Disease: Malabsorption, 20
   胃肠疾病常见临床表现：吸收不良，21

4. Common Clinical Manifestations of Gastrointestinal Disease: Diarrhea, 34
   胃肠疾病常见临床表现：腹泻，35

5. Endoscopic and Imaging Procedures, 44
   内镜与影像学检查，45

6. Esophageal Disorders, 58
   食管疾病，59

7. Diseases of the Stomach and Duodenum, 76
   胃和十二指肠疾病，77

8. Inflammatory Bowel Disease, 102
   炎症性肠病，103

9. Diseases of the Pancreas, 122
   胰腺疾病，123

第2篇　肝脏与胆道系统疾病　Diseases of the Liver and Biliary System

10. Laboratory Tests in Liver Diseases, 152
    肝脏疾病的实验室检查，153

11. Jaundice, 158
    黄疸，159

12. Acute and Chronic Hepatitis, 170
    急性和慢性肝炎，171

13. Acute Liver Failure, 186
    急性肝衰竭，187

14 Cirrhosis of the Liver and Its Complications, 192
    肝硬化及其并发症，193

15 Disorders of the Gallbladder and Biliary Tract, 214
    胆囊和胆道疾病，215

索引 Index，230

CECIL ESSENTIALS OF MEDICINE

Gastrointestinal Disease
Diseases of the Liver and Biliary System

SECTION I

Gastrointestinal Disease

1 Common Clinical Manifestations of Gastrointestinal Disease: Abdominal Pain, 4

2 Common Clinical Manifestations of Gastrointestinal Disease: Gastrointestinal Hemorrhage, 12

3 Common Clinical Manifestations of Gastrointestinal Disease: Malabsorption, 20

4 Common Clinical Manifestations of Gastrointestinal Disease: Diarrhea, 34

5 Endoscopic and Imaging Procedures, 44

6 Esophageal Disorders, 58

7 Diseases of the Stomach and Duodenum, 76

8 Inflammatory Bowel Disease, 102

9 Diseases of the Pancreas, 122

第1篇

胃肠疾病

1 胃肠疾病常见临床表现：腹痛，5

2 胃肠疾病常见临床表现：消化道出血，13

3 胃肠疾病常见临床表现：吸收不良，21

4 胃肠疾病常见临床表现：腹泻，35

5 内镜与影像学检查，45

6 食管疾病，59

7 胃和十二指肠疾病，77

8 炎症性肠病，103

9 胰腺疾病，123

1

Common Clinical Manifestations of Gastrointestinal Disease: Abdominal Pain

Charles M. Bliss, Jr.

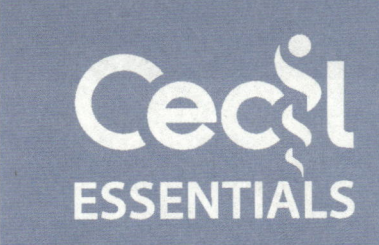

DEFINITION AND EPIDEMIOLOGY

Abdominal pain is a frequent manifestation of intra-abdominal disease. However, abdominal pain is difficult to localize or grade because the sensation of pain often is colored by emotional and physical factors. Abdominal pain may be classified as acute or chronic. Acute pain occurs suddenly and more often suggests serious physiologic alterations. Chronic pain may be present for several months; although it does not mandate immediate attention, chronic pain may lead to prolonged evaluation. According to a recent survey of 71,812 patients, 25% of the respondents reported abdominal pain within the past week. Appropriate evaluation of abdominal pain requires knowledge of pain mechanisms, close attention to history and physical examination findings, and recognition of important accompanying symptoms as well as awareness of the strengths and weaknesses of the tests that might be used.

PHYSIOLOGY

Abdominal pain results from stimulation of receptors specific for thermal, mechanical, or chemical stimuli. Once these receptors are excited, pain impulses travel through sympathetic fibers. Abdominal pain can be characterized as somatic or visceral. Somatic pain originates from the abdominal wall and parietal peritoneum, whereas visceral pain originates in internal organs and from the visceral peritoneum. Two types of neurons carry pain: *A fibers*, which have rapid conduction, and *C fibers*, which have slow conduction. Most visceral neurons are of the C type, and the pain resulting from their stimulation tends to be variable with regard to sensation and localization. In contrast, both A and C fibers originate from the parietal peritoneum and abdominal wall, and somatic pain tends to be sharp and distinctly localized.

Because of this pattern of innervation, abdominal viscera are not sensitive to cutting, tearing, burning, or crushing. However, visceral pain results from stretching of the walls of hollow organs or of the capsule of solid organs, as well as from inflammation or ischemia.

CAUSES OF ABDOMINAL PAIN

Multiple intra-abdominal and extra-abdominal disorders can produce abdominal pain. Distinguishing acute from chronic symptoms is helpful. The approach varies with each specific cause, but acute abdominal pain usually demands prompt intervention.

CLINICAL PRESENTATION

History

The differential diagnosis of abdominal pain, whether acute or chronic, requires thorough history taking with regard to pain characteristics, location and radiation, timing, and the presence of any accompanying symptoms. Recognition of characteristic patterns is essential to narrowing the differential diagnosis.

Pain location often indicates the organ responsible for the problem. For instance, epigastric pain is usually typical of peptic ulcer or dyspepsia, whereas right upper quadrant pain is more suggestive of cholecystitis and other biliary disorders. Early in the course of illness, pain may be perceived in one location and subsequently felt in another; this pattern of progression may be suggestive of specific pain syndromes. In acute cases, abdominal pain tends to be sharp and severe. The pain of a perforated viscus is intense, and the pain from a dissecting aneurysm may be described as tearing or crushing. Chronic pain may be less severe; pain from irritable bowel or dyspepsia is constant and dull, and the pain of chronic peptic ulcer is described as gnawing or hunger pain. The pattern of pain relief is helpful for diagnosing some conditions. The physician should also inquire about whether the pain is steady or intermittent and whether it occurs at night. For nocturnal pain, a distinction should be made between pain that awakens the patient and pain that is felt when the patient wakes up for other reasons.

Table 1.1 outlines characteristics, location, and radiation of pain for a few common acute and chronic abdominal conditions.

Physical Examination

Examination of the abdomen provides valuable clues to the diagnosis, but the examination should start with the general appearance of the patient. A patient who is writhing in bed and unable to find a comfortable position may be suffering from obstruction. In contrast, a patient lying with the lower extremities flexed and avoiding any motion may be suffering from peritonitis because movement makes peritoneal pain worse. Abdominal distention indicates obstruction or ascites. Visual inspection for peristalsis is helpful for the diagnosis of small bowel obstruction, but this sign is present only in the early stages. Focal areas of distention may indicate hernias; notice should also be taken of any scars from prior surgeries.

Auscultation should be performed in several areas to evaluate the timbre and pattern of bowel sounds and to search for bruits or hums. Absence of bowel sounds suggests ileus, whereas the presence of hyperactive, high-pitched sounds may indicate obstruction. Multiple bruits

胃肠疾病常见临床表现：腹痛

陈慧敏 译　肖英莲 陈旻晅 审校　房静远 通审

定义和流行病学

腹痛是腹腔内疾病的常见表现。由于疼痛的感觉常受情绪和躯体因素的影响，因此很难进行定位或分级。腹痛可分为急性或慢性。急性腹痛突然发生，常提示严重的生理学变化。慢性腹痛可持续数月；尽管慢性腹痛无须立即关注，但需要持续评估。根据对71 812名患者的调查，25%的应答者报告在过去1周内出现腹痛。正确评估腹痛需要了解疼痛的发生机制，密切关注病史和体格检查结果，识别重要的伴随症状，以及了解可能采用的检测的优缺点。

生理学

腹痛是由热刺激、机械性刺激或化学性刺激激活特异性受体所致。一旦这些受体被激活，疼痛冲动就会通过交感神经纤维传递。腹痛可分为躯体疼痛和内脏疼痛。躯体疼痛源自腹壁和腹膜壁层，而内脏疼痛则源自内脏器官和腹膜脏层。两种类型的神经元参与疼痛传导：A型纤维传导速度快，C型纤维传导速度慢。大多数内脏神经元属于C型，它们受到刺激后引起的疼痛在感觉和定位方面往往是可变的。相反，A型和C型纤维都源自腹膜壁层和腹壁，躯体疼痛往往剧烈，并且定位明确。

基于这种神经支配模式，腹腔脏器对切割、撕裂、烧灼或挤压不敏感。但是，内脏疼痛可由牵拉空腔脏器壁或实体脏器包膜，以及炎症或缺血而引起。

病因

多种腹腔内和腹腔外疾病可引起腹痛。需要甄别急慢性症状。治疗方法因具体病因而异，但急性腹痛通常需要及时干预。

临床表现

病史

无论是急性还是慢性腹痛，都需要对患者进行详细的病史采集，包括疼痛的特点、部位及放射痛、发作时机和伴随症状，以便进行鉴别诊断。识别腹痛的特点对缩小鉴别诊断的范围至关重要。

疼痛部位通常可提示疾病起源的脏器。例如，上腹部疼痛通常是消化性溃疡或消化不良的典型症状，而右上腹疼痛更可能提示胆囊炎和其他胆道疾病。在疾病早期，疼痛可能在某个部位被感知，随后又出现在另一个部位；这种进展模式可能提示特定的疼痛综合征。急性病例的腹痛通常剧烈且严重。内脏穿孔的疼痛剧烈，而夹层动脉瘤可表现为撕裂样痛或挤压痛。慢性疼痛的程度略低；肠易激综合征或消化不良引起的疼痛为持续钝痛，而慢性消化性溃疡的疼痛则被描述为啃咬痛或饥饿痛。疼痛缓解的模式有助于某些疾病的诊断。医生还应询问疼痛是持续还是间歇，是否发生在夜间。对于夜间痛，应区分患者是被疼痛唤醒还是因其他原因而在醒来时感觉疼痛。

表1.1概述了一些常见的急慢性腹部疾病的疼痛特征、定位和放射痛情况。

体格检查

腹部查体可为诊断提供有价值的线索，但检查应从患者的一般表现开始。例如，患者在床上翻滚无法找到舒适的姿势提示可能存在梗阻。相反，由于运动可加剧腹膜性疼痛，如患者下肢屈曲并避免任何运动提示腹膜炎。腹部膨隆提示梗阻或腹腔积液。视诊可见肠蠕动有助于诊断小肠梗阻，但该体征仅在早期出现。局部膨隆提示疝；还应注意是否有既往手术遗留的瘢痕。

应在多个区域听诊，评估肠鸣音的音色和模式，同时寻找有无异常血流杂音（收缩期杂音、静脉杂音）。肠鸣音消失提示肠闭塞，过度活跃、高调的肠鸣

TABLE 1.1 Key Abdominal Pain Syndromes

Condition	Type	Location	Radiation
Acute Abdominal Pain			
Appendicitis	Crampy, steady	Periumbilical, RLQ	Back
Cholecystitis	Intermittent, steady	Epigastric, RUQ	Right scapula
Pancreatitis	Steady	Epigastric, periumbilical	Back
Perforation	Sudden, severe	Epigastric	Entire abdomen
Obstruction	Crampy	Periumbilical	Back
Infarction	Severe, diffuse	Periumbilical	Entire abdomen
Chronic Abdominal Pain			
Esophagitis	Burning	Retrosternal	Left arm, back
Peptic ulcer	Gnawing	Epigastric	Back
Dyspepsia	Bloating, dull	Epigastric	None
IBS	Crampy	LLQ, RLQ	None

IBS, Irritable bowel syndrome; *LLQ*, left lower quadrant; *RLQ*, right lower quadrant; *RUQ*, right upper quadrant.

alert the examiner to the possibility of significant vascular disease, suggesting ischemia.

The abdomen should be palpated gently, starting in an area away from the pain. The examiner searches for areas of localized tenderness and rebound as well as for masses and enlarged organs. Percussion is performed to identify the size of organs or to determine the presence of ascites. Pain on percussion of the abdomen indicates peritoneal reaction, as does severe rebound tenderness.

A rectal examination is important for identifying a rectal tumor in the case of colon obstruction or tenderness high in the rectum in acute appendicitis. A pelvic examination should be performed in women to rule out pelvic inflammatory disease, or masses.

ACUTE ABDOMEN

The evaluation of a patient with an acute abdomen is a challenge in medical practice. The acute abdomen is caused by sudden inflammation, perforation, obstruction, or infarction of an intra-abdominal organ. The urgent question to be answered is whether immediate surgery is needed; a quick but complete evaluation is necessary to avoid undue delay in intervention for patients who require surgery. The physician must assess for abdominal tenderness, rebound, and guarding. Early surgical consultation should be obtained, even in doubtful cases, rather than awaiting confirmation of the diagnosis via laboratory or radiologic studies. However, many extra-abdominal conditions such as pneumonia, myocardial infarction, nephrolithiasis, and metabolic disorders can cause acute abdominal pain.

In some instances of the acute abdomen in its early stages, there are few findings. The examiner should be aware that patients with benign chronic conditions may have severe pain at presentation that is out of proportion to any physical findings. The context provided by the medical history, particularly previous abdominal surgery, is very valuable. Indeed, a patient with sudden crampy pain and abdominal distention may have an intestinal obstruction caused by adhesions or an incarcerated hernia. Therefore, examination of the entire patient, looking for jaundice, skin lesions, evidence of prior surgery, or evidence of chronic liver disease, is important.

In evaluating a patient with acute abdominal symptoms, a complete blood cell count with differential, a urinalysis, and measurements of serum amylase, lipase, bilirubin, and electrolytes are necessary components of the laboratory examination. Additional studies may be done but usually do not aid in the rapid decision making required. An elevated white blood cell count may indicate inflammatory disease, and extremely high values are typical of acute intestinal ischemia. An elevated serum amylase concentration usually indicates acute pancreatitis, although a perforated ulcer or mesenteric thrombosis can also cause hyperamylasemia.

Radiographic examination with an abdominal film is important to reveal the intra-abdominal gas pattern, and an upright film that includes the diaphragm or a left lateral decubitus film may identify intra-abdominal air suggesting perforation of a hollow viscus. Ultrasonography can be helpful in the diagnosis of acute cholecystitis or appendicitis. Computed tomography (CT) scans have become more helpful with technologic improvements in scanners; early CT scans allow prompt diagnosis of sometimes unsuspected abdominal diseases. Examination with a radiopaque medium should be used judiciously, especially if surgery is anticipated.

CHRONIC ABDOMINAL PAIN

In the evaluation of chronic abdominal pain, it can be challenging to distinguish between organic pain resulting from a specific pathologic process and functional pain. The location and characteristics of pain, as already discussed, serve as important guides, as do other accompanying symptoms. The presence of postprandial nausea and vomiting suggests chronic peptic ulcer, disorders of gastric emptying, or outlet obstruction. Documentation of weight loss mandates the search for an organic cause, such as inflammatory bowel disease or celiac disease. If anorexia accompanies weight loss, particularly in elderly patients, cancer must be excluded. If no cancer can be found and all objective tests are normal, the possibility of chronic depression must be entertained.

The most frequent causes of chronic abdominal pain are functional. Dyspepsia is characterized by chronic intermittent epigastric discomfort, sometimes accompanied by nausea or bloating. These symptoms are not always relieved by acid suppression and may be the result of an underlying motor disorder. Furthermore, when *Helicobacter pylori* is found in a patient with dyspeptic symptoms, its eradication may not necessarily lead to the resolution of symptoms. Controversy exists regarding the most effective strategy for the treatment of dyspepsia when *H. pylori* organisms are found in the absence of peptic ulcer disease.

Irritable bowel syndrome (IBS) is a very common disorder. Estimates are that 15% of Americans suffer from IBS on a regular basis and that 40% to 50% of referrals to gastroenterologists are related to IBS. The syndrome consists of abdominal distention, flatulence, and disordered bowel function. There are two important variants of IBS: constipation predominant IBS (IBS-C) is characterized by pain in the setting of constipation, and diarrhea predominant IBS (IBS-D) involves pain in the setting of diarrhea. IBS with both diarrhea and constipation is sometimes denoted as IBS mixed. The abdominal pain of IBS tends to be in the left lower quadrant, but it can be located elsewhere or be more generalized. Any patient with weight loss, anemia, nocturnal symptoms, steatorrhea, or onset of symptoms after age 50 years should be evaluated carefully for organic disease because these symptoms are not associated with IBS.

The Rome criteria, developed for research studies, may be helpful in the diagnosis of IBS. These criteria include pain that is associated with change in bowel habits, relieved with defecation, or accompanied by distention or bloating. Patients are reassured, counseled, and treated with anticholinergic agents and stool softeners. Although serotonin (5-HT) agonists such as alosetron and

表 1.1	重要的腹痛综合征		
疾病	疼痛类型	疼痛部位	放射痛部位
急性腹痛			
阑尾炎	痉挛痛、持续	脐周、右下腹	背部
胆囊炎	间歇痛、持续	上腹部、右上腹	右侧肩胛骨
胰腺炎	持续	上腹部、脐周	背部
穿孔	突发疼痛、严重	上腹部	全腹
梗阻	痉挛痛	脐周	背部
梗死	严重、弥漫	脐周	全腹
慢性腹痛			
食管炎	烧灼痛	胸骨后	左臂、背部
消化性溃疡	进食相关痛	上腹部	背部
消化不良	腹胀、钝痛	上腹部	无
肠易激综合征	痉挛痛	左下腹、右下腹	无

音则提示肠梗阻。存在多种杂音提示患者可能存在严重血管疾病引起的缺血。

触诊时应轻触，从远离疼痛的区域开始触诊。检查者应寻找有无局部压痛及反跳痛，同时注意有无包块及脏器肿大。叩诊可确定脏器大小及是否存在腹腔积液。腹部叩击痛及严重反跳痛提示腹膜反应。

直肠检查有助于识别由直肠肿瘤导致的肠梗阻或由急性阑尾炎所致的直肠压痛（常位于直肠右前方）。应对女性进行盆腔检查以排除盆腔炎或包块。

急腹症

急腹症患者的评估是临床实践中的一项挑战。急腹症由腹腔脏器突发炎症、穿孔、梗阻或梗死引起。迫切需要决定是否有必要立即手术，因此必须快速而全面地评估病情，以避免延误对需手术患者的处理。医生应评估腹部压痛、反跳痛和肌紧张。即便是可疑病例也应尽早进行外科会诊，而不是等待实验室或影像学检查结果确认诊断。但是，许多腹外疾病，如肺炎、心肌梗死、肾结石和代谢紊乱，也会引起急性腹痛。

部分急腹症在早期几乎没有异常发现。检查者应注意，良性慢性疾病患者就诊时可能会出现与体征不成比例的剧烈疼痛。询问病史（尤其是既往腹部手术史）极有价值。例如，突发痉挛性腹痛和腹部膨隆可能是粘连或嵌顿疝引起的肠梗阻。因此，对患者进行全身检查，寻找黄疸、皮肤病变、既往手术或慢性肝病的证据非常重要。

在评估急腹症患者时，全血细胞计数和分类、尿液分析，以及血清淀粉酶、脂肪酶、胆红素和电解质测定是必要的实验室检查。还可进行其他检查，但对快速决策通常并无益处。白细胞计数升高提示患者可能有炎症性疾病，而白细胞水平极高是急性肠缺血的典型表现。尽管溃疡穿孔或肠系膜血栓也可引起高淀粉酶血症，但血清淀粉酶浓度升高通常提示急性胰腺炎。

腹部 X 线检查对于显示腹腔内气体非常重要，包括膈肌的立位片及左侧卧位片可识别腹腔气体，提示空腔脏器穿孔。超声检查有助于诊断急性胆囊炎或阑尾炎。随着技术的进步，计算机断层成像（CT）更有助于疾病诊断；早期行 CT 可及时诊断有时未被察觉的腹部疾病。应谨慎使用射线不透性造影剂进行检查，尤其是在拟行手术的情况下。

慢性腹痛

评估慢性腹痛时，区分特定病理学过程引起的器质性疼痛和功能性疼痛的难度较大。如前所述，疼痛的位置、特征及伴随症状是重要提示。餐后恶心和呕吐提示慢性消化性溃疡、胃排空障碍或出口梗阻。明确的体重减轻需寻找器质性因素，如炎症性肠病或乳糜泻。若厌食伴体重减轻，特别是老年患者，必须排除癌症。如果未发现癌症且所有客观检查均正常，则需考虑慢性抑郁症的可能。

慢性腹痛最常见的原因是功能性腹痛。消化不良以慢性间歇性上腹部不适为特征，有时伴恶心或腹胀。这些症状通过抑酸治疗缓解不佳时，动力障碍也是可能的病因。此外，有消化不良症状的患者合并幽门螺杆菌感染时，根除幽门螺杆菌并不一定会使症状消失。无消化性溃疡但合并幽门螺杆菌感染的消化不良患者，其最佳治疗策略存在争议。

肠易激综合征（IBS）非常常见。据估计，15% 的美国人经常受到 IBS 的困扰，40%～50% 的胃肠疾病转诊与 IBS 有关。该综合征包括腹部膨隆、胀气和肠道功能紊乱。IBS 有两种重要的亚型：便秘型 IBS（IBS-C）的特征是便秘伴腹痛；腹泻型 IBS（IBS-D）的特征为腹泻伴腹痛。腹泻和便秘并存被称为混合型 IBS。IBS 引起的腹痛常见于左下腹，但也可发生在其他部位或更大范围。由于体重减轻、贫血、夜间症状、脂肪泻或发病年龄 > 50 岁通常与 IBS 无关，因此合并以上情况者应仔细评估是否存在器质性疾病。

罗马标准是为研究而制定的，有助于诊断 IBS。这些标准包括疼痛与排便习惯改变有关、排便后腹痛可缓解，可伴有腹部膨隆或腹部胀气。应对患者进行安慰、解释，并使用抗胆碱能药物和大便软化剂治疗。尽管阿洛司琼和替加色罗等 5- 羟色胺（5-HT）激动剂最初显示出良好的应用前景，但由于不可接受的副作

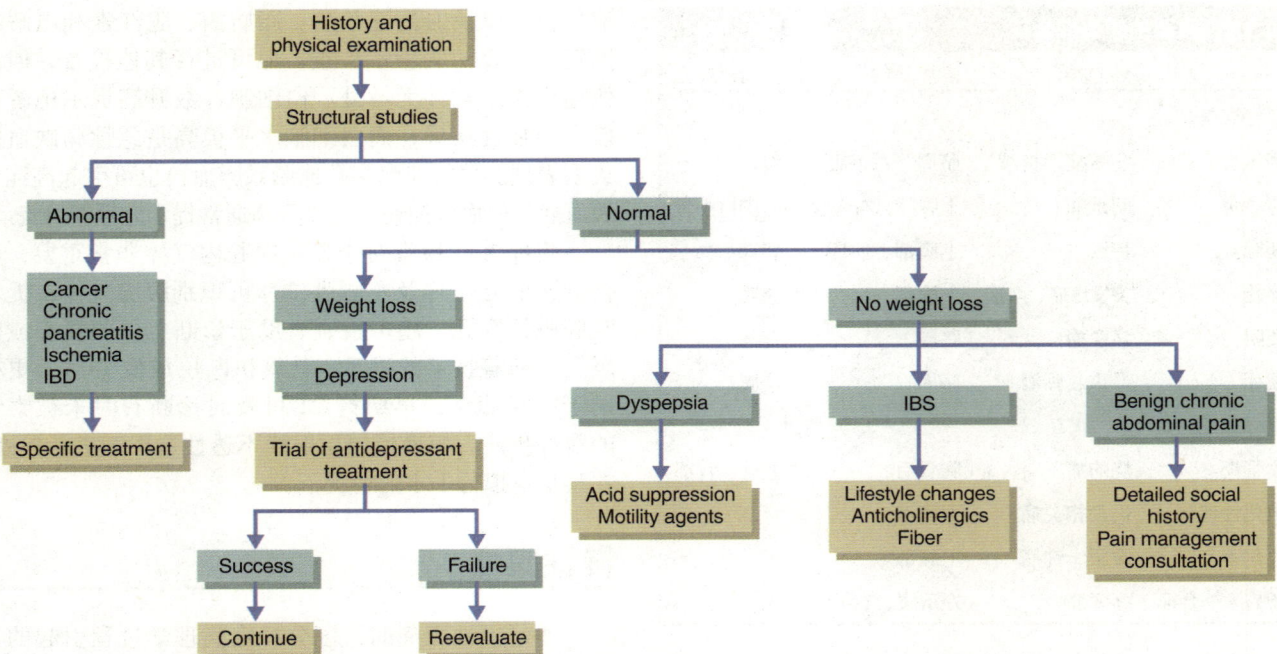

Fig. 1.1 Approach to the patient with chronic abdominal pain. *IBD*, Inflammatory bowel disease; *IBS*, irritable bowel syndrome.

tegaserod showed promise initially, they have been relegated to limited use due to unacceptable side effects. Eluxadoline, which targets opioid receptors, has been helpful in some cases of IBS-D in controlling pain and diarrhea in patients who have failed loperamide. Linaclotide causes increased secretion of chloride and bicarbonate into the intestinal lumen via a cyclic guanosine monophosphate (cGMP) pathway. This pathway also may be responsible for relief of visceral pain in patients with IBS-C. However, its use has been limited by unacceptable side effects, though a lower 72 mcg dose is now available. A new member of this class, plecanatide, has shown promise in initial studies but has not yet proved to be more effective than linaclotide. Tenapanor is a member of a new class of small molecule medications that act by inhibiting transport of sodium from the lumen of the large intestine, leading to improvements in constipation and pain in patients with IBS-C. This medication is still in the process of study but has been approved by the FDA. It represents a new method of treatment.

The more challenging clinical problem is *functional abdominal pain syndrome*. This term describes a condition in which the pain has been present for months or years. The complaints of pain often are not related to eating, defecation, or menses, unlike other causes of chronic pain. The patient is most likely to be a woman who has undergone numerous examinations and diagnostic studies with negative findings and, in many cases, surgical operations without any relief. Lengthy or repeated diagnostic work-ups are counterproductive and only convince the patient that one more test is what is needed to determine the source of the pain. The physician must establish that organic disease is not present and must also realize that the pain is real. These patients are not malingerers despite the fact that the pain does not fit any familiar pattern. Depression may be the result rather than the cause of the pain.

Management of chronic abdominal pain is demanding and requires as much tact, diplomacy, and compassion as scientific knowledge. An effort should be made to inquire about social factors, including history of physical and sexual abuse, particularly in women. Psychiatric evaluation may be necessary, but the suggestion for such a consultation may be interpreted by the patient as evidence that the physician believes "the pain is in my head." Referral to a competent pain management specialist is helpful in some cases. This approach offers the possibility of providing relief with nerve blocks if the pain is localized or with other pain-relieving devices. If this approach fails, referral to a psychologist or psychiatrist may be acceptable to the patient.

Because of the challenges involved with chronic pain treatment, especially in light of the current issues with opioids, new approaches using less traditional methods are being tried.

A new study done in the Netherlands showed that use of tetrahydrocannabinol, one of the active substances in marijuana, is not effective in the treatment of chronic pain from prior surgery or chronic pancreatitis.

Fig. 1.1 presents a practical approach to chronic abdominal pain.

For further information, please see Chapter 128, "Functional Gastrointestinal Disorders," in *Goldman-Cecil Medicine*, 26th Edition. ❖

SUGGESTED READINGS

Almario CV, Ballal ML, Chey WD, et al: Burden of gastrointestinal symptoms in the United States: results of a nationally representative survey of over 71,000 Americans, Am J Gastroenterol 113:1701–1710, 2018.

Brenner DM, Fogel R, Dorn SD, et al: Efficacy, safety, and tolerability of plecanatide in patients with irritable bowel syndrome with constipation: results of two phase 3 randomized clinical trials, Am J Gastroenterol 113:735–745, 2018.

Brenner DM, Sayuk GS, Gutman CR, et al: Efficacy and safety of eluxadoline in patients with irritable bowel syndrome with diarrhea who report inadequate symptom control with loperamide: RELIEF phase 4 study, Am J Gastroenterol 114:1502–1511, 2019.

Chang L, Lembo A, Sultan S: American gastroenterological association institute technical review on the pharmacological management of irritable bowel syndrome, Gastroenterology 147:1149–1172, 2014.

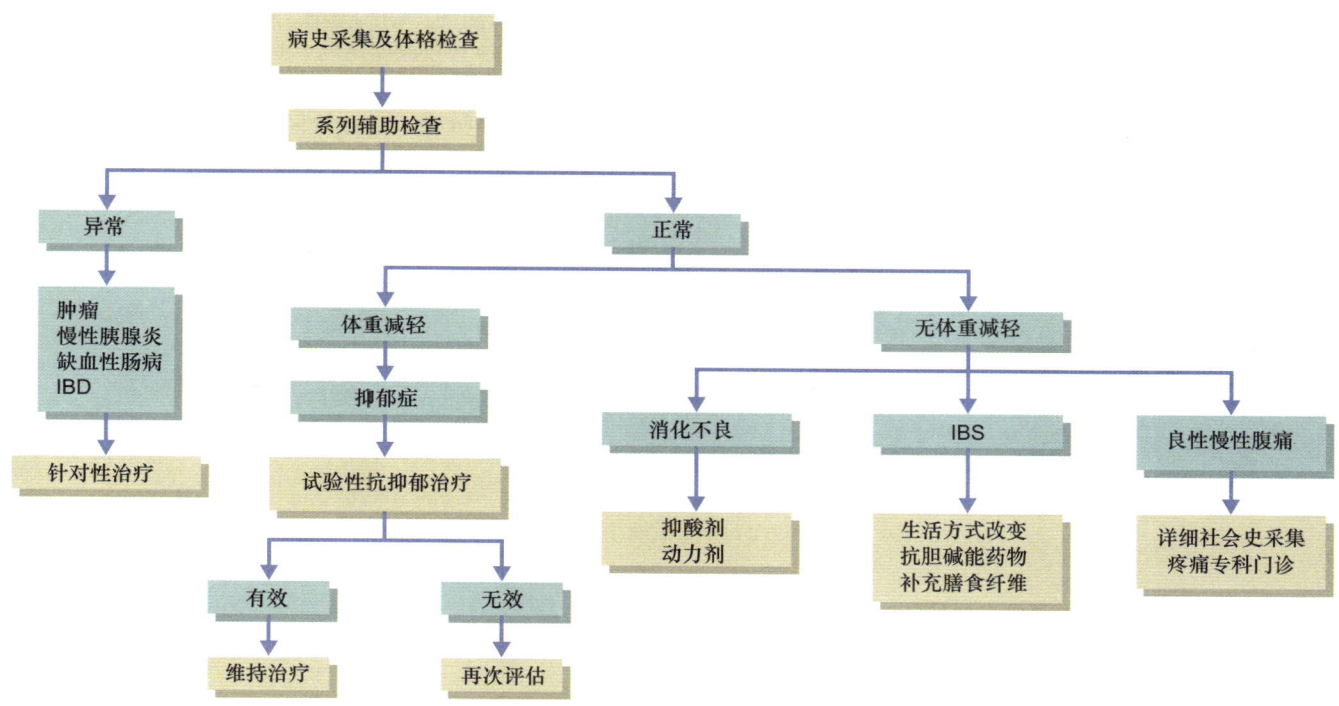

图 1.1 慢性腹痛患者的接诊。IBD，炎症性肠病；IBS，肠易激综合征

用，这些药物的使用受到限制。艾沙杜林以阿片类受体为靶点，在部分洛哌丁胺治疗失败的 IBS-D 患者中，艾沙杜林有助于控制腹痛和腹泻。利那洛肽可通过环磷酸鸟苷（cGMP）通路增加氯化物和碳酸氢盐在肠腔的分泌。该作用机制也可缓解 IBS-C 患者的内脏痛，但由于不可接受的副作用，其使用受到限制，目前可使用 72 μg 的较低剂量（译者注：利那洛肽尚未报道不可接受的不良反应，且无使用限制的报道。较低剂量主要是为了维持治疗）。普卡那肽是该类药物的新成员，在初步研究中显示出良好的应用前景，但尚未证明其比利那洛肽更有效。替那帕诺是一种新型小分子药物，其作用机制是抑制钠从大肠的肠腔内转运，从而改善 IBS-C 患者的便秘和腹痛。该药物仍在研究中，但已获得美国食品药品监督管理局（FDA）批准。它代表了一种新的治疗方法。

临床上更具挑战性的问题是功能性腹痛综合征，其是指持续数月或数年的腹痛。与其他慢性疼痛的原因不同，功能性腹痛综合征的腹痛通常与进食、排便或月经无关。常见于女性，既往多次检查和诊断性试验均为阴性，且通常在手术后症状也不能缓解。冗长或重复的检查适得其反，只会让患者相信需要再做一次检查才能确定腹痛的来源。医生必须确定没有器质性疾病，且必须意识到疼痛是真实的。尽管该病的腹痛不符合任何常见的模式，但这些患者确实不是诈病者，抑郁症可能是疼痛的结果，而不是原因。

慢性腹痛的管理要求很高，除科学知识外，还要结合一定的策略、交流技巧及同情心。应尽可能询问社会因素，包括有无躯体虐待和性虐待病史，尤其是女性患者。精神评估是必要的，但该建议可能会被患者解读为"医生认为疼痛是我自己想出来的"。部分病例需转诊至经验丰富的疼痛管理专家，从而通过神经阻滞或其他止痛装置来缓解局部疼痛。如果仍然无效，患者可转诊至心理学家或精神科医生。

由于慢性腹痛治疗所面临的挑战，尤其是当前阿片类药物使用的问题，人们正在尝试使用非传统治疗的新方法。

荷兰的一项研究表明，使用四氢大麻酚（大麻的一种活性物质）对治疗既往手术或慢性胰腺炎引起的慢性腹痛无效。

图 1.1 展示了慢性腹痛的诊疗方法。

有关此专题的深入讨论，请参阅 *Goldman-Cecil Medicine* 第 26 版第 128 章"功能性胃肠疾病"。

推荐阅读

Almario CV, Ballal ML, Chey WD, et al: Burden of gastrointestinal symptoms in the United States: results of a nationally representative survey of over 71,000 Americans, Am J Gastroenterol 113:1701–1710, 2018.

Brenner DM, Fogel R, Dorn SD, et al: Efficacy, safety, and tolerability of plecanatide in patients with irritable bowel syndrome with constipation: results of two phase 3 randomized clinical trials, Am J Gastroenterol 113:735–745, 2018.

Brenner DM, Sayuk GS, Gutman CR, et al: Efficacy and safety of eluxadoline in patients with irritable bowel syndrome with diarrhea who report inadequate symptom control with loperamide: RELIEF phase 4 study, Am J Gastroenterol 114:1502–1511, 2019.

Chang L, Lembo A, Sultan S: American gastroenterological association institute technical review on the pharmacological management of irritable bowel syndrome, Gastroenterology 147:1149–1172, 2014.

Chey WD, Lembo AJ, Rosenbaum DP: Tenapanor treatment of patients with constipation-predominant irritable bowel syndrome: a phase 2, randomised, placebo-controlled efficacy and safety trial, Am J Gastroenterol 112:763–774, 2017.

De Vries M, van Rijckevorsel DCM, Vissers KCP, et al: Tetrahydrocannabinol does not reduce pain in patients with chronic abdominal pain in a phase 2 placebo-controlled study, Clin Gastroenterol Hepatol 15:1079–1086, 2017.

Lacy BE, Chey WD, Cash BD, et al: Eluxadoline efficacy in IBS-D patients who report prior loperamide use, Am J Gastroenterol 112:924–932, 2017.

Schoenfeld P, Lacey BE, Chey WD, et al: Low dose linaclotide (72 µg) for chronic idiopathic constipation: a 12-week, randomized, double-blind, placebo-controlled trial, Am J Gastroenterol 113:105–114, 2017.

Shah ED, Kim HM, Shoenfeld P: Efficacy and tolerability of guanylate cyclase-c agonists for irritable bowel syndrome with constipation and chronic idiopathic constipation: a systematic review and meta-analysis, Am J Gastroenterol 113:329–338, 2018.

Sperber AD, Drossman D: The functional abdominal pain syndrome, Aliment Pharmacol Ther 33:514–524, 2011.

Chey WD, Lembo AJ, Rosenbaum DP: Tenapanor treatment of patients with constipation-predominant irritable bowel syndrome: a phase 2, randomised, placebo-controlled efficacy and safety trial, Am J Gastroenterol 112:763–774, 2017.

De Vries M, van Rijckevorsel DCM, Vissers KCP, et al: Tetrahydrocannabinol does not reduce pain in patients with chronic abdominal pain in a phase 2 placebo-controlled study, Clin Gastroenterol Hepatol 15:1079–1086, 2017.

Lacy BE, Chey WD, Cash BD, et al: Eluxadoline efficacy in IBS-D patients who report prior loperamide use, Am J Gastroenterol 112:924–932, 2017.

Schoenfeld P, Lacey BE, Chey WD, et al: Low dose linaclotide (72 μg) for chronic idiopathic constipation: a 12-week, randomized, double-blind, placebo-controlled trial, Am J Gastroenterol 113:105–114, 2017.

Shah ED, Kim HM, Shoenfeld P: Efficacy and tolerability of guanylate cyclase-c agonists for irritable bowel syndrome with constipation and chronic idiopathic constipation: a systematic review and meta-analysis, Am J Gastroenterol 113:329–338, 2018.

Sperber AD, Drossman D: The functional abdominal pain syndrome, Aliment Pharmacol Ther 33:514–524, 2011.

2

Common Clinical Manifestations of Gastrointestinal Disease: Gastrointestinal Hemorrhage

Waihong Chung, Abbas Rupawala

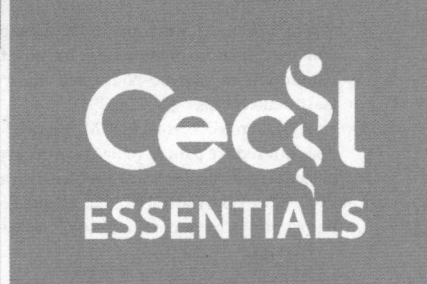

INTRODUCTION

Gastrointestinal bleeding (GIB) is a major cause of morbidity, accounting for over 844,000 emergency department visits and 513,000 hospitalizations in the United States in 2014. GIB also accounts for over 2.2 million days of productivity loss and $5 billion in direct cost annually. Despite increasing costs of care, mortality due to GIB has declined in recent years in part due to increased rates of endoscopy and improved endoscopic therapy. GIB can result from a variety of etiologies (Table 2.1), its presentation can vary greatly depending on age and comorbidity, and its clinical course can evolve rapidly over time and in response to treatment. It is, therefore, essential to apply a systematic approach to the management of all cases of suspected GIB. We advocate a four-step approach that can be encapsulated by a simple mnemonic *PRET*: *P*rioritize, *R*esuscitate, *E*valuate, and *T*reat.

APPROACH TO PATIENTS WITH GASTROINTESTINAL BLEEDING

Prioritize

The first step in the approach to GIB is to prioritize and triage patients based on acuity and severity of blood loss. The objective of this step is to guide the pace of evaluation and ensure that the patient is managed in a timely and cost-effective manner.

GIB can be broadly classified as overt GIB, when patients present with hematemesis, coffee-ground emesis, melena, or hematochezia (Table 2.2), and occult GIB, when symptoms of overt bleeding are absent but patients are anemic with heme (occult blood) positive stools. In addition to symptoms of bleeding, patients may also present with some combination of weakness, dizziness, lightheadedness, shortness of breath, postural changes in blood pressure or pulse, cramping abdominal pain, and diarrhea. Intuitively, overt GIB likely represents faster or higher volume blood loss; thus, patients presenting with overt GIB should be prioritized to receive an expedited work-up in the emergency room or in the inpatient setting. Meanwhile, patients with occult GIB, who are otherwise asymptomatic, may be evaluated safely and more efficiently in the outpatient setting.

GIB can also be classified into acute GIB, arbitrarily defined as bleeding duration of less than 3 days, and chronic GIB. The authors, however, find this classification less useful in guiding prioritization because it fails to convey the difference in severity between protracted or continual occult GIB versus ongoing or recurrent overt GIB.

Resuscitate

The second step is to resuscitate and stabilize the patient's hemodynamic parameters and to alleviate symptoms. The objective of this step is to prevent and reverse the complications of blood loss and restore end-organ perfusion. It is worth emphasizing that adequate resuscitation is *the most important step* in the management of GIB and must take priority over the subsequent steps of evaluation and treatment.

In cases of overt GIB, the resuscitative effort should follow the basic principle of airway, breathing, and circulation. Airway management and respiratory support should be considered in patients presenting with massive or recurrent hematemesis as well as those with altered mental status to minimize risk of aspiration. Restoration of normal circulatory function should be achieved by rapid infusion of an isotonic crystalloid fluid, such as normal saline or lactated Ringer's solution. Concerns regarding volume overload and pulmonary edema in patients with heart failure or renal failure should not delay initiation of fluid resuscitation but may necessitate the use of positive-pressure ventilation. A restrictive transfusion threshold of hemoglobin less than 7 g/dL has been shown to improve survival (95% vs. 91%) and decreased rebleeding (10% vs. 16%) compared to a threshold of 9 g/dL. This is especially true in cirrhotic patients presenting with suspected variceal bleeding where over-transfusion may increase portal hypertension, bleeding and mortality.

In cases of occult GIB, resuscitation should aim at relieving the symptoms of anemia. Those with severe, symptomatic anemia and signs of end-organ ischemia, such as angina or renal insufficiency, may be transfused. Those with nonsevere symptoms of anemia, such as weakness, fatigue, exercise intolerance, or exertional dyspnea, can receive oral or parenteral iron replacement therapy.

Evaluate

The third step is performing a focused history and physical exam and obtaining relevant laboratory and imaging tests (Table 2.3). The goal of this step is to localize the potential bleeding site and identify the most likely etiology of the bleed.

From a diagnostic and therapeutic perspective, it is most useful to distinguish GIB into upper GIB (UGIB), historically defined as bleeding emanating from a source proximal to the ligament of Treitz, and lower GIB (LGIB). LGIB can be further subdivided into small bowel bleeding, originating proximal to the terminal ileum, and colonic bleeding. UGIB has traditionally been considered to account for 76% to 82% of GIB cases and is associated with a significantly higher emergency room to hospital admission rate (78% vs. 40%) as well as in-hospital mortality (1.5% vs. 0.5%) compared to LGIB. Patients with suspected UGIB should, therefore, be managed more aggressively, including offering an early endoscopy within 24 hours of presentation, while those with self-limiting LGIB may be observed clinically. Up to 15% of patients presenting with presumed LGIB may have UGIB. The term *obscure*

胃肠疾病常见临床表现：消化道出血

蒋青伟 译　吴晰 谭蓓 审校　杨爱明 通审

引言

消化道出血（GIB）是消化系统常见的并发症，2014年美国超过 844 000 人次和 513 000 人次因 GIB 而急诊就诊和住院治疗。GIB 每年造成超过 220 万天的生产力损失和 50 亿美元的直接成本。尽管医疗成本逐年增加，但近年来 GIB 的死亡率有所下降，部分原因是内镜检查率的提高和内镜治疗的进步。GIB 可由多种病因引起（表 2.1），因年龄和合并症情况不同，患者的临床表现差异很大，其临床病程可随时间推移和治疗反应而迅速演化。因此，采用系统路径化管理所有疑诊 GIB 的患者尤为重要。目前主张采用四步法（概括为"PRET"）：确定优先级（**P**rioritize）、复苏（**R**esuscitate）、评估（**E**valuate）和治疗（**T**reat）。

消化道出血患者的接诊

确定优先级

GIB 的处理首先应根据出血速度和严重程度对患者进行优先排序和分流，旨在指导评估进度和确保患者得到及时且经济有效的诊疗。

GIB 大致可分为显性和隐性 GIB，前者是指患者出现呕血、呕吐咖啡渣样物、黑便或便血（表 2.2），后者是指患者没有显性出血的症状，但有贫血且粪便血红素（隐血）阳性。除出血症状外，患者还可能伴有乏力、头晕、眩晕、气短、体位性血压或脉搏变化、腹部痉挛痛和腹泻等症状。从直观上看，显性 GIB 通常意味着失血较快或失血量较大，因此这些患者应优先在急诊室或住院部接受加急处理。隐性 GIB 患者如果没有症状，可以安全高效地在门诊进行评估。

GIB 还可分为急性 GIB（定义为出血持续时间 < 3 天）和慢性 GIB。但这种分类方法在指导优先级方面作用不大，因为它无法区分长期/持续隐性 GIB 与活动性/复发性显性 GIB 的严重程度。

复苏

第二步是复苏和稳定患者的血流动力学参数并缓解症状。这一步的目标是避免和逆转失血并发症，恢复内脏器官的灌注。需要强调的是，充分复苏是管理 GIB 最重要的步骤，必须优先于随后的评估和治疗环节。

对于显性 GIB 患者，复苏工作应遵循气道、呼吸和循环的基本原则。对于出现大量或反复呕血及意识状态改变的患者，应考虑进行气道管理和呼吸支持，以减小误吸风险。恢复正常循环功能应通过快速输注等渗晶体溶液（如生理盐水或乳酸盐林格液）。对心力衰竭或肾衰竭患者出现容量超负荷和肺水肿的担忧不应延迟液体复苏的启动，但可能需要正压通气。相比于血红蛋白阈值 < 9 g/dl 的限制性输血，血红蛋白阈值 < 7 g/dl 的限制性输血可改善生存率（95% *vs.* 91%）并降低再出血率（10% *vs.* 16%）。尤其是对于疑似静脉曲张出血的肝硬化患者，过度输血可能会增加门静脉高压、出血，使死亡率升高。

对于隐性 GIB 患者，复苏的目的是缓解贫血相关症状。对于有重度症状性贫血和内脏器官缺血症状（如心绞痛或肾功能不全）的患者，可进行输血。贫血症状不严重（如乏力、疲劳、运动不耐受或劳力性呼吸困难）的患者，可接受口服或静脉输注铁剂替代治疗。

评估

第三步是询问重点病史和体格检查，并进行相关的实验室检查和影像学检查（表 2.3）。这一步的目的是确定可能的出血部位和病因。

从诊断和治疗的角度看，最有用的方法是将 GIB 区分为上消化道出血（UGIB）和下消化道出血（LGIB）。UGIB 的定义为来自十二指肠悬韧带（屈氏韧带）以上部位的 GIB。LGIB 又可进一步分为小肠出血（出血位于末端回肠的近端）和结肠出血。UGIB 占全部 GIB 病例的 76%～82%，与 LGIB 相比，UGIB 的急诊入院率（78% *vs.* 40%）和院内死亡率（1.5% *vs.* 0.5%）明显更高。因此，对于疑似 UGIB 的患者，应采取更积极的措施，包括在出血 24 h 内尽早进行内镜检查，而自限性 LGIB 患者可进行临床观察。多达 15% 疑诊 LGIB 的患者实际上可能是 UGIB。"不明原因消化道出血"一词

TABLE 2.1 Common Etiologies of GIB

Source	Associated Clinical Features	Management
Upper Gastrointestinal Tract		
Esophagitis/esophageal ulcer	Reflux, dysphagia, odynophagia	Acid suppression, antireflux surgery
Esophageal cancer	Dysphagia, weight loss	Chemoradiation, surgery
Gastroesophageal varices/portal gastropathy	Chronic liver disease, portal hypertension	Octreotide, endoscopic therapy, antibiotics
Mallory-Weiss tear	Repeated retching, vomiting, alcoholics	Supportive care, endoscopy
Gastritis/gastric ulcer/duodenitis/duodenal ulcer	NSAIDs, alcohol, *Helicobacter pylori*, epigastric pain	Hold NSAIDs, treat *H. pylori*, acid suppression, endoscopic therapy
Gastric cancer	Early satiety, weight loss, abdominal pain	Surgery, chemotherapy
Gastric antral vascular ectasia	Cirrhosis, systemic sclerosis	Endoscopic therapy
Angioectasias	Painless bleeding, may be present throughout GI tract, aortic stenosis (Heyde syndrome)	Endoscopic therapy
Cameron lesion	Hiatal hernia	Surgery for hiatal hernia repair
Dieulafoy lesion	Cardiovascular disease, chronic kidney disease, NSAIDs, alcohol	Endoscopic therapy
Aortoenteric fistula	History of open abdominal aortic aneurysm repair, sentinel bleed, large-volume bleeding	Surgery
Hemobilia	History of biliary tract instrumentation, biliary malignancy	Repeat endoscopy, vascular interventional radiology (VIR), surgery
Hemosuccus pancreaticus	Pancreatic pseudocyst, pancreatic tumor	VIR
Lower Gastrointestinal Tract		
Diverticular bleed	Diverticulosis, painless hematochezia in older patients	Endoscopic therapy, VIR
Infectious colitis	History of exposure, diarrhea, abdominal pain	Treat underlying infection
Inflammatory bowel disease	History of colitis, diarrhea, abdominal pain, fever, tenesmus	Treat underlying inflammation
Ischemic colitis	History of profound hypotension, abdominal pain, followed by bleeding	Supportive care, surgery
Angioectasia	Obscure overt or occult bleeding	Endoscopic therapy
Radiation-induced telangiectasia	Pelvic radiation	Endoscopic therapy
Meckel's diverticulum	Painless hematochezia in younger patients	Surgery
Colorectal cancer	Weight loss, change in bowel habits, anemia	Surgery, chemotherapy
Colon polyp	Painless hematochezia	Endoscopic resection
Post-polypectomy bleed	Recent colonoscopy with polypectomy	Endoscopic therapy
Hemorrhoidal bleed	Hematochezia with bowel movement	Supportive care, surgery, banding
Stercoral ulcer	Severe constipation	Supportive care, treat constipation

TABLE 2.2 Definitions of Overt GIB

Hematemesis
Vomiting of bright red blood or partially digested blood that resembles coffee grounds.
Source of bleeding is likely to be proximal to the ligament of Treitz.
Consider swallowed blood from nasopharynx (e.g., epistaxis) or the respiratory tract (hemoptysis).

Melena
Passing of black, tarry, and usually foul-smelling stool, representing digested blood.
Source of bleeding is likely to be in the upper gastrointestinal tract, the small bowel, or occasionally the proximal colon.
As little as 50-100 mL of blood can result in melena.

Hematochezia
Passing of bright red blood or maroon stool per rectum.
Source of bleeding is likely to be in the lower gastrointestinal tract (small bowel and colon).
10-15% of severe UGIB with brisk bleeding may present with hematochezia.

GIB, which was previously used interchangeably with small intestinal bleeding, is now reserved to describe cases of overt or occult GIB where the bleeding source is not readily identified after complete evaluation of the entire GI tract including the small bowel.

Signs and symptoms that are strongly predictive of an UGIB include the presence of bright red blood or coffee-ground emesis as well as a markedly elevated blood urea nitrogen (BUN)-to-creatinine ratio in a patient without chronic kidney disease. Melena refers to black, tarry, foul-smelling stools formed as a result of blood being altered by gastric acid, digestive enzymes, and intestinal bacteria. Although the presence of melena is often indicative of UGIB, it can also be seen in cases of small intestinal as well as right-sided colonic bleed. The use of nasogastric lavage for ruling out UGIB has largely fallen out of favor due to its poor negative likelihood ratio and its association with significant patient discomfort.

A critical decision point in the evaluation step is assessing the odds of variceal bleeding being the etiology, as it is a serious gastrointestinal emergency that is associated with a high (>30%) mortality rate and is managed somewhat differently than other etiologies of GIB. Any patients with known varices, acute alcoholic hepatitis, or cirrhosis of any etiologies, especially those with signs and symptoms of portal

表 2.1 GIB 的常见病因

出血来源	相关临床特征	管理方案
上消化道		
食管炎/食管溃疡	反流、吞咽困难、吞咽疼痛	抑酸治疗、抗反流手术
食管癌	吞咽困难、体重减轻	放化疗、手术
胃食管静脉曲张/门静脉高压性胃病	慢性肝病、门静脉高压	奥曲肽、内镜治疗、抗生素
食管贲门黏膜撕裂（Mallory-Weiss 撕裂）	反复干呕、呕吐、酒瘾者	支持治疗、内镜
胃炎/胃溃疡/十二指肠炎/十二指肠溃疡	非甾体抗炎药、酒精、幽门螺杆菌、上腹痛	停用非甾体抗炎药、根除幽门螺杆菌、抑酸治疗、内镜治疗
胃癌	早饱、体重减轻、腹痛	手术、化疗
胃窦血管扩张症	肝硬化、系统性硬化症	内镜治疗
血管扩张症	无痛性出血（可出现在整个消化道）、主动脉狭窄（Heyde 综合征）	内镜治疗
Cameron 病变	食管裂孔疝	食管裂孔疝修补术
胃恒径动脉病（Dieulafoy 病变）	心血管疾病、慢性肾脏病、非甾体抗炎药、酒精	内镜治疗
主动脉肠瘘	开腹主动脉瘤修补术史、前哨出血、大量出血	手术
胆道出血	胆道器械操作史、胆道恶性肿瘤	复查内镜、血管放射介入治疗（VIR）、手术
胰管出血	胰腺假性囊肿、胰腺肿瘤	VIR
下消化道		
憩室出血	憩室病、老年患者无痛性便血	内镜治疗、VIR
感染性结肠炎	暴露史、腹泻、腹痛	治疗潜在感染
炎症性肠病	结肠炎史、腹泻、腹痛、发热、里急后重	治疗潜在炎症
缺血性结肠炎	严重低血压史、腹痛伴继发出血	支持治疗、手术
血管扩张症	原因不明的显性或隐性出血	内镜治疗
放疗继发毛细血管扩张症	盆腔放疗	内镜治疗
梅克尔憩室	年轻患者无痛性便血	手术
结直肠癌	体重减轻、排便习惯改变、贫血	手术、化疗
结肠息肉	无痛性便血	内镜下切除
息肉切除后出血	近期结肠镜下息肉切除	内镜治疗
痔疮出血	排便时便血	支持治疗、手术、套扎治疗
粪性溃疡	严重便秘	支持治疗、治疗便秘

表 2.2 显性 GIB 的定义

呕血
呕吐鲜红色血液或部分消化的咖啡渣样血液
出血部位多位于十二指肠悬韧带近端
应考虑吞咽来自鼻咽（如鼻出血）或呼吸道（咯血）的血液

黑便
排出黑色柏油样且常伴恶臭的粪便，即消化后的血液
出血部位可能在上消化道、小肠或近端结肠
仅 50～100 ml 血液即可导致黑便

便血
经直肠排出鲜红色血便或褐红色粪便
出血部位可能在下消化道（小肠和结肠）
10%～15% 严重活动性 UGIB 患者可能出现便血

既往等同于小肠出血，现在仅用于描述对整个消化道（包括小肠）进行全面评估后仍无法确定出血部位的显性或隐性 GIB。

对 UGIB 有重要提示意义的体征和症状包括出现呕鲜红色血液或咖啡渣样呕吐物，以及无慢性肾脏病患者血尿素氮（BUN）/肌酐比值明显升高。黑便是血液被胃酸、消化酶和肠道细菌作用后形成的黑色柏油样伴恶臭的粪便。虽然出现黑便通常提示 UGIB，但其也可见于小肠和右半结肠出血患者。通过鼻胃管灌洗来排除 UGIB 的阴性似然比欠佳，且患者有明显不适感，故已逐渐被弃用。

评估步骤中的一个关键决策点是评估静脉曲张导致出血的概率，因其为严重的胃肠道急症，且死亡率高（＞30%），其处理方法与其他病因引起的 GIB 有所不同。任何已知患有静脉曲张、急性酒精性肝炎或任何病因的肝硬化患者，尤其是有门静脉高压症状和

TABLE 2.3	Key Information in the Evaluation of GIB	
History	Physical Exam	Laboratory Test

• Nature of bleeding (hematemesis, melena, hematochezia)
• Other gastrointestinal symptoms
• Systemic (cardiopulmonary, constitutional, and other) symptoms
• Medications: NSAIDs, corticosteroids, bisphosphonates, anticoagulants, and antiplatelets
• Illicit drug and alcohol exposure
• Surgical history
• Past medical history
  • Peptic ulcer disease
  • *Helicobacter pylori* infection and treatment
  • Gastrointestinal bleed
  • Chronic liver disease
  • Inflammatory bowel disease
  • Malignancy
  • Pelvic radiation
  • Recent endoscopic interventions (e.g., polypectomy)
	• Vital signs
	• Presence of gross blood in oropharynx
	• Presence of abdominal tenderness
	• Digital rectal exam
		• Complete blood count
		• Basic metabolic panel
		• Hepatic function panel
		• Prothrombin Time/INR
		• Blood type and cross match

hypertension as evident by the presence of *caput medusa*, jaundice, splenomegaly, and/or ascites on exam as well as coagulopathy and thrombocytopenia on laboratory tests, should be managed as a potential variceal hemorrhage.

Older patients and those with significant comorbidities, continued bleeding, and hemodynamic instability are also at higher risk of poor outcomes and should be managed more aggressively and monitored in the intensive care setting. Prognostic scores such as the Glasgow-Blatchford score, Rockall scale, and AIMS65 score may help identify high-risk patients in need of more urgent evaluation and treatment.

Treat

The fourth step in the management of GIB is to confirm the location and etiology of bleeding and to deliver treatment both locally and systemically. The goal of this step is to achieve adequate hemostasis and minimize the risk of rebleeding. A comprehensive treatment plan for GIB may consist of up to six components that can be summarized by another simple mnemonic CAMPER: *C*oagulopathy, *A*cid suppression, *M*edical therapy, *P*reprocedural preparation, *E*ndoscopy, and *R*escue technique.

Coagulopathy

Coagulopathy should be addressed in any patient presenting with overt GIB. In general, pharmacologic anticoagulation and antiplatelets should be held, unless otherwise contraindicated due to another medical condition such as recent vascular stent placement, until hemostasis is achieved. In patients presenting with hemodynamically significant GIB, reversal of warfarin using intravenous vitamin K as well as inactivated 4-factor prothrombin complex concentrate (PCC) should be considered. Fresh frozen plasma has fallen out of favor due to its higher risk of adverse reactions and volume overload but may be an option when PCC is not available. Patients on direct oral anticoagulants do not typically require reversal due to their shorter half-life, although the use of antifibrinolytic agents can be considered in those with significant comorbidities or worsening bleeding symptoms. Specific reversal agents for the direct oral anticoagulants are reserved for those at imminent risk of death from bleeding. Cirrhotic patients are not necessarily hypocoagulable despite the elevated INR due to impaired synthesis of both anticoagulants and procoagulants. Platelet transfusion should be considered in those with a platelet level less than 50,000/μL but has limited benefit in individuals continuing on antiplatelet agents. Desmopressin can be considered in patients with uremic platelet dysfunction or von Willebrand disease.

Acid Suppression

Acid suppression with an intravenous proton pump inhibitor (PPI) should be initiated on admission in patients with suspected UGIB. It primarily helps with clot stabilization and is associated with reduced rates of high-risk stigmata identified on endoscopy, the need for endoscopic therapy in patients with peptic ulcer bleeding, and the risk of ulcer rebleeding. The optimal dose of preprocedure PPI has not been determined, although intermittent PPI therapy was found to be comparable to continuous therapy in patients with endoscopically treated high-risk bleeding ulcers.

Medical Therapy

Medical therapy plays an important role in the management of GIB in cirrhotic patients. Prophylactic antibiotics, intravenous ceftriaxone or a quinolone, may be administered to any cirrhotic patients with GIB for 7 days to decrease the risk of bacterial infections and mortality. Vasoactive medications, such as octreotide, terlipressin, and vasopressin, should be initiated as soon as possible in any patients presenting with suspected variceal bleeding and continued for 3 days if the etiology is confirmed on endoscopy.

Preprocedural Preparation

Preprocedural preparation is essential to achieving adequate endoscopic hemostasis while minimizing procedure-related complications. Prokinetic agents, such as erythromycin or metoclopramide, should be considered in patients presenting with ongoing or recurrent hematemesis in order to clear the stomach of food and blood clots, which may obscure potential bleeding sources and increase the risk of aspiration. Similarly, adequate colon cleansing using a polyethylene glycol-based solution until the colon is clear of stool and blood clots is preferred prior to colonoscopy and associated with higher cecal intubation rate, improved diagnostic yield, and lower risk of perforation.

Endoscopy

Endoscopy serves a diagnostic and therapeutic role in the management of GIB after adequate resuscitation. Urgent upper endoscopy should be performed within 12 hours of hospitalization in any patients with suspected variceal bleeding, and early upper endoscopy within 24 hours of hospitalization is recommended in patients with nonvariceal overt UGIB. Patients with ulcers and stigmata of recent bleeding may need endoscopic therapy to reduce risk of rebleeding. Examples of endoscopic hemostatic techniques include epinephrine injection, contact thermal coagulation for visible vessels, as well as through-the-scope clip and over-the-scope clip as methods to achieve physical tamponade of a bleeding site. In cases of variceal bleeding, band ligation and

表2.3 评估 GIB 的关键信息

病史	体格检查	实验室检查

• 出血性质（呕血、黑便、便血）
• 其他消化道症状
• 全身（心肺、一般状况、其他）症状
• 服用药物：非甾体抗炎药、糖皮质激素、双膦酸盐、抗凝剂、抗血小板药
• 毒品及饮酒
• 手术史
• 既往史
  • 消化性溃疡
  • 幽门螺杆菌感染和治疗
  • 消化道出血
  • 慢性肝病
  • 炎症性肠病
  • 恶性肿瘤
  • 盆腔放疗
  • 近期内镜治疗（如息肉切除）
	• 生命体征
	• 口咽部大量血液
	• 腹部压痛
	• 直肠指检
		• 全血细胞计数
		• 基础代谢检测
		• 肝功能检测
		• 凝血酶原时间/INR
		• 血型和交叉配型

INR，国际标准化比值。

体征［如海蛇头样腹壁静脉曲张、黄疸、脾大和（或）腹腔积液，以及实验室检查发现凝血功能障碍和血小板减少］的患者，均应作为潜在静脉曲张出血处理。

老年、伴严重并发症、持续出血和血流动力学不稳定的患者，预后不良的风险较高，应在重症监护病房进行更积极的治疗和监测。预后评分［如 Glasgow-Blatchford 评分、Rockall 评分和 AIMS65 评分］有助于识别需要进行更紧急评估和治疗的高风险患者。

治疗

管理 GIB 的第四步是确认出血部位和病因，并进行局部和全身治疗。这一步的目标是实现充分止血，降低再出血风险。GIB 的综合治疗计划由六部分组成（可概括为"CAMPER"）：纠正凝血功能障碍（**C**oagulopathy）、抑酸（**A**cid suppression）、药物治疗（**M**edical therapy）、操作前准备（**P**reprocedural preparation）、内镜检查（**E**ndoscopy）和补救技术（**R**escue technique）。

纠正凝血功能障碍

所有显性 GIB 患者均应治疗凝血功能障碍。一般来说，应停用抗凝剂和抗血小板药物，直至出血停止，除非因其他疾病而无法停用（如近期置入血管支架）。对于有明显血流动力学异常的 GIB 患者，应考虑静脉注射维生素 K 及无活性的四因子凝血酶原复合体浓缩物（PCC）来逆转华法林导致的出血。新鲜冰冻血浆因其导致不良反应和容量超负荷的风险较高而不作为首选，但在无法使用 PCC 时也不失为一种选择。服用直接口服抗凝剂（DOAC）的患者由于药物半衰期较短，通常不需要拮抗，但对于有明显合并症或出血症状恶化的患者，可考虑使用抗纤溶药物。DOAC 的特异性拮抗剂仅用于因出血面临死亡风险的急症患者。肝硬化患者由于抗凝因子和促凝因子的合成同时受损，尽管国际标准化比值（INR）升高，但并不一定是低凝状态。血小板计数 < 50 000/μl 的患者应考虑血小板输注，但对于继续服用抗血小板药物的患者，输注血小板的获益有限。尿毒症性血小板功能障碍或血管性血友病（vWD）患者可考虑使用去氨加压素。

抑酸

疑诊 UGIB 的患者在入院时即应开始静脉输注质子泵抑制剂（PPI）抑制胃酸，其有助于稳定血凝块，并能降低内镜检查发现高危病灶的概率、消化性溃疡出血患者对内镜治疗的需求及溃疡再出血的风险。虽然在需要内镜治疗的高危出血性溃疡患者中，间歇 PPI 治疗与持续治疗效果相当，但操作前 PPI 的最佳剂量尚未确定。

药物治疗

药物治疗在肝硬化合并 GIB 患者的治疗中发挥重要作用。所有肝硬化合并 GIB 患者可予以 7 天的预防性抗生素治疗（静脉注射头孢曲松或喹诺酮类药物），以降低细菌感染风险和死亡率。疑诊静脉曲张出血的患者均应尽快开始使用血管活性药物（如奥曲肽、特利加压素和血管升压素），在内镜检查确认病因后应继续用药 3 天。

操作前准备

操作前准备对于实现充分的镜下止血并减少操作相关并发症至关重要。对于正在呕血或反复呕血的患者，应考虑使用促动力药（如红霉素或甲氧氯普胺），以清理胃腔中的食物和血凝块，避免其掩盖出血来源并增加误吸风险。同样，结肠镜检查前适当应用聚乙二醇溶液清除结肠内的粪便和血凝块，可以提高达盲率和诊断率，并降低穿孔风险。

内镜检查

经过充分复苏后，内镜检查在 GIB 的管理中具有诊断和治疗作用。对于疑诊静脉曲张出血的患者，应在住院 12 h 内进行急诊上消化道内镜检查；对于非静脉曲张性显性 UGIB 患者，建议在住院 24 h 内进行早期上消化道内镜检查。有溃疡和近期出血征象的患者可能需要内镜治疗，以降低再次出血的风险。内镜止血技术包括肾上腺素注射、针对可见血管进行接触式热凝，以及经活检孔道止血夹或经镜身外止血夹

injection of sclerosing agents for esophageal varices and injection of cyanoacrylate and other tissue glue in gastric varices can be performed. Other techniques include argon plasma coagulation for superficial vascular lesions and hemostatic topical powders as temporizing measures. The optimal timing of colonoscopy for overt LGIB is less well defined. Urgent colonoscopy, defined variably as within 12 to 24 hours of hospitalization, may improve diagnostic yield but does not improve rebleeding risk, need for surgery, or length of stay compared to elective colonoscopy. In general, it is reasonable to prioritize patients with ongoing or recurrent overt LGIB for an inpatient colonoscopy whereas those with self-limiting bleed may be evaluated electively. Hemodynamically unstable patients with suspected LGIB should also undergo upper endoscopy to rule out a brisk UGIB. Presence of blood in terminal ileum may be indicative of a proximal or small bowel bleeding source. Video capsule endoscopy (VCE) is a valuable tool for diagnosing a small bowel bleeding source, especially when performed within 72 hours of index bleeding episode. Patients with occult GIB should undergo endoscopy and colonoscopy, followed by VCE if necessary, electively once they are medically optimized. Enteroscopy techniques such as push, balloon, or spiral enteroscopy can be used for diagnosis and treatment of small bowel pathology detected on capsule endoscopy. Computed tomography (CT) and magnetic resonance (MR) enterography techniques have largely replaced fluoroscopy and can be used to diagnose small bowel pathology when VCE is not available.

Rescue Technique

Rescue techniques are sometimes necessary, for both diagnostic and therapeutic purposes, in patients who fail endoscopic management or are unable to tolerate endoscopy. CT angiography or multidetector row CT is a reasonable first-line imaging test to facilitate localization of GIB in patients presenting with hemodynamically significant overt GIB. Angiography relies on active bleeding and may be falsely negative in cases of intermittent bleeding. Tagged red blood cell scintigraphy, although less readily available and more logistically cumbersome than CT angiography, is ideally suited for evaluation of intermittent, obscure GIB because of its higher sensitivity and the ability to perform repeated scans after initial injection of tagged cells. Super-selective angiographic embolization can be successful in achieving immediate hemostasis in many cases of GIB, including large penetrating duodenal ulcers, small bowel tumor bleed, and colonic diverticular bleed. In cases of uncontrollable variceal bleeding, balloon tamponade or esophageal stenting can be used as a bridge to more definitive treatment such as transjugular intrahepatic portosystemic shunt (TIPS) or balloon-occluded retrograde transvenous obliteration (BRTO) for esophageal and gastric varices, respectively. Hemostatic spray consists of an inorganic powder that may be used endoscopically in cases of severe ulcer or cancer-related bleeding or other nonvariceal bleeding where directed therapy may not be possible. Ultimately, surgery may be necessary in a small proportion of patients with severe or recurrent bleeding, such as bleeding associated with tumors, perforated ulcers, recurrent ulcer bleeding or severe colitis that is refractory to endoscopic or interventional radiologic therapies.

SUGGESTED READINGS

ASGE Standards of Practice Committee, et al.: The role of endoscopy in the management of suspected small-bowel bleeding, *Gastrointest Endosc* 85:22–31, 2017.

Gerson LB, Fidler JL, Cave DR, Leighton JA: ACG clinical guideline: diagnosis and management of small bowel bleeding, *Am J Gastroenterol* 110:1265–1287, 2015.

Hwang JH, Fisher DA, Ben-Menachem T, et al.: The role of endoscopy in the management of acute non-variceal upper GI bleeding, *Gastrointest Endosc* 75:1132–1138, 2012.

Kim BS, Li BT, Engel A, et al.: Diagnosis of gastrointestinal bleeding: A practical guide for clinicians, *World J Gastrointest Pathophysiol* 5:467–478, 2014.

O'Leary JG, Greenberg CS, Patton HM, Caldwell SH: AGA clinical practice update: coagulation in cirrhosis, *Gastroenterology* 157:34–43, 2019.

Stanley AJ, Laine L: Management of acute upper gastrointestinal bleeding, *BMJ* 364:l536, 2019.

Strate LL, Gralnek IM: ACG clinical guideline: management of patients with acute lower gastrointestinal bleeding, *Am J Gastroenterol* 111:459–474, 2016.

Villanueva C, Colomo A, Bosch A, et al.: Transfusion strategies for acute upper gastrointestinal bleeding, *N Engl J Med* 368:11–21, 2013.

（OTSC）对出血灶血管采取物理夹闭止血。对于静脉曲张出血，可采用套扎和注射硬化剂治疗食管静脉曲张，注射氰基丙烯酸酯和其他组织胶治疗胃底静脉曲张。其他技术包括针对浅表血管病变的氩等离子体凝固（APC）和局部止血粉（作为临时措施）。对于显性LGIB，结肠镜检查的最佳时机尚不明确。与择期结肠镜检查相比，急诊结肠镜检查（定义不尽相同，范围为住院后12～24 h）可提高诊断率，但并不能改善再出血风险、对外科手术的需求或住院时间。一般来说，对于持续性出血或复发性显性LGIB的患者，优先安排住院行结肠镜检查是合理的，而自限性出血的患者可以择期进行评估。疑诊LGIB且血流动力学不稳定的患者也应接受上消化道内镜检查，以排除活动性UGIB。回肠末端出现新鲜血液提示近端或小肠出血。视频胶囊内镜检查（VCE）是诊断小肠出血来源的重要工具，尤其是在出血后72 h内进行。隐性GIB患者应接受胃镜和结肠镜检查，必要时接受VCE。推进式、气囊式或螺旋式小肠镜等检查技术可用于诊断和治疗胶囊内镜检查发现的小肠病变。CT和磁共振（MR）小肠成像已在很大程度上取代了透视检查，在无法使用VCE时可用于诊断小肠病变。

补救技术

对于内镜治疗失败或无法耐受的患者，有时需要采用补救技术进行诊断和治疗。CT血管成像或多排螺旋CT是合理的一线影像学检查，可对血流动力学异常的显性GIB患者进行出血定位。血管造影依赖于活动性出血，在间歇性出血患者中可能出现假阴性。标记红细胞闪烁成像虽然不如CT血管成像普及，操作流程上也更加繁琐，但由于其敏感性更高，且能够在首次注射标记红细胞后进行重复扫描，因此非常适合用于评估不明原因的间歇性GIB。超选择性血管栓塞术可为许多GIB患者成功快速止血，包括大面积穿透性十二指肠溃疡、小肠肿瘤出血和结肠憩室出血。对于无法控制的静脉曲张出血，气囊压迫止血或食管支架置入术可作为食管静脉曲张和胃静脉曲张的桥接治疗，后续分别进行经颈静脉肝内门体静脉分流术（TIPS）或气囊封堵逆行静脉阻塞术（BRTO）等治疗。止血喷雾剂由一种无机粉末组成，可用于无法进行直接内镜治疗的严重溃疡或癌症相关出血或其他非静脉曲张出血患者。少数严重或复发性出血（如肿瘤相关出血、溃疡穿孔、反复溃疡出血，以及内镜或放射介入治疗无效的重症结肠炎）的患者可能需要进行手术治疗。

推荐阅读

ASGE Standards of Practice Committee, et al.: The role of endoscopy in the management of suspected small-bowel bleeding, *Gastrointest Endosc* 85:22–31, 2017.

Gerson LB, Fidler JL, Cave DR, Leighton JA: ACG clinical guideline: diagnosis and management of small bowel bleeding, *Am J Gastroenterol* 110:1265–1287, 2015.

Hwang JH, Fisher DA, Ben-Menachem T, et al.: The role of endoscopy in the management of acute non-variceal upper GI bleeding, *Gastrointest Endosc* 75:1132–1138, 2012.

Kim BS, Li BT, Engel A, et al.: Diagnosis of gastrointestinal bleeding: A practical guide for clinicians, *World J Gastrointest Pathophysiol* 5:467–478, 2014.

O'Leary JG, Greenberg CS, Patton HM, Caldwell SH: AGA clinical practice update: coagulation in cirrhosis, *Gastroenterology* 157:34–43, 2019.

Stanley AJ, Laine L: Management of acute upper gastrointestinal bleeding, *BMJ* 364:l536, 2019.

Strate LL, Gralnek IM: ACG clinical guideline: management of patients with acute lower gastrointestinal bleeding, *Am J Gastroenterol* 111:459–474, 2016.

Villanueva C, Colomo A, Bosch A, et al.: Transfusion strategies for acute upper gastrointestinal bleeding, *N Engl J Med* 368:11–21, 2013.

Common Clinical Manifestations of Gastrointestinal Disease: Malabsorption

Brisas M. Flores, Sharmeel K. Wasan

DEFINITION AND EPIDEMIOLOGY

The main purpose of the gastrointestinal (GI) tract is to digest and absorb major nutrients (fats, carbohydrates, and proteins), essential micronutrients (vitamins and trace minerals), water, and electrolytes. Impaired absorption of these nutrients is defined as malabsorption. Under normal conditions, the digestion and absorption of nutrients requires both mechanical and enzymatic breakdown of food. Mechanical processes include chewing, gastric churning, and the to-and-fro mixing in the small intestine. Enzymatic hydrolysis is initiated by intraluminal processes requiring salivary, gastric, pancreatic, and biliary secretions and is completed at the intestinal brush border. The final products of digestion are then absorbed through the intestinal epithelial cells and transported into the portal circulation. The coordinated regulation of gastric emptying, normal intestinal progression, and the presence of adequate intestinal surface area are all important factors. The human gut microbiome, which comprises the communities of microorganisms that inhabit the GI tract, has been recognized to play an important role in nutrient utilization as well. From birth, interactions between the microbiota and the intestinal mucosa contribute to maturation of the host immune system. Disruptions to the homeostasis between the microbiota and the host immune system can lead to increased inflammation and decreased absorption.

Most dietary components can be absorbed anywhere along the length of the small intestine, but there are important exceptions in which absorption is limited to specific areas (e.g., vitamin B_{12} and cholesterol are absorbed only in the terminal ileum). Diseases associated with diffuse mucosal involvement, such as celiac disease, can lead to impaired absorption of many nutrients, whereas diseases affecting only the terminal ileum can lead to decreased vitamin B_{12} absorption. Bile acids are necessary for fat absorption; they undergo an enterohepatic circulation with release into bile and reabsorption from the terminal small intestine. Diseases interfering with this mechanism deplete the bile acid pool and can lead to fat malabsorption. Water and electrolytes are absorbed primarily by the colon. In addition, there is caloric salvage of much of the carbohydrate from indigestible fiber through bacterial enzymatic activity in the colon. The following sections discuss normal assimilation of the major nutrients and the approach to evaluation of patients with suspected malabsorption.

DIGESTION AND ABSORPTION OF FAT

Dietary fat is composed predominantly of triglycerides (≈95%) with long-chain fatty acids (16- and 18-carbon molecules). In animal fat, the constituent fatty acids are mostly saturated (e.g., palmitic acid, stearic acid), whereas those of vegetable origin are rich in unsaturated fatty acids (i.e., having one or more double bonds in the carbon chain, such as oleic and linoleic acids). Fats are insoluble in water (hydrophobic), and digestion begins with a process of emulsification, wherein larger fat droplets are dispersed in the aqueous medium of the lumen. In the proximal small intestine, bile salts from liver and pancreatic enzymes are released into the intestinal lumen; there, they mix with and bind to the surface of these globules, where colipase activity results in the release of fatty acids and a monoglyceride. These are taken up as mixed micelles with bile salts, and these hydrophobic particles cross the unstirred water layer that overlies the epithelial brush border.

Within the cell, fatty acids are resynthesized into triglycerides, and, together with cholesterol and phospholipids, they are packaged into chylomicrons and very-low-density lipoproteins to be exported via lymphatic channels. Bile salts remain in the intestinal lumen, are recycled into new micelles, and are finally reabsorbed in the terminal ileum with 95% efficiency. Most dietary lipids are absorbed in the jejunum, together with the fat-soluble vitamins A, D, E, and K. It is recommended that dietary fat account for no more than 35% of calories because higher levels are associated with increased risk of cardiac disease, obesity, and some cancers. The recommended intake is 20% to 35% of daily dietary intake.

DIGESTION AND ABSORPTION OF CARBOHYDRATES

Most dietary carbohydrates consist of starch (a glucose polymer) and the disaccharides sucrose and lactose, but only monosaccharides are absorbed. Salivary and pancreatic amylases release oligosaccharides from starch. The final hydrolysis to glucose monomers occurs at the brush border and includes disaccharide hydrolysis by sucrase and lactase. Glucose and galactose are actively transported in conjunction with sodium, whereas fructose absorption occurs by facilitated diffusion. About one half of dietary energy is derived from carbohydrate, with a nutritional goal of 45% to 65% and an increased component of insoluble fiber (i.e., that which is indigestible by mammalian enzymes but variably broken down by colonic bacteria).

DIGESTION AND ABSORPTION OF PROTEINS

Dietary proteins are the major source for amino acids and the only source for the essential amino acids. Digestion starts in the stomach with pepsins secreted by the gastric mucosa, but most of the hydrolysis is accomplished by pancreatic enzymes in the proximal small bowel. The pancreas secretes the proteases trypsin, elastase, chymotrypsin, and carboxypeptidase as inactive proenzymes. Enterokinase (more properly, enteropeptidase) is secreted by the intestinal brush border; it splits trypsinogen to its active form, trypsin, which in turn converts the other proenzymes to their active forms. The products of luminal brush border peptidase digestion consist of amino acids and oligopeptides,

胃肠疾病常见临床表现：吸收不良

谢元鸿 译 陈倩 陈萦晅 审校 房静远 通审

定义和流行病学

胃肠道的主要功能是消化和吸收主要营养成分（脂肪、碳水化合物及蛋白质）、必需微量营养素（维生素及微量矿物质）、水和电解质。这些营养物质的吸收障碍被定义为吸收不良。正常情况下，营养物质的消化和吸收需要经过食物的机械降解和酶水解。机械降解过程包括口腔咀嚼、胃内蠕动及小肠内反复混合。酶水解过程始于消化道腔内，依赖于唾液、胃液、胰液及胆汁的分泌，最终在小肠刷状缘完成。消化的终产物通过小肠上皮细胞吸收并转运至门静脉循环。协调的胃排空、正常的肠道推动及足够的肠道表面积均为消化和吸收的重要因素。人类肠道菌群是胃肠道微生物系统的组成部分，其在机体营养吸收中亦发挥重要作用。从出生开始，肠道黏膜与肠道菌群的相互作用就促进了机体免疫系统的成熟。破坏肠道菌群与宿主免疫系统的平衡稳态可导致炎症增加和吸收减少。

大部分食物成分在小肠吸收，但部分营养物质例外，其吸收部位仅限于特定区域，如维生素 B_{12} 及胆固醇仅在回肠末端被吸收。弥漫性黏膜受累的疾病（如乳糜泻）通常会引起许多营养物质的吸收障碍，而仅累及末端回肠的疾病可导致维生素 B_{12} 吸收减少。胆汁酸在脂肪吸收中不可或缺。胆汁酸随胆汁分泌至肠腔，并在小肠末端重吸收，这一过程被称为肠肝循环。破坏肠肝循环的疾病可导致胆汁酸池耗竭，从而引起脂肪吸收不良。水和电解质的吸收主要在结肠。此外，结肠中的细菌酶可酵解难以消化的食物纤维，并重吸收大部分碳水化合物。下文将讨论主要营养物质的正常消化吸收及对疑诊吸收不良患者的评估方法。

脂肪的消化和吸收

饮食中的脂肪主要由长链脂肪酸（16-碳和18-碳）组成的甘油三酯（约占95%）构成。动物脂肪主要由饱和脂肪酸（如棕榈酸、硬脂酸）构成，而植物来源的脂肪富含不饱和脂肪酸（即碳链中有1个或多个双键，如油酸和亚油酸）。脂肪不溶于水（疏水性），因此其消化始于乳化，这一过程使较大的脂肪颗粒分散至肠腔内的水介质中形成液滴。在近端小肠，肝产生的胆盐和胰酶被释放至肠腔，两者与这些脂肪液滴混合，在辅脂肪酶的作用下产生脂肪酸和单甘油酯。它们与胆盐形成疏水性混合胶粒后透过肠道上皮刷状缘表面的静水层而被吸收。

进入细胞内，脂肪酸被重新合成为甘油三酯，并与胆固醇和磷脂一起被包装成乳糜微粒和极低密度脂蛋白，并通过淋巴管转运。胆盐仍留在肠腔内，形成新的微粒再循环利用，95%最终在回肠末端被重吸收。大部分膳食脂肪在空肠与脂溶性维生素A、D、E、K一起被吸收。由于与心脏病、肥胖症及部分癌症的风险增加有关，饮食中脂肪在整体热量构成中的占比不应超过35%，推荐占比为20%～35%。

碳水化合物的消化和吸收

饮食中大部分的碳水化合物由淀粉（葡萄糖聚合物）、二糖及乳糖构成，但只有单糖能被吸收。唾液淀粉酶及胰淀粉酶可将淀粉降解为寡糖。最终产生单糖的水解过程发生在刷状缘，该过程也包括通过蔗糖酶和乳糖酶的二糖水解过程。葡萄糖及半乳糖通过与钠结合而进行主动转运，而果糖吸收则依赖易化扩散作用。近1/2的膳食能量由碳水化合物提供，因此建议其在饮食中的占比为45%～65%，并增加不溶性纤维（即哺乳动物无法酶解但可被肠道菌群降解的纤维）的摄入。

蛋白质的消化和吸收

饮食中的蛋白质是氨基酸的主要来源，也是必需氨基酸的唯一来源。蛋白质的消化过程始于胃（胃黏膜分泌的胃蛋白酶进行初步降解），而主要水解过程是在近端小肠内由胰酶完成。胰腺以非活性酶原的形式分泌胰蛋白酶、弹性蛋白酶、糜蛋白酶及羧肽酶。肠激酶（更确切地说是肠肽酶）由小肠刷状缘分泌，其将胰蛋白酶原裂解为具有生物活性的胰蛋白酶，后者进一步将其他酶原转化成活性形式。肠道刷状缘肽酶消化产物由氨基

which are transported across the epithelial cell. The transfer of most amino acids is sodium dependent and takes place in the proximal small bowel. Dietary requirements for amino acid nitrogen are met with about 10% to 35% of calories from protein.

MECHANISMS OF MALABSORPTION

The term *maldigestion* refers to defective hydrolysis of nutrients, whereas *malabsorption* refers to impaired mucosal absorption. In clinical practice, however, *malabsorption* refers to all aspects of impaired nutrient assimilation. Malabsorption can involve multiple nutrients, or it can be more selective. Therefore, the clinical manifestations of malabsorption are highly variable. The complete process of absorption consists of a *luminal phase*, in which various nutrients are hydrolyzed and solubilized; a *mucosal phase*, in which further processing takes place at the brush border of the epithelial cell with subsequent transfer into the cell; and a *transport phase*, in which nutrients are moved from the epithelium to the portal venous or lymphatic circulation. Impairment in any of these phases can result in malabsorption (Table 3.1).

Luminal Phase

Digestion is accomplished for the most part by pancreatic enzymes, particularly lipase, colipase, and trypsin; the gastric digestive enzymes do not play a major role. As a consequence, chronic pancreatitis can result in malabsorption, particularly for fat and protein. Deficiency in bile salts also contributes to fat malabsorption and may result from cholestatic liver disorders (impaired secretion of bile), bacterial overgrowth (resulting in luminal bile salt deconjugation), or ileal disease or resection with loss of effective enterohepatic circulation of the bile acids. The major part of the luminal phase of digestion occurs in the duodenum and the proximal jejunum.

Mucosal Phase

Mucosal disease is a more common cause of malabsorption. It can result from diffuse small intestinal diseases such as celiac disease or Crohn's disease, or from a decrease in surface area (e.g., after surgical resection for small bowel infarction). The net effect is a smaller effective mucosal surface and a relative loss of mucosal absorption. Selective defects in an otherwise normal intestine may result in specific entities such as lactase deficiency or abetalipoproteinemia.

Transport Phase

After absorption, nutrients leave the cells through venous or lymphatic channels. Consequently, malabsorption may be associated with mesenteric venous obstruction, lymphangiectasia, or lymphatic obstruction due to malignancy or infiltrative processes such as Whipple disease.

The absorptive process can be impaired at many stages. For example, patients with subtotal gastrectomy or bariatric surgery often experience malabsorption. There are resultant defects at all phases: impaired gastric churning, premature emptying, and impaired mixing (in the jejunum) of food with bile and pancreatic enzymes. The impaired mixing is a consequence of anatomic changes (gastrojejunostomy bypassing the duodenum) and reduced production of pancreatic enzymes (because cholecystokinin and secretin release is blunted when gastric contents bypass the duodenum). Moreover, stasis may lead to bacterial overgrowth in the afferent loop with changes in the bile acids needed for fat absorption. Another example of manifold mechanisms is diabetes mellitus, which may lead to delayed gastric emptying, abnormal intestinal motility, bacterial overgrowth, and pancreatic exocrine insufficiency.

CLINICAL PRESENTATION

The clinical manifestations of malabsorption are usually nonspecific, particularly in the early stages. A change in bowel movements, usually with diarrhea, and weight loss despite adequate food intake may occur in more severe cases. Usually, however, patients have relatively mild symptoms such as bloating and flatulence. Clinical manifestations related to a specific micronutrient deficiency can occur. For example, iron deficiency anemia may be the only manifestation of celiac disease

TABLE 3.1 Pathophysiologic Mechanisms in Malabsorption

Luminal Phase	Mucosal Phase	Transport Phase
Reduced nutrient availability	Extensive mucosal loss (resection or infarction)	Vascular conditions (vasculitis; atheroma)
Cofactor deficiency (pernicious anemia; gastric surgery)	Diffuse mucosal disease (celiac disease)	Lymphatic conditions (lymphangiectasia; irradiation; nodal tumor, cavitation, or infiltrations)
Nutrient consumption (bacterial overgrowth)	Crohn's disease; irradiation; infection; infiltrations; drugs: alcohol, colchicine, neomycin, iron salts	
Impaired fat solubilization	Brush border hydrolase deficiency (lactase deficiency)	
Reduced bile salt synthesis (hepatocellular disease)	Transport defects (Hartnup cystinuria; vitamin B_{12} and folate uptake)	
Impaired bile salt secretion (chronic cholestasis)	Epithelial processing (abetalipoproteinemia)	
Bile salt inactivation (bacterial overgrowth)		
Impaired cholecystokinin release (mucosal disease)		
Increased bile salt losses (terminal ileal disease or resection)		
Defective nutrient hydrolysis		
Lipase inactivation (Zollinger-Ellison syndrome)		
Enzyme deficiency (pancreatic insufficiency or cancer)		
Improper mixing or rapid transit (resection; bypass; hyperthyroidism)		

Modified from Riley SA, Marsh MN: Maldigestion and malabsorption. In Feldman M, Scharschmidt BF, Sleisenger MH, editors: Sleisenger and Fordtran's Gastrointestinal and Liver Disease: Pathophysiology/Diagnosis/Management, ed 6, Philadelphia, 1998, WB Saunders, pp 1501-1522.

酸及寡肽构成，并通过肠上皮转运吸收。大部分氨基酸在近端小肠的转运依赖于钠。饮食中蛋白质的摄入量占总热量的 10%～35% 可满足机体所需的氨基酸态氮。

吸收不良的机制

消化不良是指营养物质水解障碍，而吸收不良是指黏膜吸收障碍。然而，在临床实践中，吸收不良指各种原因引起的营养物质利用障碍。吸收不良可涉及多种营养物质，也可仅涉及其中的几种。因此，吸收不良的临床表现差异很大。完整的吸收过程包括：①腔内期：营养物质水解并溶解的过程。②黏膜期：肠上皮细胞刷状缘进一步处理并转运至细胞内的过程。③转运期：营养物质由上皮细胞转运至门静脉或淋巴循环的过程。上述任何一个过程受损均会导致吸收不良（表 3.1）。

腔内期

消化过程大部分由胰酶完成，尤其是脂肪酶、辅脂肪酶及胰蛋白酶，胃消化酶在这一过程中发挥次要作用。因此，慢性胰腺炎会导致吸收不良，尤其是对脂肪和蛋白质的吸收。胆盐缺乏亦可引起脂肪吸收不良，病因可能为胆汁淤积性肝病（胆汁分泌障碍）、细菌过度生长（肠腔内胆盐解离）、回肠疾病或切除引起胆汁酸丧失有效的肠肝循环。腔内期主要发生在十二指肠及近端空肠。

黏膜期

黏膜疾病是吸收不良更为常见的原因。通常见于广泛累及小肠的疾病，如乳糜泻、克罗恩病或肠道表面积减少（手术切除梗阻小肠）等，导致有效黏膜表面积减小及黏膜吸收能力的相应下降。部分选择性缺陷（即便肠道功能正常）亦可能导致特殊类型的吸收不良，如乳糖酶缺乏症或 β-脂蛋白缺乏症。

转运期

经吸收后，营养物质一般通过静脉或淋巴管离开细胞。因此，吸收不良与肠系膜静脉阻塞、淋巴管扩张症或淋巴管梗阻［由恶性或浸润性疾病（如 Whipple 病）所致］有关。

吸收过程的各个阶段均可受影响。例如，胃次全切除术或减重术后患者常发生吸收不良。其各阶段均存在异常：胃蠕动受损、胃排空过早、食物与胆汁及胰酶（在空肠中）的混合过程受损。食物与胆汁及胰酶的混合异常是由于解剖改变（胃空肠吻合十二指肠旁路术）及胰酶产生减少（因为当胃内容物不经过十二指肠时，胆囊收缩素和促胰液素释放减少）。此外，肠淤积亦会引起输入袢细菌过度生长，同时伴随脂肪吸收所需的胆汁酸的变化。另一个累及多阶段的例子是糖尿病，其可能引起胃排空延迟、肠道动力异常、细菌过度生长和胰腺外分泌功能不全。

临床表现

吸收不良的临床表现常为非特异性，尤其在早期阶段。患者可表现为排便习惯改变，通常以腹泻为主，严重患者可出现摄入足够食物后体重仍下降。然而，患者的症状通常相对较轻，可表现为腹胀和胀气等。特定微量营养素缺乏可引起相关的临床表现，如缺铁性贫血可能是部分乳糜泻患者唯一的表现。蛋白质吸

表 3.1　吸收不良的病理生理学机制		
腔内期	黏膜期	转运期
营养物质供应减少	广泛黏膜缺失（切除或梗死）	血管病变（血管炎；动脉粥样硬化）
辅因子缺乏（恶性贫血；胃部手术）	弥漫性黏膜病变（乳糜泻）	淋巴病变（淋巴管扩张症；放疗；淋巴结肿瘤、空洞或浸润性病变）
营养消耗（细菌过度生长）	克罗恩病；放疗；感染；浸润性病变；药物（酒精、秋水仙碱、新霉素、铁盐）	
脂肪溶解受损	刷状缘水解酶缺乏（乳糖酶缺乏）	
胆盐合成减少（肝细胞病）	转运障碍［色氨酸加氧酶缺乏症（Hartnup 病）相关胱氨酸尿症、摄入维生素 B_{12} 及叶酸］	
胆盐分泌障碍（慢性胆汁淤积）	上皮细胞功能异常（β-脂蛋白缺乏症）	
胆盐失活（细菌过度生长）		
胆囊收缩素释放受损（黏膜疾病）		
胆盐丢失增加（末端回肠疾病或切除）		
营养物质水解缺陷		
脂肪酶失活（胃泌素瘤）		
酶缺乏（胰腺功能不全或胰腺癌）		
食糜混合不当或传输过快（切除术；旁路术；甲状腺功能亢进症）		

改编自 Riley SA, Marsh MN: Maldigestion and malabsorption. In Feldman M, Scharschmidt BF, Sleisenger MH, editors: Sleisenger and Fordtran's Gastrointestinal and Liver Disease: Pathophysiology/Diagnosis/Management, ed 6, Philadelphia, 1998, WB Saunders, pp 1501-1522.

in some patients. Muscle wasting and edema result from protein malabsorption. Nutritional anemia, caused by deficiencies of iron, folate, and vitamin B_{12}, contributes to fatigue. Bleeding tendency (e.g., ecchymosis) may be attributed to prolonged prothrombin time resulting from vitamin K deficiency related to fat malabsorption. Bulky, oily stools are the hallmark of steatorrhea resulting from fat malabsorption, whereas bloating (abdominal distention) and soft diarrheal movements occur as a result of carbohydrate malabsorption. Signs associated with malabsorption are presented in Table 3.2.

DIAGNOSIS

Malabsorption can be caused by a large number of disorders, some of the more common of which are listed in Table 3.2. The cause of malabsorption can often be determined by a very detailed patient history. However, because the clinical symptoms are varied, more specific assays of albumin, cobalamin, iron, cholesterol, calcium, folic acid, and prothrombin time are useful to support the diagnosis of malabsorption. These tests are helpful in assessing the severity of malabsorption, but they are not specific for the differential diagnosis. Many tests are available in the work-up of malabsorption; those that have been most useful clinically are discussed in the following sections (Fig. 3.1).

Fecal Fat Analysis

If fat malabsorption is suspected, the simplest qualitative method for detecting fat in stool is microscopic examination with Sudan staining of a drop of stool. Sensitivity varies anywhere from 80% to 99%, but the test is quick and easy. The result correlates well with the quantitative measurement of fecal fat when moderate to severe steatorrhea is present. To quantify fat, stool is collected for three consecutive days while the patient is on a diet containing 60 g to 100 g of fat per day, and the specimen is analyzed for fat content. If the fecal fat amount is

TABLE 3.2 Signs Associated With Malabsorption Syndromes

Signs	Associated Syndromes
Gastrointestinal	
Mass	Crohn's disease, lymphoma, tuberculosis, glands
Distention	Intestinal obstruction, gas, ascites, pseudocyst (pancreatic), motility disorder
Steatorrheic stool	Mucosal disease, bacterial overgrowth, pancreatic insufficiency, infective or inflammatory, drug induced
Extraintestinal	
Skin	
Nonspecific	Pigmentation, thinning, inelasticity, reduced subcutaneous fat
Specific	Blisters (dermatitis herpetiformis), erythema nodosum (Crohn's disease), petechiae (vitamin K deficiency), edema (hypoproteinemia)
Hair	
Alopecia	Gluten sensitivity
Loss or thinning	Generalized inanition, hypothyroidism, gluten sensitivity
Eyes	
Conjunctivitis, episcleritis	Crohn's disease, Behçet's syndrome
Paleness	Severe anemia
Mouth	
Aphthous ulcers	Crohn's disease, gluten sensitivity, Behçet's syndrome
Glossitis	Deficiencies of vitamin B_{12}, iron, folate, niacin
Angular cheilosis	Deficiencies of vitamin B_{12}, iron, folate, B complex
Dental hypoplasia (pitting, dystrophy)	Gluten sensitivity
Hands	
Raynaud's phenomenon	Scleroderma
Finger clubbing	Crohn's disease, lymphoma
Koilonychia	Iron deficiency
Leukonychia	Inanition
Musculoskeletal	
Monoarthropathy and polyarthropathy	Crohn's disease, gluten sensitivity, Whipple disease, Behçet's syndrome
Back pain (osteomalacia, osteoporosis, sacroiliitis)	Crohn's disease, malnutrition, gluten sensitivity
Muscle weakness (low potassium, magnesium, vitamin D; generalized inanition)	Diffuse mucosal disease, bacterial overgrowth, lymphoma
Nervous System	
Peripheral neuropathy (weakness, paresthesias, numbness)	Vitamin B_{12} deficiency
Cerebral (seizures, dementia, intracerebral calcification, meningitis, pseudotumor, cranial nerve palsies)	Whipple disease, gluten sensitivity, diffuse lymphoma

From Riley SA, Marsh MN: Maldigestion and malabsorption. In Feldman M, Scharschmidt BF, Sleisenger MH, editors: Sleisenger and Fordtran's Gastrointestinal and Liver Disease: Pathophysiology/Diagnosis/Management, ed 6, Philadelphia, 1998, WB Saunders, pp 1501-1522.

收不良可引起肌肉萎缩和水肿。缺乏铁、叶酸、维生素B_{12}可导致营养不良性贫血，从而引起疲劳。脂肪吸收不良导致的维生素K缺乏可引起凝血酶原时间（PT）延长，进而表现为出血倾向（如皮肤瘀斑）。粪便量大且呈油脂状是脂肪吸收不良引起脂肪泻的特征性表现，而胀气（腹部膨隆）和以软便为主的排便次数增多则提示碳水化合物吸收不良。吸收不良相关的主要临床表现见表3.2。

诊断

很多疾病可引起吸收不良（常见疾病见表3.2）。吸收不良的病因往往可通过详尽的病史询问来确定。然而，由于患者的临床症状各异，因此进一步检测白蛋白、维生素B_{12}、铁、胆固醇、钙、叶酸和凝血酶原时间有助于吸收不良的诊断，以及评估吸收不良的严重程度，但对鉴别诊断的作用有限。多项检查可用于吸收不良的诊断，下文将介绍在临床中较有价值的方法（图3.1）。

粪便脂肪检测

怀疑脂肪吸收不良时，最简便的定性方法是显微镜下粪便液滴苏丹红染色检查。该方法快速、简便，敏感性为80%~99%。对于中重度脂肪泻，该检查与粪便脂肪含量的定量检测结果相关性较好。定量检测需要患者在每日膳食摄入60~100 g脂肪的基础上连续收集3天的粪便，然后对粪便样本进行脂肪测定。若粪便脂肪含量＞7 g/d，则考虑脂肪吸收不良。脂肪

表3.2　吸收不良综合征的相关临床表现

临床表现	相关疾病和综合征
胃肠道表现	
腹部包块	克罗恩病、淋巴瘤、结核病、增生或突出腺体
腹胀	肠梗阻、积气、腹腔积液、胰腺假性囊肿、动力障碍
脂肪泻	黏膜病变、细菌过度生长、胰腺功能不全、感染或炎症、药物作用
肠外表现	
皮肤	
非特异性表现	皮肤色素沉着、变薄、缺乏弹性、皮下脂肪减少
特异性表现	水疱（疱疹样皮炎）、结节性红斑（克罗恩病）、瘀点（维生素K缺乏）、水肿（低蛋白血症）
头发	
脱发	麸质过敏
减少或稀疏	全身性营养不良、甲状腺功能减退症、麸质过敏
眼	
结膜炎、巩膜外层炎	克罗恩病、白塞综合征
结膜苍白	重度贫血
口腔	
阿弗他溃疡（口疮样溃疡）	克罗恩病、麸质过敏、白塞综合征
舌炎	维生素B_{12}、铁、叶酸、烟酸缺乏
口角干裂	维生素B_{12}、铁、叶酸、B族维生素缺乏
牙发育不全（釉质凹陷、营养不良）	麸质过敏
手	
雷诺现象	硬皮病
杵状指	克罗恩病、淋巴瘤
反甲（匙状甲）	铁缺乏
白甲	营养不足
肌肉骨骼	
单关节病和多关节病	克罗恩病、麸质过敏、Whipple病、白塞综合征
背痛（骨软化、骨质疏松、骶髂关节炎）	克罗恩病、营养不良、麸质过敏
肌无力（低钾、低镁、维生素D缺乏；全身性营养不良）	弥漫性黏膜病变、细菌过度生长、淋巴瘤
神经系统	
周围神经病（乏力、感觉异常、麻木）	维生素B_{12}缺乏
脑病（癫痫、痴呆、颅内钙化、脑膜炎、假性肿瘤、脑神经麻痹）	Whipple病、麸质过敏、弥漫性淋巴瘤

引自Riley SA，Marsh MN：Maldigestion and malabsorption. In Feldman M，Scharschmidt BF，Sleisenger MH，editors：Sleisenger and Fordtran's Gastrointestinal and Liver Disease：Pathophysiology/Diagnosis/Management，ed 6，Philadelphia，1998，WB Saunders，pp 1501-1522.

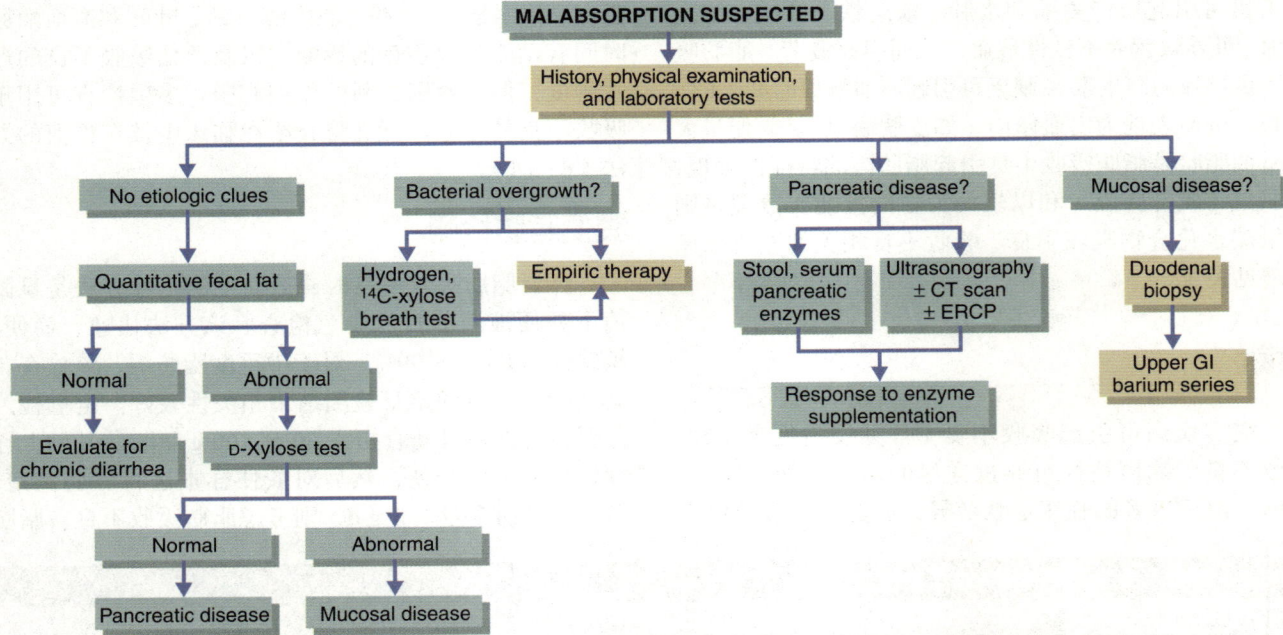

Fig. 3.1 Approach to the patient with suspected malabsorption. *CT*, Computed tomography; *ERCP*, endoscopic retrograde cholangiopancreatography; *GI*, gastrointestinal. (Modified from Riley SA, Marsh MN: Maldigestion and malabsorption. In Feldman M, Scharschmidt BF, Sleisenger MH, editors: Sleisenger and Fordtran's Gastrointestinal and Liver Disease: Pathophysiology/Diagnosis/Management, ed 6, Philadelphia, 1998, WB Saunders, pp 1501-1522.)

greater than 7 g per day, it is suggestive of fat malabsorption. Patients with steatorrhea (excess fat in the stool) often have results with greater than 20 g per day. Values ranging from 7 to 14 g per day are suggestive of fat malabsorption, but values should be interpreted judiciously as diarrheal illnesses can also produce these results. This test is cumbersome and nonspecific, but it offers an accurate quantification of fecal fat excretion provided fat consumption is appropriate. Near-infrared reflectance spectroscopy may produce similar results, but this is not often utilized in the United States.

Tests of Pancreatic Exocrine Function
Aspiration of duodenal contents for evaluation of bicarbonate and enzyme output after stimulation of the pancreas may be the best index of pancreatic exocrine function. However, the test is invasive, time-consuming, and performed only in a few specialized centers. The measurement of pancreatic enzymes (i.e., fecal elastase 1) in the stool is simple and provides helpful laboratory evidence for the diagnosis of moderate to severe pancreatic insufficiency. Pancreatic calcifications seen on abdominal films or computed tomography (CT) scans indicate the presence of chronic pancreatitis. Magnetic resonance cholangiopancreatography (MRCP) and endoscopic retrograde cholangiopancreatography (ERCP) can help outline abnormal duct anatomy and may supplement CT scanning for diagnostic purposes to evaluate the sequelae of chronic pancreatitis. However, normal findings on pancreatography do not exclude the presence of pancreatic exocrine insufficiency.

Small Intestinal Biopsy
Whereas the gross appearance of the mucosa during upper GI endoscopy can provide some clues regarding the presence of a disease causing malabsorption, biopsy of the small intestinal mucosa is a key diagnostic test for diseases that affect the cellular phase of absorption. In some diseases, the histologic features are diagnostic; in others, the findings may be highly suggestive (Table 3.3). Several tissue samples should be taken from the duodenal bulb and from the distal duodenum to enhance the diagnostic accuracy.

Imaging Studies
In patients with malabsorption, barium studies of the small bowel are usually nonspecific. Occasionally, however, distinct anatomic changes are seen, such as in jejunal diverticulosis, lymphoma, Crohn's disease, strictures, or enteric fistulas. Also, there may be a distinctive barium pattern of thin-walled, dilated loops suggestive of celiac disease. CT and magnetic resonance enterography provide a more detailed imaging of the small intestine and are more sensitive in identifying abnormalities such as active bowel inflammation, mesenteric stranding and edema, strictures, fibrofatty proliferation of the mesentery, and fistula formation.

Wireless capsule endoscopy is a noninvasive method that permits direct visualization of the small bowel mucosa and can provide a more detailed evaluation of small bowel disease compared with radiographic studies. However, capsule endoscopy should be avoided in patients in whom a stricture is suspected because of the risk of retention. The detection of mucosal lesions by the capsule endoscopy can often be followed by deep enteroscopy (double-balloon endoscopy, single-balloon endoscopy, or spiral enteroscopy), allowing for tissue biopsy, tattoo placement before surgery, balloon dilatation, and foreign body retrieval.

Schilling Test
Vitamin B_{12} is an essential micronutrient, and its absorption requires several steps. First, the ingested vitamin binds to salivary R-factor protein. In the stomach, gastric parietal cells secrete intrinsic factor, which mixes with the ingested meal. In the duodenum, pancreatic trypsin

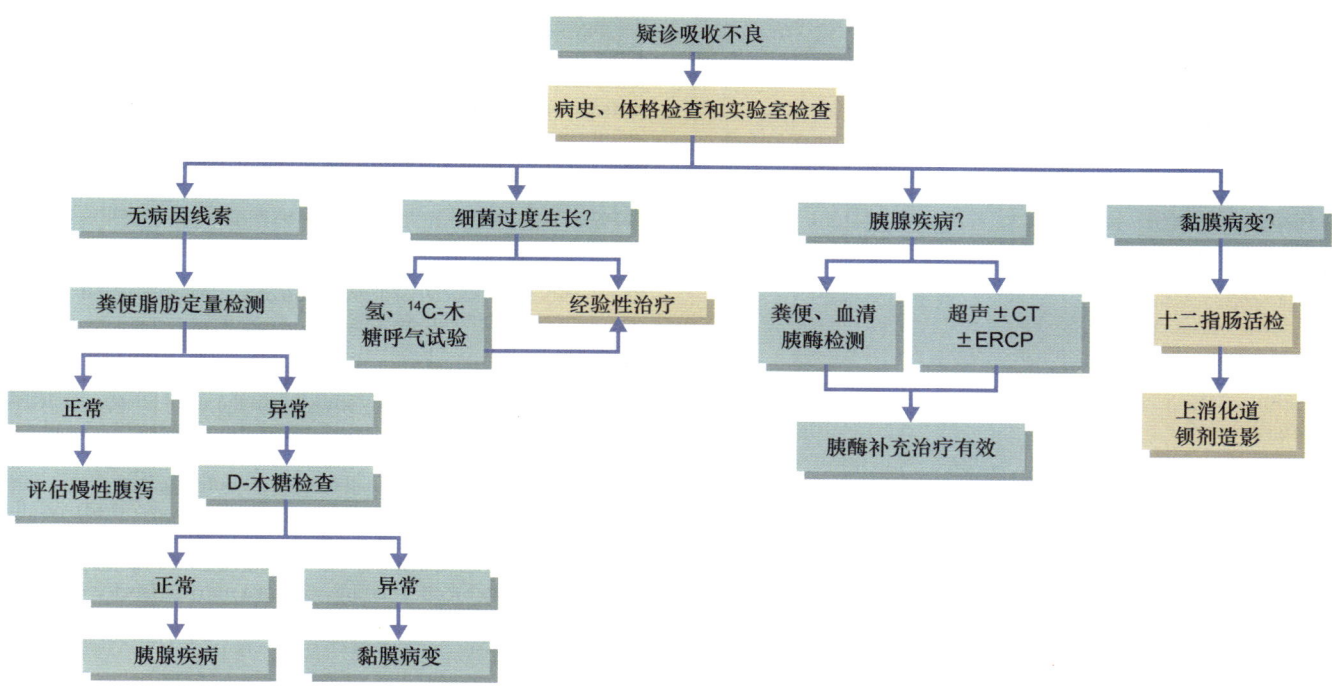

图3.1 疑诊吸收不良患者的接诊。CT，计算机断层成像；ERCP，内镜逆行胰胆管造影（改编自 Riley SA，Marsh MN：Maldigestion and malabsorption. In Feldman M，Scharschmidt BF，Sleisenger MH，editors：Sleisenger and Fordtran's Gastrointestinal and Liver Disease：Pathophysiology/Diagnosis/Management，ed 6，Philadelphia，1998，WB Saunders，pp 1501-1522.）

泻患者（粪便脂肪过量）粪便脂肪通常＞20 g/d。粪便脂肪为 7～14 g/d 高度提示脂肪吸收不良，但应结合患者情况审慎地解释这些数值，因为其他腹泻性疾病亦可产生类似结果。虽然这一检查耗时且特异性有限，但它可在脂肪摄入适当的情况下准确定量粪便脂肪排泄。近红外光谱检测法亦可得到相似结果，但在美国不常用。

胰腺外分泌功能检测

抽吸十二指肠内容物评估刺激胰腺后碳酸氢盐及酶的产生可能是胰腺外分泌功能的最佳检测方法。然而，该检查为侵入性且耗时，仅有少数机构能够开展。粪便检测胰酶（如粪弹性蛋白酶1）操作简便，有助于诊断中重度胰腺功能不全。腹部X线检查或CT可见胰腺钙化，提示可能存在慢性胰腺炎。磁共振胰胆管成像（MRCP）及内镜逆行胰胆管造影（ERCP）可发现异常胰管结构，结合CT结果可评估慢性胰腺炎的预后。然而，胰腺影像学检查结果正常并不能排除胰腺外分泌功能不全。

小肠黏膜活检

上消化道内镜检查所见的消化道黏膜大体外观可为诊断吸收不良提供部分线索，而小肠黏膜活检是诊断累及细胞层面而引起吸收不良的疾病的关键检测方法。在某些疾病中，组织学特征具有关键的诊断价值，而在另一些疾病中则具有高度提示作用（表3.3）。为提高诊断准确性，应在十二指肠球部及远端多点活检。

影像学检查

对于吸收不良患者，小肠钡剂造影通常是非特异性的。然而，该检查偶尔可发现一些明确的解剖学异常，如空肠憩室、淋巴瘤、克罗恩病、肠腔狭窄或肠瘘。此外，钡剂造影发现特征性的肠壁变薄、管腔扩张可提示乳糜泻。肠道CT及磁共振小肠成像可提供更详细的小肠影像，对识别肠道异常（如活动性肠炎、肠系膜扭转及水肿、肠腔狭窄、肠系膜纤维脂肪性增生及瘘道形成）更为敏感。

无线胶囊内镜是一种非侵入性检查，可对小肠黏膜进行直视检查，相比于影像学检查，其能提供更为详细的小肠疾病评估。然而，因存在胶囊滞留的风险，应避免在怀疑肠道狭窄的患者中使用。胶囊内镜发现黏膜病变后，可进一步行深度内镜检查（单气囊及双气囊小肠镜、螺旋式小肠镜），以进行组织活检、术前标记、气囊扩张及异物取出等。

希林试验（维生素 B_{12} 吸收试验）

维生素 B_{12} 是必需微量营养素，其吸收需要多步骤来完成。首先，摄入的维生素与唾液R-因子蛋白结合。在胃内，胃壁细胞分泌内因子，内因子与食物混合。在十二指肠，胰蛋白酶水解R-蛋白，将维生素释

TABLE 3.3 Utility of Small Bowel Biopsy Specimens in Malabsorption
Findings Often Diagnostic
Whipple disease
Amyloidosis
Eosinophilic enteritis
Lymphangiectasia
Primary intestinal lymphoma
Giardiasis
Abetalipoproteinemia
Agammaglobulinemia
Mastocytosis
Findings Abnormal But Not Diagnostic
Celiac disease
Systemic sclerosis
Radiation enteritis
Bacterial overgrowth syndrome
Tropical sprue
Crohn's disease

Data from Trier JS: Diagnostic value of peroral biopsy of the proximal small intestine. N Engl J Med 285:1470, 1971.

hydrolyzes the R-protein, freeing the vitamin to bind with intrinsic factor. The vitamin B_{12}–intrinsic factor complex is then absorbed by specific receptors that are found only on enterocytes in the distal ileum. Malabsorption of vitamin B_{12} can occur because of lack of intrinsic factor (e.g., pernicious anemia, gastric resection), pancreatic insufficiency, bacterial overgrowth, or ileal resection or mucosal disease (e.g., Crohn's disease).

The Schilling test quantifies vitamin B_{12} absorption using radiolabeled vitamin B_{12} as a marker. The test may be expanded to several stages to amplify its diagnostic spectrum. In stage 1, after the injection of 1000 μg of unlabeled vitamin B_{12} to saturate hepatic storage, the patient ingests 0.5 μg of radiolabeled vitamin. Urine is then collected for the measurement of radioactivity; reduced radioactivity suggests B_{12} malabsorption. The test is repeated (stage 2) with the addition of oral intrinsic factor to the ingested vitamin B_{12}. If urinary excretion of the radiolabel is corrected, pernicious anemia is diagnosed. If malabsorption is still present, the patient is given a short course of oral antibiotics (stage 3), and the test is repeated; correction of radiolabeled B_{12} excretion establishes bacterial overgrowth. If the test result remains abnormal, oral pancreatic enzymes are given (stage 4) and the test is repeated; correction of the abnormality at this stage implies pancreatic deficiency. Finally, if all these interventions fail, ileal disease or absence of transcobalamin protein is determined by other diagnostic tests, including assessment for intrinsic factor antibodies or *Helicobacter pylori* infection. This long outline serves merely as an example of an algorithm of clinical analysis; the usual routine in clinical settings is to administer parenteral vitamin B_{12} while the etiology is delineated by other modalities.

D-Xylose Test

The D-xylose test serves as an indicator of mucosal absorption in the proximal small bowel and is used to determine whether defects in the epithelium of the intestine are responsible for malabsorption. D-Xylose is a 5-carbon monosaccharide that is transported across the intestinal mucosa largely by passive diffusion. In this test, the subject ingests 25 g of D-xylose, and urine is collected for the next 5 hours. Healthy subjects excrete more than 4.5 g of D-xylose in 5 hours (or ≥20% of the ingested load). Excretion of a lower amount of D-xylose suggests abnormal absorption. However, an abnormally low (false-positive) result may occur in the presence of impaired renal excretory function, gastroparesis, massive peripheral edema, ascites, aspirin, neomycin, indomethacin, and glipizide. Abnormal results can also be seen in the presence of bacterial overgrowth as a result of bacterial degradation of D-xylose in the lumen, but this "pseudomalabsorption" may be corrected after treatment with antibiotics serving as a therapeutic trial.

Breath Tests

Breath tests rely on bacterial degradation of luminal compounds, which releases metabolic byproduct gases (e.g., hydrogen, methane, carbon dioxide) that can be measured in the exhaled breath. In the case of disaccharidase deficiency, a specific disaccharide (e.g., lactose) that is orally ingested but not properly absorbed in the small intestine is delivered to the colon, where bacterial fermentation liberates metabolites; hydrogen gas is the marker assayed in the breath. In the presence of bacterial overgrowth of the small intestine, orally ingested glucose ferments in the proximal small bowel (instead of being absorbed), resulting in increased hydrogen in the breath; here, the timing of exhaled hydrogen aids in the diagnosis. The measurement of radioactive carbon dioxide in the breath after ingestion of a nutrient labeled with carbon 14 (^{14}C) has been used to estimate the malabsorption of fat or bile acids and for measurement of bacterial overgrowth (^{14}C-xylose).

Summary

The overlap of symptoms and the large number of diagnostic tests available for evaluation of malabsorption necessitate the use of a systematic approach and a rational algorithm (see Fig. 3.1). The most accurate test for fat malabsorption remains the 72-hour fecal fat analysis; however, the test is difficult to carry out in clinical practice. Surrogate screening for steatorrhea is done with the qualitative stool fat examination (Sudan stain) and measurement of serum carotene. If the stool fat content is normal, the patient may still have selective impairment of absorption of a specific carbohydrate. This latter condition should be suspected if the primary symptoms are cramps, flatulence, and diarrhea. The most common example of carbohydrate malabsorption is lactose intolerance; specific tests include the oral lactose tolerance test, but measurement of breath hydrogen is more sensitive and more specific.

More generally, an *osmotic gap in fecal water* suggests a dietary (rather than a secretory) cause of the diarrhea related to luminal short-chain fatty acids or carbohydrates. The osmotic gap is calculated by the following formula:

$$\text{Osmotic gap} = \text{Plasma osmolality} - [2 \times (\text{fecal }[Na^+] + \text{fecal }[K^+])]$$

The osmotic gap is not calculated by directly measuring stool osmolality, because it increases with time in the specimen container. In addition, luminal osmolality is equal to serum osmolality because the colon cannot establish a gradient against the serum concentration of solutes.

When fat malabsorption is demonstrated (>7 g/24 hours, or increased qualitative stool fat and decreased serum carotene), a D-xylose absorption-excretion test should be performed next. A normal D-xylose test result makes diffuse mucosal disease unlikely and suggests maldigestion, principally pancreatic enzyme or bile salt deficiency. Clues to chronic pancreatitis include a history of alcohol abuse or previous episodes of pancreatitis. Unusual causes of pancreatic malabsorption, such as cystic fibrosis, microlithiasis,

表 3.3　小肠黏膜活检在吸收不良中的诊断作用
结果具备诊断意义
Whipple 病
淀粉样变性
嗜酸细胞性小肠炎
淋巴管扩张
原发性肠淋巴瘤
贾第鞭毛虫病
β-脂蛋白缺乏症
无丙种球蛋白血症
肥大细胞增多症
结果异常但无诊断意义
乳糜泻
系统性硬皮病
放射性肠炎
细菌过度生长
热带口炎性腹泻
克罗恩病

数据引自 Trier JS: Diagnostic value of peroral biopsy of the proximal small intestine. N Engl J Med 285：1470，1971.

放出来并与内因子结合。维生素 B_{12}-内因子聚合物被特异性受体（仅存在于远端回肠的肠细胞上）吸收。缺乏内因子（如恶性贫血、胃切除术后），胰腺功能不全，细菌过度生长，回肠切除或黏膜病变（如克罗恩病），均可导致维生素 B_{12} 吸收不良。

希林试验可通过放射性核素标记维生素 B_{12}，定量检测维生素 B_{12} 的吸收。该试验可通过多步骤检查扩大其诊断范围。第一步，注射 1000 μg 未标记的维生素 B_{12} 以达到肝饱和储存量，然后患者口服 0.5 μg 标记的维生素 B_{12}。收集患者尿液，以备放射性检测；放射性减弱提示维生素 B_{12} 吸收不良。第二步，在摄入的维生素 B_{12} 中添加口服内因子，并重复上述检测。若尿液中放射性标记的维生素 B_{12} 排出量恢复正常，则考虑恶性贫血。若仍存在吸收不良，则给予患者短期口服抗生素，并重复检查（第三步）。若尿液维生素 B_{12} 排出量被纠正，则考虑维生素 B_{12} 吸收不良是由细菌过度生长所致。若仍存在异常，则给予口服胰酶后重复检查（第四步）。若尿液排出量恢复，则考虑胰腺功能不全。第五步，若上述干预后仍存在排出量减少，则需要完善其他检查以明确是否有回肠疾病或钴胺素转运蛋白缺失，包括内因子抗体检测或幽门螺杆菌检测。上述一系列检查过程只是展示临床分析的一个例子，临床实践中通常是注射维生素 B_{12}，同时进行检查以寻找病因。

D-木糖检测

D-木糖检测常用于评估近端小肠的黏膜吸收功能，可用于明确是否存在肠上皮缺陷造成的吸收不良。D-木糖是一种五碳单糖，主要通过被动扩散跨肠黏膜运输。该检查中，给予受试者口服 25 g D-木糖，并收集随后 5 h 内的尿液。健康受试者 5 h 内排泄的 D-木糖应 > 4.5 g（或≥摄入量的 20%）。D-木糖排出量减少则考虑吸收异常。然而，肾排泄功能受损、胃轻瘫、广泛外周水肿、腹腔积液、服用药物（如阿司匹林、新霉素、吲哚美辛及格列吡嗪）可引起 D-木糖异常低值（假阳性）。细菌过度生长亦可引起异常结果，因为肠道内细菌可降解 D-木糖，但这种"假性吸收不良"可通过应用抗生素试验性治疗而纠正。

呼气试验

呼气试验主要测定呼出气体中细菌降解肠腔内混合物产生的气体代谢产物（如氢、甲烷、二氧化碳）。当双糖酶缺乏时，口服摄入但不能在小肠内被正常吸收的特定二糖（如乳糖）会被转运至结肠，从而在结肠内由细菌发酵产生代谢产物；氢是呼气检测中的标志物。当小肠细菌过度生长时，口服摄入的葡萄糖在近端小肠发酵（而不是被吸收），导致呼气中氢增多；此时，呼出氢的时间有助于诊断。摄入碳-14（^{14}C）标记的营养素后，检测呼出气体中具有放射性的二氧化碳，可用于评估脂肪或胆汁酸吸收不良，并可检测细菌过度生长（^{14}C-木糖）。

总结

吸收不良的不同症状相互重叠，且有多种检测手段，因此有必要建立系统的评估方法和合理的诊断流程（图 3.1）。测定脂肪吸收不良最准确的方法是 72 h 粪便脂肪分析，然而临床上其可行性欠佳。替代方法是定性粪便脂肪检测（苏丹染色）和血清胡萝卜素测定。即使粪便脂肪含量正常，患者仍可能存在特定碳水化合物的选择性吸收障碍，尤其是以肠痉挛、肠胀气和腹泻为主要症状时。碳水化合物吸收不良最常见的例子是乳糖不耐受，特异性检测方法包括口服乳糖耐量试验，但氢呼气试验更为敏感和特异。

一般来说，粪便液体渗透压差可提示与肠道短链脂肪酸或碳水化合物相关的饮食原因导致的腹泻（而不是分泌性腹泻）。渗透压差可通过下列公式计算：

渗透压差 = 血浆渗透压 − 2 × （粪便 Na^+ + 粪便 K^+）

渗透压差并不是通过直接检测粪便渗透压来计算，因为粪便渗透压会随标本盒内保存时间的延长而增大。此外，由于结肠不能产生与血清溶质浓度相对应的梯度，因此肠腔内渗透压与血清渗透压相等。

当存在脂肪吸收不良时（> 7 g/24 h；或粪便脂肪定性阳性、血清胡萝卜素水平降低），应进一步行 D-木糖吸收−排泄试验。D-木糖试验正常可排除弥漫性黏膜病变，提示可能为胰酶或胆盐缺乏引起的消化不良。需要考虑慢性胰腺炎的线索包括酗酒史或既往胰腺炎发作史。胰源性吸收不良的少见原因包括囊性纤维化、微小结石及药物毒性作用，需行特异性检查和细致的

or drug toxicity, require specific testing and a detailed history. Serum enzyme tests and abdominal imaging (plain films or, with much greater sensitivity, abdominal CT scans) can be obtained next to identify pancreatic disease. If the urinary D-xylose excretion is abnormal, the breath hydrogen test may be used to diagnose bacterial overgrowth using glucose for the carbohydrate load. If no bacterial overgrowth is present, a mucosal biopsy should be performed (see Table 3.3). Imaging studies of the small bowel may be helpful on occasion.

If the cause of malabsorption remains unclear, other considerations should include parasitic infection, such as *Giardia lamblia*, or ascariasis involvement of the pancreatic duct (more common in undeveloped countries). These diagnoses require a careful stool examination for ova and parasites or fecal antigen studies.

TREATMENT

The specific treatment of malabsorption depends on identification of the underlying condition. Occasionally, therapeutic trials for treatable conditions should be instituted, such as a gluten-free diet for celiac disease, pancreatic enzyme replacement for pancreatic exocrine malfunction, metronidazole for *G. lamblia* infection, or broad-spectrum antibiotics for suspected bacterial overgrowth. Parenteral nutrition may have a role in maintaining adequate nutritional status. Treatment modalities are discussed in later chapters focusing on specific diseases. Two disorders, celiac disease and bacterial overgrowth, are discussed here as illustrative of the pathophysiology.

Celiac Disease

Celiac disease (also called celiac sprue, nontropical sprue, or gluten-sensitive enteropathy) is characterized by intestinal mucosal injury resulting from gluten-related immunologic damage in persons genetically predisposed to this condition. The prevalence is estimated at about 1% in Western countries and has notably been rising across the world over the past 20 years. There is about an 80% concordance rate in monozygotic twins and less than 20% concordance rate in dizygotic twins. The prevalence of the disease among relatives of patients with celiac disease is approximately 10%. There is a strong association of celiac disease with human leukocyte antigen (HLA) class II molecules, particularly HLA-DQ2 and HLA-DQ8. However, in Western countries about 40% of the population possess either HLA-DQ2 or DQ8, notably different than the estimated celiac disease prevalence of 1%.

The disease is induced by exposure to storage proteins found in grain plants such as wheat (which contains gliadin), barley, and rye and their products. Oats are implicated, not because of gliadin, but because of contamination with wheat during packaging and transportation. The exposure initiates a cellular immune response that results in mucosal damage, particularly in the proximal intestine. Results of investigations suggest that an enzyme, tissue transglutaminase, may be the autoantigen of celiac disease.

Clinical Presentation

Celiac disease can manifest with the classic constellation of symptoms and signs of a malabsorption syndrome. Not uncommonly, however, the manifestation is atypical, with nonspecific GI symptoms such as bloating, chronic diarrhea (with or without steatorrhea), flatulence, lactose intolerance, or deficiencies of a single micronutrient (e.g., iron deficiency anemia). Extraintestinal complaints such as depression, weakness, fatigue, arthralgias, osteoporosis, or osteomalacia may predominate. A number of diseases, including dermatitis herpetiformis, type 1 diabetes mellitus, autoimmune thyroid disease, and selective immunoglobulin A (IgA) deficiency, are found in significant association with celiac disease.

Diagnosis

Celiac disease is a leading consideration in every patient with the malabsorption syndrome. It should be included as well in the differential of atypical manifestations, such as iron deficiency anemia, metabolic bone disease, neuropsychiatric symptoms, and intestinal lymphoma. Fiberoptic or capsule endoscopy may show the typical features of broad and flattened villi; with the former instrument, tissue can be sampled for histologic analysis. Intestinal biopsy is the most valuable test in establishing the diagnosis. The spectrum of pathologic changes ranges from normal villous architecture with an increase in mucosal lymphocytes and plasma cells (the infiltrative lesion) to partial blunting or total villous flattening. Although abnormal biopsy findings are not specific, they are highly suggestive, particularly because most other conditions that can mimic celiac disease (e.g., Crohn's disease, gastrinoma, lymphoma, tropical sprue, graft-versus-host disease, immune deficiency) may be distinguished clinically. A clinical response to a gluten-free diet establishes the diagnosis and precludes the need, in adults, to document healing by repeated biopsies. Serologic blood tests (antigliadin, antiendomysial, antireticulin, and tissue transglutaminase IgA antibodies) are helpful in screening of patients with atypical symptoms and asymptomatic relatives of patients with celiac disease. HLA genotyping has a high negative predictive value but low positive predictive value and is not routinely ordered.

Treatment

Strict, lifelong adherence to a gluten-free diet is the only treatment for celiac disease. Specific nutritional supplementation should be provided to correct deficiencies, particularly those of iron, vitamins, and calcium. A clinical response may be seen within a few weeks. Follow-up monitoring with serologic testing should be done after 3 to 6 months in the first year and then yearly thereafter in stable patients clinically responding to a gluten-free diet. Repeat biopsies should be considered for those who are seronegative or have persistent symptoms despite a gluten-free diet. The long-term prognosis is excellent for patients who adhere to the diet, although there may be a slight increase in the incidence of malignancies, particularly lymphoma.

Nonresponsive and Refractory Celiac Disease

Patients with ongoing symptoms more often than not are not truly adhering to a gluten-free diet. There may also be presence of an additional disease process, such as inflammatory bowel disease, microscopic colitis, lactose intolerance, pancreatic insufficiency, and ulcerative jejunitis.

Patients with persistent celiac disease activity despite adherence to a strict gluten-free diet for 12 months are deemed to have refractory celiac disease (RCD). Type 1 RCD is characterized by normal intraepithelial lymphocytes and a polyclonal T-cell receptor population. Type 2 RCD is described as having aberrant intraepithelial lymphocytes with monoclonal T-cell receptors. The overall prognosis for type 1 RCD is good, with a 5-year survival rate of 80%. Type 2 RCD, on the other hand, has a 5-year mortality rate of 50%. Type 2 RCD is strongly associated with ulcerative jejunitis and enteropathy-associated T-cell lymphoma (EATL). MR enterography, CT enterography, capsule endoscopy, and device-assisted enteroscopy may all be helpful in the diagnosis. PET CT is useful in diagnosing associated malignancy. Treatment options for type 2 RCD include azathioprine, steroids, methotrexate, cyclosporine, alemtuzumab, cladribine or fludarabine with or without autologous stem cell transplant.

病史询问。血清酶检测及腹部影像学检查（腹部X线平片或敏感性更高的腹部CT）有助于识别胰腺疾病。如果尿D-木糖排泄异常，则需以葡萄糖作为碳水化合物负荷进行氢呼气试验，以确定细菌过度生长。若无细菌过度生长，则推荐进行黏膜活检（表3.3）。小肠影像学检查有时亦具有诊断价值。

如果吸收不良的病因仍未明确，则需要考虑其他可能，包括寄生虫感染，如蓝氏贾第鞭毛虫或侵入胰腺导管的蛔虫（欠发达国家多见）。以上诊断需进行粪便虫卵及虫体检查或粪便抗原检测。

治疗

吸收不良的具体治疗有赖于病因诊断。某些情况下，应针对可治疗的疾病进行试验性治疗，如去麸质饮食治疗乳糜泻、胰酶替代治疗胰腺外分泌功能不全、甲硝唑治疗蓝氏贾第鞭毛虫感染、广谱抗生素治疗疑似细菌过度生长。肠外营养可维持足够的营养状态。特定疾病的具体治疗方法详见相应章节，本章以两种疾病（即乳糜泻和细菌过度生长）为例对病理生理学加以讨论。

乳糜泻

乳糜泻（又称口炎性腹泻、非热带口炎性腹泻或麸质敏感性肠病）的主要特征是在遗传易感人群中发生的由麸质相关免疫损害引起的肠黏膜损伤。据统计，西方国家乳糜泻的患病率约为1%，在过去20年里，全球患病率显著上升。同卵双胞胎中患病一致率约为80%，异卵双胞胎则低于20%。乳糜泻患者亲属的患病率约为10%。乳糜泻与人类白细胞抗原（HLA）Ⅱ类分子（尤其是HLA-DQ2和HLA-DQ8）有很强的相关性。然而，约40%的西方国家人群存在HLA-DQ2或HLA-DQ8，但其乳糜泻患病率却仅有1%。

该病由暴露于谷物植物［如小麦（含麦醇溶蛋白）、大麦、黑麦及其副产品］中的贮存蛋白质引起。燕麦也涵盖其中，但不是因为它含有麦醇溶蛋白，而是其运输包装过程中受到小麦污染。暴露于这些物质后机体会启动细胞免疫反应，导致黏膜损伤，尤其是近端小肠。研究表明，组织转谷氨酰胺酶可能是乳糜泻的自身抗原。

临床表现

乳糜泻可表现为吸收不良综合征的典型症状与体征。但是，不典型表现亦不少见，即非特异性胃肠道症状，如腹胀、慢性腹泻（伴或不伴脂肪泻）、胃肠胀气、乳糖不耐受或单种微量营养素缺乏（如缺铁性贫血）。患者可能以肠外表现为主，如抑郁、乏力、疲劳、关节痛、骨质疏松或骨软化。多种疾病与乳糜泻密切相关，包括疱疹样皮炎、1型糖尿病、自身免疫性甲状腺疾病和选择性免疫球蛋白A（IgA）缺乏。

诊断

吸收不良综合征患者均应首先考虑乳糜泻。此外，在对一些不典型表现的鉴别诊断中，亦应考虑乳糜泻，如缺铁性贫血、代谢性骨病、神经精神症状、肠道淋巴瘤等。纤维内镜或胶囊内镜可显示宽大低平的绒毛等典型特征。纤维内镜检查可获得组织标本进行病理组织学分析。肠道活检是最具诊断价值的检查方法。病理学表现范围较广，可从正常绒毛结构伴黏膜淋巴细胞和浆细胞增多（浸润性病变）到绒毛部分变钝或完全变平。虽然活检结果通常为非特异性，但仍具有较高的诊断价值，因为大多数与乳糜泻类似的其他疾病（如克罗恩病、胃泌素瘤、淋巴瘤、热带口炎性腹泻、移植物抗宿主病、免疫缺陷）在临床上是可以鉴别的。去麸质饮食治疗有效可确诊，在成人中以此可避免重复活检来证实黏膜愈合。血清学检查（抗麦醇溶蛋白抗体、抗肌内膜抗体、抗网状蛋白抗体及组织转谷氨酰胺酶IgA抗体）有助于筛查症状不典型的患者及无明显症状的乳糜泻患者亲属。HLA基因分型有较高的阴性预测值，但阳性预测值较低，因此不常规推荐。

治疗

严格的终身无麸质饮食是目前治疗乳糜泻的唯一方法。应补充特定的营养素以纠正营养缺乏，尤其是铁、维生素和钙。一般可在数周内观察到疗效。对于无麸质饮食治疗有效的稳定患者，第一年应在接受治疗后3～6个月内进行随访并完善血清学检查，此后每年随访复查。对于血清学检查阴性或无麸质饮食后仍持续有症状的患者，需考虑重复黏膜活检。严格遵循无麸质饮食的患者长期预后很好，但恶性疾病（特别是淋巴瘤）的发生率可能略升高。

治疗无效的乳糜泻及难治性乳糜泻

症状持续存在的患者可能并没有严格遵循无麸质饮食，同时也需考虑存在其他疾病的可能，如炎症性肠病、显微镜下结肠炎、乳糖不耐受、胰腺功能不全及溃疡性空肠炎。

严格坚持无麸质饮食12个月但乳糜泻仍持续活动的患者即为难治性乳糜泻（RCD）。1型RCD的特征是正常的上皮内淋巴细胞及多克隆T细胞受体群。2型RCD的特征是异常的上皮内淋巴细胞和单抗隆T细胞受体。1型RCD的总体预后较好，5年生存率约为80%；而2型RCD的5年死亡率为50%。2型RCD与溃疡性空肠炎、肠病相关性T细胞淋巴瘤（EATL）密切相关。磁共振小肠成像、CT小肠成像、胶囊内镜、气囊辅助小肠镜有助于诊断。正电子发射计算机断层成像（PET/CT）可用于诊断相关恶性肿瘤。2型RCD的治疗选择包括硫唑嘌呤、类固醇、甲氨蝶呤、环孢素、阿仑单抗、克拉立滨、氟达拉滨，可联合或不联合自体干细胞移植。

Bacterial Overgrowth Syndrome

The proximal small bowel normally contains fewer than 10^4 bacteria per milliliter of fluid, with no anaerobic *Bacteroides* organisms and few coliforms. Overgrowth of luminal bacteria can result in diarrhea and malabsorption by a number of mechanisms, including (1) deconjugation of bile salts, which leads to impaired micelle formation and impaired uptake of fat; (2) patchy injury to the enterocytes (small intestinal epithelial cells); (3) direct competition for the use of nutrients (e.g., uptake of vitamin B_{12} by gram-negative bacteria or the fish tapeworm *Diphyllobothrium latum*); and (4) stimulated secretion of water and electrolytes by products of bacterial metabolism, such as hydroxylated bile acids and short-chain (volatile) organic acids.

Conditions Associated With Bacterial Overgrowth

The most important factors maintaining the relative sterility of the upper gut are gastric acidity, peristalsis, and intestinal immunoglobulins (IgA). Conditions that impair these functions can result in bacterial overgrowth. Impaired peristalsis may be caused by motility disorders (e.g., scleroderma, amyloidosis, diabetes mellitus) or by anatomic changes (e.g., surgically created blind loops, obstruction, jejunal diverticulosis). Achlorhydria, pancreatic insufficiency, and hypogammaglobulinemia are also associated with bacterial overgrowth but uncommonly result in clinical steatorrhea. One should have particular suspicion for bacterial overgrowth in patients with chronic pancreatitis and associated diabetes mellitus, low zinc levels, and opiate use with ongoing weight loss or steatorrhea despite enzyme replacement therapy.

Diagnosis

Direct culture of jejunal aspirate is the most definitive diagnostic test, but it is invasive, uncomfortable, and costly. The ^{14}C-xylose breath test is an accurate and sensitive laboratory test; measurement of breath hydrogen after an oral challenge with glucose is simpler but not as sensitive or as specific. Adding methane to the hydrogen breath test may capture up to 20% to 30% of the population who produce methane as the byproduct of carbohydrate fermentation. An empirical therapeutic trial with antibiotics is an acceptable alternative to diagnostic testing.

Treatment

When appropriate, specific therapy, such as surgery for intestinal obstruction, should be provided. More commonly, patients are treated with antibiotics, most appropriately those that are effective against aerobic and anaerobic enteric organisms. Rifaximin, amoxicillin-clavulanate, quinolone, metronidazole with a cephalosporin or trimethroprim-sulfamethoxazole are suitable agents. A single course of therapy for 7 to 10 days may be therapeutic for months. In other patients, intermittent therapy (1 week of every 4) or even an extended period of continuous therapy may be effective, although data are limited.

MALABSORPTIVE THERAPY

Cardiovascular disease and other consequences of obesity have reached epidemic proportions in the United States, and one approach to this problem has been the deliberate induction of malabsorption (primarily of fats) to reduce a patient's lipid levels and body mass index. Medications used for this purpose include bile acid–binding resins, such as cholestyramine and colestipol, and the lipase inhibitors orlistat (Xenical) and ezetimibe (Zetia). Surgical treatment (bariatric operations) usually consists of gastric partition combined with some degree of small intestinal bypass, which induces significant weight loss by several proposed mechanisms, including malabsorption, improved nutrient deposition, and enhanced satiety. Recent data suggest that the malabsorption itself contributes less to overall weight loss from bariatric surgery than the latter two mechanisms and that it is fat malabsorption, rather than carbohydrate or protein malabsorption, that predominates.

SUGGESTED READINGS

Bai JC, Ciacci C; World Gastroenterology Organisation Global Guidelines: Celiac Disease February 2017. J Clin Gastroenterol. 2017 Oct;51(9):755-768. Erratum in: J Clin Gastroenterol. 2019 Apr;53(4):313.

Dye CK, Gaffney RR, Dykes TM, et al: Endoscopic and radiographic evaluation of the small bowel in 2012, *Am J Med* 125:1228.e1–1228.e12, 2012.

Forsmark CE: Management of chronic pancreatitis, *Gastroenterology* 144:1282–1291, 2013.

Goulet O, Ruemmele F: Causes and management of intestinal failure in children, *Gastroenterology* 2(Suppl 1):S16–S28, 2006.

Lee AA, Baker JR, Wamsteker EJ, Saad R, DiMagno MJ: Small intestinal bacterial overgrowth is common in chronic pancreatitis and associated with diabetes, chronic pancreatitis severity, low zinc Levels, and opiate use, *Am J Gastroenterol* 114(7):1163–1171, 2019.

Mueller K, Ash C, Pennisi E, et al: The gut microbiota: introduction, *Science* 336:1245, 2012.

Nasr I, Nasr I, Campling H, Ciclitira PJ. Approach to patients with refractory coeliac disease. F1000Res. 2016 Oct 20;5. pii: F1000 Faculty Rev-2544. eCollection 2016. Review.

Shannahan S, Leffler DA: Diagnosis and updates in Celiac disease, *Gastrointest Endosc Clin N Am* 27(1):79–92, 2017.

Siddiqui I, Ahmed S, Abid S: Update on diagnostic value of breath test in gastrointestinal and liver diseases, *World J Gastrointest Pathophysiol* 7(3):256–265, 2016.

细菌过度生长综合征

正常情况下，近端小肠每毫升小肠液的细菌量≤10^4，无厌氧拟杆菌，大肠菌群很少。肠腔内细菌过度生长可通过多种机制引起腹泻和吸收不良，包括：①胆盐的解偶联，导致微粒形成受损和脂肪吸收障碍；②小肠上皮细胞屏障功能受损；③营养素的直接竞争性利用（革兰氏阴性菌、鱼带绦虫及阔节裂头绦虫摄取维生素B_{12}）；④细菌代谢产物［如羟基化胆汁酸、短链（挥发性）有机酸］刺激肠道分泌水和电解质。

细菌过度生长相关疾病

胃酸、胃肠蠕动及肠道免疫球蛋白（IgA）是维持上消化道相对无菌环境的最重要因素。引起这些功能受损的疾病可导致细菌过度生长。胃肠道动力异常（如硬皮病、淀粉样变性、糖尿病）或解剖学改变（如手术造成的盲襻、梗阻、空肠憩室）可引起蠕动不良。胃酸缺乏、胰腺功能不全及低丙种球蛋白血症也与细菌过度生长相关，但很少引起脂肪泻。在慢性胰腺炎患者合并糖尿病、低锌、应用阿片类药物等情况下，且接受胰酶替代治疗后仍有体重减轻和脂肪泻时，需高度怀疑细菌过度生长。

诊断

空肠抽取物直接培养是最明确的诊断方法，但其为侵入性检查，且患者舒适度低、费用高。^{14}C-木糖呼气试验的准确性和敏感性高，口服葡萄糖后氢呼气试验更为简便，但其敏感性和特异性欠佳。氢呼气试验中增加甲烷可检出20%～30%其碳水化合物在肠菌发酵后产生甲烷的人群。抗生素经验性治疗也是可接受的试验性诊断方法。

治疗

建议在合适的时机进行特定治疗，如手术治疗肠梗阻。抗生素治疗更为常用，最合适的选择是可有效抗需氧和厌氧肠道微生物的抗生素。利福昔明、阿莫西林-克拉维酸钾、喹诺酮类、甲硝唑联合头孢菌素、甲氧苄啶-磺胺甲噁唑均为合适的药物。7～10天的单疗程治疗可维持数月疗效。对于一些患者，间歇治疗（每4周治疗1周）或长期持续治疗也有一定效果，虽然研究数据有限。

吸收不良疗法

在美国，心血管疾病和肥胖导致的其他疾病已达到流行病的程度，解决这一问题的办法之一是有意诱导吸收不良（主要是脂肪），以降低患者的血脂水平和体重指数。用于这一疗法的主要药物包括胆汁酸结合树脂（如考来烯胺和考来替泊）和脂酶抑制剂［奥利司他（Xenical）和依折麦布（Zetia）］。外科手术治疗（减重术）通常包括胃隔间术联合一定程度的小肠旁路手术，从而通过多种机制显著降低体重，包括吸收不良、改善营养存储及增加饱腹感。近期研究表明，相比于其他两种机制，吸收不良本身在减重术引起的体重减轻中的作用较小，且主要是脂肪吸收不良，而不是碳水化合物或蛋白质吸收不良。

推荐阅读

Bai JC, Ciacci C; World Gastroenterology Organisation Global Guidelines: Celiac Disease February 2017. J Clin Gastroenterol. 2017 Oct;51(9):755-768. Erratum in: J Clin Gastroenterol. 2019 Apr;53(4):313.

Dye CK, Gaffney RR, Dykes TM, et al: Endoscopic and radiographic evaluation of the small bowel in 2012, *Am J Med* 125:1228.e1–1228.e12, 2012.

Forsmark CE: Management of chronic pancreatitis, *Gastroenterology* 144:1282–1291, 2013.

Goulet O, Ruemmele F: Causes and management of intestinal failure in children, *Gastroenterology* 2(Suppl 1):S16–S28, 2006.

Lee AA, Baker JR, Wamsteker EJ, Saad R, DiMagno MJ: Small intestinal bacterial overgrowth is common in chronic pancreatitis and associated with diabetes, chronic pancreatitis severity, low zinc Levels, and opiate use, *Am J Gastroenterol* 114(7):1163–1171, 2019.

Mueller K, Ash C, Pennisi E, et al: The gut microbiota: introduction, *Science* 336:1245, 2012.

Nasr I, Nasr I, Campling H, Ciclitira PJ. Approach to patients with refractory coeliac disease. F1000Res. 2016 Oct 20;5. pii: F1000 Faculty Rev-2544. eCollection 2016. Review.

Shannahan S, Leffler DA: Diagnosis and updates in Celiac disease, *Gastrointest Endosc Clin N Am* 27(1):79–92, 2017.

Siddiqui I, Ahmed S, Abid S: Update on diagnostic value of breath test in gastrointestinal and liver diseases, *World J Gastrointest Pathophysiol* 7(3):256–265, 2016.

4

Common Clinical Manifestations of Gastrointestinal Disease: Diarrhea

Ronan Farrell, Sean Fine

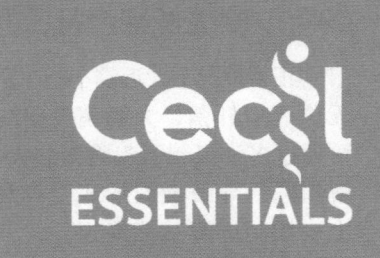

DEFINITION

Diarrhea can range from a mild self-limiting illness to a chronic debilitating disease. Although many definitions of diarrhea exist, the most clinically relevant definition is the passage of a greater number of stools of decreased form from a patient's baseline. The average number of bowel movements for a normal adult can range from three per day to three per week. Therefore, it remains crucial to establish through history a normal, baseline bowel habit prior to making the diagnosis. Once a diagnosis is made, diarrhea is initially classified into acute or chronic. Acute diarrhea has a duration of less than 4 weeks and is commonly infectious, whereas chronic diarrhea is diagnosed when symptoms have been ongoing for more than 4 weeks.

PATHOPHYSIOLOGY

Each day, as we consume water and food, the fluid ingested is added to the many secretions produced in our body, including salivary, pancreatic, and biliary secretions. Approximately 9 L of fluid eventually enters the small bowel, of which 90% is absorbed, leaving 1 L of fluid to pass into the colon. Ninety percent of this fluid is absorbed in the colon, leaving 100 mL to be excreted each day in feces. Any disease process in the gut that interferes with the absorption of water or the excretion of electrolytes can result in excess water in the gut lumen and diarrhea. The colon can overcome excess water excreted into its lumen by absorbing up to 4000 mL/24 hr, although 100 mL of excess water beyond this compensation is enough to cause diarrhea.

EVALUATION OF ACUTE DIARRHEA

The majority of acute diarrheal illnesses are infectious in nature. Acute infectious diarrhea can have an abrupt onset with clinical features including cramps, fevers, vomiting, bloody stools, and urgency. Outbreaks can be found in groups of people who travel or work closely together (daycare centers, nursing facilities, college dorms, hospital wards). For these reasons, it is important to take a detailed travel and exposure history from all patients who present with acute diarrhea. Most cases of infectious diarrhea are self-limiting, requiring only supportive treatment, and do not require further investigation. However, infants, elderly, immunosuppressed, and pregnant patients are at a greater risk for potential complications and may need closer attention to hydration status and electrolyte disturbances in a hospital setting. Other indicators of severe disease that may warrant a more robust clinical evaluation (Table 4.1) and treatment include diarrhea lasting longer than 72 hr, fever, bloody or mucoid stools, severe abdominal pain or signs of sepsis.

Acute Infectious Diarrhea

Clinically, acute infectious diarrhea can be classified into milder noninflammatory diarrhea and the more severe inflammatory diarrhea (Table 4.2). Noninflammatory diarrhea is usually a mild illness but can still result in severe electrolyte disturbances. These microorganisms act by disrupting the absorptive or secretory mechanisms of the small bowel and do not typically invade the mucosa, thus fecal leukocytes are usually absent. Noninflammatory acute diarrhea is mostly caused by viral illness such as rotavirus and norovirus. These viral illnesses are passed easily from person to person and can occur in large outbreaks. Symptoms can last 2 to 3 days before fully resolving. Bacteria that act in a similar way include Enterotoxigenic *Escherichia coli* and *Vibrio cholera*. Enterotoxigenic *Escherichia coli* is a common cause of travelers' diarrhea than can last up to 7 days. *Vibrio cholera* is less common in industrialized nations and can present with extreme diarrhea and can cause large epidemics in countries with unclean drinking water or poor sanitation.

Noninflammatory acute diarrhea caused by bacteria that use preformed toxin to mediate small bowel mucosal disruption is commonly referred to as "food poisoning." These bacteria use preformed toxin to mediate mucosal disruption that leads to an abrupt onset of illness, almost within 6 hours of eating contaminated food. *Staphylococcus aureus* is typically found in stale dairy products or processed meats. *Clostridioides perfringens* forms a toxin that is heat-labile and therefore found in meats that have not been reheated or cooked properly, whereas *Bacillus cereus* is classically implicated in acute diarrheal illness after eating reheated rice.

Protozoal infections are a rare cause of noninflammatory acute diarrhea. Giardia, a protozoal infection, can present as an acute illness often with abdominal bloating but is more commonly associated with chronic diarrhea and found in hikers who drink stream water. Cryptosporidia is a waterborne and self-limiting diarrhea but can also cause chronic diarrhea in the immunocompromised. It is important to note that although the above infectious agents may be implicated, often no diagnosis is found in self-limiting noninflammatory diarrhea and extensive investigation can be avoided.

Inflammatory diarrhea is caused by microorganisms that invade or release toxins that disrupt the intestinal barrier. This leads to the presence of elevated numbers of fecal leukocytes. These acute diarrheal illnesses are usually less voluminous and associated with bloody diarrhea, high fevers, cramping, and tenesmus. Risk factors include food consumption and preparation of undercooked meats, vegetables, and dairy products. In the United States, *Salmonella* and *Campylobacter jejuni* are the two most commonly isolated bacterial agents. Both are associated with undercooked poultry and stale, unpasteurized dairy products. *Shigella* is an invasive bacteria that can result in grossly bloody diarrhea. Enteroinvasive and enterohemorrhagic *Escherichia*

胃肠疾病常见临床表现：腹泻

苏文雨 译　陈煐晅 肖英莲 审校　房静远 通审

定义

腹泻既可表现为轻微的自限性疾病，亦可迁延为慢性消耗性疾病。虽然腹泻有许多定义，但临床最常用的定义是患者较平素排出更多性状稀薄的粪便。正常成人的平均排便次数为每天 3 次到每周 3 次不等，因此在诊断前了解患者的基础排便习惯至关重要。腹泻可分为急性腹泻和慢性腹泻。急性腹泻多为感染性腹泻，病程 < 4 周；慢性腹泻的病程 > 4 周。

病理生理学机制

人体每天都会摄入水和食物，摄入的液体与体内的消化液（由唾液腺、胰腺和胆汁分泌）混合。最终进入小肠的液体总量约 9 L，其中 90% 被吸收，其余 1 L 进入结肠。在结肠，90% 的液体被吸收，剩余 100 ml 每天随粪便排出。任何影响水分吸收或电解质排泄的疾病都会引起肠腔中水分过多和腹泻。结肠的最大吸收量为 4000 ml/24 h，超过此限量则可使结肠内的水分过多，超过 100 ml 就足以导致腹泻。

急性腹泻的评估

绝大多数急性腹泻为感染性疾病。急性感染性腹泻呈急性起病，临床特点包括痉挛痛、发热、呕吐、血便、腹泻，病情较紧急。多在集体旅行或工作（如日托中心、护理机构、大学宿舍、医院病房）的人群中暴发。因此，对于急性腹泻患者，明确详细的旅行和接触史非常重要。大多数感染性腹泻呈自限性，予以对症支持治疗即可，无须进一步检查。然而，婴儿、老年人、免疫抑制人群和孕妇发生潜在并发症的风险较大，应在医院内密切监测水和电解质紊乱。对于腹泻持续时间 > 72 h、发热、血便或黏液样便、重度腹痛及感染中毒症体征等提示重症腹泻的情况，均需要临床密切监测评估（表 4.1）和治疗。

急性感染性腹泻

在临床上，急性感染性腹泻可分为较轻微的非炎症性腹泻和较严重的炎症性腹泻（表 4.2）。非炎症性腹泻通常病情较轻，但仍可导致严重的电解质紊乱。这些微生物通过破坏小肠的吸收或分泌机制而发挥作用，通常不会侵入黏膜，因此粪便检测中一般没有白细胞。非炎症性急性腹泻多由病毒感染（如轮状病毒和诺如病毒）等引起，这些病毒感染易在人与人之间传播，引起大规模暴发。腹泻症状可持续 2～3 天，直至完全缓解。具有类似作用的细菌包括肠产毒性大肠埃希菌和霍乱弧菌。肠产毒性大肠埃希菌是旅行者腹泻的常见原因，腹泻症状可持续 7 天。霍乱弧菌在经济发达国家不太常见，可表现为严重腹泻，在饮用水不洁或卫生条件差的国家可能会引起大规模流行。

由细菌引起的非炎症性急性腹泻通常被称为"食物中毒"，这些细菌利用形成的毒素介导小肠黏膜破坏，患者几乎均在进食受污染食物后 6 h 内快速起病。金黄色葡萄球菌通常存在于不新鲜的乳制品或加工肉类中。产气荚膜梭状芽孢杆菌可形成一种热敏性毒素，因此会出现在未经加热或烹饪不当的肉类中，而蜡样芽孢杆菌则多与食用再加热米饭后的急性腹泻有关。

原虫感染是非炎症性急性腹泻的少见病因。贾第鞭毛虫感染可表现为急性腹泻伴腹胀，但更常见慢性腹泻，多发生于有饮用溪水史的徒步旅行者。隐孢子虫病是一种经水源传染的自限性腹泻，但也会在免疫力低下的人群中引起慢性腹泻。值得注意的是，上述病原体虽然可能与自限性非炎症性腹泻有关，但通常无法明确病因，也不建议过度检查。

炎症性腹泻是由微生物入侵或释放毒素破坏肠道屏障引起，因此患者粪便中可检出较多白细胞。急性炎症性腹泻患者一般排便量较少，常伴有血便、高热、痉挛痛及里急后重感。食用和制作未煮熟的肉类、蔬菜和乳制品是主要的诱因。在美国，沙门菌和空肠弯曲菌是两种常见的病原体，存在于未煮熟的禽肉、不新鲜或未经严格消毒的乳制品中。志贺菌是一种侵袭性细菌，可导致严重的血性腹泻。未煮熟的肉类或未

coli, found in undercooked meats or raw produce, can also cause bloody diarrhea. *Yersinia enterocolitica* is associated with undercooked pork and may present as a "pseudo-appendicitis" from mesenteric adenitis. When acute diarrhea is the presenting symptom in pregnant women, *Listeria monocytogenes* found in unpasteurized dairy products should always be considered in the differential diagnosis. *Vibrio parahaemolyticus* is commonly found in brackish water or in coastal areas and in contaminated shellfish.

Although rare, and usually only in the immunosuppressed, cytomegalovirus can cause invasion and ulceration of the colon resulting in inflammatory diarrhea. *Entamoeba histolytica* is a parasite that can cause severe diarrhea. It is found mostly in tropical countries with poor sanitation and may also seed to liver and brain resulting in abscess formation.

Another rare form of infectious diarrhea is Whipple disease, caused by the actinomycete *Tropheryma whipplei*, which causes malabsorption that results in weight loss, diarrhea, joint pain, and cognitive problems. Tropical sprue also causes malabsorption and is found in tropical climates of the Caribbean, South America, and Asia. The causative organism has not been identified, but symptoms respond to antibiotic treatment and therefore are highly suspected to be infectious.

Clostridioides difficile infection (CDI) is a common cause of severe hospital-acquired diarrheal infection resulting in a pseudomembranous colitis. *Clostridioides difficile* can colonize the human GI tract but usually does not cause clinical symptoms unless the normal gut flora is altered, therefore allowing *C. difficile* to grow uncontrolled. CDI should be considered in all hospitalized patients that develop diarrhea or have a history of antibiotic use. Other high-risk patients include the elderly, immunosuppressed patients, and patients with inflammatory bowel disease. CDI can result in large, voluminous, watery diarrhea, usually with significant leukocytosis, that can be a major cause of morbidity and mortality. Testing for CDI is commonly done using molecular tests for the toxins associated with CDI such as polymerase chain reaction and is highly sensitive but does not differentiate between colonization and infection. This can result in high false-positive testing; therefore, it is important to only send CDI testing in patients with symptoms of infectious diarrhea. This will increase the positive predictive value of the test.

Treatment

Volume depletion is the main consideration when evaluating a person with acute diarrhea. By evaluating the volume status of patients and their ability to maintain adequate oral intake, a decision can be made whether to treat with oral rehydration or if admission to hospital and intravenous fluids are needed. The objective of rehydration and electrolyte replacement is to prevent hypotension and electrolyte disturbances that can be a major cause of morbidity and mortality, especially in the elderly and very young. For most people with acute diarrhea, fluid replacement can be achieved with sports drinks and eating saltine crackers. Some people with more severe disease or the elderly and infants may require a more balanced commercially available oral rehydration solution. In patients with mild illness, who are afebrile and do not have bloody diarrhea, symptomatic relief agents such as loperamide or diphenoxylate can be used to reduce the volume of diarrhea. These antimotility drugs reduce gut motility, therefore allowing slower passage of water through the gut and allowing greater reabsorption of fluid. Another class of agents that can be used are antisecretory drugs such as bismuth subsalicylates.

The decision to treat with antibiotics is a common one faced by physicians who are evaluating patients with acute diarrhea. In the community, most diarrheal illnesses are viral and therefore empiric treatment with antibiotics is not recommended. In a returning traveler who is being evaluated for diarrhea, the severity of the illness will guide treatment. Mild travelers' diarrhea should not be treated with antibiotics. Antibiotics have been shown to be effective in reducing the duration of moderate to severe travelers' diarrhea by 1 to 3 days when compared to no treatment. Moderate to severe travelers' diarrhea

TABLE 4.1 Diagnostic Evaluation of Acute Severe Diarrhea

Lab	Complete blood count, basic metabolic panel, C-reactive protein, blood cultures
Stool studies	*Salmonella, Shigella, Campylobacter, Yersinia*, enterohemorrhagic *Escherichia coli* and *Clostridioides difficile*
Imaging	1. Radiograph abdomen for evaluation of intra-abdominal free air or toxic megacolon 2. Computed tomography for signs and symptoms of peritonitis or if there is sustained fever or bacteremia despite treatment with appropriate antibiotics

TABLE 4.2 Acute Diarrhea Lasting Less Than 2 Weeks

Noninflammatory		Inflammatory	
Mild watery diarrhea		Severe bloody diarrhea	
Disruption of small bowel transport		Invasion and destruction of gut mucosa	
Fecal leukocytes (-)		Fecal leukocytes (+)	
Preformed toxin "food poisoning"	*Staphylococcus aureus* *Bacillius cereus* *C. perfringens*	Bacterial	*Campylobacter* *Salmonella* *Shigella* *E. coli* *Clostridioides difficile* *Vibrio parahaemolyticus*
Viral	Norovirus Rotavirus	Viral	Cytomegalovirus (CMV)
Bacterial	*Escherichia coli* *Vibrio cholera*	Parasitic	*Entamoeba histolytica*
Parasitic	Giardia Cryptosporidium Cyclospora		

加工的农产品中的肠侵袭性大肠埃希菌和肠出血性大肠埃希菌也会导致血性腹泻。小肠结肠炎耶尔森菌与未煮熟的猪肉有关，其感染可表现为由肠系膜炎引起的"假性阑尾炎"。当孕妇出现急性腹泻时，鉴别诊断时应注意未经严格消毒乳制品中的单核细胞性李斯特菌。副溶血性弧菌常存在于半咸水、沿海地区和受污染的贝类中。

巨细胞病毒感染的发生率低，多发生于免疫抑制患者中；巨细胞病毒感染可导致结肠溃疡，继而引起炎症性腹泻。溶组织内阿米巴是阿米巴痢疾的病原体，易引起严重腹泻，也会累及肝和脑，形成脓肿。其主要存在于卫生条件较差的热带国家。

另一种罕见的感染性腹泻是由感染放线菌惠普尔养障体引起的惠普尔病（Whipple病），患者会因吸收不良而出现体重减轻、腹泻、关节痛和认知障碍。热带口炎性腹泻也会引起吸收不良，多见于加勒比海、南美洲和亚洲的热带气候地区。虽然该病的致病菌尚未明确，但经抗生素治疗有效，因此被认为是一种感染性疾病。

艰难梭菌感染（CDI）是严重的院内获得性感染性腹泻的常见原因，可导致假膜性结肠炎。艰难梭菌可在人体胃肠道内定植，但通常不引起临床症状。当正常肠道菌群失调时，艰难梭菌可大量生长而致病。所有出现腹泻的住院患者或有抗生素使用史者，应考虑CDI。CDI的其他高危人群包括老年人、免疫抑制患者和炎症性肠病患者。CDI可引起严重的水样便，伴白细胞明显增多，是导致并发症发生率和死亡率升高的主要原因。CDI的检测通常采用分子检测，如聚合酶链反应（PCR）检测CDI相关毒素，其敏感性很高，但易出现假阳性，且不能区分定植和感染。因此，应仅对有感染性腹泻症状的患者进行CDI检测，以提高检测的阳性预测值。

治疗

液体丢失量是评估急性腹泻患者的主要考虑因素。通过评估患者的血容量和口服摄入的能力，可决定采用口服补液治疗还是入院静脉输液治疗。补液和补充电解质的目的是预防低血压和电解质紊乱，其是引起患者（尤其是儿童和老年患者）死亡的主要原因。对于大多数急性腹泻患者，可通过饮用运动饮料和食用苏打饼干来补充丢失的液体和电解质；病情较重的患者、婴儿或老人需要补充更均衡的市售口服补液溶液；无发热、无血便等病情较轻的患者，可使用洛哌丁胺或地芬诺酯，这些抗动力药物可抑制肠蠕动，减缓水通过肠道的速度，并促进肠液的再吸收，从而缓解腹泻症状。另一类可以使用的药物是抗分泌药物，如次水杨酸铋。

抗生素的使用也是医生在处理急性腹泻时经常面临的问题。在社区，大多数腹泻由病毒引起，不建议使用抗生素进行经验性治疗。对于旅行者腹泻，需根据病情的严重程度选择：轻度患者不需要使用抗生素；中重度患者使用抗生素可使病程缩短 1～3 天。中重度旅行者腹泻多表现为发热、腹痛、便血和感染中毒症。

表 4.1 急性严重腹泻的诊断性评估

实验室检查	全血细胞计数、基础代谢检查、C反应蛋白、血培养
粪便检查	沙门菌、志贺菌、弯曲菌、耶尔森菌、肠出血性大肠埃希菌和艰难梭菌
影像学检查	1. 腹部X线检查用于评估腹内游离空气或中毒性巨结肠 2. CT用于评估腹膜炎的症状和体征，或抗生素治疗后仍发热或出现菌血症的情况

表 4.2 病程少于 2 周的急性腹泻

非炎症性		炎症性	
轻度水样便		重度血便	
小肠转运障碍		肠黏膜侵袭和破坏	
粪便白细胞（－）		粪便白细胞（＋）	
"食物中毒"的毒素	金黄色葡萄球菌 蜡样芽孢杆菌 产气荚膜梭菌	细菌	弯曲菌 沙门菌 志贺菌 大肠埃希菌 艰难梭菌 副溶血性弧菌
病毒	诺如病毒 轮状病毒	病毒	巨细胞病毒（CMV）
细菌	大肠埃希菌 霍乱弧菌	寄生虫	溶组织内阿米巴
寄生虫	贾弟鞭毛虫 隐孢子虫 环孢子虫		

includes patients with fever, abdominal pain, bloody stool, and sepsis. The most common pathogen identified in travelers' diarrhea is enterotoxigenic *Escherichia coli*, followed by *Campylobacter jejuni*, *Shigella*, and *Salmonella*. Fluoroquinolones, such as ciprofloxacin, are the antibiotics of choice for most cases of travelers' diarrhea. Rifaximin also has been shown to be as effective as ciprofloxacin for noninvasive travelers' diarrhea. However, the resistance of *Campylobacter* to fluoroquinolones is increasing, and in such cases, treatment with a macrolide such as azithromycin should be used. Antibiotics should be avoided in enterohemorrhagic *Escherichia coli* because there may be an increased risk of hemolytic-uremic syndrome related to increased release of Shiga-like toxin.

The recommended treatment of initial CDI is with oral vancomycin or fidaxomicin for 10 days. Patients who have a repeat CDI should be treated with oral vancomycin therapy using a tapered and pulsed regimen. Finally, patients who have more than one recurrence of CDI should be considered for fecal microbiota transplant. Although numerous studies and meta-analyses have been performed on the benefits of probiotics in CDI, currently there is insufficient evidence to recommend their use for the primary prevention of CDI.

CHRONIC DIARRHEA

Chronic diarrhea can be defined as an increase in stool frequency, reduced consistency, and duration longer than 4 weeks. Patient symptoms may include loose stools, increased stool frequency, change of consistency or incontinence. These symptoms can be disabling, and patients will often describe a fear of leaving the house or avoiding long trips without immediate access to a toilet. Though acute diarrhea is commonly infectious in nature, the differential diagnosis of chronic diarrhea is vast and includes intestinal inflammation, colonic neoplasia, malabsorption due to small bowel mucosal disorders, maldigestion due to pancreatic insufficiency, motility disorders, and functional bowel disorders.

Evaluation of Chronic Diarrhea

A thorough history is essential in narrowing down the diagnosis in chronic diarrhea. History should focus on travel and exposures, stool characteristics, prior surgeries, current medications, and over-the-counter supplements. Infectious causes of chronic diarrhea are uncommon in the United States but should be considered in newly arrived immigrants, returned travelers, and people with exposure to farm animals or unclean drinking water. The characteristics of the patient's stool should be described because the presence of blood may suggest malignancy or inflammatory bowel disease (IBD), oily or sticky stools may suggest malabsorption or maldigestion, and watery stools point to an osmotic or secretory process. Associated symptoms such as fevers, abdominal pain, bloating, and cramps should be noted, as should the relationship of defecation to meals and periods of fasting. Nocturnal symptoms and weight loss can strongly suggest an organic etiology. In patients who are of colon cancer screening age or have alarm features, endoscopic evaluation should be performed. Alarm features include microcytic anemia, bloody diarrhea, fevers, weight loss, nocturnal symptoms, or family history of IBD or colorectal cancer. It is helpful to classify chronic diarrhea into inflammatory, watery or fatty (Table 4.3).

Laboratory Testing

Routine laboratory testing can be used to provide clues to the etiology or severity of chronic diarrhea. A microcytic anemia may point towards chronic blood loss or iron malabsorption seen in an inflammatory process. Macrocytic anemia may point towards a vitamin B_{12} deficiency that can be seen in IBD or in patients who have had small bowel or gastric resection.

Leukocytosis, elevated inflammatory markers such as C-reactive protein, and fecal calprotectin can be seen in inflammatory diarrhea. Serology testing for antitissue transglutaminase antibodies can be performed to rule out celiac disease. Finally, hormone-secreting tumors are rare and should only be tested for in highly selected patients.

Further Evaluation of Chronic Diarrhea

Due to clustering of symptoms, one of the most practical tasks facing a physician in evaluating chronic diarrhea is to try and make the distinction between functional and organic etiologies.

Irritable bowel syndrome (IBS) is common and can present with an array of symptoms that can include diarrhea, bloating, cramping, and abdominal pain associated with defecation. The Rome IV consensus, formed by a worldwide committee to set criteria for the diagnosis of functional gastrointestinal disorders, may help establish the diagnosis. The most recent criteria focuses on abdominal pain in relation to defecation, change in frequency or change in consistency of stool (Table 4.4). The majority of patients who present with classic symptoms of IBS do not need further diagnostic testing and the focus should be on treatment through diet or available medicines approved for IBS.

When a specific etiology is strongly suspected in the work-up of chronic diarrhea that has no confirmatory testing or testing may be invasive or expensive, an empirical trial of treatment may be pursued. Examples include patients with a history of small bowel resection or

TABLE 4.3 Causes of Chronic Diarrhea

Watery Diarrhea		Inflammatory Diarrhea	Fatty Diarrhea
Osmotic	**Secretory**	• IBD: Crohn's disease, ulcerative colitis	**Malabsorption**
• Osmotic laxatives: Lactulose, magnesium sulphate (milk of magnesia), polyethylene glycol (Miralax)	• IBD: Crohn's disease, ulcerative colitis	• Diverticulitis	• Celiac disease
	• Microscopic colitis	• Pseudomembranous colitis	• Whipple's disease
	• Hyperthyroidism	• Ischemic colitis	• Short bowel syndrome
	• Medication	• Radiation colitis	• Mesenteric ischemia
• Carbohydrate malabsorption (lactase deficiency)	• Bacterial toxins	• Bacterial infection: tuberculosis, yersiniosis	• Small intestinal bacterial overgrowth
	• Irritable bowel syndrome	• Viral infection: cytomegalovirus, herpes simplex	**Maldigestion**
	• Neoplasm: colon carcinoma, lymphoma	• Parasitic infection: strongyloides	• Exocrine pancreatic insufficiency
	• Bile acid malabsorption	• Neoplasm: colon carcinoma, lymphoma	• Reduced bile acid secretion (primary biliary cholangitis)
	• Neuroendocrine tumors		

IBD, Inflammatory bowel disease.

最常见的病原体是肠产毒性大肠埃希菌，其次是空肠弯曲菌、志贺菌和沙门菌。氟喹诺酮类（如环丙沙星）是大多数旅行者腹泻患者的首选抗生素。利福昔明对非侵袭性旅行者腹泻的疗效与环丙沙星相当。然而，弯曲菌对氟喹诺酮类药物的耐药性正在增加，在这种情况下，应使用阿奇霉素等大环内酯类药物治疗。肠出血性大肠埃希菌感染者应避免使用抗生素，因为类志贺毒素释放增加可能会增加溶血性尿毒综合征的风险。

初诊CDI患者建议口服万古霉素或非达米星，疗程为10天；复发CDI患者可口服万古霉素，并采用逐渐减量配合脉冲式给药方案。对于CDI反复复发者，应考虑粪菌移植。虽然已有大量研究和荟萃分析证实了益生菌对治疗CDI的益处，但目前尚无足够的证据推荐将其用于CDI的一级预防。

慢性腹泻

慢性腹泻是指排便次数增加、粪质减少，持续时间>4周。症状包括粪便松散、排便次数增多、粪质稀薄或大便失禁。患者常因担心离开家或旅途中找不到厕所而避免长途旅行。急性腹泻多为感染性，而慢性腹泻的鉴别诊断范围更广，包括肠道炎症、结肠肿瘤、小肠黏膜病变引起的吸收不良、胰腺功能不全引起的消化不良、肠蠕动异常和功能性肠病。

慢性腹泻的评估

详尽的病史对缩小慢性腹泻的鉴别诊断范围至关重要。病史采集应重点关注旅行和暴露因素、粪便特征、既往手术史、当前用药史及非处方营养补充剂。在美国，由感染引起的慢性腹泻并不常见，但新移民、回国旅行者及接触过农场动物或不洁饮用水的患者，应考虑感染性病因。患者的粪便性状应加以描述，血便可能提示恶性肿瘤或炎症性肠病（IBD）；油性便或粘性便可能提示吸收不良或消化不良；水样便多见于渗透性或分泌性腹泻。此外，还应关注发热、腹痛、腹胀和痉挛痛等伴随症状，以及排便与进食的时间关系。出现夜间症状和体重减轻强烈提示器质性病因。对于达到结肠癌筛查年龄或有报警症状的患者，建议进一步完善内镜检查。报警症状包括小细胞性贫血、血便、发热、体重减轻、夜间症状、IBD或结直肠癌家族史等。将慢性腹泻分为炎症性腹泻、水样便和脂肪泻有助于临床诊断和评估病情（表4.3）。

实验室检查

常规实验室检查可为慢性腹泻的病因或严重程度提供线索。小细胞性贫血可能与慢性失血或炎症过程中铁吸收不良有关。大细胞性贫血可能与维生素B_{12}缺乏有关，而维生素B_{12}缺乏也可见于IBD或接受过小肠或胃切除术的患者。

白细胞增多、炎症标志物（如C反应蛋白）和粪便钙卫蛋白水平升高可见于炎症性腹泻。血清学检测抗组织转谷氨酰胺酶抗体可排除乳糜泻；由于激素分泌性肿瘤较为罕见，应仅在高度选择的患者中进行检测。

慢性腹泻的进一步评估

由于症状的聚集性，临床医生在评估慢性腹泻时最实际的任务之一是区分功能性和器质性病因。

肠易激综合征（IBS）是以腹泻、腹胀、痉挛痛和排便相关腹痛为主要症状的常见综合征。由国际功能性胃肠病专家委员会制定的罗马Ⅳ共识有助于IBS的诊断。最新的标准侧重于与排便相关的腹痛、排便频率或粪便性状改变（表4.4）。绝大多数具有典型IBS症状的患者无须进一步检查，主要通过饮食调整或已获批的药物进行治疗。

如果在针对慢性腹泻的检查中强烈怀疑有特定病因，但又没有确诊的检查方法或相关检查可能具有侵入性或费用昂贵，则可以进行经验性治疗。例如，有小肠切除术或胆囊切除术病史的患者可以经验性给予抑制

表4.3 慢性腹泻的原因

水样便		炎症性腹泻	脂肪泻
渗透性腹泻	分泌性腹泻	• IBD：克罗恩病、溃疡性结肠炎	吸收障碍
• 渗透性泻药：乳果糖、硫酸镁（氢氧化镁）聚乙二醇、（Miralax）	• IBD：克罗恩病、溃疡性结肠炎	• 憩室炎	• 乳糜泻
• 碳水化合物吸收不良（乳糖酶缺乏症）	• 显微镜下结肠炎	• 假膜性结肠炎	• Whipple病
	• 甲状腺功能亢进症	• 缺血性结肠炎	• 短肠综合征
	• 药物	• 放射性结肠炎	• 肠系膜缺血
	• 细菌毒素	• 细菌感染：结核病、耶尔森菌病	• 小肠细菌过度生长
	• 肠易激综合征	• 病毒感染：巨细胞病毒、单纯疱疹病毒	消化不良
	• 肿瘤：结肠癌、淋巴瘤	• 寄生虫感染：类圆线虫	• 胰腺外分泌功能不全
	• 胆汁酸吸收不良	• 肿瘤：结肠癌、淋巴瘤	• 胆汁酸分泌减少（原发性胆汁性胆管炎）
	• 神经内分泌肿瘤		

IBD，炎症性肠病。

TABLE 4.4	Criteria for Diagnosis of IBS
Recurrent abdominal pain on average at least 1 day/week in the last 3 months, associated with two or more of the following: Related to defecation Associated with change in the frequency of stool Associated with a change in stool consistency	

TABLE 4.5	Chronic Watery Diarrhea	
	Osmotic	Secretory
Stool volume (L/day)	<1 L	>1 L
Effect on fasting	Reduced	Continued
Fecal osmotic gap	>100 mOsm/kg	<50 mOsm/kg
pH	Usually <5	Usually >6

cholecystectomy who may be empirically treated for bacterial overgrowth or started on a bile acid binder. In such patients who fail empiric treatment or in which the diagnosis remains broad and elusive, a colonoscopy with biopsies should be performed.

Chronic Inflammatory Diarrhea

Chronic inflammatory diarrhea typically presents with bloody diarrhea associated with abdominal pain. Any disease process that can disrupt or inflame the mucosa of the gut should be considered, including infections, inflammatory bowel disease, ischemia, neoplasm or radiation enteritis. Direct visualization with colonoscopy is the best next diagnostic step. Biopsies should be taken to characterize the inflammation. Ischemic colitis should be suspected in elderly patients with underlying vascular disease and a recent hypotensive episode. Characteristic findings on colonoscopy show rectal sparing that is not seen with ulcerative colitis and well-demarcated, segmental inflammation, usually in the watershed area of the splenic flexure. Inflammatory bowel disease, which includes both Crohn's disease or ulcerative colitis, is a more common cause of chronic inflammatory diarrhea. Crohn's disease can involve any part of the GI tract and the presentation may not include bloody diarrhea and can be more varied. Typical symptoms include abdominal pain, weight loss, and diarrhea. However, oral ulcers, fistulous openings or perianal disease in the setting of chronic inflammatory diarrhea are also strong indicators pointing towards Crohn's disease. During colonoscopy, the terminal ileum should be evaluated for ulcers and strictures, which would be consistent with Crohn's disease. In contrast, ulcerative colitis involves only the colon. Clinical presentation and severity are dependent on the location and extent of colonic involvement. When the rectum or rectosigmoid region is involved, patients can present with mild intermittent bloody diarrhea, rectal urgency, and tenesmus. Rarely, patients with isolated severe rectal inflammation may also present with constipation and an inability to pass stools. Pancolitis and left-sided colitis typically have more profound presentations with severe abdominal pain, fevers, anemia, and frequent bloody diarrhea.

Chronic Watery Diarrhea

Chronic watery diarrhea should be subdivided into secretory and osmotic types, based on fecal osmotic gap. The fecal osmotic gap is calculated as 290 mOsm/kg − 2 × (stool Na + stool K). When the calculated fecal osmotic gap is greater than 100 mOsm/kg, it is consistent with osmotic diarrhea, while a gap of less than 50 mOsm/kg is suggestive of a secretory etiology of diarrhea such as infection, inflammation, or circulating secretagogues (Table 4.5).

Osmotic diarrhea may be caused by magnesium ingestion or malabsorption of carbohydrates. Both result in water retention in the lumen of the gut and therefore a high osmotic gap. High magnesium concentration in the stool is commonly seen in patients who use laxatives or high doses of antacids. For this reason, it is important to review medication lists. Lactose intolerance due to lactase deficiency or ingestion of other poorly absorbed sugars can also pull water into the lumen of the gut, resulting in diarrhea. As these malabsorbed carbohydrates ferment, the stool becomes more acidic. Therefore, a pH less than 7.0 can point to excess carbohydrates in the stool. Common dietary sugar substitutes that cause osmotic diarrhea include sorbitol and high-fructose corn syrup. For this reason, osmotic diarrhea should disappear with fasting.

Secretory diarrhea can result from any process that impairs or disrupts the absorption of salt and water in the gut. Often an overlap of secretory and inflammatory diarrhea may be seen.

Although rare in developed countries, infectious organisms can cause chronic diarrhea and should be ruled out, especially in returned travelers. Parasites such as *Cryptosporidium*, *Microsporidia*, *Cyclospora*, and *Giardia* can all cause chronic secretory diarrhea. Testing of stool for ova and parasites should be performed if there is a travel history or recent immigration from a high-risk area. Giardia testing using ELISA is recommended in all patients with chronic diarrhea.

More commonly, mucosal disease as seen in IBD or structural disease as seen in short bowel syndrome or neoplasm is the cause of chronic secretory diarrhea. Imaging with small bowel radiograph or computerized tomography (CT) should be used to assess for tumors, strictures, fistulas or inflammation. Further examination with colonoscopy should be performed for direct visualization and biopsies of the mucosa.

Microscopic colitis is characterized by chronic watery diarrhea and is commonly seen in women older than 60 years old, although men and women of any age can be affected. Typical symptoms include more than 10 watery stools/day that can be accompanied by abdominal cramping and even mild weight loss. Nocturnal symptoms are common. There are two subtypes of microcytic colitis, lymphocytic and collagenous. The cause of microscopic colitis is unknown but there is a strong association with other autoimmune diseases and certain medications such as proton pump inhibitors and nonsteroidal anti-inflammatory drugs. Direct visualization with colonoscopy typically shows no mucosal inflammation, so biopsies of the left and right colon are needed to make this histologic diagnosis. Budesonide is recommended as first-line treatment for microscopic colitis; however, this medication may be cost prohibitive, and alternative treatments include bismuth subsalicylate or aminosalicylates.

Patients who are post cholecystectomy or have ileal disease or resection may have bile acid malabsorption. This can result when excess bile acid is passed into the colon resulting in electrolyte absorption impairment. In such cases, a trial of bile acid–sequestering resins should be tried.

Peptide-secreting neuroendocrine tumors are rare and should only be investigated when the work-up has been unrevealing for chronic diarrhea. Plasma peptides such as gastrin and vasoactive intestinal peptide (VIP) can be used to help diagnose Zollinger-Ellison syndrome or VIPoma respectively. Elevated levels of gastrin can be seen in patients taking acid suppressing medications such as proton pump inhibitors; however, in Zollinger-Ellison syndrome, gastrin levels are often 10 times the upper limit of normal. CT, MRI, or endoscopic ultrasound of the liver and pancreas should be performed to identify tumors. Zollinger-Ellison syndrome can have characteristic multiple gastric

表 4.4	IBS 的诊断标准
在过去 3 个月中，平均每周至少有 1 天反复腹痛，并与以下两种或两种以上情况有关： 　　与排便有关 　　与排便频率改变有关 　　与粪便性状改变有关	

表 4.5　慢性水样腹泻		
	渗透性腹泻	分泌性腹泻
粪便量（L/d）	< 1	> 1
禁食的影响	减轻	无变化
粪便渗透压（mOsm/kg）	> 100	< 50
pH 值	通常 < 5	通常 > 6

细菌过度生长的治疗或胆汁酸螯合剂。对于经验性治疗失败或诊断仍不明确患者，应进行结肠镜检查和活检。

慢性炎症性腹泻

慢性炎症性腹泻主要表现为伴有腹痛的血性腹泻。感染、炎症性肠病、缺血、肿瘤或放射性肠炎等任何引起肠道黏膜损伤或炎症的疾病，均可导致慢性炎症性腹泻。结肠镜检查直视下观察肠黏膜是进一步诊断的最佳方法，并应行活检明确炎症性质。有基础血管疾病和近期低血压发作的老年患者应考虑缺血性结肠炎，其结肠镜的特征性表现是肠道界限清楚的节段性炎症，通常位于脾区分水岭区域，与溃疡性结肠炎的不同点是直肠黏膜一般正常。炎症性肠病（包括克罗恩病和溃疡性结肠炎）是慢性炎症性腹泻更常见的病因。克罗恩病可累及消化道的任何部位，可不伴有血便，症状多样。典型症状包括腹痛、体重减轻和腹泻。慢性炎症性腹泻患者出现口腔溃疡、瘘管开口或肛周疾病时多提示克罗恩病。结肠镜检查时应评估回肠末端是否有溃疡和狭窄。相比之下，溃疡性结肠炎只累及结肠，临床表现和严重程度取决于结肠受累的部位和范围。当直肠或直肠乙状结肠受累时，患者表现为轻度间歇性血便、直肠紧迫感和里急后重。极少数情况下，严重的孤立性直肠炎患者会出现便秘和无法排便。全结肠炎和左侧结肠炎通常表现为剧烈腹痛、发热、贫血和频繁的血便。

慢性水样腹泻

根据粪便渗透压的不同，慢性水样腹泻可分为分泌性和渗透性。粪便渗透压差的计算公式为 290 mOsm/kg − 2×（粪便 Na^+ + 粪便 K^+）。当计算得出的粪便渗透压差 > 100 mOsm/kg 时，考虑渗透性腹泻；< 50 mOsm/kg 时，则提示由感染、炎症或循环中促分泌物引起的分泌性腹泻（表 4.5）。

渗透性腹泻可能由摄入镁或碳水化合物吸收不良引起，这两种情况都会引起肠腔内水潴留，造成高渗透压差。服用泻药或大剂量抗酸剂的患者粪便中可检出高浓度的镁，因此，回顾患者用药史非常重要。由乳糖酶缺乏或摄入其他不易吸收的糖类导致的乳糖不耐受也会将水吸入肠腔，导致腹泻。当这些吸收不良的碳水化合物发酵时，粪便的酸性会增强。因此，粪便 pH 值 < 7.0 提示粪便中含有过量的碳水化合物。常见的膳食代糖可引起渗透性腹泻，包括山梨醇和高果糖玉米糖浆。因此，禁食后腹泻会消失。

分泌性腹泻由肠道对盐和水的吸收受损或障碍引起。分泌性腹泻和炎症性腹泻常重叠出现。

病原体感染引起的慢性腹泻在发达国家很少见，但也应注意排除相关的病原体感染，尤其是旅行者腹泻。隐孢子虫、微孢子虫、环孢子虫和贾第鞭毛虫等寄生虫感染均会引起慢性分泌性腹泻。若有旅行史或近期从高危地区入境，应进行粪便虫卵和寄生虫检测。建议所有慢性腹泻患者行 ELISA 法检测贾第鞭毛虫。

IBD 中的黏膜病变和短肠综合征或肿瘤导致的结构异常也是慢性分泌性腹泻的较常见原因。小肠 X 线检查或 CT 可用于评估肿瘤、肠腔狭窄、瘘管或炎症情况，进一步完善结肠镜检查并活检可直接观察肠黏膜病变。

显微镜下结肠炎以慢性水样腹泻为特征，任何年龄人群均可发病，但多见于 60 岁以上的女性。典型症状包括水样便 > 10 次 / 天，可伴有腹部痉挛痛，甚至轻度体重减轻。夜间症状很常见。显微镜下结肠炎包括淋巴细胞性结肠炎和胶原性结肠炎两种亚型。尽管病因不明，但其与部分自身免疫病和药物（如质子泵抑制剂和非甾体抗炎药）密切相关。结肠镜检查可见黏膜基本正常，需要左半结肠和右半结肠活检以进行组织学诊断。布地奈德是治疗显微镜下结肠炎的一线药物，但该药费用较高，可将次水杨酸铋或氨基水杨酸盐作为替代治疗。

胆囊切除术后、回肠疾病或接受回肠切除术的患者会出现胆汁酸吸收不良。过量的胆汁酸进入结肠可引起电解质吸收障碍，此时可试用胆酸螯合树脂治疗腹泻。

由于神经内分泌肿瘤较为罕见，应仅在慢性腹泻患者反复检查仍未能明确病因时考虑完善神经内分泌瘤的相关检查。血浆中的胃泌素和血管活性肠肽（VIP）分别有助于诊断佐林格-埃利森综合征或 VIP 瘤。服用质子泵抑制剂等抑酸剂的患者可出现胃泌素水平升高，但在佐林格-埃利森综合征（Zollinger-Ellison 综合征）中，胃泌素水平通常是正常值上限的 10 倍。应进一步完善肝和胰腺 CT、MRI 或超声内镜，以明确肿瘤病灶。佐林格-埃利森综合征胃镜下可见特

ulcers seen on endoscopy whereas VIPoma can have profound hypokalemia when electrolytes are checked.

Carcinoid syndrome is characterized by secretory diarrhea resulting from the release of excess serotonin from a neuroendocrine tumor. Serotonin syndrome should be suspected in patients with unexplained chronic diarrhea who have symptoms such as flushing of the skin, wheezing, and heart murmurs. Urine should be tested for elevated 5-HIAA.

Chronic Fatty Diarrhea

Chronic fatty diarrhea or steatorrhea can often be described as oily, floating, or sticky stool. Such characteristic stool often implies malabsorption or maldigestion from pancreatic or small bowel mucosal disease. In many cases the cause of fatty diarrhea may be obvious, such as a patient with chronic pancreatitis or severe biliary disease. In other cases, the etiology may not be so obvious and Sudan stain of fecal smear or fecal fat concentration can be obtained. A high concentration of fat in the stool greater than 9.5 g/100 g suggests maldigestion as seen in exocrine pancreatic insufficiency and lack of bile. A low concentration of fecal fat can be seen in mucosal disease that results in the malabsorption of fat and carbohydrates together (see below). CT or MRI of the pancreas, biliary system, and small bowel should be obtained to further assess structural disease and pancreatic disease.

Malabsorption of fat and carbohydrates can result in excess fluid being pulled into the lumen of the gut, therefore diluting the concentration of fecal fat. Such conditions include celiac disease, short bowel syndrome, and small intestine bacterial overgrowth (SIBO). Celiac disease is caused by gluten intolerance and is mainly seen in people of European descent. Presentation can vary from iron deficiency anemia and weight loss to mild abnormalities in liver function tests. Testing for antitissue transglutaminase antibodies with an IgA level can be used to screen for the disease. If suspicions remain high despite negative serologic testing, endoscopy with duodenal biopsies can be performed for definitive diagnosis. The treatment is complete gluten avoidance. SIBO results when the small bowel is colonized by excessive microbes. Patients with motility disorders such as gastroparesis or structural disease such as blind intestinal loops are at risk. SIBO should be considered in such patients who complain of bloating, abdominal pain, and chronic diarrhea. Hydrogen breath testing can be used to confirm the diagnosis. Treatment with a course of antibiotics can be initiated following a positive test.

Maldigestion is seen in patients who have insufficient amounts of bile to break down fats, such as in primary biliary cholangitis or exocrine pancreatic insufficiency due to lack of pancreatic enzymes. In such cases, measuring stool chymotrypsin and stool elastase can be performed to confirm suspicions of this disorder. In other cases, imaging with MRI, CT or endoscopic ultrasound should be obtained to confirm pancreatic disease. Patients who are strongly suspected of having pancreatic insufficiency are best served with a trial of pancreatic enzymes and evaluating their response.

SUGGESTED READINGS

Camilleri M, Sellin JH, Barrett KE: Pathophysiology, evaluation, and management of chronic watery diarrhea, Gastroenterology 152(3):515–532.e2, 2017.

Riddle MS, DuPont HL, Connor BA: ACG clinical guideline: diagnosis, treatment, and prevention of acute diarrheal infections in adults, Am J Gastroenterol 111(5):602–622, 2016.

Schiller LR, Pardi DS, Sellin JH: Chronic diarrhea: diagnosis and management, Clin Gastroenterol Hepatol 15:182–193, 2016.

Shane AL, Mody RK, Crump JA, et al: 2017 Infectious diseases society of america clinical practice guidelines for the diagnosis and management of infectious diarrhea, Clin Infect Dis 65(12):e45–e80, 2017.

Smalley W, Falck-Ytter C, Carrasco-Labra A, et al.: AGA clinical practice guidelines on the laboratory evaluation of functional diarrhea and diarrhea-predominant irritable bowel syndrome in adults (IBS-D), Gastroenterology 157(3):851–854, 2019.

Steffen R, Hill DR, DuPont HL: Traveler's diarrhea: a clinical review, JAMA 313(1):71–80, 2015.

征性的多发性胃溃疡，而 VIP 瘤患者血清电解质检查可提示重度低钾血症。

类癌综合征腹泻的特征是分泌性腹泻，这是由于神经内分泌肿瘤释放过量的 5- 羟色胺。当不明原因的腹泻患者出现皮肤潮红、喘息和心脏杂音等症状时，需要考虑血 5- 羟色胺综合征，应检测尿液 5- 羟基吲哚乙酸（5-HIAA）水平是否升高。

慢性脂肪泻

慢性脂肪泻通常表现为粪便含有油脂、常浮于水面、糊状黏稠，提示胰腺或小肠黏膜病变引起的吸收不良或消化不良。多数情况下，脂肪泻的病因是明确的，如慢性胰腺炎或严重胆道疾病。对于病因不明确的患者，可行粪便涂片苏丹染色或检测粪便脂肪浓度。粪便中脂肪浓度升高（＞9.5 g/100 g）提示存在胰腺外分泌功能不全和胆汁缺乏等引起的消化不良。粪便脂肪浓度较低提示存在黏膜病变引起的脂肪和碳水化合物吸收不良（见下文）。完善胰腺、胆道系统和小肠 CT 或 MRI 检查，有助于进一步评估结构性病变和胰腺疾病。

脂肪和碳水化合物吸收不良会导致过多液体进入肠腔，使粪便中的脂肪浓度因被稀释而降低。这种情况可由乳糜泻、短肠综合征和小肠细菌过度生长（SIBO）等疾病引起。乳糜泻由麸质不耐受引起，多见于欧裔人群，临床表现多样，可从缺铁性贫血、体重减轻到肝功能指标轻度异常。抗组织转谷氨酰胺酶抗体 IgA 水平可用于筛查该病，如果高度怀疑但血清学检测呈阴性，可进行内镜检查并行十二指肠活检以明确诊断。主要的治疗方法是完全避免麸质食物。过多微生物定植于小肠时可引起 SIBO，多见于动力障碍（如胃轻瘫）或结构性疾病（如盲肠袢）的患者。这类患者如果出现腹胀、腹痛和慢性腹泻，则应考虑 SIBO。氢呼气试验有助于 SIBO 的诊断，呼气试验结果呈阳性时，即可使用抗生素治疗。

消化不良见于胆汁分泌不足以分解脂肪（如原发性胆汁性胆管炎）或因缺乏胰酶而导致胰腺外分泌功能不全的患者。检测粪便糜蛋白酶和弹性蛋白酶有助于明确诊断。MRI、CT 或超声内镜检查可确诊胰腺疾病。强烈怀疑胰腺功能不全的患者最好试验性补充胰酶，并评估治疗效果。

推荐阅读

Camilleri M, Sellin JH, Barrett KE: Pathophysiology, evaluation, and management of chronic watery diarrhea, Gastroenterology 152(3):515–532.e2, 2017.

Riddle MS, DuPont HL, Connor BA: ACG clinical guideline: diagnosis, treatment, and prevention of acute diarrheal infections in adults, Am J Gastroenterol 111(5):602–622, 2016.

Schiller LR, Pardi DS, Sellin JH: Chronic diarrhea: diagnosis and management, Clin Gastroenterol Hepatol 15:182–193, 2016.

Shane AL, Mody RK, Crump JA, et al: 2017 Infectious diseases society of america clinical practice guidelines for the diagnosis and management of infectious diarrhea, Clin Infect Dis 65(12):e45–e80, 2017.

Smalley W, Falck-Ytter C, Carrasco-Labra A, et al.: AGA clinical practice guidelines on the laboratory evaluation of functional diarrhea and diarrhea-predominant irritable bowel syndrome in adults (IBS-D), Gastroenterology 157(3):851–854, 2019.

Steffen R, Hill DR, DuPont HL: Traveler's diarrhea: a clinical review, JAMA 313(1):71–80, 2015.

5
Endoscopic and Imaging Procedures

Andrew Canakis, Christopher S. Huang

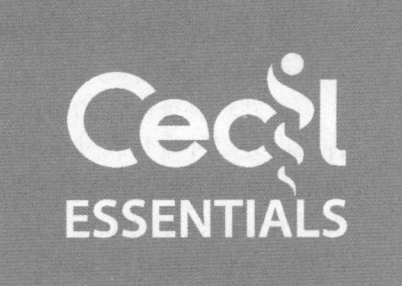

INTRODUCTION

Since Mikulicz first used a prototype esophagoscope to visualize the lumen of the esophagus in 1880, physicians have been attempting to peer into every portion of the gastrointestinal (GI) tract in an attempt to understand disease and to restore their patients to health. This goal has become more achievable than ever, thanks to the wide variety of both invasive and noninvasive endoscopic and imaging procedures that are currently available. This chapter reviews the various endoscopic and radiographic procedures currently in use, including their indications and basic information regarding their performance.

GASTROINTESTINAL ENDOSCOPY

Gastrointestinal endoscopy is the primary modality for directly visualizing the GI tract, as well as obtaining tissue samples to establish definitive diagnoses. Moreover, a wide variety of therapeutic maneuvers can be performed endoscopically to deal with a host of disease processes, such as hemostasis for bleeding ulcers or varices, resection or ablation of neoplastic tissue, dilation or stenting of strictures, and removal of bile duct stones, to name just a few.

Over the years, endoscopes have evolved from early rigid designs with limited capabilities to more sophisticated flexible instruments with advanced imaging capabilities, specialized features for therapeutic maneuvers, and different designs to enable examination of specific areas of the GI tract and biliopancreatic systems. Endoscopes come in varying lengths and diameters ranging from 3.1 mm to 15 mm (Fig. 5.1) and consist of a control handle, insertion tube, and connector section that attaches to the light source and image processing units. The control handle comprises dials that deflect the scope tip in all directions, as well as buttons for suction, air/water insufflation, and image capture. The control handle also includes the entry port to the "working channel" that runs down the length of the insertion tube, through which a wide array of accessories such as biopsy forceps, snares, and balloon dilators can be passed. The tip of the insertion tube houses a charge-coupled device for color image generation, a light guide illumination system, and an objective lens, which may be oriented for forward viewing, side viewing, or oblique viewing, depending on the type of endoscope.

Technologic advances continue to improve the quality of endoscopic imaging, such as the recent introduction of high-definition instruments, magnification endoscopy (from baseline of 30 to 35× to up to 150×), and enhanced imaging technologies such as narrow band imaging (NBI) and multiband imaging.

GI endoscopy can be performed in dedicated endoscopy suites or at a patient's bedside in emergency situations. After positioning the patient appropriately and providing sedation, if necessary, the lubricated endoscope is passed through the intended orifice and advanced manually by the endoscopist. The angulations of the GI lumen are navigated by deflecting the endoscope tip and by applying torque to the instrument shaft (i.e., rotating the shaft along the long axis of the instrument). Endoscopy is generally safe, with complications that include bleeding (0.3% to 1% after colonoscopic polypectomy), perforation (0.05% in general, but 0.1% to 0.5% after polypectomy), and sedation-associated hypotension and hypoxia (1% to 5%). Death related to endoscopic procedures is exceedingly rare (0% to 0.01%).

Esophagogastroduodenoscopy

Esophagogastroduodenoscopy (EGD), often referred to as *upper endoscopy*, is performed with a *gastroscope* and allows the endoscopist to visualize the esophagus, stomach, and duodenum to its third and sometimes fourth portions (Fig. 5.2). Common indications for EGD include evaluation of upper GI symptoms (such as dyspepsia, heartburn, nausea, vomiting, dysphagia and odynophagia), screening for and surveillance of Barrett esophagus, screening for gastroesophageal varices, suspected upper GI bleeding (acute or chronic), and investigation of malabsorptive diarrhea (e.g., celiac sprue or protein-losing enteropathy). A partial list of the therapeutic interventions that can be performed during EGD include the treatment of esophageal varices; dilation of esophageal strictures, rings, and webs; removal or ablation of neoplastic tissue; hemostasis therapy for upper GI bleeding; and the placement of palliative stents for malignant obstruction of the esophagus, pylorus, or duodenum.

Enteroscopy

Examination of the small intestine beyond the ligament of Treitz is not feasible with a standard gastroscope. More recently, greater strides have been made to gain direct visualization of the 6 m or so of the small intestine. *Push* enteroscopy using a long (>200 cm) endoscope allows the endoscopist to both image and biopsy or cauterize lesions in the small intestine, but due to looping of the endoscope and tortuosity of the small intestine, advancing this instrument beyond the first 50 cm of jejunum can be difficult. Balloon-assisted enteroscopy is a newer technique that provides endoscopic access to most of the small bowel. Double balloon enteroscopy (DBE) was initially introduced in 2001 and has emerged as the primary modality for extensive examination of the small bowel. This method employs balloons, incorporated into overtubes or the endoscope itself, to permit pleating of the small bowel onto the endoscope. By inflating and deflating the balloons in sequence, the enteroscope can be advanced through extremely long stretches of small intestine. Combining an anterograde (through the mouth) and retrograde (through the anus) approach may potentially allow for complete examination of the entire small intestine. However, its use is limited to high volume tertiary centers due to its technical difficulties and long procedure times. As a result, single balloon

内镜与影像学检查

冯云路 译　郭涛　谭蓓 审校　杨爱明 通审

引言

自1880年Mikulicz首次使用食管镜原型观察到食管管腔后，医生们一直在尝试窥视消化道的每个部分，从而理解疾病，使患者重获健康。如今，得益于各种侵入性内镜检查和非侵入性影像学检查的广泛应用，距离实现理想已经越来越接近。本章综述了目前应用的各种内镜和影像学检查的适应证及其性能的基本信息。

胃肠镜

胃肠镜检查是直接观察胃肠道的主要方法，同时可获取组织样本以明确诊断。此外，内镜下还可进行各种操作来治疗多种疾病，如溃疡或静脉曲张出血的止血治疗、切除或消融肿瘤组织、在狭窄部位进行扩张或置入支架，以及取出胆管结石等。

多年来，内镜已经从早期功能有限的硬镜演变为更复杂的软镜，具有先进的成像功能、实现治疗性操作的特殊功能，以及能够检查胃肠道和胆胰系统特殊部位的不同设计。内镜的长度和直径从3.1 mm到15 mm不等（图5.1），由控制手柄、插入部和连接部分（连接到光源和图像处理器）组成。控制手柄包括可使内镜前端在各个方向上弯曲的旋钮，以及用于吸引、注气/注水和捕捉图像的按钮，还包括"工作通道"的入口，该通道沿插入部的长轴延伸，通过该通道可送入各种配件，如活检钳、圈套器和扩张气囊。插入部的前端装有生成彩色图像的电荷耦合器件、光导照明系统和物镜。根据内镜类型，物镜的方向可以是前视、侧视或斜视。

技术进步使内镜成像的质量不断提升，如高分辨率内镜、放大内镜（从基础的30～35倍放大提升至150倍放大）、增强成像技术［如窄带成像（NBI）］和多波段成像。

胃肠镜通常在专门的内镜检查室进行，紧急情况下也可在患者床旁进行。在患者摆好体位和镇静（必要时）后，内镜医生将润滑过的内镜穿过目标开口并手动推进。通过弯曲内镜前端并对镜身施加扭力（如沿镜身的长轴旋转内镜）来调整胃肠道管腔的走向。内镜检查通常是安全的，但也有一些并发症，包括出血（结肠镜下息肉切除后的发生率为0.3%～1%）、穿孔（通常为0.05%，息肉切除后的发生率为0.1%～0.5%），以及镇静相关的低血压和低氧（1%～5%）。内镜检查相关死亡极为罕见（0%～0.01%）。

食管胃十二指肠镜

食管胃十二指肠镜（EGD）通常被称为上消化道内镜，使用胃镜进行，内镜医生可观察到食管、胃和十二指肠的前三段，有时包括第四段（图5.2）。常见的EGD适应证包括评估上消化道症状（如消化不良、烧心、恶心、呕吐、吞咽困难和吞咽疼痛），筛查和监测巴雷特食管（Barrett食管），筛查胃食管静脉曲张，疑诊（急性或慢性）上消化道出血，寻找吸收不良性腹泻的病因（如乳糜泻或蛋白丢失性肠病）。EGD下可开展部分治疗性干预，包括食管静脉曲张治疗、扩张食管狭窄/食管环/食管蹼、切除或消融肿瘤组织、上消化道出血的止血治疗，以及置入姑息性支架以解除食管、幽门或十二指肠的恶性梗阻。

小肠镜

使用标准胃镜无法检查十二指肠悬韧带（屈氏韧带）以远的小肠。目前，人们已经能够通过内镜对长达6 m的小肠进行直接观察。使用长内镜（>200 cm）进行推进式小肠镜使得内镜医生可以观察、活检或烧灼小肠病变，但由于内镜成祥和小肠成角，进镜至空肠50 cm以远的区域很困难。气囊辅助小肠镜检查可使内镜到达小肠的大部分区域。双气囊小肠镜（DBE）自2001年应用以来，已成为广泛检查小肠的主要方式。该方法利用装在外套管上或内镜本身的气囊，将气囊依次充气和放气，使小肠套在内镜上，从而让内镜可以深入到更长的肠段。结合顺行（经口）和逆行（经肛）进镜可对整个小肠进行全面检查。然而，由于技术难度大、操作时间长，该技术仅限于较大的医学中心使用。因此，单气囊小肠镜（SBE）于2007年被

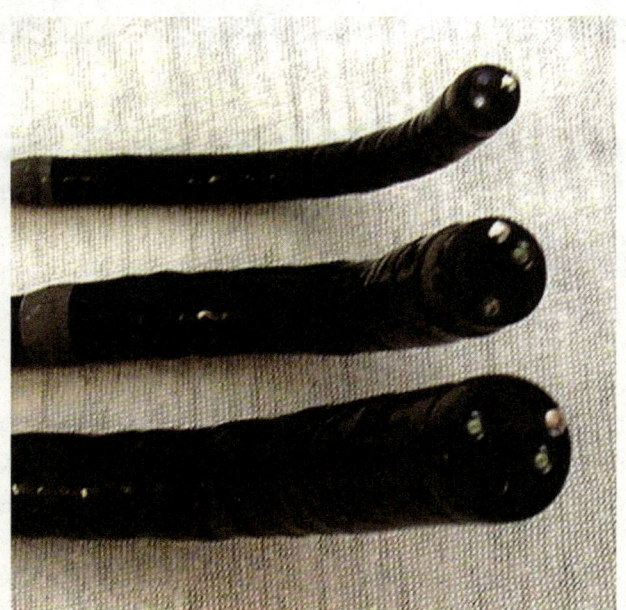

Fig. 5.1 Endoscopes used for upper GI endoscopy. Endoscopes of varying sizes are available for use in different situations. The uppermost endoscope (6-mm diameter) can be used for unsedated endoscopy. The middle endoscope (9-mm diameter) is used for standard diagnostic endoscopy. The lowermost endoscope (12-mm diameter) is used for therapeutic endoscopy, such as the placement of enteral stents. (Courtesy of Brian C. Jacobson.)

enteroscopy (SBE) was developed in 2007 as a means to shorten procedure times, though the chances of total enteroscopy are limited by its single balloon design. A meta-analysis comparing DBE and SBE found that both modalities had similar diagnostic/therapeutic yields, adverse events, and failure rates.

Spiral enteroscopy represents a different technique that utilizes rotational energy of a spiral overtube device that retracts the small bowel over the scope, allowing for deep enteroscopy. Recently, the novel use of a motorized spiral endoscope was developed as a means to improve scope maneuverability, decrease procedure times, and limit the cumbersome nature of balloon enteroscopy (which often requires two operators). Through the use of a foot-switch-operator motor, an overtube equipped with spiral-shaped fins can smoothly advance through the small bowel. Additionally, the system is equipped with high-definition imaging and a 3.2-mm channel that may offer versatile diagnostic and therapeutic modalities in the near future.

Intraoperative enteroscopy is the final means for obtaining visualization of the entire small bowel, although this is obviously the most invasive approach and is now uncommonly performed given the development of device-assisted enteroscopy procedures. In this procedure, a surgeon will make an incision in the patient's abdomen and then pleat the small bowel onto the enteroscope while the endoscopist visualizes the lumen. Once a lesion is identified, the surgeon may elect to proceed directly to a resection of the affected segment of small intestine if the lesion is not amenable to endoscopic treatment.

Video Capsule Endoscopy

The desire to obtain visualization of the GI lumen in the least invasive way has resulted in the development of video capsule endoscopy, the use of pill-sized wireless cameras that the patient swallows. Currently, capsule endoscopes are available for the evaluation of the esophagus, small intestine, and the colon. Capsule endoscopes are swallowed or deployed endoscopically and transmit images wirelessly to a data recorder as they travel through a patient's GI tract, without the need for sedation. At the end of the study, the data recorder allows for stored images to be uploaded into a computer for viewing while the capsule is ultimately passed in the patient's stool. The esophageal capsule is helpful in patients being screened for esophageal varices or individuals with suspected complications of acid reflux, such as reflux esophagitis or Barrett esophagus. The small bowel capsule has become the gold standard for visualizing the small intestine, most commonly for the purpose of investigating obscure GI bleeding and suspected inflammatory bowel disease. Colon capsule endoscopy (CCE) is typically used in patients with a prior colonoscopy failure or suspected lower GI bleeding and may even offer a role in monitoring disease activity in inflammatory bowel disease (IBD) patients. Recent technologic advancements in second-generation CCE now offers clinicians with high-resolution, nearly 360-degree views of the colon with adaptive frame rates that improve battery life and visualization during rapid motions. Additionally, its adjunctive software can estimate polyp size and provide flexible spectral imaging color enhancement to further differentiate neoplastic versus non-neoplastic lesions. Although rare, the main potential complication of capsule endoscopy is retention within the small bowel, usually at a site of pathology.

Sigmoidoscopy and Colonoscopy

Flexible sigmoidoscopy allows visualization of the rectum, sigmoid colon, and descending colon to the level of the splenic flexure. Enemas are given before the procedure to clear stool from the distal colon. Because sigmoidoscopy is generally a brief procedure and not particularly painful, sedation is typically not necessary, making it a convenient tool for colorectal cancer screening. Sigmoidoscopy may also be useful for evaluating symptoms such as chronic diarrhea and rectal bleeding suspected to be arising from the distal colon or rectum, as well as assessing response to therapy in patients with inflammatory bowel disease involving the rectosigmoid colon.

Colonoscopy allows direct visualization of the entire large bowel and the terminal ileum. Bowel cleansing for colonoscopy requires the ingestion of osmotically active solutions, such as polyethylene glycol, coupled with a clear liquid diet for 24 hours before the procedure. Colonoscopy can be more uncomfortable for the patient than sigmoidoscopy due to stretching and distension of the colon, so sedation and analgesia are typically provided. Colonoscopy has become widely performed as a first-line colorectal cancer screening test because of its ability to not only detect early cancers but also *prevent* colon cancer (through the removal of premalignant polyps). Other indications for colonoscopy include evaluation of chronic diarrhea, iron deficiency anemia, overt and occult GI blood loss, and assessing inflammatory bowel disease, including surveillance for dysplasia. Therapeutic interventions possible during colonoscopy include polypectomy, endoscopic mucosal resection of neoplastic lesions, thermal ablation of vascular ectasias, decompression of colonic dilation associated with pseudo-obstruction, stenting of malignant obstruction, and control of lower GI bleeding.

Endoscopic Retrograde Cholangiopancreatography

Endoscopic retrograde cholangiopancreatography (ERCP) is a combined endoscopic and radiographic procedure for imaging and intervening within the biliary and pancreatic ducts. A *duodenoscope* is a specially designed instrument for use during ERCP that includes an imaging lens oriented on the side of the endoscope's tip (as opposed to the front), allowing a direct view of the ampulla of Vater on the medial wall of the second

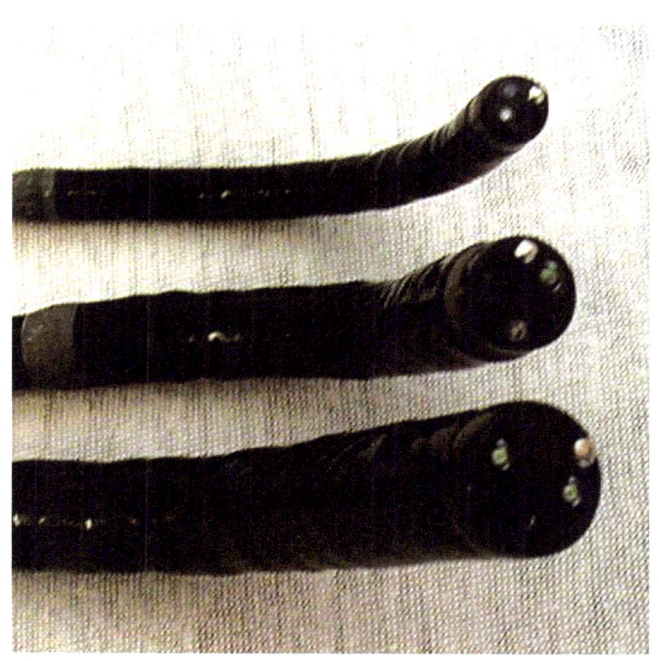

图 5.1　用于上消化道检查的内镜。根据不同情况使用不同尺寸的内镜。最上方的内镜（直径 6 mm）可用于非镇静状态下的内镜检查。中间的内镜（直径 9 mm）用于常规诊断的内镜检查。最下方的内镜（直径 12 mm）用于治疗性内镜操作，如置入肠道支架（授权自 Brian C. Jacobson.）

研发出来，尽管单气囊设计降低了全小肠检查率，但可以明显缩短操作时间。一项比较 DBE 和 SBE 的荟萃分析显示，两种方法的诊断/治疗获益、不良事件发生率和失败率相近。

螺旋式小肠镜代表了另一种技术，其利用旋转螺旋套管产生的作用力，将小肠套在内镜上，从而进入小肠深部。近期已开发出了一种新型动力螺旋式小肠镜，以提高内镜的可操作性、缩短操作时间，并降低了气囊小肠镜检查（通常需要两名操作者）的繁琐程度。通过脚踏开关操作电机，配备螺旋形鳍片的套管可以平稳地进入小肠。此外，该设备还配备了高清成像系统和 3.2 mm 钳道，未来可提供多种诊断和治疗功能。

术中小肠镜是对全小肠进行检查的终极手段，但这种方法显然最具侵入性。由于设备辅助小肠镜技术的发展，术中小肠镜目前在临床并不常用。在这种操作中，外科医生会在患者腹部做一个切口，然后将小肠套在肠镜上，同时由内镜医生观察肠腔。一旦发现病变，如果病变不适合内镜治疗，外科医生可以选择直接切除病变肠段。

胶囊内镜

为了尽可能以侵入性最小的方式获得胃肠道腔内图像，胶囊内镜应运而生，即患者吞下胶囊大小的无线摄像头进行检查。目前，胶囊内镜可用于评估食管、小肠和结肠。胶囊内镜被吞下或被内镜送入体内后，能将患者的胃肠道图像传输到数据记录器，且患者无须镇静。在检查结束时，数据记录器将存储的图像上传至计算机以供查看，而胶囊最终随患者的粪便排出体外。食管胶囊有助于筛查食管静脉曲张或疑诊胃酸反流并发症（如反流性食管炎或巴雷特食管）的患者。小肠胶囊已成为观察小肠的金标准，最常用于诊断不明原因的消化道出血和疑诊炎症性肠病（IBD）的患者。结肠胶囊内镜（CCE）通常用于既往结肠镜检查失败或疑诊下消化道出血的患者，甚至可以在监测 IBD 患者的疾病活动度方面发挥作用。第二代 CCE 的新技术进步，为临床医生提供了高分辨率、接近 360° 的结肠视图，且具有自适应帧率这一特性，可在快速运动中延长电池寿命和改善图像质量。此外，其辅助软件可以估算息肉大小，并提供灵活的光谱成像和颜色增强效果，以进一步区分肿瘤性和非肿瘤性病变。尽管较为罕见，胶囊内镜的主要并发症是胶囊滞留在小肠内，且通常滞留在病变部位。

乙状结肠镜和结肠镜

乙状结肠软镜可用于观察直肠、乙状结肠，直至降结肠脾曲。在操作前，需要进行灌肠以清除远端结肠中的粪便。由于乙状结肠镜检查时间通常较短，且不会引起强烈疼痛，患者通常无须镇静，这使其成为结直肠癌筛查的便捷工具。乙状结肠镜还可用于评估症状，如疑似来自远端结肠或直肠的慢性腹泻和出血，以及评估累及直肠乙状结肠的 IBD 患者的治疗反应。

结肠镜可直接观察整个大肠和末段回肠。结肠镜需要在检查前 24 h 清洁肠道，服用渗透性溶液（如聚乙二醇）并严格清流质饮食。由于对结肠的拉伸和扩张，结肠镜检查对患者来说可能比乙状结肠镜更不舒服，因此通常需要对患者进行镇静和镇痛。结肠镜能够筛查早期结肠癌并（通过去除癌前病变息肉）预防结肠癌，因此被广泛用于结直肠癌的一线筛查。结肠镜的其他适应证包括寻找慢性腹泻、缺铁性贫血、显性或隐性消化道出血的原因，以及评估 IBD 的活动度（包括对黏膜异型增生的监测）。结肠镜检查中可能进行的治疗性干预包括息肉切除、内镜下黏膜切除术（肿瘤性病变）、热消融（毛细血管扩张症）、结肠扩张的减压（假性肠梗阻）、支架置入（恶性肠梗阻）和止血（下消化道出血）。

内镜逆行胰胆管造影

内镜逆行胰胆管造影（ERCP）是一种结合内镜和放射影像技术的操作，用于对胆胰管病变的显影和治疗。十二指肠镜是专门设计用于 ERCP 的设备，其成像镜头位于内镜前端的侧面（而不是正面），可以直

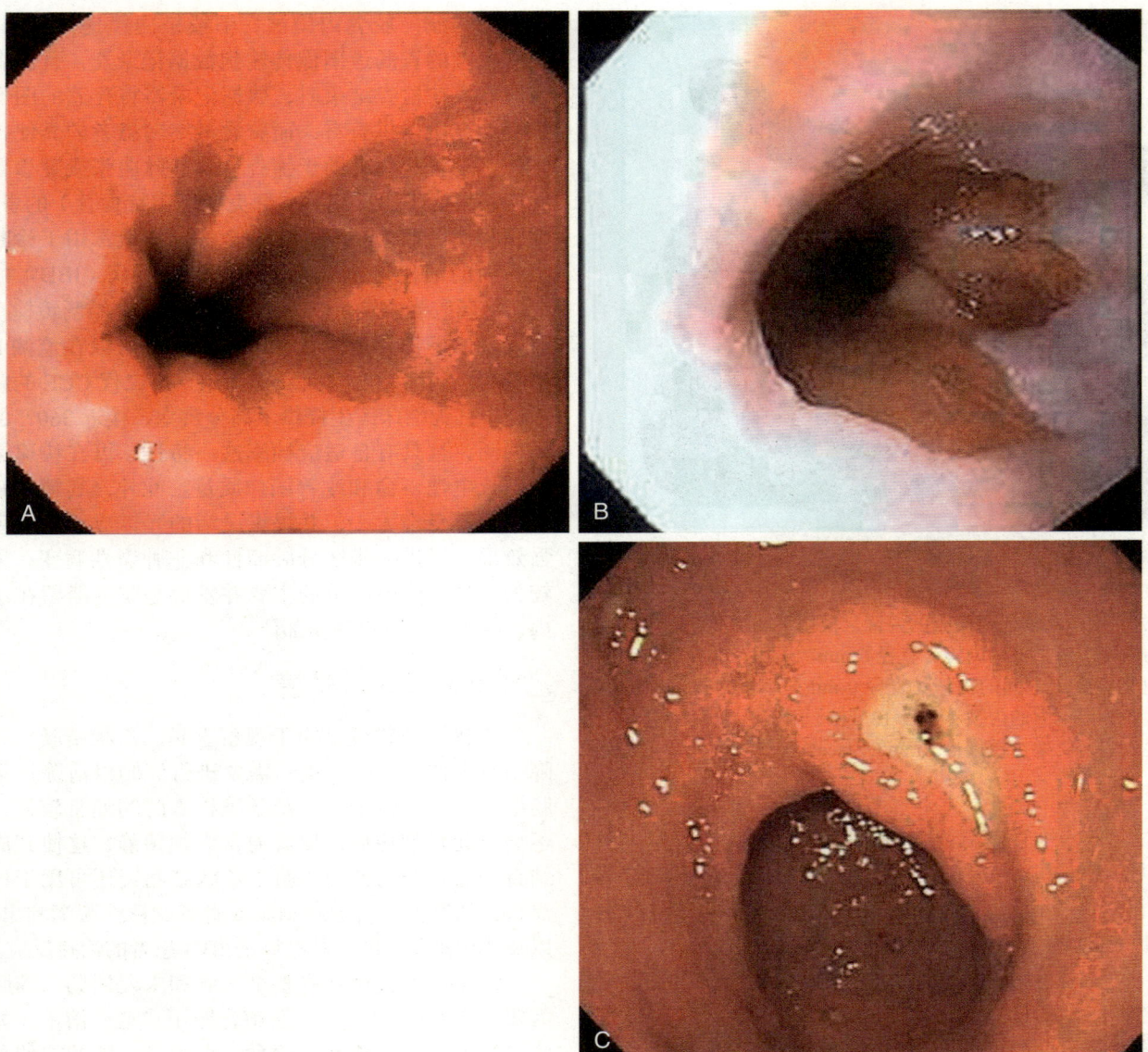

Fig. 5.2 (A) Endoscopic view of the distal esophagus. The distal esophagus contains an abrupt transition between its squamous-lined mucosa and the columnar-lined mucosa of the stomach. (B) Endoscopic view of Barrett esophagus, in which the squamous epithelium of the distal esophagus is replaced by columnar-lined epithelium. Evident in this view is a tongue of columnar-lined mucosa extending proximally into the esophagus. (C) Endoscopic view of a gastric ulcer. A yellow-based ulceration with a pigmented spot is visualized on the gastric wall at the transition between the corpus and the antrum. (Courtesy of M. Michael Wolfe.)

portion of the duodenum. An adjustable instrument *elevator* located at the tip of the duodenoscope helps the endoscopist guide a catheter and other accessories into the duct of interest. Contrast is then injected through the catheter, filling the duct, and fluoroscopic images are obtained (Fig. 5.3). Indications for ERCP include evaluation and treatment of bile duct obstruction due to benign or malignant causes (e.g., bile duct stones, strictures, and bile duct or pancreatic malignancies), cholangitis, postoperative or traumatic bile leaks and pancreatic duct leaks, and transpapillary drainage of pseudocysts. Therapeutic interventions possible during ERCP include sphincterotomy (an incision through the sphincter of Oddi using a catheter with an electrocautery cutting wire), removal of bile duct stones, and placement of biliary or pancreatic duct stents to alleviate signs and symptoms of obstruction or to promote healing of duct leaks. ERCP carries a significant (5%) risk for complications, including pancreatitis, postsphincterotomy bleeding, and perforation. Therefore, ERCP should only be performed when therapeutic benefits are anticipated.

Choledochoscopy and *pancreatoscopy* are techniques in which an endoscope 3 mm or less in diameter is passed through the accessory channel of a duodenoscope and into the bile or pancreatic ducts. The use of this small endoscope permits direct visualization of ductal abnormalities, guides electrohydraulic lithotripsy of large stones, and allows for direct sampling of ductal lesions.

Endoscopic Ultrasound

Endoscopic ultrasound (EUS) or endosonography is performed with an endoscope containing an ultrasound transducer in its tip. Because

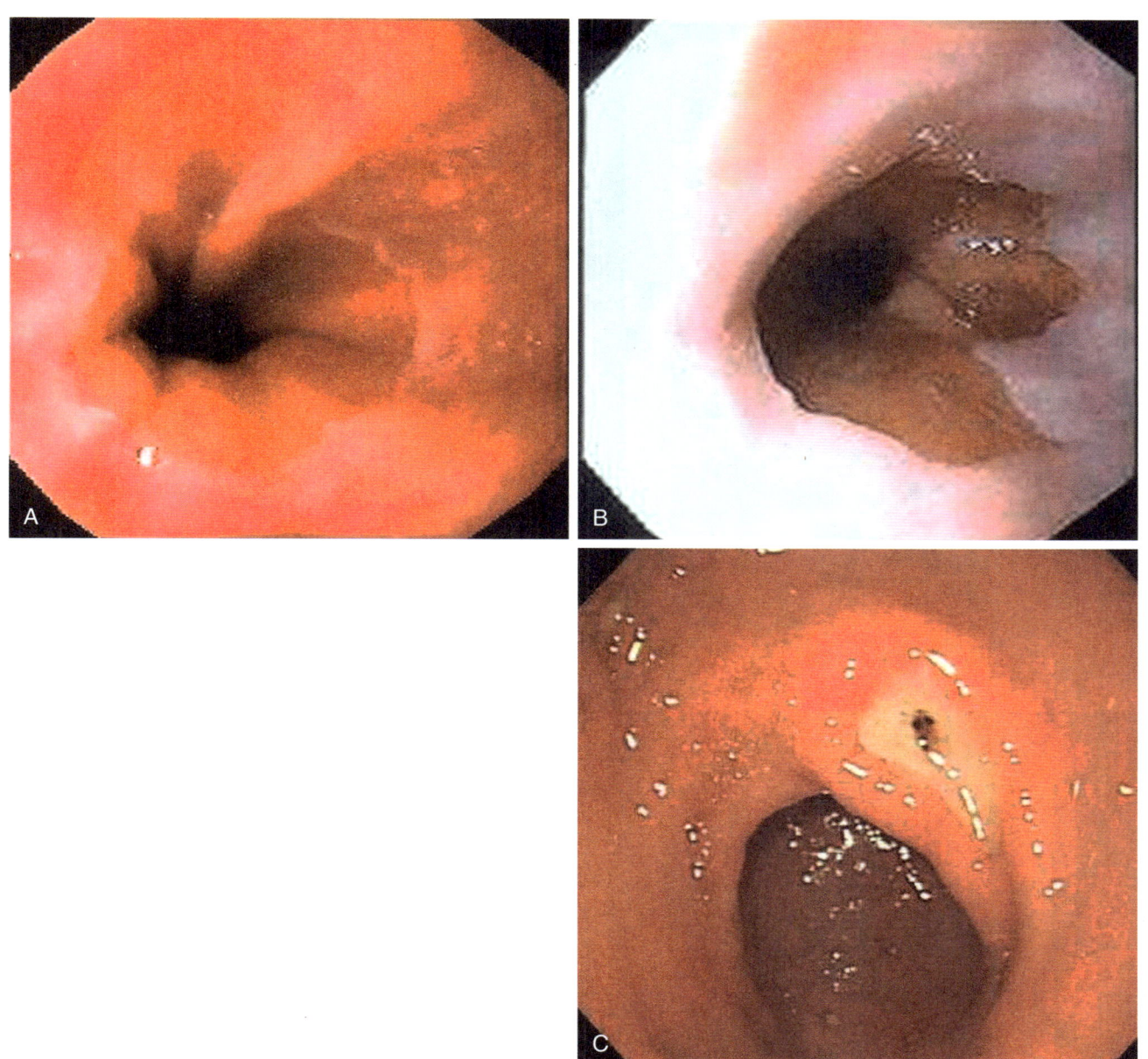

图 5.2　A. 远端食管的内镜图像。远端食管包含鳞状上皮与柱状上皮的分界。B. 巴雷特食管的内镜图像，其中远端食管的鳞状上皮被柱状上皮取代。图中可明显观察到一条柱状上皮黏膜延伸至食管近端。C. 胃溃疡的内镜图像。在胃体和胃窦交界处可见胃壁上一枚带有咖啡斑的黄色基底溃疡（授权自 M. Michael Wolfe.）

接观察到十二指肠降部内侧壁上的肝胰壶腹（Vater 壶腹）。十二指肠镜前端的可变角度的抬钳器可协助内镜医生将导管和其他配件插入目标管腔。然后经导管注入造影剂，造影剂充满管腔并在 X 线透视下成像（图 5.3）。ERCP 的适应证包括诊断和治疗由良性或恶性病因导致的胆管梗阻（如胆管结石、狭窄，以及胆管或胰腺恶性肿瘤），胆管炎，术后或外伤性胆漏和胰漏，以及经乳头的假性囊肿引流。ERCP 中可进行的治疗包括括约肌切开术［使用带有电切功能的导管切开奥迪括约肌（Oddi 括约肌）］、胆管结石取石，以及置入胆管或胰管支架以缓解梗阻症状或促进瘘口愈合。ERCP 具有明显的并发症风险（约 5%），包括胰腺炎、括约肌切开后出血和穿孔。因此，ERCP 应仅在预期有治疗获益时进行。

胆道镜和胰管镜是指将直径 ≤ 3 mm 的内镜通过十二指肠镜钳道插入胆管或胰管。这种小型内镜可以对管腔内病变进行直接观察，辅助巨大结石的液电碎石，还可在直视下对腔内病变进行活检。

超声内镜

超声内镜（EUS）是在内镜前端整合超声换能器的特殊设备。由于该换能器可以进入胃肠道腔内，

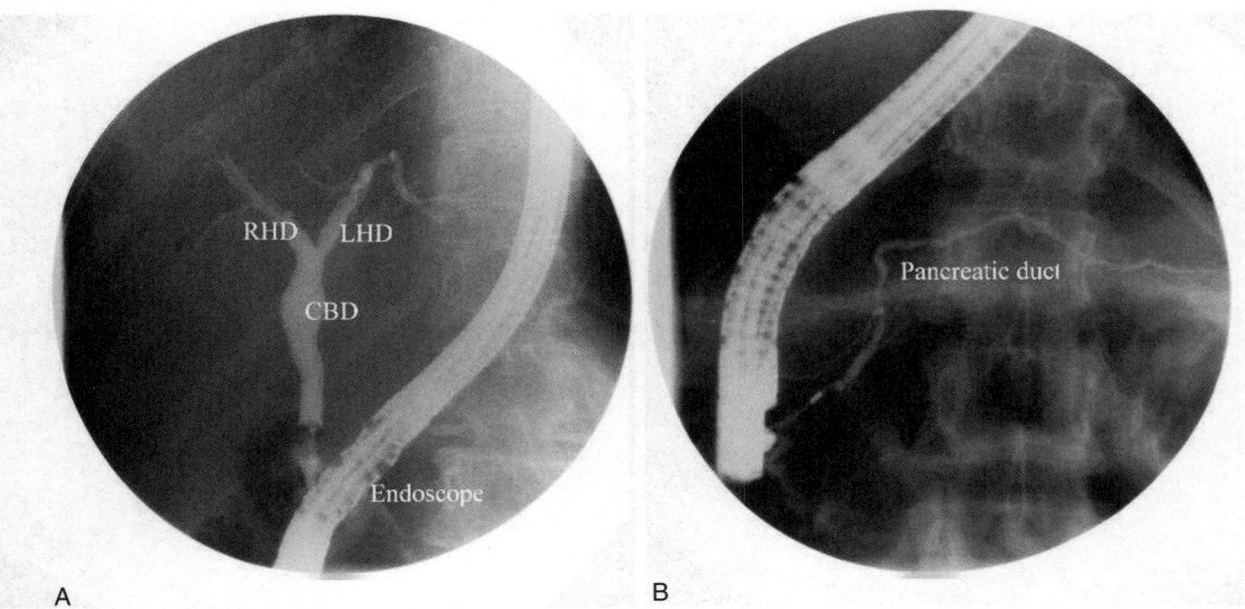

Fig. 5.3 Endoscopic retrograde cholangiopancreatography (ERCP). (A) Normal cholangiogram. Contrast injected into the biliary tree during ERCP demonstrates the intraductal anatomy of the common bile duct *(CBD)*, right hepatic duct *(RHD)*, left hepatic duct *(LHD)*, and smaller intrahepatic biliary radicals. (B) Normal pancreatogram. Contrast injected into the pancreatic duct during ERCP defines the intraductal anatomy throughout the length of the pancreas. (Courtesy of Brian C. Jacobson.)

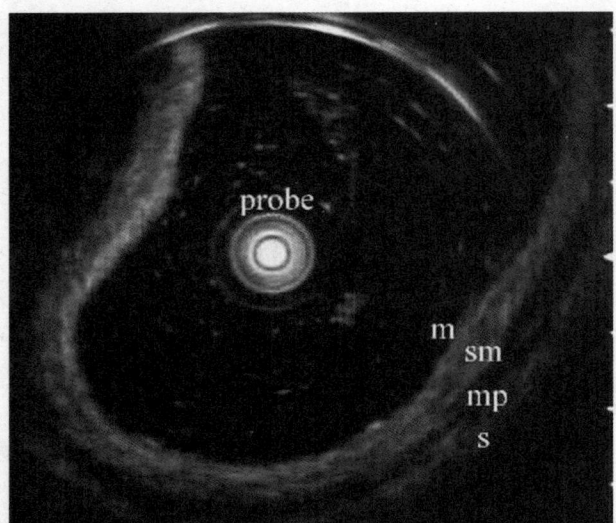

Fig. 5.4 Endoscopic ultrasound of the gastrointestinal wall. A 12-MHz ultrasound probe, passed through the accessory channel of an endoscope, demonstrates the normal layers of the rectal wall. The mucosa *(m)* appears as a superficial, hyperechoic *(white)* band and a deeper hypoechoic *(black)* band. The submucosa *(sm)* appears as the next hyperechoic layer. The muscularis propria *(mp)* appears hypoechoic, and the serosa *(s)* appears as the outermost, hyperechoic layer. (Courtesy of Brian C. Jacobson.)

this transducer can be placed within the GI lumen, high-resolution images of the bowel wall can be obtained, revealing distinct layers that correspond to the mucosa, submucosa, muscularis propria, and serosa (Fig. 5.4). This technique allows the endoscopist to stage tumor depths and determine the layer of origin of subepithelial masses. In addition, EUS can image beyond the gastrointestinal tract wall, providing sonographic images of adjacent structures within the mediastinum and upper abdomen, including the pancreas, liver, gallbladder, mesenteric vessels, lymph nodes, and adrenal glands. High-frequency EUS catheter probes can be passed through the accessory channel of a duodenoscope and into the biliary and pancreatic ducts to provide sonographic images of small tumors and stones. They can likewise be used through a standard endoscope to evaluate diminutive subepithelial lesions and stage obstructing esophageal cancers. Fine-needle aspiration (FNA) as well as core biopsy can be performed under EUS guidance and is the preferred approach to obtaining a tissue diagnosis in many circumstances (e.g., pancreatic masses or cysts, subepithelial lesions of the GI tract, and intra-abdominal or paraesophageal lymphadenopathy). Technologic advancements such as elastography and contrast-enhanced harmonic EUS have further enhanced the diagnostic capability of EUS, particularly in terms of distinguishing malignancy from benign processes. Furthermore, EUS-guided vascular access provides a unique modality for portal vein sampling and portal pressure measurements. However, EUS is more than just a diagnostic modality, and the spectrum of EUS-guided therapies is rapidly expanding. Therapeutic maneuvers that can be performed via EUS guidance include transluminal drainage of pseudocysts and walled-off pancreatic necrosis, pancreatic cyst ablation, celiac axis neurolysis, fiducial (technical) placement into solid tumors to guide stereotactic radiotherapy, and achieving bile duct access or biliary drainage (when initial attempts at ERCP have failed or surgically altered anatomy precludes standard ERCP.)

"Second Space" and "Third Space" Endoscopy

Recent advancements in endoscopic techniques and equipment have led to the development of so-called "second-space" and "third-space" endoscopy procedures within the peritoneal cavity and intramural/submucosal tissue planes, respectively.

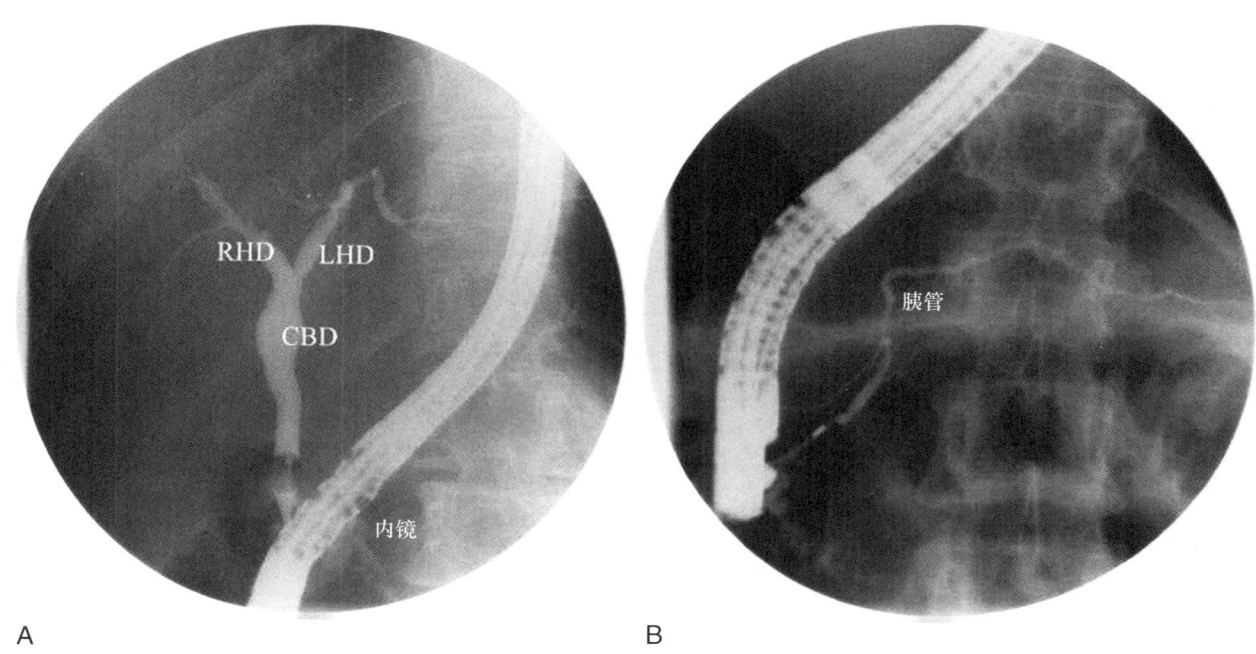

图 5.3　内镜逆行胰胆管造影（ERCP）。**A**. 正常胆管造影图。在 ERCP 期间注入胆管造影剂后显示胆总管（CBD）、右肝管（RHD）、左肝管（LHD）和较小的肝内胆管的腔内解剖。**B**. 正常胰管造影图。在 ERCP 期间注入胰管造影剂后显示胰管全程的解剖（授权自 Brian C. Jacobson.）

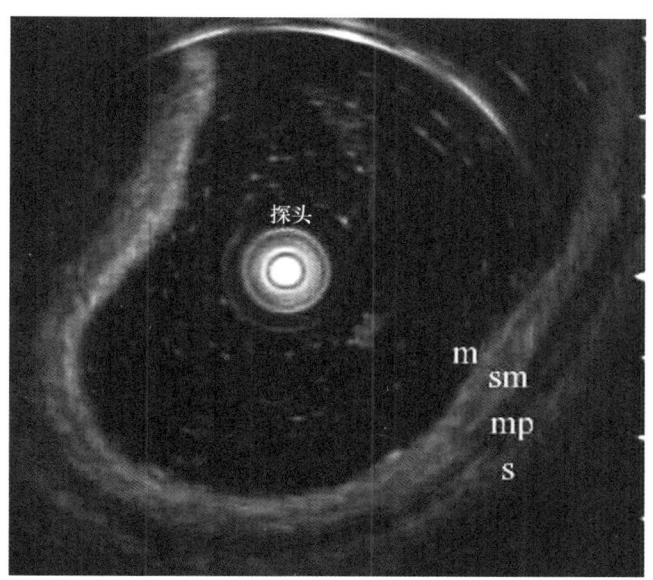

图 5.4　消化道管壁超声内镜检查。通过内镜钳道插入 12 MHz 超声探头显示直肠壁的正常层次结构。黏膜层（m）表现为浅表的强回声带（白色）和较深的低回声带（黑色）。黏膜下层（sm）表现为下一个强回声层。固有肌层（mp）表现为低回声。浆膜层（s）表现为最外层的强回声（授权自 Brian C. Jacobson.）

因此能获得高分辨率的消化道管壁图像，显示与黏膜、黏膜下层、固有肌层和浆膜相对应的不同层次结构（图 5.4）。内镜医生可以借此评估肿瘤深度并确定黏膜下肿物的起源。此外，EUS 可以透过胃肠道管壁，提供纵隔和上腹部邻近结构的超声图像，包括胰腺、肝、胆囊、肠系膜血管、淋巴结和肾上腺。高频 EUS 微探头可通过十二指肠镜钳道进入胆管和胰管，提供较小肿瘤和结石的超声图像。同样，它们也可以配合标准内镜使用，以评估较小的黏膜下病变，或对梗阻型食管癌进行分期。EUS 引导下可进行细针穿刺抽吸（FNA）和组织活检，这是很多情况获得组织学诊断的首选方法（如胰腺肿块或囊肿、胃肠道黏膜下病变、腹腔内或食管旁淋巴结肿大）。超声弹性成像和谐波成像 EUS 等技术进一步增强了 EUS 的诊断能力，特别是在区分恶性肿瘤和良性病变方面。此外，EUS 引导的血管穿刺为门静脉采血和门静脉压力测定提供了一种特殊方式。EUS 不仅是一种诊断工具，EUS 引导的治疗范围也正在迅速扩大。EUS 引导下的治疗性操作包括：假性囊肿和胰腺坏死性包裹的引流、胰腺囊肿消融、腹腔干神经毁损、实体肿瘤内植入粒子辅助立体定向放射治疗，以及在 ERCP 失败或因手术改变解剖结构而无法进行标准 ERCP 时进行胆管引流。

"第二间隙"和"第三间隙"内镜

内镜技术和设备的进展促进了"第二间隙"和"第三间隙"内镜操作的发展，两者分别位于腹腔和消化道壁内 / 黏膜下层组织。

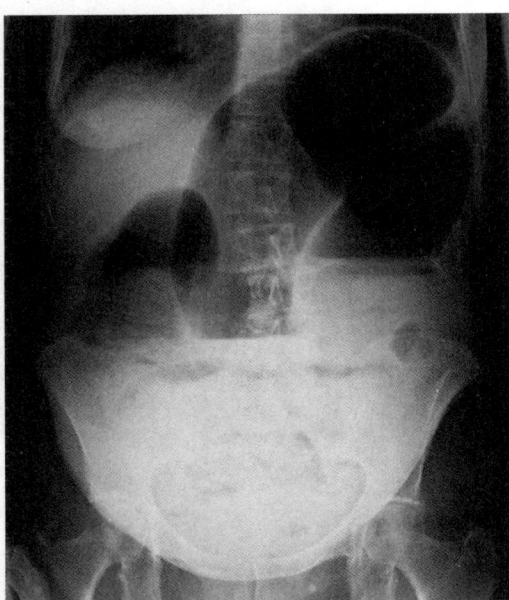

Fig. 5.5 Upright plain radiograph of the abdomen. Air in dilated loops of colon and air-fluid levels can be seen in this patient with a sigmoid volvulus. (Courtesy of Brian C. Jacobson.)

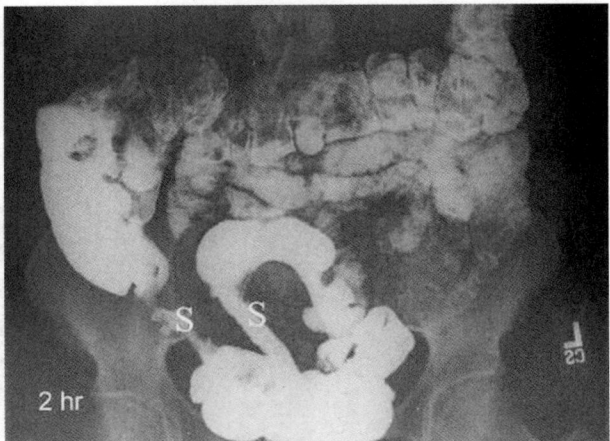

Fig. 5.6 Small bowel follow-through. Ingested barium defines the contours of the small and large bowel lumen. A long stricture (S) of the terminal ileum can be seen in this patient with Crohn's disease. (Courtesy of Brian C. Jacobson.)

Natural orifice transluminal endoscopic surgery (NOTES) is an evolving, minimally invasive field that combines endoscopic and surgical approaches to access the peritoneal cavity. Through the use of an endoscope, a clinician can access a desired target or organ through a transgastric, transcolonic, transvaginal or transurethral approach. Examples of NOTES procedures include cholecystectomy, appendectomy, sleeve gastrectomy, hysterectomy, and hernia repair.

The success and promise of NOTES procedures has led to the development of "third space" endoscopic interventions within the intramural tissue planes of the gastrointestinal tract. Such procedures include full-thickness resection of subepithelial tumors of the GI tract, as well as peroral endoscopic myotomy (POEM) to treat achalasia and esophageal motility disorders. By utilizing submucosal endoscopy, the POEM procedure consists of four steps involving a mucosal incision, submucosal tunneling, subsequent myotomy, and finally mucosal closure through the placement of clips or sutures. POEM has become a very popular modality in treating achalasia, due to its long-term efficacy, lack of abdominal incisions, and rapid recovery.

The same principles and techniques of POEM have been used in the treatment of pyloric dysfunction in patients with gastroparesis in what is known as gastric POEM (G-POEM). Lately, there has been a growing body of evidence proposing that pyloric dysfunction may indeed be a significant contributor to the pathogenesis and symptomatic effects related to gastroparesis. In this context, the need for an alternative, more effective, and minimally invasive therapeutic modality that can target a subset of patients who exhibit pyloric dysfunction has emerged. G-POEM has shown promise, but further long-term and head-to-head studies are needed to see if this modality can emerge as first-line therapy.

NONENDOSCOPIC IMAGING PROCEDURES

Plain Abdominal Radiographs

Plain abdominal radiographs include upright, supine, and lateral decubitus films obtained with standard radiograph equipment and without the use of contrast agents. Plain films are most useful in the initial evaluation of abdominal pain or nausea and vomiting, particularly when perforation or obstruction is suspected, and they may reveal evidence of a pneumoperitoneum, dilated bowel loops and air-fluid levels, excessive amounts of stool, or displacement of bowel loops. These findings are indicative of a perforation, obstruction or ileus, constipation or fecal impaction, and volvulus or organ enlargement, respectively (Fig. 5.5). Calcifications, such as those seen in chronic pancreatitis and gallstone disease, may also be visible on these radiographs.

Contrast Studies

Contrast agents such as barium or the water-soluble diatrizoate (e.g., Gastrografin) can be administered by mouth or rectum to detect mucosal abnormalities (ulcerations and masses), strictures, herniations, diverticula, and abnormal peristalsis. Contrast agents can be used alone *(single contrast)* or with the instillation of air or ingestion of gas-forming agents *(double contrast)*. The former method is more useful for detecting obstructing lesions and motility disturbances, whereas the latter method aids in detecting more subtle findings such as small ulcerations or polyps.

A *video esophagogram* (also known as modified barium swallow) entails the filming of a patient's oral cavity and pharynx during the ingestion of contrast materials of various thicknesses and textures. This imaging modality permits careful assessment of a patient's ability to manipulate a food bolus, swallow effectively, and avoid aspiration events. A video esophagogram is indicated for evaluating patients with oropharyngeal dysphagia and recurrent aspiration pneumonia. A standard *barium esophagogram* (barium swallow) focuses attention on the esophagus during the ingestion of a bolus of contrast. This study can detect esophageal rings, webs, strictures, and motility problems that endoscopy might miss. A barium esophagogram may be useful for evaluating esophageal dysphagia, either as a complementary test to endoscopy, or when endoscopy is contraindicated.

An *upper GI series* includes serial radiographic images as an ingested contrast agent travels through the esophagus, stomach, and duodenum. This study can define gastric abnormalities, such as masses, ulcerations, and mucosal thickening. It is indicated in evaluating abdominal pain and suspected gastric outlet obstruction. If radiographic imaging continues as the contrast agent traverses the jejunum and ileum, the study is called a *small bowel follow-through* (Fig. 5.6). Indications for a small bowel follow-through include suspected small bowel obstruction or partial obstruction from any cause, suspected small bowel mucosal diseases such as Crohn's disease, and obscure GI blood loss (although this has been

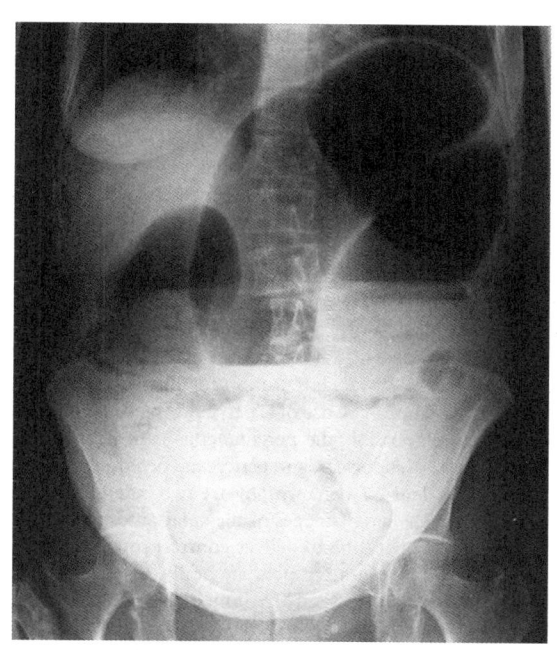

图 5.5　立位腹平片。在这位乙状结肠扭转患者中,可见结肠扩张肠袢中的气体和气液平面(授权自 Brian C. Jacobson.)

经自然腔道内镜手术(NOTES)是一种在微创领域不断发展的技术,其结合了内镜和外科手术进入腹腔的方法。临床医生可以借助内镜,经胃、经结肠、经阴道或经尿道到达目标部位或器官。NOTES 的操作可包括胆囊切除术、阑尾切除术、袖状胃切除术、子宫切除术和疝修补术等。

NOTES 的成功和应用前景推动了胃肠道壁内的"第三间隙"内镜治疗的发展,包括胃肠道黏膜下肿瘤的全层切除术,以及治疗贲门失弛缓症和食管运动功能障碍的经口内镜食管下括约肌切开术(POEM)。POEM 的操作包括 4 个步骤:黏膜切开、黏膜下隧道建立、肌切开术,以及通过夹子或缝合线闭合黏膜开口。由于 POEM 具有长期疗效稳定、无胸腹部切口和恢复快的优点,已成为目前治疗贲门失弛缓症的主流方法。

与 POEM 相同的原理和技术已被用于治疗胃轻瘫患者的幽门功能障碍,被称为胃 POEM(G-POEM)。近年来,越来越多的证据表明,幽门功能障碍确实可能是影响胃轻瘫发病机制和症状的重要因素。在这种情况下,对于幽门功能障碍的患者,需要更有效且微创的替代治疗方法。G-POEM 已显示出良好的应用前景,有望成为此类患者的一线治疗方案,但需要进一步进行长期和头对头研究以明确疗效。

非内镜影像学检查
腹平片

腹平片是应用标准 X 线设备在不使用造影剂的情况下获取,包括立位、仰卧位和侧卧位片。对于初诊腹痛或恶心和呕吐的患者,特别是当怀疑有穿孔或梗阻时,腹平片的诊断价值最大。它可显示腹腔内游离气体、扩张肠袢和气液平、大量粪便、肠袢异常。这些发现分别提示穿孔、梗阻或肠麻痹、便秘或粪便嵌顿,以及肠扭转或器官肿大(图 5.5)。慢性胰腺炎和胆石症中常见的钙化/结石,也可能在 X 线片上显示。

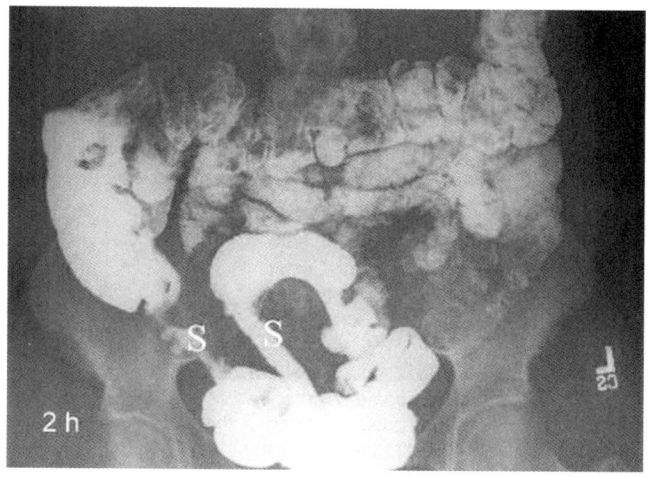

图 5.6　小肠造影。服用的钡剂勾勒出小肠和大肠的肠腔轮廓。这位克罗恩病患者可见末端回肠的长段狭窄(S)(授权自 Brian C. Jacobson.)

造影检查

造影剂[如钡剂或水溶性泛影酸(如泛影葡胺)]可通过口服或直肠灌注给药,用来诊断黏膜病变(溃疡和肿块)、狭窄、疝、憩室和异常蠕动。造影剂可以单独使用(单重对比),也可以联合口服产气剂或直肠注入空气(双重对比)。前者更适用于检测梗阻性病变和运动障碍,而后者有助于发现更微小的病变,如小溃疡或息肉。

动态食管造影(又称改良吞钡造影)是在患者吞咽不同黏稠度和质地的造影剂时,对其口腔和咽喉进行拍摄。这种成像方式可以对患者操控食团、有效吞咽及避免误吸的能力进行仔细评估。动态食管造影适用于评估有口咽吞咽困难和反复吸入性肺炎的患者。标准钡剂食管造影(钡餐)是在患者吞咽造影剂时集中关注食管,从而发现内镜检查可能遗漏的食管环、食管蹼、食管狭窄和运动障碍。用于评估食管吞咽困难时,钡剂食管造影既可作为内镜的补充,也可在有内镜禁忌证时应用。

上消化道造影包括在造影剂通过食管、胃和十二指肠时所呈现的一系列放射影像。它可以判定胃部病变,如占位、溃疡和黏膜增厚。它适用于腹痛的病因诊断和评估疑似胃出口梗阻的患者。如果在造影剂通过空肠和回肠时连续进行放射成像,则被称为小肠造影(图 5.6)。小肠造影的适应证包括不明原因的小肠完全梗阻或不全梗阻、怀疑小肠黏膜病变(如克罗恩病),以及不明原因的消化道出血(尽管目前多被胶囊

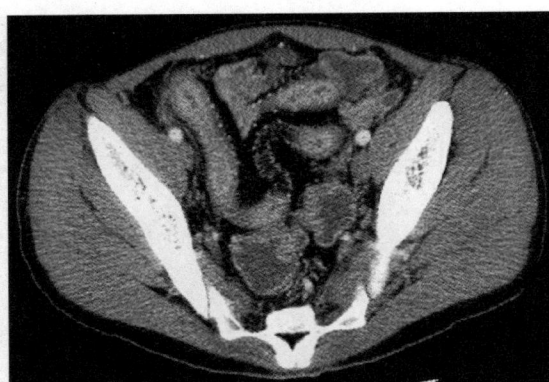

Fig. 5.7 Computed tomography enterography. A long segment of inflamed terminal ileum is demonstrated in this patient with Crohn's disease. (Courtesy of Christopher S. Huang.)

largely replaced by video capsule endoscopy). During this more involved procedure, a radiologist will obtain multiple films, including *spot films*, or close-up views of regions that appear abnormal. Fluoroscopy can be used to follow a contrast agent during the journey through the small bowel. Attention is paid not only to structural findings but also to the length of time required for contrast to reach and enter the colon. For more detailed small bowel images, *enteroclysis* can be performed. This method requires the infusion of concentrated contrast directly into the small bowel through a nasojejunal tube placed under fluoroscopic guidance. Because of its invasive nature, as well as the availability of better small bowel imaging techniques, enteroclysis is now rarely performed.

Single- and double-contrast barium enemas can detect colonic strictures, diverticula, polyps, and colonic ulcerations, and they can be therapeutic in reducing a sigmoid volvulus. Double-contrast barium enema may be used for colorectal cancer screening as a stand-alone test or in conjunction with flexible sigmoidoscopy, or it may be used to visualize the proximal colon when colonoscopy cannot be completed for various reasons. However, it is now infrequently used for these purposes given its relatively poor sensitivity, as well as availability of computed tomography colography ("virtual colonoscopy," discussed later). In general, the upper GI series and barium enema have been superseded by upper endoscopy and colonoscopy because the endoscopic procedures offer increased sensitivity for detecting mucosal abnormalities, the ability to obtain mucosal biopsies, and the potential for resection of identified lesions.

Transabdominal Ultrasound

Ultrasonography is often the first imaging study obtained in the evaluation of suspected biliary colic, jaundice, and abnormal liver tests. Its use of sound waves to create an image obviates the need for radiation exposure, and the addition of Doppler techniques permits the assessment of vascular flow. Ultrasound can detect parenchymal abnormalities, such as fatty liver or cirrhosis, focal masses or cysts, ascites, biliary ductal dilation, gallstones, and large vessel thromboses. It may detect thickening of the gut wall and areas of intussusception. Ultrasound is also used to guide needle placement for biopsies or fluid aspiration. Ultrasound cannot penetrate bone or air, preventing its use as a more general diagnostic tool for the GI tract.

Computed Tomography, Computed Tomography Enterography, and Computed Tomography Colography

Computed tomography (CT) uses computer-aided reconstruction of multiple radiographic images obtained in a circular or helical course around a patient's vertical axis. Internal organs are visualized based on their inherent tissue densities compared with their surroundings. The GI lumen is usually opacified by having the patient drink an oral contrast agent. In addition, intravenous contrast agents can be administered to highlight regions with increased blood flow, thereby improving detection of pathologic lesions, such as tumors and areas of active inflammation. CT can detect parenchymal lesions, such as tumors, cysts, and abscesses, as well as define the size, shape, and characteristics of parenchymal organs, such as the liver and spleen. Vascular abnormalities, such as perigastric varices or large vessel thromboses, and intra-abdominal fluid, such as ascites, can also be seen with CT. The caliber and contour of the GI tract wall are demonstrated by CT, aiding in the diagnosis of inflammatory lesions, such as colitis, diverticulitis, and appendicitis. CT can also be used to guide needle biopsies of abdominal masses and to place electrodes into tumors for ablative therapies such as radiofrequency ablation. The use of CT to guide placement of drainage catheters has made possible the percutaneous treatment of intra-abdominal abscesses, pseudocysts, and pancreatic necrosis.

CT enteroclysis and *CT enterography* are two emerging techniques developed to provide better images of the small intestine. CT enteroclysis uses a nasojejunal tube to deliver contrast into the small intestine, whereas CT enterography uses an orally ingested low-density intraluminal contrast to distend the lumen and highlight the small intestinal mucosa (Fig. 5.7). With the advancement of this technology and its ability to reconstruct images in multiple planes, both luminal and extraluminal information can be obtained.

CT can also be used to obtain high-resolution images of the colon. CT colonography, or *virtual colonoscopy*, makes use of special image reconstruction software to create accurate visualization of the colonic lumen, provided that the patient has completed a bowel-cleansing regimen identical to that used for colonoscopy (although techniques that do not require such preparation are being developed). These CT images are 70% to 90% sensitive for detecting polyps or masses within the colon, helping to determine which patients need therapeutic colonoscopy. CT colonography is considered an acceptable option for colorectal cancer screening in average risk individuals but is primarily used to complete colonic visualization in the setting of an incomplete colonoscopy (due to technical reasons or obstructing pathology).

Magnetic Resonance Imaging and Magnetic Resonance Cholangiopancreatography

Similar to CT, magnetic resonance imaging (MRI) provides multiple cross-sectional images of the abdomen and pelvis. These images are created using powerful field magnets to orient small numbers of nuclei within the body in such a way as to produce a measurable magnetic moment. MRI therefore avoids radiation exposure but requires the patient to lie nearly motionless, and often within a small enclosed tube, for prolonged periods. MRI can visualize parenchymal lesions such as masses and cysts and may better characterize abnormalities seen on CT, such as hemangiomas, hepatic focal nodular hyperplasia, and fatty liver. MRI is also helpful in better characterizing perirectal abscesses and fistulas in Crohn's disease. Special rectal MRI probes or coils can provide detailed images of rectal cancer used for tumor staging, as well as evaluate the anal sphincters in patients with fecal incontinence.

MRI of the biliary and pancreatic ducts (*magnetic resonance cholangiopancreatography*, MRCP) is a noninvasive method that can detect ductal dilation, strictures, stones (Fig. 5.8), pancreatic parenchymal changes in chronic pancreatitis, and congenital ductal abnormalities, such as pancreas divisum. *Magnetic resonance angiography* is a magnetic resonance method for visualizing blood vessels and serves as an important noninvasive tool for evaluating patients with suspected mesenteric ischemia, vasculitis, and other vascular anomalies.

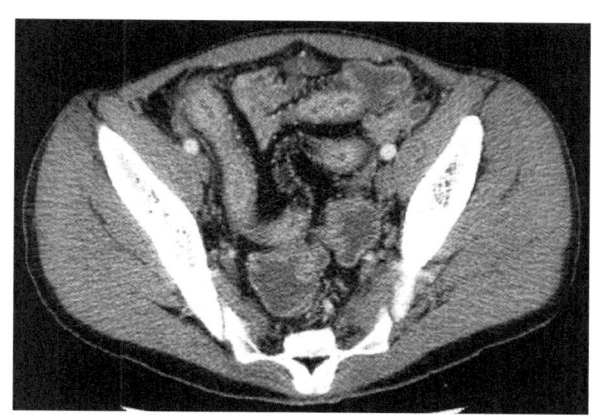

图 5.7 CT 小肠成像。该克罗恩病患者可见末端回肠的长段炎症（授权自 Christopher S. Huang.）

内镜取代）。在这种更复杂的检查中，放射科医生会获得多张胶片，包括局部影像或异常区域的特写。X 线透视可用于造影剂在小肠中的示踪，不仅可发现结构异常，还可显示造影剂到达结肠所需的时间。为了获得更清晰的小肠图像，可进行小肠灌注，即在 X 线透视引导下通过鼻空肠管直接向小肠输注高浓度造影剂。由于小肠灌注具有侵入性，且目前有效果更好的小肠成像技术，因此其应用较少。

单重对比和双重对比钡灌肠可发现结肠狭窄、憩室、息肉和结肠溃疡，在减轻乙状结肠扭转方面也有治疗作用。双重对比钡灌肠可单独应用或与乙状结肠软镜联合用于结直肠癌筛查，也可用于因各种原因无法进行全结肠镜检查时的近端结肠显影。但是，由于敏感性较低，以及 CT 结肠重建（见下文"虚拟结肠镜检查"）的广泛应用，这种方法现在已很少应用。总体而言，上消化道造影和钡灌肠已经被胃镜和结肠镜检查所取代，因为内镜检查对检测黏膜异常具有更高的敏感性，同时能够进行黏膜活检，并有可能切除已发现的病变。

经腹超声

当患者疑似胆绞痛、黄疸和肝功能异常时，超声通常是首选的影像学检查。其利用声波成像，无需辐射暴露，且多普勒技术能够评估血流情况。超声可发现实质病变（如脂肪肝或肝硬化）、局灶性肿块或囊肿、腹腔积液、胆管扩张、胆石症和大血管血栓。经腹超声还可以诊断肠壁增厚和肠套叠。超声还能引导穿刺活检或液体抽吸。但超声波无法穿透骨骼或空气，因此无法被用作更普遍的胃肠道疾病诊断工具。

CT、CT 小肠成像和 CT 结肠成像

CT 通过围绕患者纵轴以环形或螺旋形轨迹扫描而获得多个放射图像，并利用计算机进行重建。基于器官相对于周围环境的固有组织密度而使器官成像，并通过让患者口服造影剂使胃肠腔显影。此外，可通过静脉注射造影剂以强化富血供区域，从而辅助预测病理类型（如肿瘤和活动性炎症）。CT 不仅可发现占位性病变（如肿瘤、囊肿和脓肿），并判定实质器官（如肝和脾）的大小、形状和特征，还可发现胃周静脉曲张或大血管血栓等血管异常，以及观察腹腔内液体（如腹腔积液）。CT 可显示消化道管壁的厚度和轮廓，有助于诊断结肠炎、憩室炎和阑尾炎等炎症性病变。CT 还可引导腹腔占位穿刺和肿瘤内置入电极行消融治疗（如射频消融），也可引导置管经皮引流腹腔脓肿、假性囊肿和胰腺坏死。

CT 小肠灌注成像和 CT 小肠成像是两种新兴技术，均能提供更好的小肠图像。CT 小肠灌注成像是通过鼻空肠管将造影剂输送到小肠，而 CT 小肠成像是通过口服低密度造影剂来充盈肠腔使小肠黏膜清晰显示（图 5.7）。由于这项技术可以重建多平面图像，因此能够同时获得小肠腔内和腔外的信息。

CT 还可用于获得结肠的高分辨率图像。CT 结肠成像（又称虚拟结肠镜检查）利用特殊的图像重建软件精确创建结肠肠腔可视化，但患者需要进行与结肠镜检查类似的肠道准备（尽管正在开发无需肠道准备的相关技术）。CT 结肠成像对于结肠息肉或占位的敏感性为 70%～90%，有助于判断哪些患者需要接受治疗性结肠镜检查。CT 结肠成像可作为筛查工具用于结直肠癌风险不高的个体，临床多用于因技术原因或肠腔阻塞而无法进行全结肠镜检查的患者。

MRI 和磁共振胰胆管成像（MRCP）

与 CT 类似，MRI 可提供腹盆腔多个横断面图像。其成像是通过高能磁场影响体内少量原子核的排列，从而产生可测量的磁矩。MRI 可避免辐射暴露，但要求患者长时间几乎静止不动地躺在一个较小的封闭空间内。MRI 可显示实质性病变（如肿块和囊肿），并能更好地呈现 CT 所观察到的异常，如血管瘤、肝局灶性结节性增生和脂肪肝。MRI 能更清晰地显示克罗恩病的直肠周围脓肿和瘘管。特殊的直肠 MRI 探头或线圈可以对直肠癌进行肿瘤分期，以及评估大便失禁患者的肛门括约肌。

MRCP 是一种非侵入性检查，可检测胰胆管扩张、狭窄、结石（图 5.8）、慢性胰腺炎的胰腺实质性改变，以及胰胆管先天性异常（如胰腺分裂）。磁共振血管成像是一种用于可视化血管的磁共振方法，是评估疑诊肠系膜缺血、血管炎和其他血管异常患者的重要无创性诊断工具。

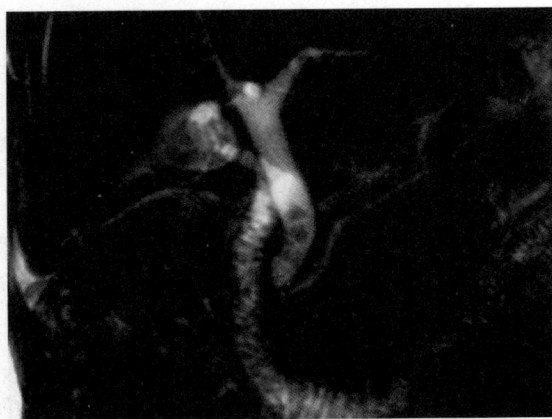

Fig. 5.8 Magnetic resonance cholangiopancreatography. Several stones are visualized within the common bile duct, appearing as hypointense filling defects on T2-weighted images. (Courtesy of Christopher S. Huang.)

Visceral Angiography

Angiography is an invasive technique whereby a catheter is introduced into a blood vessel, and intravascular contrast is injected during fluoroscopic imaging to visualize the vessel's lumen. Visceral angiography is used for evaluating mesenteric vessels in the setting of GI bleeding and suspected mesenteric ischemia. For GI bleeding, angiography is sensitive enough to detect 1 to 1.5 mL per minute of blood loss. Once the site of bleeding has been localized, the radiologist can infuse vasopressin (a vasoconstrictor) or embolize the vessel using tiny coils or gelatin sponges to ensure hemostasis. In the setting of mesenteric ischemia, angiography permits localization of a vascular stenosis or obstruction, followed by possible therapeutic interventions (e.g., balloon angioplasty, stent placement, infusion of vasodilators and thrombolytics). Other indications for angiography include the placement of transjugular intrahepatic portosystemic shunts (TIPS) in cirrhotic patients with intractable variceal bleeding or refractory ascites and for chemoembolization of liver tumors.

Radionuclide Imaging

Technetium-99m (^{99m}Tc) is currently the major radionuclide used in GI imaging. Its 6-hour half-life and ready availability make it ideal for clinical use. ^{99m}Tc is used to label various substances for use in several imaging techniques. ^{99m}Tc-sulfur colloid scanning and ^{99m}Tc-labeled red blood cell scanning are two distinct methods that can be used to detect active GI bleeding. The latter uses the patient's own blood cells to carry the radionuclide throughout the body. These methods can detect as little as 0.05 to 0.4 mL per minute of blood loss. However, localization of the site of bleeding is less accurate with these methods compared with angiography. ^{99m}Tc scans are often performed before angiography to document ongoing bleeding before subjecting a patient to the more invasive, less sensitive study. A ^{99m}Tc-labeled red blood cell scan can also be used to diagnose a hepatic hemangioma with an almost 100% positive predictive value.

Cholescintigraphy using ^{99m}Tc-iminodiacetic acid (IDA) analogs is the most commonly performed liver study in nuclear medicine. The radionuclide is taken up by the liver, is excreted into bile, and passes through the biliary tree into the gallbladder and duodenum. Failure to visualize the gallbladder during a hepatobiliary IDA scan may indicate cholecystitis secondary to cystic duct obstruction by a gallstone. Meckel's diverticulum can be a source of abdominal pain and bleeding, but it can be difficult to visualize with standard endoscopic and radiographic imaging. The agent ^{99m}Tc-pertechnetate has a high affinity for gastric mucosa and is therefore used to demonstrate the presence of this congenital anomaly.

Gastric emptying studies are useful for the evaluation of patients with suspected gastroparesis. Patients are given a ^{99m}Tc-sulfur colloid-labeled standardized meal (consisting of liquid egg whites, toast, jam/jelly, and water) and are imaged at 0, 1, 2, and 4 hours after meal ingestion. Gastric retention of greater than 10% at 4 hours is highly sensitive and specific for delayed gastric emptying.

Radionuclide imaging studies are also useful for the detection, staging, and monitoring of certain neoplasms such as neuroendocrine tumors (NETs). Most well-differentiated NETs express somatostatin receptors and can therefore be detected with radiolabeled somatostatin analogues such as 111-In pentetreotide and 68-Ga DOTATATE.

PROSPECTUS FOR THE FUTURE

Through continued technologic advances, improvements in both endoscopic and radiologic image quality and resolution will also continue. In addition, the gastrointestinal lumen will no longer be regarded as a boundary to therapeutic endoscopy. Examples of expected innovations include the following:
- *The continued expansion of endoscopic procedures beyond the walls of the GI tract*, providing a less invasive approach to treatment of diseases traditionally managed surgically.
- "Second-space" and "third-space" endoscopy techniques are likely to be refined further, and bariatric endoscopy techniques are likely to become more widely performed.
- Further development of computer-aided diagnosis (or "artificial intelligence") for colonoscopy with automated polyp detection and characterization.

SUGGESTED READINGS

ASGE Technology Committee, Aslanian HR, Sethi A, et al.: ASGE guideline for endoscopic full-thickness resection and submucosal tunnel endoscopic resection, *VideoGIE* 4(8):343–350, 2019.

Byrne MF, Jowell PS: Gastrointestinal imaging: Endoscopic ultrasound, *Gastroenterology* 122:1631–1648, 2002.

DiSario JA, Petersen BT, Tierney WM, et al.: Enteroscopes, *Gastrointest Endosc* 66:872–880, 2007.

Fletcher JG, Huprich J, Loftus EV, et al.: Computerized tomography enterography and its role in small-bowel imaging, *Clin Gastroenterol Hepatol* 6:283–289, 2008.

Gore RM, Levine MS: *Textbook of gastrointestinal radiology*, ed 2, Philadelphia, 2000, Saunders.

Mishkin DS, Chuttani R, Croffie J, et al.: ASGE Technology Status Evaluation Report: Wireless capsule endoscopy, *Gastrointest Endosc* 63:539–545, 2006.

Muguruma N, Tanaka K, Teramae S, Takayama T: Colon capsule endoscopy: toward the future, *Clin J Gastroenterol* 10(1):1–6, 2017.

Riff BP, DiMaio CJ: Exploring the small bowel: update on deep enteroscopy, *Curr Gastroenterol Rep* 18(6):28, 2016.

Schneider M, Höllerich J, Beyna T: Device-assisted enteroscopy: A review of available techniques and upcoming new technologies, *World J Gastroenterol* 25(27):3538–3545, 2019.

Shah SL, Perez-Miranda M, Kahaleh M, Tyberg A: Updates in Therapeutic Endoscopic Ultrasonography, *J Clin Gastroenterol* 52(9):765–772, 2018.

Thrall JH, Ziessman HA: *Nuclear Medicine: The Requisites*, ed 2, St. Louis, 2000, Mosby.

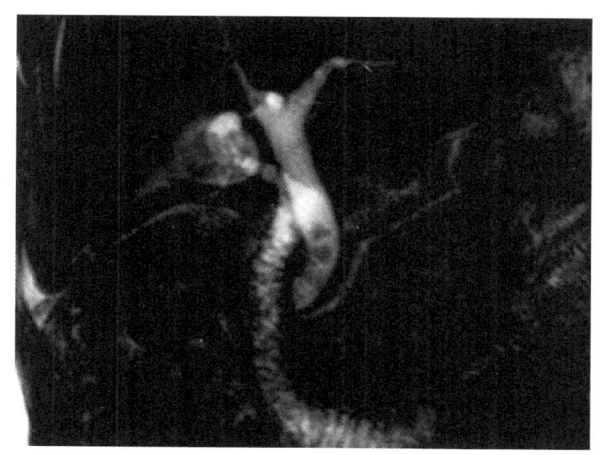

图 5.8　MRCP。T2 加权像中，胆总管结石显示为多发低信号充盈缺损（授权自 Christopher S. Huang.）

腹部血管造影

血管造影是一种侵入性技术，通过将导管插入血管，并在 X 线透视下注射血管内造影剂以观察血管腔。腹部血管造影可用于在消化道出血和疑似肠系膜缺血时评估肠系膜血管。在消化道出血的情况下，血管造影的敏感性足以检测到 1～1.5 ml/min 的失血。一旦确定出血部位，放射科医生可注射血管升压素（血管收缩剂）或使用弹簧圈或明胶海绵进行血管栓塞止血。在肠系膜缺血的情况下，血管造影可定位血管狭窄或阻塞部位，从而酌情进行治疗性干预（如气囊血管成形术、支架置入、输注血管扩张剂和溶栓剂）。血管造影还可用于对肝硬化患者难治性静脉曲张出血或顽固性腹腔积液行经颈静脉肝内门体静脉分流术（TIPS），以及进行肝肿瘤的栓塞化疗。

放射性核素显像

锝-99m（^{99m}Tc）是目前胃肠成像中使用的主要放射性核素，半衰期为 6 h 且易制备使其非常适合临床使用。^{99m}Tc 可标记不同物质，用于多种成像技术。^{99m}Tc-硫胶体扫描和 ^{99m}Tc 标记红细胞扫描均可用于诊断活动性消化道出血，后者借助患者自身的红细胞将放射性核素遍布全身。这些方法可以检测到 0.05～0.4 ml/min 的出血。但与血管造影相比，核素显像在出血部位定位方面不够精确。因此，患者通常在接受更具侵入性和敏感性较低的检查（如血管造影）前进行 ^{99m}Tc 扫描评估，以发现活动性出血。^{99m}Tc 标记红细胞扫描还可用于诊断肝血管瘤，阳性预测值接近 100%。

使用 ^{99m}Tc-亚氨基二乙酸（IDA）类似物进行胆道显像是核医学最常用的肝脏检查。该放射性核素被肝摄取，通过胆汁排出，经过胆道进入胆囊和十二指肠。在肝胆 IDA 扫描中，胆囊不显影提示胆结石阻塞胆囊管继发胆囊炎。梅克尔憩室可能是导致腹痛和出血的原因，但通过常规内镜和放射成像手段难以发现。^{99m}Tc-过锝酸盐对胃黏膜具有高亲和力，可以诊断这种先天性异常。

胃排空试验可用于评估疑诊胃轻瘫的患者。患者接受 ^{99m}Tc-硫胶体标记的标准餐（包括液态蛋白、烤面包、果酱/果冻和水），并在进餐后 0 h、1 h、2 h 和 4 h 进行成像。如果在 4 h 后胃内残留超过 10%，其诊断胃排空延迟的敏感性和特异性均很高。

放射性核素显像还可用于特定肿瘤的检测、分期和监测，如神经内分泌肿瘤（NET）。大多数分化良好的 NET 表达生长抑素受体，因此可通过放射性同位素标记的生长抑素类似物（如 111-铟五肽酰胺和 68-镓 DOTATATE）检测这些肿瘤。

未来展望

随着技术的不断进步，内镜和影像学检查的质量和分辨率也将持续提高。此外，消化道壁不再是内镜治疗的边界。预期的创新包括以下几个方面：

- 内镜手术将继续扩展到消化道壁以外，为以往需要传统手术治疗的疾病提供微创治疗选择。
- "第二间隙"和"第三间隙"内镜技术将进一步完善，内镜减重治疗将得到更广泛的应用。
- 计算机辅助诊断（或"人工智能"）在结肠镜检查中将得到进一步发展，包括自动息肉检测和类型识别。

推荐阅读

ASGE Technology Committee, Aslanian HR, Sethi A, et al.: ASGE guideline for endoscopic full-thickness resection and submucosal tunnel endoscopic resection, *VideoGIE* 4(8):343–350, 2019.

Byrne MF, Jowell PS: Gastrointestinal imaging: Endoscopic ultrasound, *Gastroenterology* 122:1631–1648, 2002.

DiSario JA, Petersen BT, Tierney WM, et al.: Enteroscopes, *Gastrointest Endosc* 66:872–880, 2007.

Fletcher JG, Huprich J, Loftus EV, et al.: Computerized tomography enterography and its role in small-bowel imaging, *Clin Gastroenterol Hepatol* 6:283–289, 2008.

Gore RM, Levine MS: *Textbook of gastrointestinal radiology*, ed 2, Philadelphia, 2000, Saunders.

Mishkin DS, Chuttani R, Croffie J, et al.: ASGE Technology Status Evaluation Report: Wireless capsule endoscopy, *Gastrointest Endosc* 63:539–545, 2006.

Muguruma N, Tanaka K, Teramae S, Takayama T: Colon capsule endoscopy: toward the future, *Clin J Gastroenterol* 10(1):1–6, 2017.

Riff BP, DiMaio CJ: Exploring the small bowel: update on deep enteroscopy, *Curr Gastroenterol Rep* 18(6):28, 2016.

Schneider M, Höllerich J, Beyna T: Device-assisted enteroscopy: A review of available techniques and upcoming new technologies, *World J Gastroenterol* 25(27):3538–3545, 2019.

Shah SL, Perez-Miranda M, Kahaleh M, Tyberg A: Updates in Therapeutic Endoscopic Ultrasonography, *J Clin Gastroenterol* 52(9):765–772, 2018.

Thrall JH, Ziessman HA: *Nuclear Medicine: The Requisites*, ed 2, St. Louis, 2000, Mosby.

6

Esophageal Disorders

Harlan Rich, Zilla Hussain, Neal D. Dharmadhikari

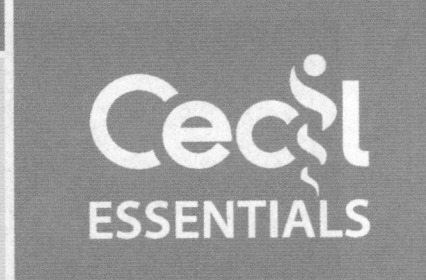

INTRODUCTION

The esophagus is a muscular tube that serves as conduit for the passage of solids and liquids into the stomach. It averages 23 to 25 cm in length and descends from the pharynx, at the lower border of the cricoid cartilage, to the stomach, at the cardiac orifice. Its descent is generally vertical and follows anterior to the vertebral column through the diaphragm and into the abdomen.

The esophagus is made up of four strata: mucosa, submucosa, muscularis externa, and adventitia. The stratified squamous nonkeratinized mucosa also contains the lamina propria and smooth muscle muscularis mucosae. Esophageal cardiac glands, in the lamina propria, produce mucous secretions that coat the lining of the esophagus. The submucosal layer contains esophageal glands, mucous and serous cells, and the Meissner, or submucosal, plexus. The muscularis externa is composed of an inner circular and outer longitudinal muscle layer. The upper third is mostly skeletal muscle innervated by the vagus nerve, while the lowest third is predominantly smooth muscle innervated by the enteric nervous system. The middle third is a mix of both skeletal and smooth muscle. The Auerbach, or myenteric, plexus is located between the inner circular and outer longitudinal layers. The outermost layer of the esophagus is the adventitia. A serosal layer covers the short segment of the abdominal esophagus across the diaphragm to the gastric cardia.

Sphincters are found at each end of the esophagus: the upper esophageal sphincter (UES) and the lower esophageal sphincter (LES). The UES is composed of three striated skeletal muscles: cricopharyngeus, thyropharyngeus, and cranial cervical esophagus. It maintains a degree of muscular activity at rest and relaxes during swallowing, vomiting, or belching. Opening of the UES occurs both via relaxation of these muscles and the pulling open of the sphincter via the superior and inferior hyoid and posterior pharyngeal muscles. The LES is a zone of circular, smooth muscle that maintains tonic contraction at rest and relaxes during swallowing, vomiting, and belching. The LES is supported by a functional external sphincter composed of the right crus of the diaphragm, which surrounds the esophagus as it enters the abdomen. Together, the LES and the functional external sphincter contribute to a high-pressure zone, preventing the regurgitation of gastric contents. Relaxation of the LES occurs when vagal efferent impulses activate myenteric neurons that release nonadrenergic, noncholinergic neurotransmitters, predominantly nitric oxide, and vasoactive intestinal polypeptide.

Swallowing requires the synchronization of voluntary and involuntary processes. Food mixes with saliva in the mouth and then is pushed back into the oral pharynx by the tongue. Once food enters the oral pharynx the glottis closes, protecting the airway. The bolus is then pushed to the esophagus where the UES is located. The UES relaxes, allowing food to enter the esophagus and then immediately closes, preventing the regurgitation of food. The bolus spends 8 to 13 seconds in the esophagus. Primary peristaltic waves, activated by central sequential firing mechanisms in the striated esophagus, and a latency gradient through the smooth muscle esophagus activated by vagal impulses, allow the bolus to travel through the esophagus. The pressure created by these waves ranges from 40 to 180 mm Hg. The pressure varies by the bolus's location in the esophagus, consistency, volume, and temperature. The LES relaxes and peristaltic waves push the bolus into the stomach.

SYMPTOMS OF ESOPHAGEAL DISEASE

Heartburn and regurgitation are two of the most common symptoms of esophageal disease and are defining features of gastroesophageal reflux disease (GERD). Heartburn is described as a burning sensation in the chest but can also be described as chest pain. Regurgitation is the sensation of food or liquid moving up and down the esophagus or as a sour taste in the mouth.

Dysphagia describes difficulty swallowing and can be characterized by trouble initiating a swallow or a bolus of material feeling stuck in the neck or chest while swallowing. The etiology of dysphagia can be mechanical or functional in nature. Odynophagia is pain with swallowing. Globus sensation is the feeling of something "stuck" or "tightness" in the esophagus. This symptom may be unrelated to swallowing, separating it from dysphagia.

Chest pain can be a manifestation of esophageal disease, but cardiac disease should always be considered. Chest pain related to cardiac disease, or angina, can have characteristics similar to those associated with esophageal-related chest pain. A careful history and physical examination with appropriate diagnostic studies can help distinguish the etiology of chest pain.

DIAGNOSTIC STUDIES OF THE ESOPHAGUS

Radiology

Barium esophagography, a video fluoroscopic procedure, can be used to assess dysphagia and can diagnose structural abnormalities in the esophagus or altered motility. When performed with a speech therapist (a modified barium swallow), it can be used to study the swallowing mechanism in more detail. A timed barium esophagogram can be used to assess esophageal emptying.

Computed tomography (CT) and magnetic resonance imaging (MRI) can often be used to define anatomy further and assess disease outside the lumen and beyond the mucosa. Positron emission tomography (PET) can be used to evaluate the esophagus but is typically used to evaluate malignant pathology when there is concern for metastasis.

食管疾病

李晓青 译　费贵军　谭蓓 审校　杨爱明 通审

引言

食管是一条肌性管状结构，是固体和液体进入胃部的通道。食管的平均长度为 23～25 cm，从咽部（环状软骨下缘）延伸到胃部（贲门口）。食管通常呈垂直下降，沿脊柱前方穿过横膈进入腹部。

食管由 4 层组成：黏膜层、黏膜下层、外肌层和外膜。复层鳞状非角化黏膜层还包含固有层和平滑肌性的黏膜肌层。食管贲门腺位于固有层，可产生覆盖食管内壁的黏液分泌物。黏膜下层包含食管腺、黏液细胞和浆液细胞，以及黏膜下神经丛（Meissner 神经丛）。外肌层由内侧的环行肌层和外侧的纵行肌层组成。食管上 1/3 主要是迷走神经支配的骨骼肌，而下 1/3 主要是由肠神经系统支配的平滑肌，中间 1/3 由骨骼肌和平滑肌混合组成。肌间神经丛（Auerbach 神经丛）位于内侧环行肌层和外侧纵行肌层之间。食管的最外层是外膜。浆膜层覆盖横跨横膈至贲门的一小段腹腔段食管。

食管两端均有括约肌：食管上括约肌（UES）和食管下括约肌（LES）。UES 由 3 块骨骼肌组成：环咽肌、咽下缩肌甲咽部和颈段食管。UES 在静息时保持一定程度的肌肉活动，在吞咽、呕吐或打嗝时松弛。UES 的打开既可通过这些肌肉的放松来实现，也可通过舌骨上肌、舌骨下肌和咽后肌将括约肌拉开来实现。LES 是一个环形的平滑肌带，它在静息时保持张力性收缩，在吞咽、呕吐或打嗝时松弛。LES 由功能性外括约肌（由右膈脚组成，在食管进入腹腔时环绕食管）支撑，并与其共同形成一个高压区，防止胃内容物反流。当迷走神经传出冲动激活肌间神经丛神经元，释放非肾上腺素能-非胆碱能神经递质（主要是一氧化氮）和血管活性肠肽时，LES 即松弛。

吞咽需要自主和非自主过程的同步进行。食团在口腔中与唾液混合，然后被舌推向口咽部。食团一旦进入口咽部，声门就会关闭，以保护气道。然后，食团被推向 UES，UES 松弛，使食团进入食管，然后立即关闭，防止反流。食团在食管中停留 8～13 s。由横纹肌食管的中枢序贯放电机制激活的原发蠕动波，以及由迷走神经冲动激活的平滑肌食管的延时梯度，使食团能够通过食管。这些蠕动波产生的压力范围为 40～180 mmHg。压力因食团在食管中的位置、稠度、体积和温度而异。随后，LES 松弛，蠕动波将食团推入胃内。

食管疾病的症状

烧心和反流是食管疾病最常见的两个症状，也是胃食管反流病（GERD）的典型特征。烧心被描述为胸部烧灼感，也可表现为胸痛。反流是指食物或液体在食管上下移动或口腔有酸味的感觉。

吞咽困难是指咽下困难，其特征是开始吞咽时感到困难或咽下后感觉有团块卡在颈部或胸部。吞咽困难可能由机械性病因或功能性病因引起。吞咽疼痛是伴随吞咽产生的疼痛。癔球症是指食管内有东西"卡住"或"紧绷"的感觉。该症状可能与吞咽无关，从而可与吞咽困难区分开来。

胸痛可能是食管疾病的一种表现，但始终需要考虑心脏病。心脏病或心绞痛相关的胸痛可能与食管源性胸痛有相似的特征。仔细的病史询问和体格检查，以及适当的诊断性检查有助于胸痛病因的鉴别。

食管疾病的诊断性检查方法

影像学检查

食管钡剂造影是一种视频 X 线透视检查，可用于评估吞咽困难，并诊断食管结构异常或动力改变。当与言语治疗师一起进行检查（改良吞钡造影）时，可更详细地研究吞咽机制。食管定时钡剂造影可用于评估食管排空。

CT 和 MRI 通常用于进一步明确解剖结构，并评估腔外或黏膜层以下的病变。正电子发射断层成像（PET）可用于评估食管，但通常用于评估恶性病变是否转移。

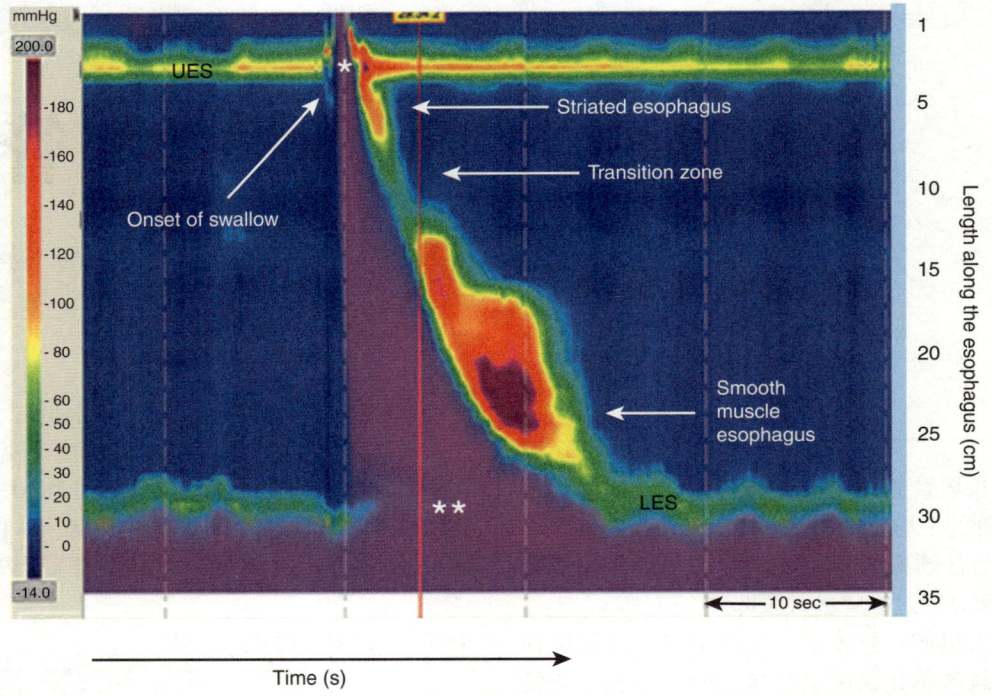

Fig. 6.1 High-resolution manometry (HRM) of normal esophageal peristalsis. HRM catheter consisting of 36 pressure sensors is inserted via the nares into the stomach to provide a complete physiologic pressure map of the hypopharynx, upper esophageal sphincter (UES), esophagus, lower esophageal sphincter (LES) and stomach. The Y-axis represents with sensor location; whereas the X-axis represents time. The color variation represents the different pressures along the length of the catheter at a given time and location. The resting UES and LES are shown as horizontal color bands. The relaxations of the UES (*) and LES (**) are shown as decreases in pressures (corresponding to approximately 20 mm Hg on color-pressure bar). The LES opens shortly after the UES relaxes with the onset of a wet swallow. Esophageal primary peristalsis is shown as a diagonal color band running from the UES to the LES. The onset of the swallow is seen on HRM as the high pressure contraction in the proximal, striated esophagus, followed by a lower pressure segment corresponding to the transition zone and a subsequent increase in pressure in the smooth muscle esophagus.

Endoscopy and Endoscopic Imaging

Esophagogastroduodenoscopy (EGD, upper endoscopy) allows for a direct visualization of the mucosal surface of the esophagus, stomach, and duodenum. An endoscope is a flexible fiberoptic tube with a camera that can be used for the diagnosis, screening, monitoring, and treatment of various pathologies. Endoscopes have additional channels through which a variety of endoscopic tools (i.e., forceps, dilators, injection needles, hemostatic tools) can be used to sample or treat the visualized area.

Endoscopic ultrasound (EUS) incorporates an ultrasound probe on the end of an endoscope. This ultrasound allows for imaging and biopsy across the wall of the esophagus and other nearby anatomical structures.

Manometry

Esophageal manometry is a physiologic evaluation of esophageal contractile function. High-resolution manometry is the diagnostic gold standard for the diagnosis of motility disorders. It utilizes a catheter lined with 20 to 36 pressure sensors at 1-cm intervals that is inserted via the nasal passage to the gastric body. The sensors record and compute the frequency and pressures of esophageal peristaltic waves and LES and UES function. The high-resolution manometry pressures are used to generate esophageal pressure topographies represented by color-coded, pressure-space-time plots. These objective metrics are applied to the Chicago Classification to diagnose esophageal motility disorders (Fig. 6.1).

Esophageal pH Monitoring

Esophageal wireless pH monitoring and catheter-based reflux testing are diagnostic tools used to study reflux disease. The wireless pH capsule is typically positioned 5 cm above the LES. The capsule measures the pH at the site for 24 to 48 hours in the ambulatory setting. The data are then reported as a percentage of the day the pH remains below 4. A combined impedance-pH probe measures acid and non-acid reflux as well as the direction of transit of a food or fluid bolus.

STRUCTURAL DISORDERS

Cricopharyngeal Bars

A cricopharyngeal bar is a radiographic finding consisting of a prominent posterior indentation of the esophagus at the level of the cricopharyngeus that is often asymptomatic but can contribute to dysphagia. The prominence is thought to be due to muscle spasm or impairment of muscle compliance at the UES. Cricopharyngeal bars can be managed via surgical and nonsurgical interventions. Nonsurgical options include dilation at the site or injection of botulinum toxin. Surgical management technique occurs via cricopharyngeal myotomy.

Diverticula

Diverticula of the esophagus are outpouchings contained within layers of the esophageal wall. True diverticula involve all layers to the esophageal wall, whereas false diverticula are limited to the submucosa and mucosa.

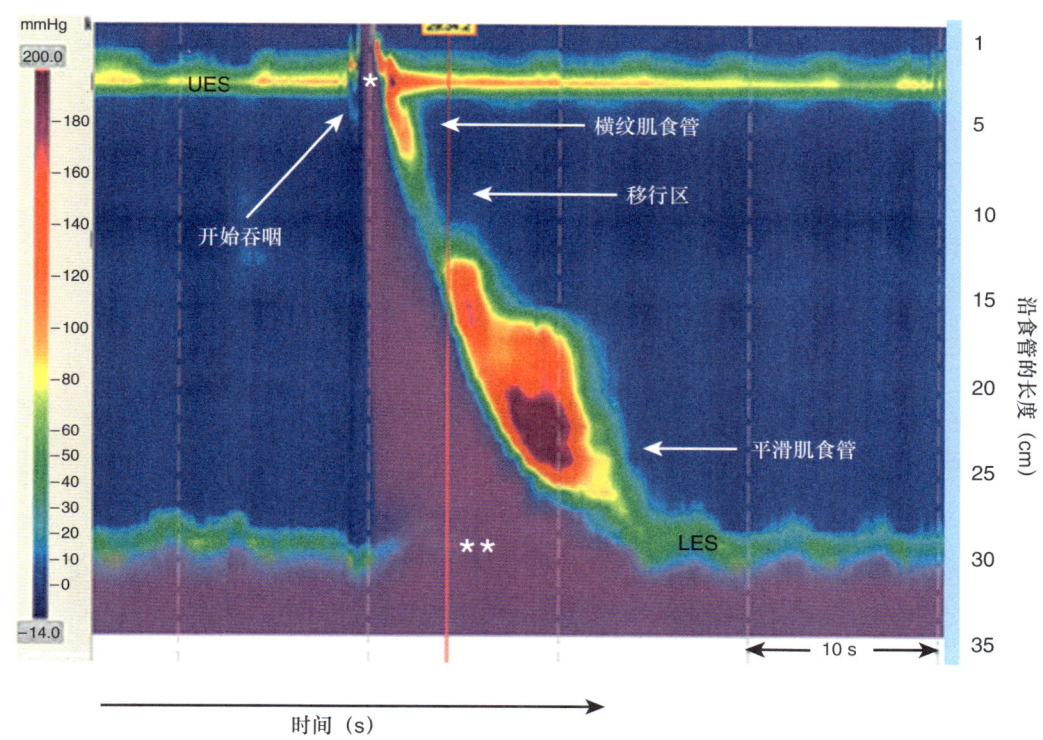

图 6.1　正常食管蠕动的高分辨率测压（HRM）。HRM 导管由 36 个压力传感器组成，经鼻插入胃内，以展示从下咽部、食管上括约肌（UES）、食管、食管下括约肌（LES）到胃的完整生理性压力图。Y 轴表示传感器位置，X 轴表示时间，颜色变化表示在特定时间和位置沿导管的不同压力。静息时的 UES 和 LES 显示为水平色带，UES（*）和 LES（**）松弛显示为压力下降（对应于彩色压力条上约 20 mmHg）。在湿吞咽开始时，UES 松弛，随即 LES 开放。食管原发蠕动显示为从 UES 到 LES 的对角线状色带。在 HRM 上，开始吞咽表现为近端横纹肌食管的高压收缩，接着是对应于食管移行区的低压带，然后是平滑肌食管的压力增大

内镜和内镜成像

食管胃十二指肠镜（EGD）可以直接观察食管、胃和十二指肠的黏膜表面。内镜是一种带有摄像装置的软光纤管，可用于诊断、筛查、监测和治疗多种疾病。此外，可通过内镜额外的通道使用内镜工具（即活检钳、扩张器、注射针、止血工具）对可视区域进行取样或治疗。

超声内镜（EUS）是在内镜末端装有超声探头。EUS 技术可对食管壁及其邻近解剖结构进行成像和活检。

测压

食管测压是评估食管收缩功能的生理学检查。高分辨率测压是诊断食管动力障碍性疾病的金标准。测压时使用一根内衬 20～36 个压力传感器（每个间隔 1 cm）的导管，经鼻腔插入胃内。传感器记录并计算食管蠕动波的频率和压力，以及 LES 和 UES 的功能。高分辨率测压以食管压力地形图（即彩色编码的压力-空间-时间图）表示。芝加哥分类标准采用这些客观指标来诊断食管动力障碍（图 6.1）。

食管 pH 值监测

食管无线 pH 值监测和导管反流监测是诊断胃食管反流病的工具。无线 pH 值胶囊通常置于 LES 上方 5 cm 处，可在所置食管位置动态监测 24～48 h 的 pH 值变化。该检查可记录数据并报告全天 pH 值＜ 4 所占的百分比。阻抗 -pH 值联合探头可监测酸性和非酸性反流，以及食物或液体的转运方向。

结构性疾病

环咽肌切迹

环咽肌切迹是一种影像学表现，即环咽肌水平处明显的突向食管后方的切迹，通常无症状，但也可能导致吞咽困难。这种突起被认为是由 UES 的肌肉痉挛或肌肉顺应性受损所致。环咽肌切迹可通过手术或非手术方法进行治疗。非手术治疗包括局部扩张或肉毒杆菌毒素注射。手术治疗为环咽肌切开术。

憩室

食管憩室是包含多层食管壁组织的膨出结构，真

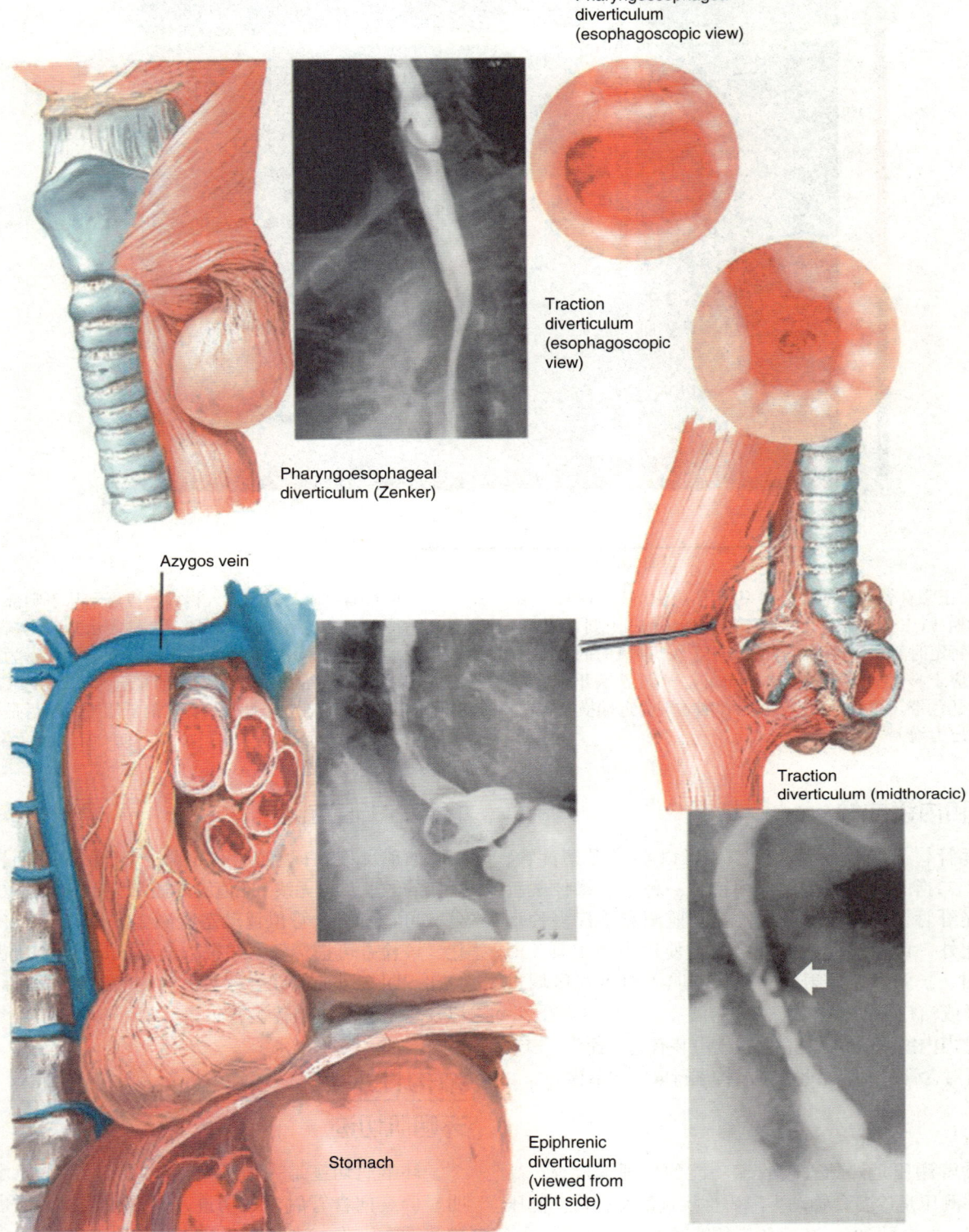

Fig. 6.2 Esophageal diverticula.

All diverticula are further categorized by their location. They are classified as proximal or pharyngoesophageal (Zenker's and Killian-Jamieson) diverticula, mid-esophageal or traction or parabronchial diverticula, and epiphrenic diverticula. The prevalence of Zenker's diverticula (ZD) ranges from 0.01% to 0.11%, and the majority of patients are diagnosed in their sixth to eighth decades of life. The prevalence of the other types of

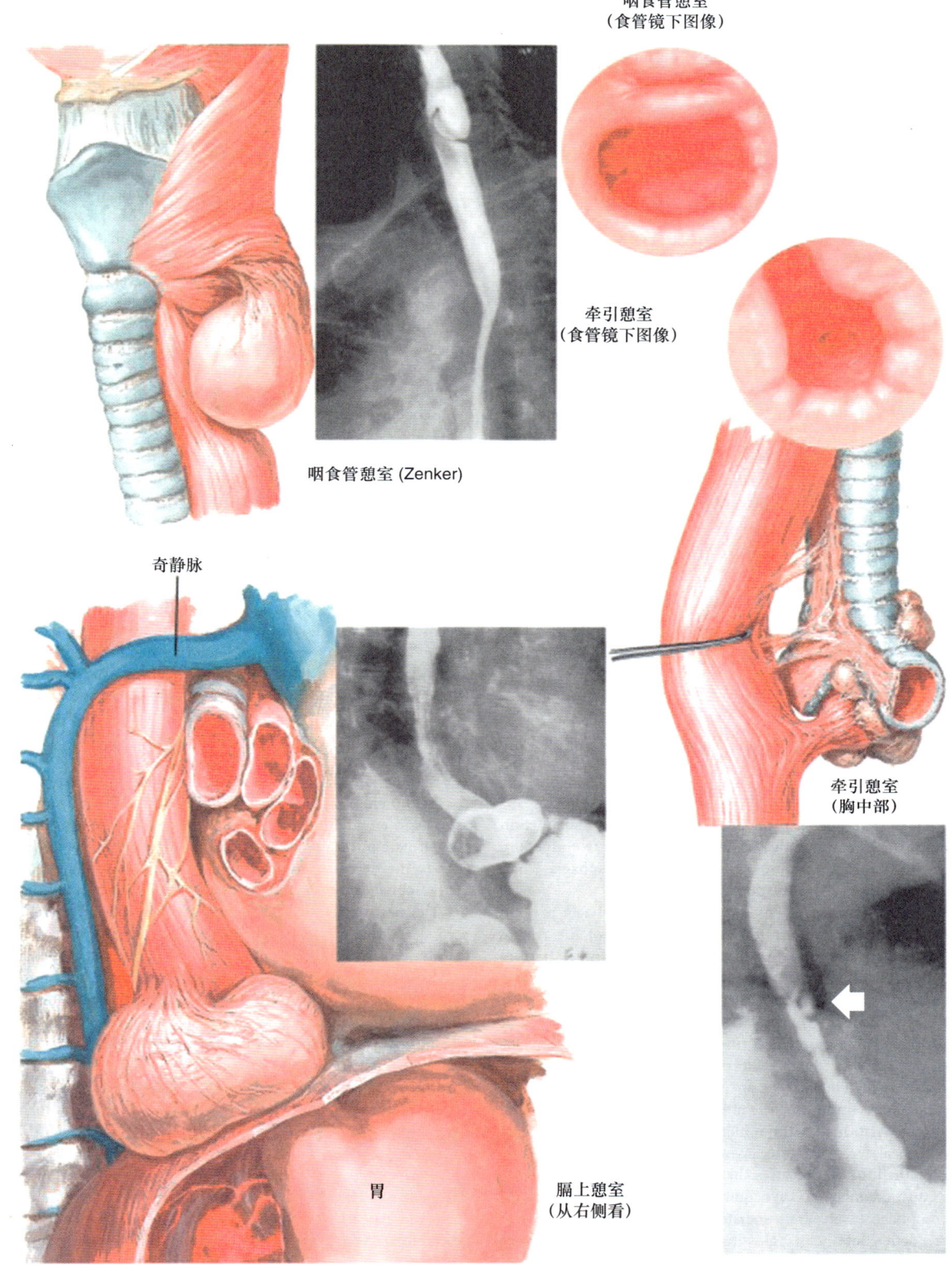

图 6.2 食管憩室

性憩室涉及食管壁的所有层,而假性憩室仅限于黏膜下层和黏膜层。根据其位置,所有憩室可进一步分为近端或咽食管憩室(Zenker 和 Killian-Jamieson 憩室)、食管中段憩室(又称牵引憩室或支气管旁食管憩室)和膈上憩室。Zenker 憩室(ZD)的患病率为 0.01%～0.11%,绝大多数患者在 50～80 岁时确诊。

diverticula are unknown but are far less common than Zenker's diverticula (Fig. 6.2).

ZD forms in the Killian triangle, an area of sparse musculature bordered by the cricopharyngeus and thyropharyngeus muscles in the posterior pharyngeal wall. As a result of diminished compliance of the cricopharyngeus muscle and the UES, the hypopharynx is exposed to increased intra-bolus pressures while swallowing, causing the ZD to form. ZD are false diverticula. Parabronchial diverticula are likely associated with mediastinal fibrosis, which is often due to inflammation of the mediastinum caused by other pathology (i.e., fungal infections, tuberculosis). Traction on the esophageal wall causes these diverticula to form. Long-standing distal esophageal obstruction can lead to the formation of pulsion diverticula either through anatomic abnormalities or motility disorders. Diffuse esophageal spasm has been associated with parabronchial diverticula, whereas achalasia has been associated with epiphrenic diverticula. The latter two are true diverticula.

Patients with ZD often present with oropharyngeal dysphagia but can also suffer from complete esophageal obstruction. Classically, these patients will complain of dysphagia with regurgitation and halitosis. Parabronchial and epiphrenic diverticula are most often asymptomatic and diagnosed as incidental findings on imaging. The complications of these diverticula are typically related to their underlying disorders (i.e., motility disorders).

Diverticula are diagnosed using barium swallow, endoscopy, and computed tomography. Manometry can also be used to diagnose underlying motility issues that contribute to diverticula formation.

Symptomatic ZD should be treated. Smaller ZD can be treated with cricopharyngeal myotomy alone. Larger ZD may need additional interventions, including diverticulum suspension or diverticulectomy. Endoscopic cricopharyngeal myotomy is an alternative to surgical approaches. Parabronchial and epiphrenic diverticula are most successfully addressed by treating the underlying disorder (i.e., motility disorders or strictures). They can also involve extended myotomy and diverticulectomy.

Rings and Webs

Esophageal rings are areas of narrowing in the esophageal lumen. An "A" ring is a muscular ring found in the upper part of the phrenic ampulla at the area of highest pressure in the LES and is defined by smooth muscle hypertrophy with normal surface epithelium. A "B" (or Schatzki) ring is a mucosal ring at the squamocolumnar junction with squamous epithelium above the ring and columnar epithelium below. This ring can lead to luminal narrowing and dysphagia. Their etiology and pathophysiology are poorly understood.

Patients with Schatzki ring often complain of dysphagia to solid food that is chronic and intermittent. The diameter of the ring is inversely associated with the incidence and symptoms. A barium swallow with a full column technique is the best modality to diagnose Schatzki rings. An endoscope can visualize Schatzki rings but can miss rings with larger diameters.

The treatment of all esophageal rings is mechanical dilation. This can be performed with Savary dilators or radial expanding balloon dilators. There is a high rate of reoccurrence after treatment and a scant 11% of patients are symptom free after 3 years. However, repeated dilations can be performed without increasing the complication rate.

An esophageal web is a thin, membranous tissue covered with squamous epithelium that reduces the size of the esophageal lumen. The webs can be congenital or acquired. Congenital webs are rare. Acquired esophageal webs are associated with Plummer-Vinson syndrome (iron deficiency anemia, glossitis, koilonychia, and esophageal/pharyngeal carcinoma).

Patients with esophageal webs will present with dysphagia. The webs are diagnosed by barium swallow or endoscopy. Lifestyle modifications are encouraged to reduced symptoms, but some patients must be treated with mechanical dilation similar to the treatment for Schatzki rings.

Malignancy

Esophageal cancer is the seventh most common cancer and the sixth leading cause of cancer-related mortality worldwide. The five-year survival rate after diagnosis is 15% to 20%. The incidence of esophageal cancer varies by region. In developed countries, the incidence of squamous cell cancer (SCC) has fallen and adenocarcinoma has become the leading type. However, SCC remains more prevalent worldwide. The major risk factors for developing SCC are alcohol and tobacco use. There are other carcinogens which, similar to alcohol and tobacco, are thought to lead to inflammation and dysplasia. Tobacco is a moderate risk factor for the adenocarcinoma. Obesity and body mass index remain the strongest risk factors for the development of esophageal adenocarcinoma. Obesity can predispose patients to GERD and Barrett esophagus, which also cause adenocarcinoma. The progression of gastrointestinal reflux disease to adenocarcinoma is described in a subsequent section (Fig. 6.3).

With esophageal cancer, patients often complain of progressive dysphagia and weight loss. Depending on the progression of symptoms, they may also present with anemia or other symptoms. The treatment of esophageal cancer depends on progression and staging but can involve chemotherapy, radiation, surgery, and/or palliative measures.

Hiatal Hernias

A hiatal hernia results in abdominal contents, such as the stomach, becoming displaced above the diaphragm. Hiatal hernias are subcategorized into four types: type I (sliding hiatal hernia), type II (paraesophageal hernia; the proximal stomach protrudes up through the diaphragm along the distal esophagus), type III (a combination of type I and type II), and type IV (herniation of other abdominal organs). Sliding hiatal hernias are the most common variety. Types II through IV are considered variations of paraesophageal hernias (Fig. 6.4).

Sliding hernias are a result of laxity in the phrenoesophageal membrane, a membrane that anchors the esophagus to the diaphragm. This results in a widening of the hiatal tunnel, allowing the gastric cardia to herniate into the thorax. Increasing age and obesity often contribute to the decreasing elasticity of the phrenoesophageal membrane. Paraesophageal hernias are caused by defects in this membrane.

Hernias may be diagnosed by plain film, barium swallow studies, cross-sectional imaging, and endoscopy. Asymptomatic hiatal hernias rarely need to be treated. If a type I hiatal hernia is associated with GERD, then medical or surgical treatment should be considered. The course of treatment would focus on treating the symptoms of GERD. Paraesophageal hernias (type II-IV) are prone to complications including volvulus, obstruction, incarceration, and perforation and should be treated expediently because continued enlargement will lead to worsening symptoms and complications.

GASTROESOPHAGEAL REFLUX DISEASE AND SEQUELAE

A consensus (the Montreal consensus, specifically) amongst a panel of world experts defined GERD as "a condition which develops when the reflux of stomach contents causes troublesome symptoms and/or complications." This definition includes symptomatic syndromes and syndromes with esophageal injury but does not include functional heartburn.

其他类型憩室的患病率不详，但远低于ZD（图6.2）。

ZD形成于Killian三角区，该区域的肌肉组织稀疏，被咽后壁的环咽肌和咽下缩肌甲咽部包围。由于环咽肌和UES的顺应性下降，吞咽时下咽部暴露于食团内的压力升高，从而形成ZD。ZD属于假性憩室。支气管旁食管憩室可能与纵隔纤维化有关，后者通常由其他病变（如真菌感染、肺结核）引起的纵隔炎症所致。食管壁受牵拉会导致这些憩室的形成。食管下段长期梗阻可通过解剖异常或运动障碍形成推压性憩室。弥漫性食管痉挛与支气管旁食管憩室有关，而贲门失弛缓症则与膈上憩室有关。后两者均为真性憩室。

ZD患者通常表现为口咽部吞咽困难，但也可能出现食管完全梗阻。这些患者通常主诉吞咽困难伴反流和口臭。支气管旁食管憩室和膈上憩室患者通常无症状，多在影像学检查时被偶然发现。这些憩室的并发症通常与其潜在疾病（即动力障碍性疾病）相关。

钡剂造影、内镜和CT可诊断憩室。食管测压可用于诊断导致憩室形成的潜在动力障碍。

症状性ZD需要治疗。较小的ZD可仅通过环咽肌切开术治疗。较大的ZD可能需要其他治疗，包括憩室悬吊术或憩室切除术。内镜环咽肌切开术是外科手术的替代方法。治疗支气管旁食管憩室或膈上憩室最有效的方法是治疗潜在疾病（即动力障碍性疾病或狭窄）。此外，还可采用扩大肌切开术和憩室切除术。

食管环和食管蹼

食管环是食管腔内狭窄的区域。"A"环是膈壶腹上部的肌肉环，位于LES压力最高的区域，其特征是平滑肌肥大，表面上皮正常。"B"（或Schatzki）环是鳞-柱交界处的黏膜环，环上方为鳞状上皮，环下方为柱状上皮。该环可导致管腔狭窄和吞咽困难。其病因和病理生理学尚不明确。

Schatzki环患者常主诉长期间歇性吞咽固体食物困难。环的直径与发病率和症状呈负相关。全食管吞钡造影是诊断Schatzki环的最佳方法。内镜可观察到Schatzki环，但可能会漏诊直径较大的环。

所有食管环的治疗方法都是机械性扩张，可使用Savary扩张器或径向膨胀气囊扩张器。治疗后复发率高，仅有11%的患者在治疗3年后仍无症状。但是，可以重复进行扩张且不会升高并发症的发生率。

食管蹼是一种表面覆盖鳞状上皮的薄膜组织，可使食管管腔缩小。食管蹼可能为先天性或获得性。先天性食管蹼很少见。获得性食管蹼与Plummer-Vinson综合征（缺铁性贫血、舌炎、反甲和食管癌/咽癌）有关。

食管蹼患者会出现吞咽困难，可通过吞钡造影或内镜确诊。应鼓励患者调整生活方式以减轻症状，但部分患者必须接受机械性扩张治疗，方法类似于Schatzki环的治疗。

恶性肿瘤

食管癌是全球第七大癌症，也是导致癌症相关死亡的第六大原因。患者确诊后5年生存率为15%～20%。食管癌的发病率因不同地区而异。在发达国家，鳞状细胞癌（SCC）的发病率下降，腺癌已成为主要类型。但是，SCC的全球发病率仍然很高。食管SCC的主要危险因素是饮酒和吸烟。此外，其他致癌物质也被认为会导致炎症和异型增生。烟草是腺癌的中度危险因素。肥胖症和体重指数（BMI）高仍然是食管腺癌发病的最强危险因素。肥胖症使患者易患GERD和巴雷特食管，这两种疾病均会导致腺癌。GERD发展为腺癌的过程详见下文（图6.3）。

食管癌患者通常主诉进行性吞咽困难和体重减轻。随着症状的进展，患者还可能出现贫血或其他表现。食管癌的治疗取决于病情进展和分期，可能涉及化疗、放疗、手术和（或）姑息治疗。

食管裂孔疝

食管裂孔疝会导致腹腔内容物（如胃）移位到横膈上方。食管裂孔疝可分为4种类型：Ⅰ型（滑动型食管裂孔疝）、Ⅱ型（食管旁疝；近端胃沿远端食管向上疝入横膈）、Ⅲ型（Ⅰ型和Ⅱ型的混合型）和Ⅳ型（其他腹腔器官疝）。Ⅰ型食管裂孔疝是最常见的类型。Ⅱ～Ⅳ型被认为是食管旁疝的不同变异类型（图6.4）。

Ⅰ型食管裂孔疝是膈食管膜（将食管固定于横膈的膜样结构）松弛的结果，这会导致食管裂孔变宽，使胃贲门疝入胸腔。年龄增大和肥胖症通常会导致膈食管膜弹性下降。食管旁疝由该膜缺陷引起。

食管裂孔疝可通过腹平片、吞钡造影、断层扫描成像技术和内镜进行诊断。无症状的食管裂孔疝很少需要治疗。如果Ⅰ型食管裂孔疝伴随GERD，则应考虑药物治疗或手术治疗，治疗过程侧重于对GERD症状的治疗。食管旁疝（Ⅱ～Ⅳ型）易发生扭转、梗阻、嵌顿和穿孔等并发症，应尽快治疗，因为裂孔疝的继续增大将导致症状和并发症的恶化。

胃食管反流病和后遗症

全球专家小组达成的共识（特别是蒙特利尔共识）将GERD定义为"胃内容物反流引起的不适症状和（或）并发症"。该定义包括症状综合征和食管损伤综合征，但不包括功能性烧心。

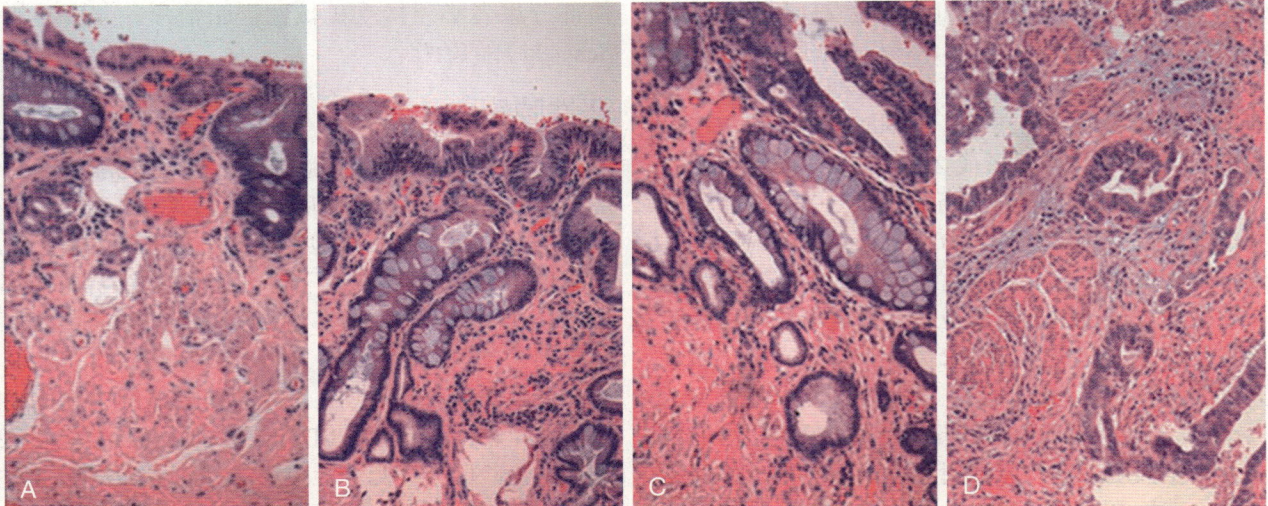

Fig. 6.3 Histologic progression of Barrett esophagus with no dysplasia (A) to low-grade (B) dysplasia, high-grade dysplasia (C), and esophageal adenocarcinoma (D).

Pathophysiology and Symptoms

The pathophysiology of GERD is determined by numerous factors including gastric acid–esophageal mucosa interaction, incompetence of the gastroesophageal junction, decrease in esophageal mucosal defenses, and altered sensory mechanisms that interpret the symptoms.

Numerous modalities can be used to help diagnose and manage GERD, but often history is enough to diagnose and begin treatment. The symptoms that are characteristic of GERD include heartburn and regurgitation. Chest pain can also be a presenting symptom but should be distinguished from cardiac chest pain. Patients can also present with less common, atypical symptoms such as dysphagia, dyspepsia, epigastric pain, bloating, nausea, and belching.

Diagnosis

The diagnosis of GERD is established using history of symptoms, objective testing (endoscopy and esophageal pH monitoring), and patient responsiveness to therapy. A proton pump inhibitor (PPI) trial is a method that may be used to diagnose GERD in patients with typical symptoms without concerning features that may include dysphagia, odynophagia, weight loss, anemia, nausea, or vomiting. A lack of response to PPIs does not exclude the diagnosis of GERD, and atypical symptoms are not as reliable at predicting response. Therefore, objective testing with endoscopy or esophageal pH monitoring should be considered in patients who do not respond to PPIs.

Endoscopy provides direct visualization of the esophageal lumen and evaluation of the esophageal mucosa in patients with suspected GERD. It can demonstrate objective findings suggestive of GERD such as erosive esophagitis, strictures, and Barrett esophagus. Not all symptomatic patients will have evidence of erosions or mucosal damage, which can limit the diagnostic specificity of endoscopy. Endoscopy allows for biopsy of the mucosa, which is helpful in screening for Barrett esophagus, but can also aid in establishing another diagnosis. Eosinophilic esophagitis may have a similar presentation and biopsy can be used to differentiate between GERD without erosions and eosinophilic esophagitis. Biopsy is not recommended to diagnose GERD in patients with heartburn and normal endoscopy.

Esophageal pH monitoring with or without impedance may objectively demonstrate the presence of abnormal esophageal acid exposure, non-acid reflux, reflux frequency, and symptoms associated with reflux.

Management

Lifestyle modifications are a part of the initial therapy for GERD. Patients are counseled on behaviors that may improve symptoms and recommendation of avoidance of foods that trigger symptoms. Weight loss is advised for overweight and obese patients. Weight gain, even in patients with normal BMI, can provoke new GERD symptoms. Other behavior modifications include tobacco cessation, raising the head of the bed, and avoiding recumbent position for at least 2 hours after a meal. The common foods that can trigger heartburn and regurgitation include coffee, alcohol, chocolate, fatty foods, citrus, and spicy foods. It is important that all lifestyle modifications be tailored to each patient's symptoms and disease course.

When lifestyle modifications fail, medical interventions should be attempted. Medications that can treat GERD include antacids, histamine-receptor antagonists (H2 blockers), and PPIs. Patients often utilize over-the-counter antacids to provide symptom relief of GERD. These antacids work to neutralize gastric hydrochloric acid and inhibit pepsin. With the advent of H2 blockers and PPIs, antacid use has declined, but a smaller cohort of patients will continue using them for heartburn. H2 blockers reversibly bind to histamine H2 receptors, preventing histamine released during a meal from binding to receptors on ECL and parietal cells. PPIs are superior to H2 blockers because they essentially irreversibly block the hydrogen-potassium ATPase that secretes hydrochloric acid from the gastric parietal cells. They have been shown to contribute to esophageal healing and have decreased relapse rates when compared to H2 blockers. In addition, PPIs have also been shown to be superior for heartburn relief.

Surgical options can be considered for GERD or esophagitis refractory to medical therapy, when patients suffer side effects of medical therapy, exhibit noncompliance, or need correction of a concomitant large hiatal hernia. The surgical options for treatment include laparoscopic fundoplication or bariatric surgery. Laparoscopic fundoplication involves "wrapping" the fundus of the stomach around the end of the esophagus to help repair and provide support to the LES. Bariatric surgery with gastric bypass in obese patients with GERD can also be used to treat GERD.

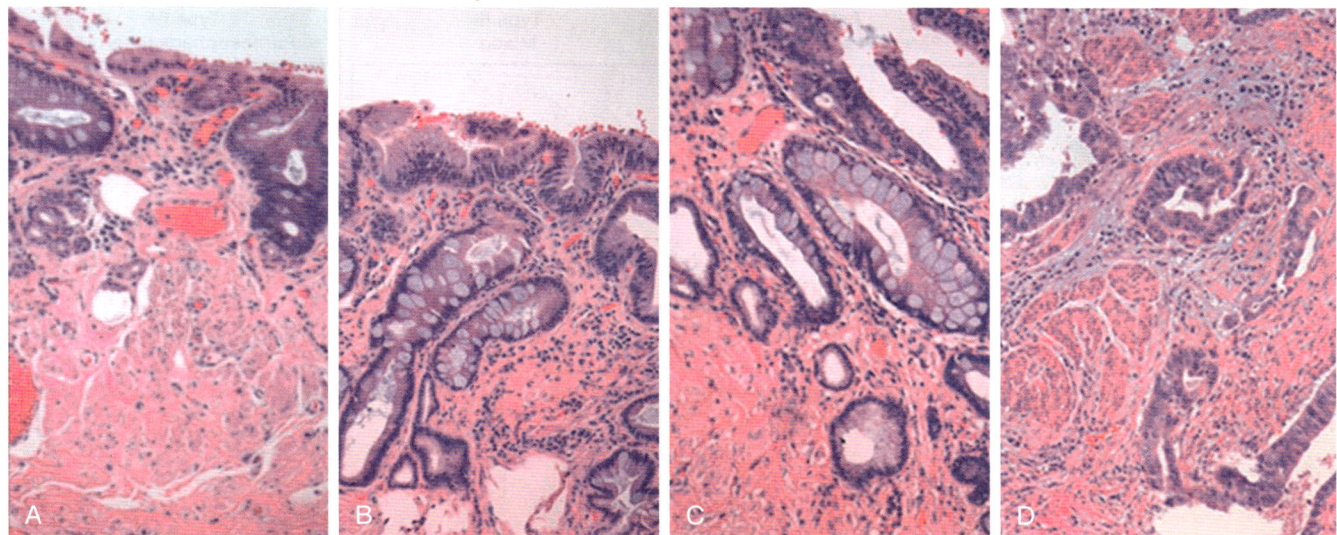

图 6.3 巴雷特食管的组织学进展，从无异型增生（**A**）到低级别异型增生（**B**）、高级别异型增生（**C**）和食管腺癌（**D**）

病理生理学和症状

GERD 的病理生理学包括多种因素：胃酸-食管黏膜相互作用、胃食管连接处功能不全、食管黏膜防御能力下降及诠释症状的食管感觉机制发生改变等。

GERD 的诊断和治疗可采用多种方法，但通过病史常足以诊断 GERD 并开始治疗。GERD 的特征性症状包括烧心和反流。患者也可能出现胸痛，但应与心源性胸痛区分开来。患者还可能出现少见的非典型症状，如吞咽困难、消化不良、上腹痛、胀气、恶心和嗳气。

诊断

GERD 的诊断应基于症状、客观检查（内镜和食管 pH 值监测）及患者对治疗的反应。质子泵抑制剂（PPI）试验可用于诊断 GERD，适用于症状典型且没有吞咽困难、吞咽疼痛、体重减轻、贫血、恶心或呕吐等症状的患者。对 PPI 无应答不能排除 GERD 的诊断，非典型症状在预测治疗反应方面并不可靠。因此，对 PPI 无应答的患者应考虑行内镜或食管 pH 值监测等客观检查。

对于疑诊 GERD 的患者，内镜可直接观察食管腔并评估食管黏膜。提示 GERD 的客观证据包括糜烂性食管炎、狭窄和巴雷特食管。并非所有症状性患者都会有糜烂或黏膜损伤的证据，这也限制了内镜的诊断特异性。内镜检查时可行黏膜活检，有助于筛查巴雷特食管和明确其他诊断。嗜酸细胞性食管炎可能引起类似的临床表现，活检可用于区分不伴有糜烂的 GERD 和嗜酸细胞性食管炎。对于有烧心症状且内镜检查结果正常的患者，不建议通过活检来诊断 GERD。

食管 pH 值监测（联合或不联合阻抗监测）可以客观地显示食管异常酸暴露、非酸性反流、反流频率及与反流相关的症状。

管理

调整生活方式是 GERD 初始治疗的一部分。应告知患者可能改善症状的行为方式，建议避免食用可引发症状的食物。建议超重和肥胖症患者减重。体重增加会诱发新的 GERD 症状，即使是 BMI 正常的患者。其他行为调整包括戒烟、抬高床头、餐后至少 2 h 避免平卧。可能诱发烧心和反流的常见食物包括咖啡、酒精、巧克力、油腻食物、柠檬和辛辣食物。重要的是，所有生活方式的改变均应根据每位患者的症状和病程进行量身定制。

当调整生活方式无效时，应尝试药物干预。治疗 GERD 的药物包括抗酸剂、组胺受体拮抗剂（H_2 受体拮抗剂）和 PPI。患者通常使用非处方抗酸剂来缓解 GERD 症状。这些抗酸剂的作用是中和胃酸并抑制胃蛋白酶。随着 H_2 受体拮抗剂和 PPI 的出现，抗酸剂的使用已逐渐减少，但仍有一小部分患者会继续使用抗酸剂来治疗烧心。H_2 受体拮抗剂可与 H_2 受体可逆性结合，阻止进餐时释放的组胺与肠嗜铬样细胞（ECL）和壁细胞上的受体结合。PPI 优于 H_2 受体拮抗剂，因为 PPI 不可逆地阻断 H^+-K^+-ATP 酶，而胃壁细胞通过该酶分泌盐酸。研究表明，与 H_2 受体拮抗剂相比，PPI 更有助于食管愈合并降低复发率。此外，PPI 还被证实在缓解烧心方面更有优势。

对于药物治疗无效的 GERD 或食管炎，如果患者出现药物副作用、不配合治疗或需要处理合并的巨大食管裂孔疝，可以考虑手术治疗。手术治疗包括腹腔镜胃底折叠术或减重术。腹腔镜胃底折叠术是将胃底"包裹"在食管末端，以帮助修复和支撑 LES。对患有 GERD 的肥胖症患者进行胃旁路减重术也可用于治疗 GERD。

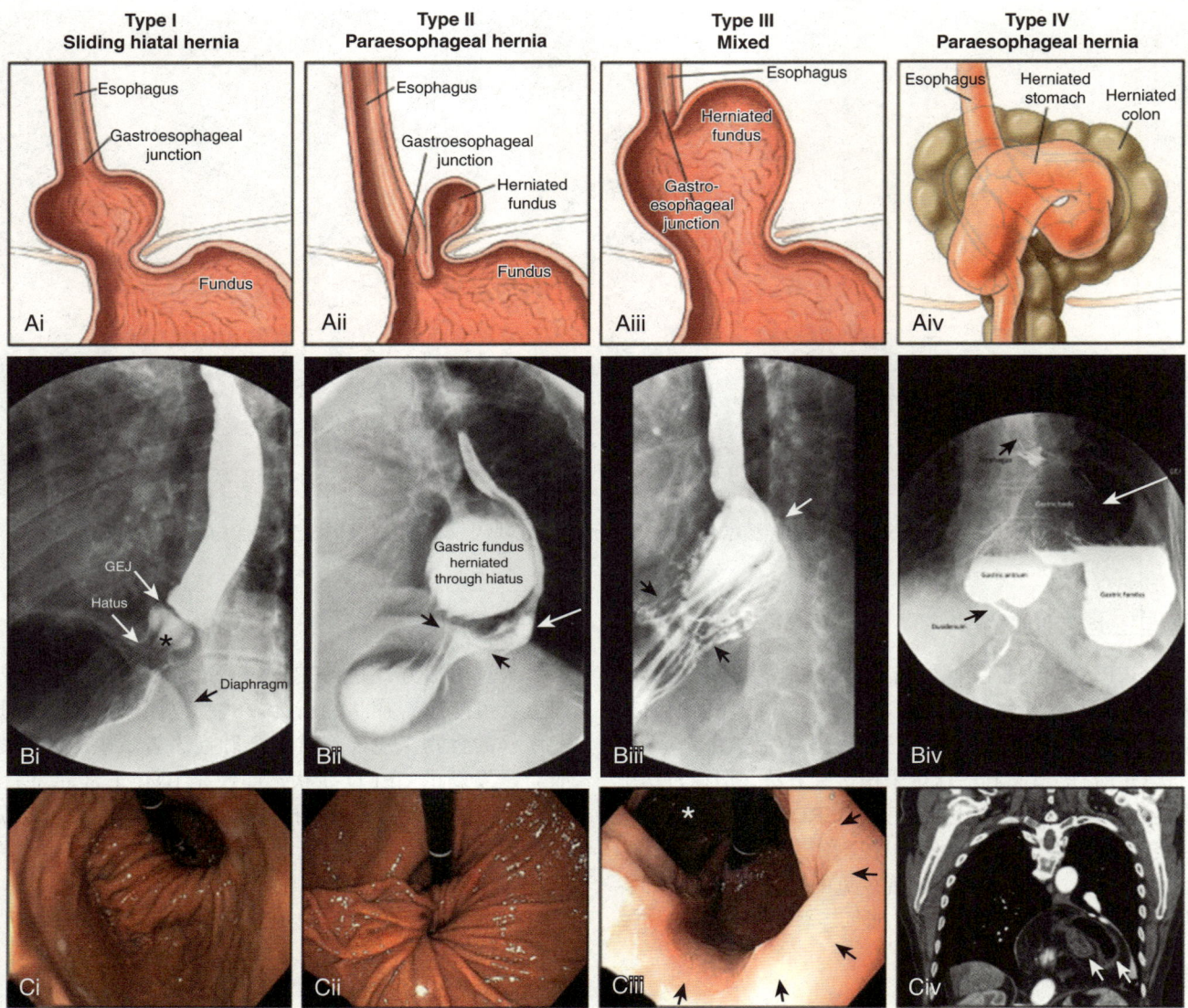

Fig. 6.4 Anatomic drawings (row A), barium contrast radiography (row B), and endoscopic (i–iii) and computed tomographic (iv) views (row C) of Type I or sliding hiatal hernia (column 1), Type II PEH (column 2), Type III PEH (column 3), and Type IV PEH (column 4). Pane Bi: *, sliding hiatal hernia. Pane Bii: True paraesophageal hernia adjacent to GEJ. Separation between GEJ and diaphragm noted, consistent with a small adjacent hiatal hernia. *White arrow:* Barium tablet present. *Black arrows:* Widened hiatus. Pane Biii: *White arrow:* Gastroesophageal junction. *Black arrows:* Widened diaphragmatic hiatus. Pane Biv: Herniated, intrathoracic stomach with herniation of duodenum. This stomach is flipped in an organoaxial rotation. Pane Ci: Sliding hiatal hernia. Pane Cii: Separate PEH present, herniated through laxity in phrenoesophageal membrane. Lax diaphragmatic hiatus also present. Pane Ciii: Image taken from the diaphragmatic hiatus *(black arrows)*. Herniation of GEJ noted with large adjacent fundus/PEH *(white asterisk)*. Pane Civ: Coronal computed tomography (CT) image of an intrathoracic stomach with herniated loops of colon *(white arrows)*. *GEJ,* Gastroesophageal junction; *PEH,* paraesophageal hernia.

Extraesophageal Manifestations of GERD

GERD contributes to several extraesophageal manifestations including respiratory, laryngopharyngeal, and dental symptoms. Respiratory symptoms include pulmonary disease (asthma, idiopathic pulmonary fibrosis, bronchitis, etc.), cough, wheezing, and shortness of breath. Laryngeal symptoms present as hoarseness, throat pain, globus, choking, postnasal drip, laryngeal and tracheal stenosis, and laryngospasm. Dental erosions can also be a result of GERD.

Non-GERD causes of extraesophageal manifestations should be considered prior to associating the symptoms with GERD. Diagnostic tools are unable to provide reliable evidence of causality between GERD and extraesophageal symptoms. In addition, PPIs have not shown a clear therapeutic benefit in the treatment of these symptoms. The diagnosis of GERD, as described previously, can help with the association, but the presence or absence of GERD cannot reliably establish it as cause of extraesophageal symptoms. Clinicians often rely on symptom association analysis to find a temporal association between reflux symptoms and other symptoms.

Acid suppression with a PPI is still used to treat extraesophageal symptoms when typical GERD symptoms are present. When typical GERD symptoms are not present, reflux monitoring is considered prior to

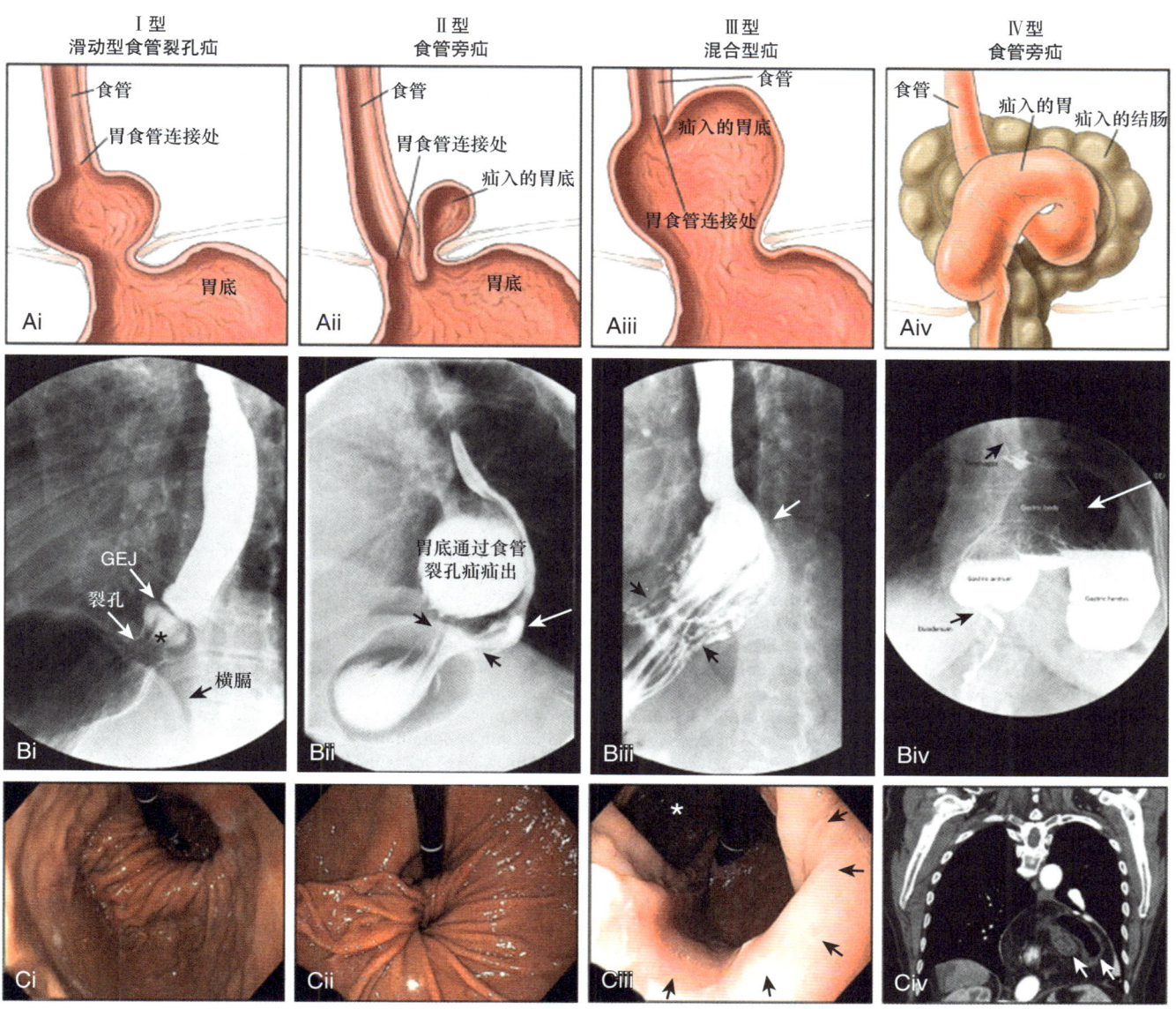

图 6.4　Ⅰ 型 (滑动型) 食管裂孔疝 (第 1 列)、Ⅱ 型食管旁疝 (第 2 列)、Ⅲ 型食管旁疝 (第 3 列) 和 Ⅳ 型食管旁疝 (第 4 列) 的解剖图示 (A 行)、钡剂造影图 (B 行)、内镜图像 (图 i ~ iii) 和 CT 图像 (图 iv) (C 行)。图 Bi.*，Ⅰ 型食管裂孔疝。图 Bii. 毗邻 GEJ 的真性食管疝。可见 GEJ 与横膈分离，符合相邻的小裂孔疝。白色箭头：钡片存留。黑色箭头：裂孔增宽。图 Biii. 白色箭头：胃食管连接处。黑色箭头：膈肌裂孔增宽。图 Biv. 疝入胸腔的胃和十二指肠。胃腔沿自身器官轴旋转翻转。图 Ci. Ⅰ 型食管裂孔疝。图 Cii. 存在单独的食管旁疝，因膈食管膜松弛而疝出，还可见松弛的膈裂孔。图 Ciii. 通过膈裂孔 (黑色箭头) 拍摄的图像。可见 GEJ 疝出，伴有邻近的大的胃底 / 食管旁疝 (白色星号)。图 Civ. 胸腔内胃和疝出的结肠肠袢 (白色箭头) 的冠状位 CT 图像。GEJ，胃食管连接处

GERD 的食管外表现

GERD 可导致多种食管外表现，包括呼吸道、咽喉和牙科症状。呼吸道症状包括肺部疾病 (哮喘、特发性肺纤维化、支气管炎等)、咳嗽、喘息和气短。咽部症状表现为声音嘶哑、咽痛、癔球症、窒息感、后鼻滴涕、喉及气管狭窄、喉痉挛。GERD 也可导致牙侵蚀症。

在确定症状与 GERD 相关之前，应考虑到非 GERD 原因导致的食管外表现。但目前的诊断方法不能提供 GERD 与食管外症状间因果关系的可靠证据。PPI 在处理这些症状时也未显示出明确的治疗获益。如前所述，GERD 的诊断有助于建立这种相关性，但 GERD 存在与否不能明确它是否是食管外症状的病因。临床医生通常依靠症状相关性分析来发现反流症状与其他症状之间的时间关联性。

如果有典型的 GERD 症状，PPI 抑酸治疗仍可用于处理食管外症状。如果没有典型 GERD 症状，应考虑在 PPI 治疗前进行反流监测。外科手术一般不用于对 PPI 无反应的患者，因为现有数据显示外科手术对这些

starting a PPI trial. Surgery is not generally considered in PPI nonresponders because the available data show no benefit in patients who have surgery.

Barrett Esophagus

Barrett esophagus (BE) is defined as the presence of at least 1 cm of metaplastic columnar epithelium in the tubular esophagus and can be described as either long-segment BE (>3 cm) or short-segment BE (<3 cm). It can further be described using the Prague classification system, which uses the circumferential extent of BE and the extent of the longest visualized segment.

BE can develop from long-standing GERD. The diagnosis of GERD is associated with a 10% to 15% risk of developing Barrett esophagus. The risk factors for developing BE are chronic GERD (>5 years), age greater than 50, male gender, tobacco use, central obesity, and Caucasian race. BE can progress to dysplasia and esophageal adenocarcinoma. The risk factors for progression include advancing age, central obesity, tobacco use, and lack of NSAID, PPI, or statin use. The majority (>90%) of patients diagnosed with BE do not die of esophageal adenocarcinoma. The risk of progression from BE to cancer is determined by the amount of dysplasia (nondysplastic is 0.2% to 0.5% risk per year, low-grade dysplasia is 0.7% risk per year, high-grade dysplasia is 7% per year).

Screening for BE should be considered in men with chronic GERD (>5 years) and/or weekly symptoms of reflux who have two additional risk factors: age greater than 50 years, Caucasian, central obesity, history of smoking, or first-degree relative with BE or adenocarcinoma. Although the progression of BE to adenocarcinoma is rare in females, they should still be screened based on the presence of the aforementioned risk factors. The endoscopist should take at least eight random biopsies to maximize yield on histology to look for intestinal metaplasia. The pathology from the biopsies is confirmed by two pathologists making the diagnosis. Alternative screening modalities include balloon cytology.

BE is treated with chemoprevention, endoscopic therapy, or surgery. All patients with BE should receive once-daily PPI for chemoprevention. Endoscopic treatment is not required in the absence of dysplasia. At initial diagnosis, if nodularity is observed in the suspected segment, the patient should undergo endoscopic mucosal resection as a diagnostic and therapeutic procedure. Endoscopic ablative therapy is used in patients with low-grade and high-grade dysplasia. Ablative techniques include radiofrequency ablation and the lesser used cryotherapy. Recurrence rates appear to be similar across different ablative modalities. Endoscopic ultrasound can also be used to evaluate the depth of invasion of nodules and adenocarcinoma, guiding definitive therapy. Antireflux surgery can be used in patients with poor control of reflux symptoms on PPI.

Endoscopic surveillance is continued to monitor for stability or progression of BE. The surveillance intervals are determined by the level of dysplasia from 3 to 5 years for patients without dysplasia, to as often as every 3 months for patients with high-grade dysplasia treated endoscopically. Surveillance endoscopy will collect four-quadrant biopsies at 2-cm intervals in patients without dysplasia and 1-cm interval in patients with prior dysplasia. Any visible abnormalities are also sampled. Virtual or chemical chromoendoscopy may enhance the yield of surveillance.

MOTILITY DISORDERS

Achalasia

Achalasia is a primary esophageal motor disorder defined as aperistalsis in the esophageal body and relaxation failure of the LES resulting in increased tone in the LES. The pathophysiology of achalasia is related to the loss of inhibitory innervation in the esophagus. Primary achalasia is caused by the failure of distal inhibitory neurons (ganglion cells) in the esophageal myenteric plexus. Denervation can also occur within the extraesophageal vagus nerve or dorsal motor nucleus of the vagus. Cholinergic innervation has also been found to remain intact and

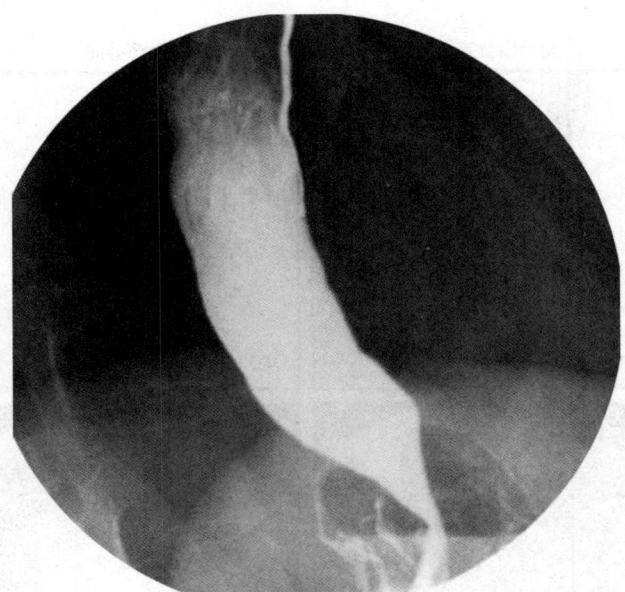

Fig. 6.5 Barium contrast radiography demonstrating narrowing at the esophagogastric junction with a bird-beak appearance and a dilated distal esophagus with retained contrast and an air-fluid level.

could possibly contribute to the increase in LES pressure. The denervation is thought to be an autoimmune process with increasing evidence, suggesting that genetic susceptibility and latent human herpes simplex virus 1 may also play a role. This is considered primary achalasia and is idiopathic by definition.

Dysphagia to solids and liquids is the classic presentation, but patients may also suffer from regurgitation, heartburn, and chest pain. Initial work-up of achalasia includes a barium swallow and/or endoscopy. A barium swallow can show esophageal dilation with a bird-beak narrowing around the gastroesophageal junction (Fig. 6.5). An endoscopy allows observation of esophageal dilation, a high-pressure LES, and the possibility of retained food in the esophagus and helps to exclude causes of secondary achalasia. The "gold standard" for the diagnosis of achalasia is high-resolution esophageal manometry. Manometry can record aperistalsis in the distal esophagus and absent LES relaxation. High-resolution manometry has defined subsets of patients with achalasia, using the Chicago Classification, who have different responses to treatment and prognoses. Type I, or classic achalasia, shows aperistalsis, incomplete or absent LES relaxation, and high resting LES pressure. Type II shows panesophageal pressurization with swallows and type III shows spastic lumen obliterating contractions of the distal esophagus with 20% or more of swallows.

The goal of treating achalasia is to promote esophageal emptying and decrease LES pressure. The initial (and most effective) treatment options include pneumatic dilation or laparoscopic surgical (Heller) myotomy. Pneumatic dilation is an endoscopic approach used to treat achalasia, involving the use of balloons to dilate the LES, theoretically breaking the fibers within. The number and the degree of dilations are determined by progression of symptom relief. Surgical (Heller) myotomy can provide a permanent solution by cutting the LES, allowing for food and liquid to pass through freely. In patients who are poor candidates for definitive therapy, endoscopy can be used to inject botulinum toxin into the gastroesophageal junction, which inhibits acetylcholine release from nerves. Acetylcholine is responsible for increased LES tone, especially when there is denervation of the inhibitory nerves. Botulinum toxin will thereby reduce the tone of the LES. If botulinum toxin therapy fails, pharmacologic therapy with nitrates and calcium-channel blockers may be considered, but the effects do not provide long-term treatment. The

患者并没有益处。

巴雷特食管

巴雷特食管（BE）被定义为食管中存在至少 1 cm 的化生性柱状上皮，可分为长段 BE（＞3 cm）和短段 BE（＜3 cm）。可应用 Prague 分类系统进一步描述，包括 BE 环周比例和最大长度。

长期 GERD 可导致 BE。诊断 GERD 后罹患 BE 的风险为 10%～15%。罹患 BE 的危险因素包括慢性 GERD（＞5 年）、年龄＞50 岁、男性、吸烟、向心性肥胖和白种人。BE 可进展为异型增生和食管腺癌。恶化的危险因素包括年龄增长、向心性肥胖、吸烟，以及未使用非甾体抗炎药（NSAID）、PPI 或他汀类药物。大多数（＞90%）被诊断为 BE 的患者不会死于食管腺癌。从 BE 发展为癌症的风险取决于异型增生的程度（无异型增生者每年风险为 0.2%～0.5%，低级别异型增生者每年风险为 0.7%，高级别异型增生者每年风险为 7%）。

对于患有慢性 GERD（＞5 年）和（或）每周出现反流症状，且至少具有以下 2 个额外危险因素（年龄＞50 岁、白种人、向心性肥胖、吸烟史、一级亲属患有 BE 或腺癌）的男性，应考虑进行 BE 筛查。虽然女性很少会从 BE 进展为腺癌，但仍应根据上述危险因素进行筛查。内镜医生应随机取至少 8 块活检组织，从而最大限度地提高组织学发现肠上皮化生的阳性率。活检的病理结果需由两名病理科医生确认后做出诊断。其他筛查方法包括气囊细胞学检查。

BE 的治疗方法包括化学预防、内镜治疗或手术。作为化学预防措施，所有 BE 患者均应接受每日 1 次的 PPI 治疗。如果没有异型增生，则无需内镜治疗。在初步诊断时，若在可疑节段观察到结节，应行内镜下黏膜切除术，以进行诊断和治疗。内镜消融治疗适用于低级别和高级别异型增生患者。消融技术包括射频消融和冷冻治疗（较少用）。不同消融方法的复发率相似。超声内镜可用于评估结节和腺癌的侵犯深度，从而指导治疗。对于服用 PPI 后反流症状控制不佳的患者，可采用抗反流手术。

应持续进行内镜监测，以评估 BE 的稳定或进展。监测的时间间隔取决于异型增生的程度，无异型增生患者的监测间隔为 3～5 年，经内镜治疗的高级别异型增生患者的监测间隔为每 3 个月 1 次。监测内镜时应收集 4 个象限的活检样本，无异型增生患者的活检间距为 2 cm，曾有异型增生患者的活检间距为 1 cm。任何可见的异常情况也应取活检。虚拟内镜或色素内镜可提高监测阳性率。

动力障碍性疾病

贲门失弛缓症

贲门失弛缓症是一种原发性食管动力障碍性疾病，其定义为食管体部蠕动消失及 LES 松弛障碍，导致 LES 张力增加。贲门失弛缓症的病理生理学与食管的抑制性神经支配缺失有关。原发性贲门失弛缓症是由远端食管肌间神经丛抑制性神经元（神经节细胞）缺失引起的。去神经支配也可发生于食管外迷走神经或迷走神经运动

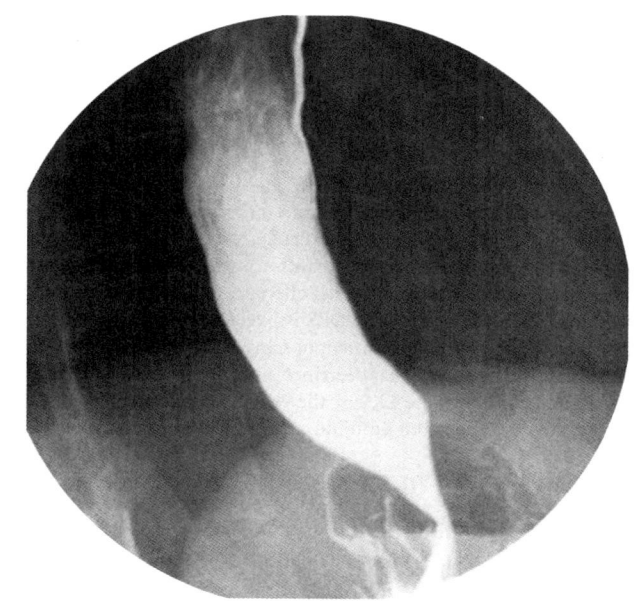

图 6.5 钡剂造影显示胃食管连接处变窄，呈鸟嘴状，远端食管扩张，并有造影剂残留和气液平

背核。胆碱能神经支配基本保持完整，且可能导致 LES 压力增加。去神经支配被认为是一种自身免疫过程，越来越多的证据表明，遗传易感性和人单纯疱疹病毒 1 潜伏性感染也可能在其中发挥作用。这被认为是原发性贲门失弛缓症，但从定义上讲是特发性的。

对固体和液体均吞咽困难是贲门失弛缓症的典型症状，但患者也可能出现反流、烧心和胸痛。贲门失弛缓症的初步检查包括钡剂造影和（或）内镜。钡剂造影可显示食管扩张，胃食管连接处周围呈鸟嘴样狭窄（图 6.5）。内镜可观察到食管扩张、LES 高压和食管内食物潴留，并有助于排除继发性贲门失弛缓症的病因。诊断贲门失弛缓症的"金标准"是高分辨率食管测压。测压可记录远端食管失蠕动和 LES 松弛缺失。通过使用芝加哥分类标准，高分辨率食管测压可进一步定义贲门失弛缓症的亚型，不同亚型的治疗反应和预后不同。Ⅰ 型（或经典型）表现为食管失蠕动、LES 松弛不全或缺失及 LES 静息压升高。Ⅱ 型表现为吞咽时全食管增压。Ⅲ 型表现为≥20% 的吞咽时远端食管呈痉挛性收缩。

贲门失弛缓症的治疗目的是促进食管排空，降低 LES 压力。初始（也是最有效的）治疗方案包括气囊扩张或腹腔镜下肌切开术（Heller 术）。气囊扩张是贲门失弛缓症的一种内镜治疗方法，即使用气囊来扩张 LES，理论上是破坏了其肌纤维。扩张的次数和程度取决于症状缓解的情况。腹腔镜下肌切开术通过切断 LES 使食物和液体顺畅通过，从而为患者提供了永久性的解决方案。对于不适合接受根治性治疗的患者，可使用内镜将肉毒杆菌毒素注射到胃食管连接处，从而抑制神经释放乙酰胆碱。乙酰胆碱可导致 LES 张力增加，尤其在抑制性神经去支配时。因此，肉毒杆菌毒素可降低 LES 张力。如果肉毒杆菌毒素治疗失败，可考虑使用硝酸盐类和钙通道阻滞剂进行药物治疗，但这些治疗的疗效不持久。最新的治疗方法是经口内镜食管下括约肌

newest approach to treatment, POEM (Per Oral Endoscopic Myotomy), uses an endoscope to tunnel below the esophageal mucosa to perform a myotomy from within, without the need for surgical incisions.

Diffuse Esophageal Spasm

Diffuse esophageal spasm (DES) is defined by uncoordinated contractions in the esophagus. Esophageal manometry provides the most specific description of the spasms. Specifically, the Chicago Classification defines DES as 20% or greater premature contractions (<4.5 seconds) with normal LES relaxation. Patients often present with dysphagia and chest pain. Similar to achalasia, DES is likely related to a decrease in inhibitory innervation. This is often observed on barium swallow.

Pharmacologic therapy has been ineffective in reliably treating DES. Pneumatic dilation of the LES or the esophageal body may alleviate some of the symptoms, but botulinum toxin is used to a better effect.

VARIANT FORMS OF ESOPHAGITIS

Eosinophilic Esophagitis

Eosinophilic esophagitis (EoE) is (likely) an allergen-mediated eosinophilic-dominant inflammation of the esophageal mucosa and is diagnosed when esophageal biopsies in symptomatic patients show 15 or greater eosinophils per high-power microscopic field. When assessing for EoE, two to four esophageal biopsies should be taken from the proximal and distal esophagus. Endoscopy can visualize fixed esophageal rings in the lumen, which are characteristic, but not diagnostic, of EoE. These rings are often referred to as trachealization of the esophagus. Other features include white eosinophilic exudates, longitudinal furrows, edema, diffuse esophageal narrowing, strictures, and lacerations secondary to the endoscope.

When EoE is diagnosed, a PPI response should be tested. Following an 8-week PPI trial, a repeat endoscopy and biopsy should be performed. If symptoms and eosinophilia have resolved then PPI-responsive esophageal eosinophilia (PPI-REE) is diagnosed. PPI-REE may be associated with GERD. If symptoms and eosinophilia persist, then EoE is diagnosed.

The goal of treatment for EoE is improvement in symptoms and decrease in esophageal inflammation. The first-line pharmacologic therapy is 8 weeks of swallowed topical corticosteroids (fluticasone or budesonide). If symptoms do not improve or rapid improvement is needed, then systemic corticosteroids (i.e., prednisone) can be used. Conversely, a specific elimination diet can also be used as initial therapy prior to the administration of topical corticosteroids. When medical and dietary therapy fail, then esophageal dilation is considered in patients with strictures.

Pill-Induced Esophagitis

Pill-induced esophagitis results in direct esophageal mucosal injury due to a pill. Patients will complain of heartburn, chest pain, odynophagia, and dysphagia. Common medications that can cause this include: tetracycline, doxycycline, clindamycin, aspirin, nonsteroidal anti-inflammatory drugs (NSAIDs), bisphosphonates, potassium chloride, quinidine preparations, iron compounds, emepronium, alprenolol, and pinaverium.

Complications include stricture, esophageal hemorrhage, and perforation. Cessation of the offending agent is often enough to treat the condition with eventual mucosal healing.

ESOPHAGEAL INFECTIONS

Infections of the esophagus are rare in immunocompetent patients. Immunocompromised individuals are typically affected, including patients on immunosuppressive medications, chemotherapy, and patients suffering from AIDS. In patients with AIDS, infectious esophagitis is more prevalent as the CD4 count declines, especially with counts below 100. The most common symptom of infectious esophagitis is odynophagia often associated with dysphagia, chest pain, and gastrointestinal bleeding. Coinfection is common and treatment is targeted by etiology. Maintenance suppressive therapy with antifungal or antiviral agents may need to be initiated in patients with AIDS.

The most common cause of infectious esophagitis is *Candida*. It typically presents with dysphagia and odynophagia, but oral thrush in patients has a high positive predictive value for esophageal candidiasis. On endoscopy, friable white patches overlying the mucosa are visualized and fungal hyphal forms are seen on histology. Patients are typically treated successfully with oral fluconazole whereas intravenous fluconazole or an echinocandin is used in patients unable to tolerate oral therapy.

Cytomegalovirus (CMV) esophagitis occurs in severely immunocompromised patients. These patients present almost identically to patients with candida esophagitis except without oropharyngeal thrush. Endoscopy reveals large (>10 cm), shallow ulcers in the middle to distal parts of the esophagus. The margins are distinct and the ulcers are often described as "punched-out." Histopathologic examination of mucosal and submucosal biopsies from the ulcer edges and bases can accurately diagnose CMV esophagitis. Histology will reveal large endothelial cells or fibroblasts with large, dense inclusion bodies. CMV esophagitis is treated with intravenous ganciclovir, foscarnet (intravenous) or valganciclovir (intravenous or oral).

Another cause of infectious esophagitis is herpes simplex virus (HSV). HSV-1 is typically the offending strain, but HSV-2 can also be a cause. HSV esophagitis is often seen in immunosuppressed individuals but can affect healthy adults. The endoscopic appearance of HSV esophagitis is multiple, small, superficial ulcers in the distal esophagus. More advanced or aggressive infections can reveal large confluent ulcers, pseudomembranous or denuded epithelium. Viral cultures can grow HSV-1 and occasionally HSV-2. The quantitative polymerase chain reaction for HSV-1 has a high sensitivity when tested in biopsy samples. Histopathologic examination reveals large intranuclear Cowdry type-A inclusion bodies along with ballooning degeneration and multinucleated giant cells. HSV esophagitis is treated with acyclovir (oral or intravenous) or valacyclovir (oral).

ESOPHAGEAL TRAUMA AND EMERGENCIES

Perforation of the Esophagus

Perforation of the esophagus can be due to numerous etiologies. The most common cause is iatrogenic but can occur due to trauma, caustic injury, malignancy, or severe vomiting. Iatrogenic perforation is often related to instrumentation from endoscopy, nasogastric tube insertion, intubation, or dilation. Boerhaave syndrome describes the spontaneous rupture of the esophagus following severe vomiting.

The most common presenting symptom is pain, which can vary depending on location of the perforation. Patients may also present with symptoms of shock or systemic infection. A physical exam can reveal palpable crepitus in the neck or chest related to subcutaneous emphysema.

Esophageal perforation should be diagnosed and treated promptly. A chest radiograph can suggest perforation by revealing mediastinal air, pleural effusion, pneumothorax, and subdiaphragmatic air. The diagnosis can be confirmed with computed tomography, Gastrografin imaging or emergency endoscopy.

The treatment of esophageal perforation starts with adequate resuscitation and early antibiotics, if needed. The perforation can be

切开术（POEM），即在内镜下通过食管黏膜下隧道技术从内部进行肌切开，无须做外科手术切口。

弥漫性食管痉挛

弥漫性食管痉挛（DES）是指食管不协调性痉挛收缩。食管测压可对这种痉挛收缩提供最具体的描述。具体来说，芝加哥分类将 DES 定义为过早收缩（< 4.5 s）≥ 20%，而 LES 松弛正常。患者常表现为吞咽困难和胸痛。与贲门失弛缓症类似，DES 可能与抑制性神经支配减少有关。DES 常在钡剂造影时被发现。

药物治疗 DES 的效果不佳。使用气囊扩张 LES 或食管体部可缓解部分症状，但使用肉毒杆菌毒素效果相对更好。

特殊类型食管炎

嗜酸细胞性食管炎

嗜酸细胞性食管炎（EoE）是一种由过敏原介导的以嗜酸性粒细胞增多为主的食管黏膜炎症，当症状性患者的食管活检结果显示嗜酸性粒细胞数量 ≥ 15 个/高倍镜视野时，即可诊断 EoE。在评估 EoE 时，应从食管近端和远端各取 2 ~ 4 块活检样本。内镜可在管腔内观察到固定的食管环，这是 EoE 的特征，但不能作为诊断依据。这些食管环常被称为食管气管化。其他特征包括白色嗜酸细胞性渗出物、纵向裂痕、水肿、弥漫性食管变窄、狭窄和继发于内镜检查的撕裂伤。

诊断 EoE 后，应观察患者对 PPI 的治疗反应。予以 8 周的 PPI 试验性治疗后，应再次进行内镜检查和活检。如果症状和嗜酸性粒细胞增多均得到缓解，则可诊断为对 PPI 有反应的食管嗜酸性粒细胞增多症（PPI-REE）。PPI-REE 可能与 GERD 有关。如果症状和嗜酸性粒细胞增多持续存在，则诊断为 EoE。

EoE 的治疗目标是改善症状和减轻食管炎症。一线药物治疗是吞服局部用皮质类固醇（氟替卡松或布地奈德）8 周。如果症状无改善或需要快速改善症状，可使用全身性皮质类固醇（如泼尼松）。相反，在使用局部用皮质类固醇前，特定的饮食剔除也可作为初始治疗措施。当药物和饮食治疗失败后，则考虑对合并狭窄的患者行食管扩张治疗。

药片引起的食管炎

药片引起的食管炎由药片直接损伤食管黏膜所致。患者常主诉烧心、胸痛、吞咽疼痛和吞咽困难。可引起这种食管炎的常见药物包括：四环素、多西环素、克林霉素、NSAID（如阿司匹林）、双膦酸盐、氯化钾、奎尼丁制剂、铁化合物、依美溴铵、阿普洛尔和匹维溴铵。

并发症包括食管狭窄、出血和穿孔。停用致病药物通常足以达到治疗目的，最终使食管黏膜愈合。

食管感染

食管感染在免疫功能正常的患者中很少出现。免疫功能低下人群可出现食管感染，包括接受免疫抑制治疗、化疗的患者及艾滋病患者。在艾滋病患者中，感染性食管炎的发病率随 CD4 细胞计数下降（尤其是计数 < 100 时）而升高。感染性食管炎最常见的症状是吞咽疼痛，常伴有吞咽困难、胸痛和消化道出血。多重感染很常见，治疗需针对病因。艾滋病患者可能需要使用抗真菌或抗病毒药物进行维持抑制治疗。

感染性食管炎最常见的病因是念珠菌感染。典型症状为吞咽困难和吞咽疼痛，鹅口疮对食管念珠菌病的阳性预测值较高。内镜可见黏膜上覆盖易碎的白色斑块，组织学检查可见真菌菌丝。患者通常可通过口服氟康唑成功治疗，无法耐受口服治疗的患者可静脉注射氟康唑或棘白菌素治疗。

巨细胞病毒（CMV）食管炎多发生于严重免疫功能低下的患者。患者的表现与念珠菌性食管炎患者几乎相同，只是没有口咽部鹅口疮。内镜可见食管中段至远段有大范围（> 10 cm）浅溃疡，溃疡边界清晰，通常被描述为"穿凿样"。于溃疡边缘和底部取黏膜及黏膜下活检样本进行组织病理学检查可确诊 CMV 食管炎。组织学检查可发现大的内皮细胞或具有大而致密包涵体的成纤维细胞。CMV 食管炎可通过更昔洛韦（静脉注射）、膦甲酸（静脉注射）、缬更昔洛韦（静脉注射或口服）治疗。

感染性食管炎的另一个病因是单纯疱疹病毒（HSV）。HSV-1 是典型的致病病毒，HSV-2 也可能是病因之一。HSV 食管炎常见于免疫抑制患者，但也可能累及健康成人。HSV 食管炎的内镜表现为远端食管多发浅小溃疡。严重或侵袭性感染可出现大片融合性溃疡、假膜或上皮剥脱。病毒培养可培养出 HSV-1，偶尔也可培养出 HSV-2。定量聚合酶链反应（qPCR）检测活检样本中的 HSV-1 的敏感性很高。组织病理学检查可显示大的核内 Cowdry A 型包涵体，以及气球样变性和多核巨细胞。HSV 食管炎的治疗方法是阿昔洛韦（口服或静脉注射）或伐昔洛韦（口服）。

食管创伤和急症

食管穿孔

食管穿孔可由多种病因引起。最常见的原因是医源性穿孔，但也可能由创伤、腐蚀性损伤、恶性肿瘤或严重呕吐引起。医源性穿孔通常与内镜检查、鼻胃管置入、插管或使用扩张器械有关。Boerhaave 综合征是指严重呕吐后食管自发性破裂。

食管穿孔最常见的症状是疼痛，疼痛程度因穿孔部位而异。患者还可出现休克或全身感染症状。体格检查可在颈部或胸部触及与皮下气肿相关的"握雪感"。

食管穿孔应及时诊断、及时治疗。胸部 X 线检查可提示穿孔，表现为纵隔积气、胸腔积液、气胸和膈下气体。可通过 CT、泛影葡胺造影或急诊内镜确诊。

食管穿孔的治疗首先应进行充分的液体复苏，必要时尽早使用抗生素。穿孔可通过手术或内镜修复。

repaired surgically or by endoscope. Surgery is indicated in unstable patients or patients with abdominal esophageal perforations. An endoscope can be used to place stents or clips. Perforations can be treated conservatively as well with medical management. This includes no oral intake for at least 7 days, parenteral nutrition, empiric antibiotics (consider antifungals), and management of complications (i.e., drainage of abscesses).

Foreign Bodies and Food Impaction

Ingestion of foreign bodies can be accidental or intentional. Symptoms depends on the object's size, shape, consistency, and location, but some patients will remain asymptomatic. Food can also become lodged in the esophagus and present with similar symptoms to foreign bodies. Food impaction is normally the result of an underlying disease process including peptic stricture, Schatzki ring, EoE, or malignancy.

Foreign bodies and food can result in complete obstruction of the esophagus. Patients will present with inability to handle secretions and severe chest pain. If the obstruction does not resolve spontaneously, emergent endoscopy is often required to resolve the obstruction. Occasionally, glucagon can be administered intravenously when food impaction is suspected prior to endoscopic intervention. Glucagon relaxes the LES and esophageal smooth muscle allowing for spontaneous passage of the bolus.

Mallory-Weiss Tear

A Mallory-Weiss tear is a mucosal or submucosal tear near the gastroesophageal junction. It results from anything that may cause a rapid increase in intra-abdominal pressure and gastric herniation. It is most often described in the setting of retching or vomiting but can also occur as a result of increased strain or forceful coughing.

Patients present with hematemesis and/or melena. They will often report excessive retching or vomiting, but the tear can also occur without this history. Endoscopy is used to diagnose a tear and rule out other causes of an upper gastrointestinal bleed.

Supportive therapy involves treating the underlying disorder and reducing instances of vomiting and retching. A Mallory-Weiss tear can be massive but is rarely fatal. Endoscopic therapies for ongoing bleeding include use of epinephrine, which can be injected locally to reduce bleeding. Cauterization, clipping, and ligation can also be used to control the site of bleeding. Patients with persistent bleeding may undergo angiographic intervention or, in rare instances, surgical intervention.

SYSTEMIC AND OTHER ILLNESSES

Scleroderma

Progressive systemic sclerosis can affect any part of the gastrointestinal tract, but more often involves the esophagus. The progressive loss of smooth muscle, collagen deposition, and fibrosis in the esophageal wall can cause reduced or absent peristalsis, GERD, and a patulous LES. Manometry is used to diagnose the esophageal disease, whereas endoscopy can be used to evaluate for complications.

Dermatologic Disorders

A wide variety of dermatologic disorders can affect the esophagus. These disorders include pemphigus vulgaris, bullous pemphigoid, erythema multiforme, Behçet's syndrome, lichen planus, dermatitis herpetiformis, and toxic epidermolysis necrosis/Stevens-Johnson syndrome. The treatment of the underlying disorder is most effective in treating the esophageal involvement and often involves glucocorticoids.

SUGGESTED READINGS

Ajani JA, D'Amico TA, Bentrem DJ, et al: Esophageal and esophagogastric junction cancers, version 2.2019, NCCN clinical practice guidelines in oncology, J Natl Compr Canc Netw 17(7):855–883, 2019.

Dellon ES, Gonsalves N, Hirano I, et al: ACG clinical guideline: evidenced based approach to the diagnosis and management of esophageal eosinophilia and eosinophilic esophagitis (EoE), Am J Gastroenterol 108(5):679–692, 2013.

Kahrilas PJ, Bredenoord AJ, Fox M, et al: The Chicago Classification of esophageal motility disorders, v3.0, Neurogastroenterol Motil 27(2):160–174, 2015.

Shaheen NJ, Falk GW, Iyer PG, Gerson LB, American College of Gastroenterology: ACG clinical guideline: diagnosis and management of Barrett's esophagus, Am J Gastroenterol 111(1):30–50, 2016.

Vakil N, van Zenten SV, Kahrilas P, et al: The Montreal definition and classification of gastroesophageal reflux disease: a global evidence-based consensus, Am J Gastroenterol 101(8):1900–1920, 2006; quiz 1943.

手术适用于病情不稳定或腹腔段食管穿孔的患者。内镜下可放置支架或缝合夹。穿孔也可通过药物保守治疗，包括避免经口摄入至少 7 天、肠外营养、经验性抗生素（可考虑抗真菌药物）和处理并发症（即脓肿引流）。

异物和食物嵌顿

吞入异物可能是意外的或故意的。症状取决于异物的大小、形状、稠度和位置，但有些患者可能没有症状。食物可能卡在食管内，出现类似食管异物的症状。食物嵌顿通常由潜在疾病引起，包括消化性狭窄、Schatzki 环、EoE 或恶性肿瘤。

异物和食物可导致食管完全梗阻。患者会出现无法处理分泌物和严重胸痛。如果梗阻不能自行缓解，通常需要急诊内镜来解决梗阻。如果怀疑食物嵌顿，有时可在内镜干预前静脉注射胰高血糖素。胰高血糖素可以松弛 LES，使食团自行通过。

Mallory-Weiss 撕裂

Mallory-Weiss 撕裂是胃食管连接处附近的黏膜或黏膜下层撕裂。任何可能导致腹内压快速升高和胃疝的因素均可造成 Mallory-Weiss 撕裂。最常在干呕或呕吐时发生，也可能在用力骤增或剧烈咳嗽时发生。

患者表现为呕血和（或）黑便。患者常报告用力干呕或呕吐，但撕裂也可能在没有相关病史的情况下发生。内镜可用于诊断 Mallory-Weiss 撕裂，并排除上消化道出血的其他原因。

支持治疗包括处理潜在疾病、减轻呕吐和干呕的情况。Mallory-Weiss 撕裂可以很严重，但很少致死。内镜下治疗活动性出血的方法包括局部注射肾上腺素，以减轻出血。出血部位的电灼、夹闭和套扎治疗也可用于止血。持续出血的患者可能需要血管造影介入治疗，极少数情况下需要接受手术干预。

系统性疾病和其他疾病

硬皮病

进行性系统性硬化症可累及胃肠道的任何部位，但最常累及食管。食管壁平滑肌的进行性丧失、胶原沉积和纤维化可导致食管蠕动减少或消失、GERD 和 LES 开放。食管测压可用于诊断食管的疾病状态，内镜可用于评估并发症。

皮肤病

多种皮肤病可影响食管，包括寻常型天疱疮、大疱性类天疱疮、多形性红斑、白塞综合征、扁平苔藓、疱疹样皮炎和中毒性表皮松解坏死/Stevens-Johnson 综合征。处理食管受累最有效的方法是治疗原发病，通常需要使用糖皮质激素。

推荐阅读

Ajani JA, D'Amico TA, Bentrem DJ, et al: Esophageal and esophagogastric junction cancers, version 2.2019, NCCN clinical practice guidelines in oncology, J Natl Compr Canc Netw 17(7):855–883, 2019.

Dellon ES, Gonsalves N, Hirano I, et al: ACG clinical guideline: evidenced based approach to the diagnosis and management of esophageal eosinophilia and eosinophilic esophagitis (EoE), Am J Gastroenterol 108(5):679–692, 2013.

Kahrilas PJ, Bredenoord AJ, Fox M, et al: The Chicago Classification of esophageal motility disorders, v3.0, Neurogastroenterol Motil 27(2):160–174, 2015.

Shaheen NJ, Falk GW, Iyer PG, Gerson LB, American College of Gastroenterology: ACG clinical guideline: diagnosis and management of Barrett's esophagus, Am J Gastroenterol 111(1):30–50, 2016.

Vakil N, van Zenten SV, Kahrilas P, et al: The Montreal definition and classification of gastroesophageal reflux disease: a global evidence-based consensus, Am J Gastroenterol 101(8):1900–1920, 2006; quiz 1943.

7

Diseases of the Stomach and Duodenum

Alma M. Guerrero Bready, Akwi W. Asombang, Steven F. Moss

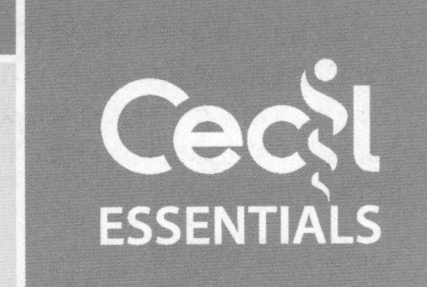

INTRODUCTION

The process of digestion begins in the mouth, with mastication. The ingested food bolus is then propelled into the esophagus, passes through the lower esophageal sphincter (LES), and enters the stomach. The stomach can hold between 1.5 and 2 L of food, which allows for intermittent feeding. While in the stomach, food is further broken down through a series of chemical and mechanical reactions into smaller particles (chyme) that travel through the pyloric channel into the beginning of the small intestine, the duodenum. This chapter reviews the normal anatomy and physiology of the stomach and duodenum and discusses the most common disease processes affecting these two organs.

ANATOMY

Anatomy of the Stomach

The stomach is a hollow organ with a superior dome-like structure on the lateral aspect (the fundus) (Fig. 7.1). The outer edge along the dome and down to the end of the stomach is called the greater curvature. On the other side is the lesser curvature. The stomach is made up of four parts: the cardia, fundus, corpus, and the pylorus. The stomach is connected proximally to the distal esophagus by the LES, a circular smooth muscle structure under parasympathetic and sympathetic control. The LES acts as a valve to prevent gastric contents from traveling in a retrograde fashion into the esophagus, thus preventing gastroesophageal reflux. The most proximal region of the stomach is the cardia, which is the area between the LES and the fundus. Below the fundus is the gastric body (also known as the corpus), which has characteristic longitudinal folds or ridges (rugae). This gastric body is where food is mainly mixed and broken down. Below a prominent circular fold (the *angulus incisura*), is the antrum, which leads into the pyloric channel. The antrum holds food until it is ready to be released through the pylorus (a circular structure made up of smooth muscle) into the duodenum. A hiatal hernia occurs when part of the stomach is pushed upward through a weakness in the diaphragm into the chest.

The stomach is innervated and controlled by both the sympathetic nervous system, via the celiac plexus, and by the parasympathetic nervous system, which is supplied by the anterior and posterior trunks of the vagus nerve. The arterial supply for the stomach originates from the celiac trunk.

Anatomy of the Duodenum

Immediately past the pylorus, the duodenum bends posteriorly to become a retroperitoneal structure and curves around the head of the pancreas in a C-shape and then re-emerges into the peritoneal cavity to join the second portion of the small intestine, the jejunum (see Fig. 7.1). The duodenum can be divided into four parts: superior (first part, or bulb), descending (second part), horizontal (third part), and ascending (fourth part). Within the descending duodenum is the ampulla of Vater, where the biliary system and the pancreatic duct unite to drain their secretions into the duodenum via the major duodenal papilla.

Similar to the stomach and the rest of the digestive tract, the duodenum is innervated by both the parasympathetic and sympathetic nervous system. The blood supply to the first half of the duodenum is from projections of the celiac trunk and to the second half of the duodenum by the superior mesenteric artery. It is this transition point that demarcates the progression from foregut to midgut.

HISTOLOGY

Histology of the Stomach

The walls of the stomach and duodenum, like the rest of the digestive system, are composed of four layers: the mucosa, submucosa, muscularis externa, and serosa. In the stomach, the mucosa is formed by a layer of simple columnar epithelial cells that invaginate to create gastric pits. These extend into millions of gastric glands that secrete gastric acid and other products. The depth and function of the gastric pits and glands differ between the various regions of the stomach. Below the mucosa is the submucosa, which houses dense connective tissue and lymphocytes, plasma cells, arterioles, venules, lymphatics, and the submucosal plexus (Meissner plexus). Deeper to this layer is the muscularis externa, which provides the contractions needed for the stomach to churn chyme. This muscle layer contains the inner oblique, middle circular, and outer longitudinal smooth muscle layers. In addition, it contains the myenteric neural plexus (Auerbach plexus). The outermost layer of the stomach is a continuation of the visceral peritoneum called the serosa.

Histology of the Duodenum

The duodenal wall is also comprised of the mucosa, submucosa, muscularis externa, and serosa. However, in the case of the duodenum, the epithelial cells contain microvilli and are arranged such that the surface of the duodenum has projections of epithelial cells called villi that are flanked by intestinal glands, called crypts of Lieberkühn. Villi and microvilli serve to increase the absorptive surface of the duodenum. In addition to its primarily absorptive function, the submucosa of the duodenum contains Brunner glands, which secrete an acid-neutralizing solution that protects the rest of the digestive tract from the effects of the acidic gastric juices.

胃和十二指肠疾病

黄志寅 译　刘苓 陈倩 审校　房静远 通审

引言

消化过程从口腔的咀嚼开始。摄入的食物随后进入食管，通过食管下括约肌（LES）进入胃。胃可容纳 1.5～2 L 的食物，并保证间歇性推送食物。食物在胃内经过一系列化学和机械反应被进一步分解成更小的颗粒（食糜），然后通过幽门进入小肠的起始部分——十二指肠。本章回顾了胃和十二指肠的正常解剖学和生理学，并讨论影响这两个器官的常见疾病。

解剖学

胃的解剖学

胃是一个中空的器官，侧上方的穹顶样结构被称为胃底（图 7.1）。沿穹顶至胃末端的外侧缘被称为大弯，另一侧为小弯。胃由 4 个部分组成：贲门、胃底、胃体和幽门。胃通过 LES 与食管远端相连。LES 是由副交感神经和交感神经支配的环形平滑肌结构，具有避免胃内容物反流进入食管的阀门作用，从而防止胃食管反流。胃的最上端是贲门，位于 LES 和胃底之间。胃底下方是胃的主体（即胃体），具有特征性的纵向皱襞。食物在胃体中主要被混合和分解。胃内突出的环形皱襞被称为胃角，下方通向胃窦和幽门。食物在胃窦储存一段时间后通过幽门（平滑肌组成的环形结构）进入十二指肠。当胃的一部分通过膈肌的薄弱处向上进入胸腔时，会形成食管裂孔疝。

胃由交感神经系统和副交感神经系统支配，交感神经通过腹腔丛分布于胃，副交感神经来自迷走神经前后干。胃的动脉供应起源于腹腔干。

十二指肠的解剖学

十二指肠在幽门以远，先向后弯曲成为腹膜后结构，呈 C 形围绕胰头，然后再次进入腹腔，与小肠的第二部分（空肠）相连（图 7.1）。十二指肠分为 4 个部分：上部（第一部分，又称球部）、降部（第二部分）、水平部（第三部分）和升部（第四部分）。十二指肠降部内有肝胰壶腹（Vater 壶腹），胆道系统和胰管在此汇合，其分泌物经十二指肠大乳头排入十二指肠。

与胃和消化道的其他部分相似，十二指肠由副交感神经和交感神经系统共同支配。十二指肠前半部分的血供来自腹腔干的分支，后半部分的血供来自肠系膜上动脉。该交界点标志着从前肠到中肠的过渡。

组织学

胃的组织学

与消化系统的其他部位类似，胃壁和十二指肠壁由 4 层组成：黏膜层、黏膜下层、外肌层和浆膜层。胃黏膜层由单层柱状上皮细胞构成，这层细胞内陷形成胃小凹，延伸成数百万个分泌胃酸和其他产物的胃腺。胃小凹和腺体的深度和功能在胃的不同区域有所不同。黏膜层的下方是黏膜下层，包含致密结缔组织和淋巴细胞、浆细胞、小动脉、小静脉、淋巴管及黏膜下神经丛（Meissner 神经丛）。其下是外肌层，提供胃搅拌食糜所需的收缩力。此肌层包含内斜行、中环行和外纵行三层平滑肌。此外，它还包含肌间神经丛（Auerbach 神经丛）。胃的最外层是脏腹膜的延续，即浆膜层。

十二指肠的组织学

十二指肠壁同样由黏膜层、黏膜下层、外肌层和浆膜层组成。然而，在十二指肠中，上皮细胞含有微绒毛，其排列方式使十二指肠表面有上皮细胞突起（绒毛），两侧有小肠腺（利伯屈恩隐窝）。绒毛和微绒毛有助于增加十二指肠的吸收面积。十二指肠的主要功能是吸收，此外，十二指肠的黏膜下层还包含布伦纳腺（Brunner 腺），该腺体分泌的液体能够中和胃酸，保护消化道的其他部分免受胃酸的影响。

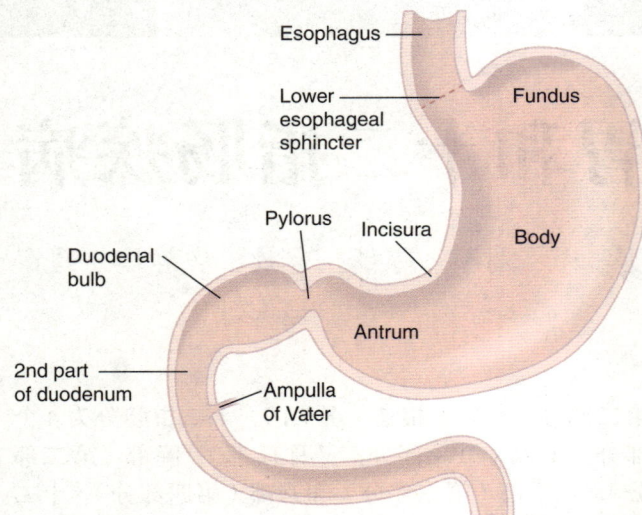

Fig. 7.1 Normal gastroduodenal anatomy.

GASTRODUODENAL SECRETIONS

Gastric secretions are responsible for breaking down food macromolecules into nutrients that can be absorbed in the gut. Gastric secretions are finely coordinated in a sophisticated system of feedback loops that ensure the balance between an acidic environment to break down food (created by parietal cells secreting hydrochloric acid) and a protective environment that defends the integrity of the gastric lumen. The latter is achieved by secretion of a bicarbonate-rich water/electrolyte/mucus solution from surface mucosal cells that buffers the gastric acid, to prevent autodigestion of the gastric epithelial cells and glands. Gastric secretions also function to protect the digestive tract from pathogenic microorganisms and aid in the absorption of calcium, iron, and vitamin B_{12}.

Parietal Cells
Acid Secretion
Gastric juice is primarily made up of hydrochloric acid (HCl), which is secreted by parietal cells at a concentration of 160 mmol/L. Parietal cells are mostly located in the gastric fundus and body, and they are stimulated to release HCl through three major pathways.

Histamine is released by specialized neuroendocrine cells called enterochromaffin-like (ECL) cells, and it is the major stimulant of H+ ion secretion. Histamine acts on H2 receptors, to activate adenylate cyclase leading to increased level of intracellular cAMP. This results in activation of the proton pumps (H+, K+-ATPases), located on the apical surface of the cell, to promote the release of HCl into the gastric lumen (Fig. 7.2).

Acetylcholine (Ach), which is released from nerve endings following vagal stimulation, also promotes acid secretion by acting on the M3 receptor on the basal aspect of parietal cells This increases intracellular Ca++, which also stimulates acid release into the stomach lumen via the apical proton pump (see Fig. 7.2).

Gastrin promotes acid release in two distinct ways (see Fig. 7.2). Gastrin is released from G cells in the antrum in response to food (especially protein) and also in response to the neural release of gastrin-related peptide, stimulated by gastric distension. Gastrin circulates in the bloodstream and may directly bind CCK2/gastrin receptors in parietal cells, stimulating the release of H+. Of greater functional consequence during feeding, gastrin also stimulates acid secretion indirectly by binding similar CCK2/gastrin receptors in ECL cells to

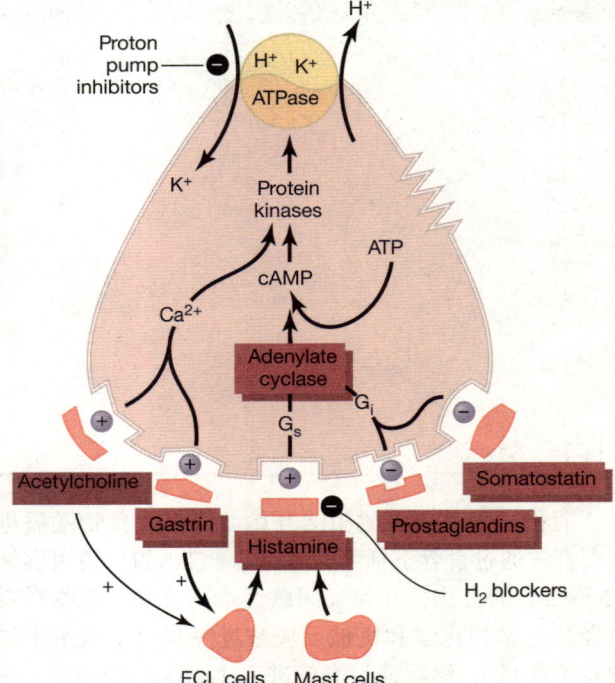

Fig. 7.2 Stimuli and mechanisms of gastric acid secretion by the parietal cell.

promote the release of histamine, which in turn acts on H2 receptors on parietal cells, as previously mentioned.

Acid secretion is inhibited by somatostatin, which is released by D cells in the gastric antrum and fundus. D cells are stimulated to secrete somatostatin when there is a high concentration of H+ ions in the gastric lumen, and they are inhibited by ACh. Somatostatin inhibits acid secretion by decreasing cAMP levels in parietal cells and by inhibiting gastrin release from G cells (see Fig. 7.2).

Intrinsic Factor
In addition to being the key cell for acid secretion, parietal cells also secrete intrinsic factor, a glycoprotein that plays a critical role in vitamin B_{12} absorption. Intrinsic factor is released from parietal cells under the same stimuli as H+ ions and binds vitamin B_{12} in the alkaline environment of the duodenum. This binding ultimately enables vitamin B_{12} absorption via specific receptors in the terminal ileum.

Chief Cells
Chief cells are zymogenic cells located deep in the gastric pits that secrete the pro-enzyme pepsinogen. Pepsinogen is converted into the active form, pepsin, under the acidic conditions created by gastric juices. Pepsin aids in digestion by breaking down proteins into peptides and amino acids, which, as mentioned above, aid in the release of gastrin as well as CCK.

Protective Factors
Gastroduodenal cells are at a high risk for damage given the very low pH of gastric juices, but these cells are well protected by several mechanisms that prevent autodigestion. The first line of defense is a mucosal barrier that consists of a thick, alkaline, aqueous mucus and HCO_3^--rich fluid that serves to lubricate the mucosa and neutralize acid at the epithelial level. This mucus is secreted in the stomach by mucus-producing cells located at the neck of gastric pits and in the

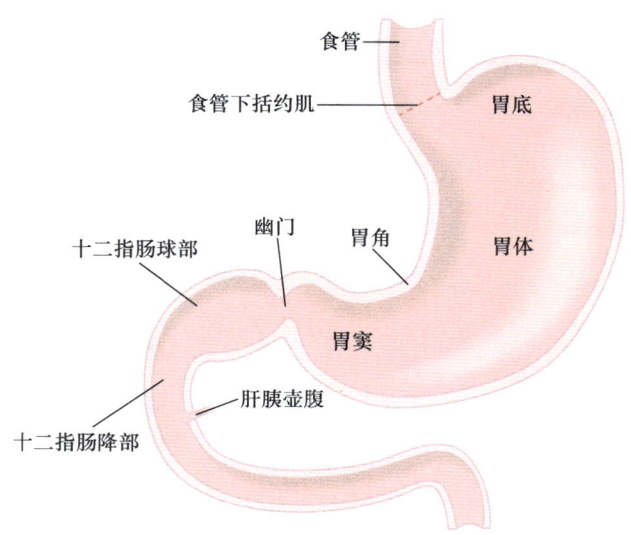

图 7.1　正常胃十二指肠解剖

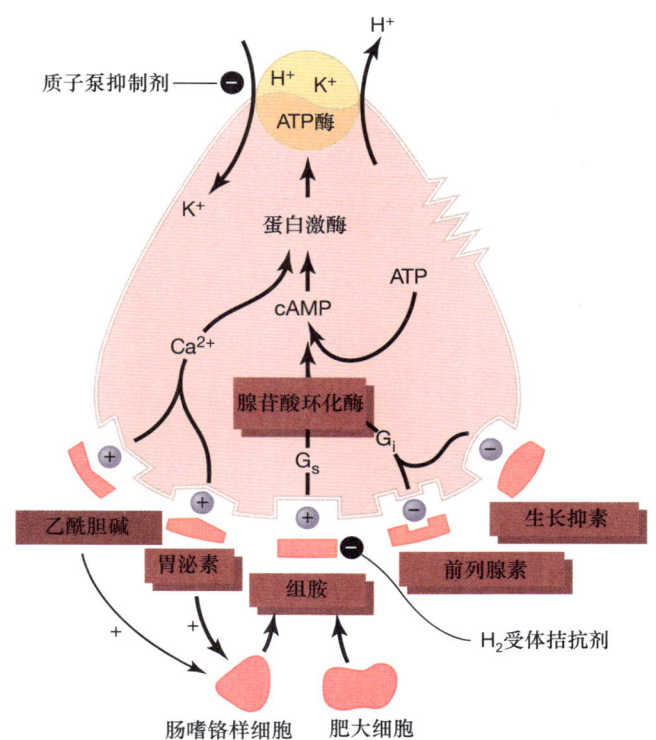

图 7.2　壁细胞胃酸分泌的刺激因素及机制

胃十二指肠的分泌

胃液将食物大分子分解成肠道可吸收的营养物质。胃液分泌受复杂反馈回路系统的精细调控，以确保在分解食物的酸性环境（由壁细胞分泌的盐酸形成）和保护胃腔完整性的环境之间保持平衡。后者通过表面黏液细胞分泌富含碳酸氢盐（HCO_3^-）的水/电解质/黏液溶液来实现，该溶液缓冲胃酸，防止胃上皮细胞和腺体的自身消化。胃液还具有保护消化道免受致病微生物侵害的功能，并促进钙、铁和维生素 B_{12} 的吸收。

壁细胞

胃酸分泌

胃液主要由盐酸（HCl）组成，其浓度为 160 mmol/L，由壁细胞分泌。壁细胞主要位于胃底和胃体，主要通过三种途径调节 HCl 的释放。

组胺由一种特殊的神经内分泌细胞肠嗜铬样细胞（ECL）释放，是氢离子（H^+）分泌的主要刺激物。组胺作用于 H_2 受体，激活腺苷酸环化酶，导致细胞内 cAMP 水平升高，继而激活位于细胞顶端表面的质子泵（H^+-K^+ ATP 酶），促进 HCl 释放到胃腔（图 7.2）。

乙酰胆碱由迷走神经受刺激后从神经末梢释放，通过作用于壁细胞基底部的 M_3 受体促进胃酸分泌。这会增加细胞内的钙离子（Ca^{2+}）浓度，通过顶端质子泵刺激胃酸分泌进入胃腔（图 7.2）。

胃泌素可通过两种方式促进胃酸分泌（图 7.2）。胃窦的 G 细胞在食物（特别是蛋白质）和胃泌素相关多肽（胃扩张引起的神经释放）的刺激下释放胃泌素。胃泌素可在血液中循环并直接与壁细胞中的缩胆囊素（CCK）2/胃泌素受体结合，刺激 H^+ 的释放。在进食过程中，胃泌素还可通过与 ECL 细胞中的 CCK2/胃泌素受体结合而促进组胺的释放，组胺作用于壁细胞上的 H_2 受体，间接刺激胃酸分泌，从而产生更大的功能性影响。

胃酸分泌受生长抑素的抑制，生长抑素由胃窦和胃底的 D 细胞释放。当胃腔中 H^+ 浓度较高时，D 细胞分泌生长抑素，而乙酰胆碱可抑制生长抑素分泌。生长抑素通过降低壁细胞内 cAMP 水平和抑制 G 细胞释放胃泌素来抑制胃酸分泌（图 7.2）。

内因子

除了作为胃酸分泌的关键细胞外，壁细胞还可分泌内因子，内因子是一种在维生素 B_{12} 吸收中发挥关键作用的糖蛋白。刺激壁细胞释放内因子的因素与刺激壁细胞释放 H^+ 的因素相同。内因子在十二指肠的碱性环境中与维生素 B_{12} 结合。结合后的维生素 B_{12} 最终通过回肠末端的特定受体被吸收。

主细胞

主细胞是位于胃小凹深处的酶原细胞，可分泌胃蛋白酶原。在胃液形成的酸性条件下，胃蛋白酶原被转化为其活性形式——胃蛋白酶。胃蛋白酶通过将蛋白质分解成多肽和氨基酸来帮助消化，进而有助于胃泌素和 CCK 的释放。

保护因素

由于胃液的 pH 值非常低，胃和十二指肠细胞受损的风险高，但这些细胞可通过多种保护机制防止自身消化。第一道防线是黏膜屏障，其由黏稠的碱性水性黏液和富含 HCO_3^- 的液体组成，能够润滑黏膜并中和上

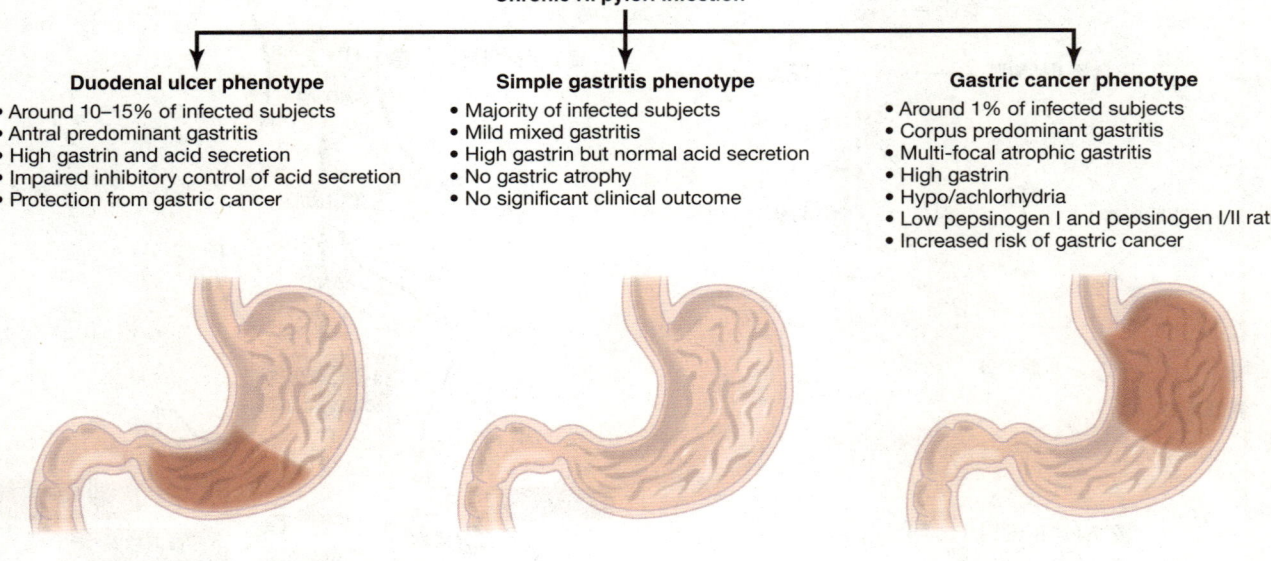

Fig. 7.3 Diverse pathologic and clinical consequences of *H. pylori*. Acid secretory status and ultimately clinical outcome are dependent upon the extent and degree of gastric inflammation in response to *H. pylori* infection. (From Amieva MR, El-Omar EM. Host-bacterial interactions in *Helicobacter pylori* infection. Gastroenterology. 2008;134:306-23.)

duodenum by mucus-producing goblet cells. Additionally, the lipid bilayer and tight junctions of the apical epithelial cell membranes serve to protect the mucosa from H+ ions diffusing into the stomach wall, thus preserving mucosal integrity. A rich submucosal blood supply enables rapid drainage of H+ ions from the mucosa and neutralizes H+ ions intravascularly with HCO_3^- and proteins. Of note, prostaglandins promote blood flow, mucus secretion, and stimulation of HCO_3^- secretion, thus prostaglandins play an important role in gastric mucosal defense.

GASTRODUODENAL MOTILITY

The physiology of gastric motility and emptying can be understood via two major gastric geographic regions. As food enters the stomach, it increases gastric intraluminal pressure, causing the fundus and proximal body to relax reflexively (a process called accommodation) in order to allow space to store recently ingested food. The proximal stomach, however, also has characteristic tonic contractions, which aid in downstream gastric emptying.

Distally in the stomach, high-pressure peristaltic contractions by the lower gastric body and the antrum grind food and liquefy it into chyme. Once food particles reach a small enough size, they are propelled through the pylorus and into the duodenum.

Gastroduodenal motility is coordinated through intrinsic and extrinsic neural and hormonal signals. Neuronal control originates from the enteric nervous system and the sympathetic and parasympathetic nervous system via gastric mechanoreceptors, whereas certain hormones, such as gastrin and cholecystokinin, serve to relax the proximal stomach and create contractions in the distal stomach.

A series of negative feedback loops initiated by the presence of chyme within the duodenum inhibit further gastric emptying into the duodenum.

PEPTIC ULCER DISEASE

Definition and Epidemiology

A peptic ulcer is a defect or defects in the mucosal layer of the stomach or duodenum measuring at least 5 mm in diameter that penetrates into the muscularis mucosa. Lesions that are smaller than 5 mm or more superficial to the muscularis mucosa are classified as erosions. Men and women are at equal risk for developing peptic ulcer disease (PUD), and in the United States the lifetime risk of suffering from PUD is about 5% to 10%.

Gastric acid plays an important role in the digestion of food. PUD development is the result of an imbalance of gastric acid and other noxious substances in the gastric lumen relative to gastric protective functions. Some persons with PUD do secrete excessive amounts of gastric acid, particularly in duodenal ulcer disease, where depletion of antral somatostatin by *Helicobacter pylori* leads predictably to gastrin and acid hypersecretion (Fig. 7.3). However, most people with PUD have normal-to-low acid secretion, suggesting that a defect in mucosal defense is the major pathophysiologic culprit.

The two most common causes of PUD are *H. pylori* infection and the use of nonsteroidal anti-inflammatory drugs (NSAIDs). These two factors compromise mucosal defense mechanisms and predispose patients to peptic ulcers. They work synergistically to increase the risk of PUD when both factors are present. The risk of developing PUD increases with age, and, given that the prevalence of *H. pylori* has been decreasing in the general population and the use of NSAIDs has been increasing among older persons, the incidence of PUD has been decreasing in younger age groups (who tend to have low rates of NSAID use and *H. pylori* infection), and increasing in persons 65 years of age and older.

Other factors also modulate the risk of developing PUD. For example, smoking impairs ulcer healing, increases the risk of recurrence, and is associated with a higher PUD-related mortality. Similarly, there

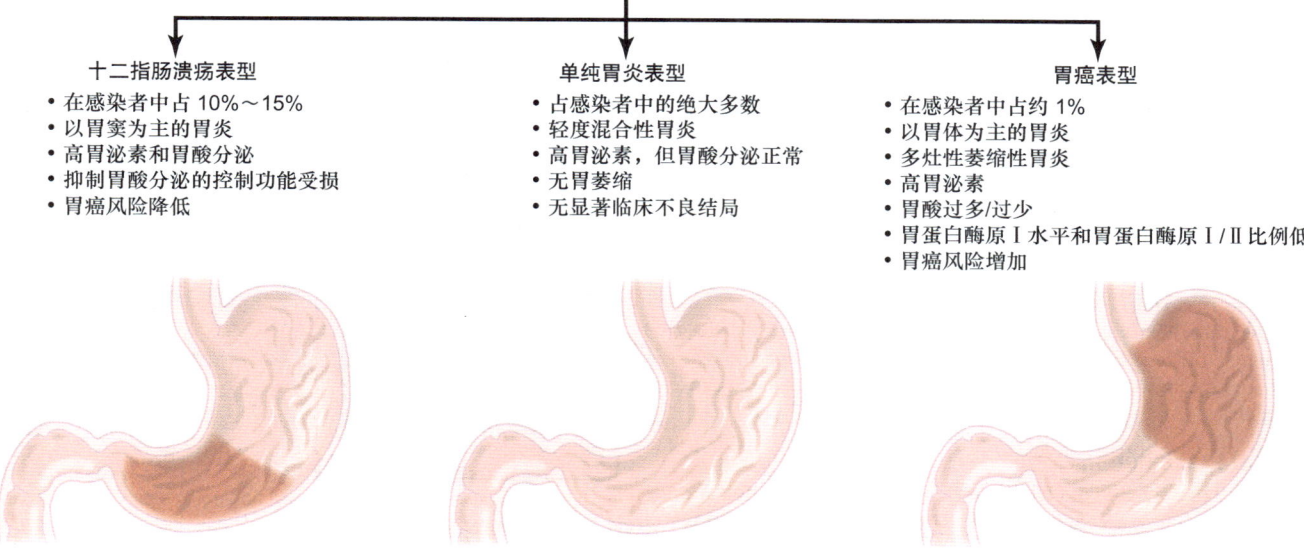

图 7.3 幽门螺杆菌引起的多种病理学改变和临床结局。胃酸分泌状况及最终的临床结局取决于幽门螺杆菌感染引起的胃炎的范围和程度（引自 Amieva MR，El-Omar EM. Host-bacterial interactions in Helicobacter pylori infection. Gastroenterology. 2008；134：306-23.）

皮层的酸性物质。这种黏液在胃中由胃小凹颈部的产黏液细胞分泌，在十二指肠中由产黏液的杯状细胞分泌。此外，顶端上皮细胞膜的脂质双层和紧密连接能够防止 H^+ 扩散到胃壁，从而保持黏膜的完整性。丰富的黏膜下层血液供应可迅速排出黏膜中的 H^+，并通过 HCO_3^- 和蛋白质在血管内中和 H^+。值得注意的是，前列腺素可促进血流、黏液分泌和 HCO_3^- 分泌，因此前列腺素在胃黏膜防御中发挥重要作用。

胃十二指肠运动

为了理解胃的运动和排空，可将胃分为两个区域。当食物进入胃内时，胃腔内的压力增加，导致胃底和近端胃体反射性舒张（这一过程被称为容受），增大容积以储存新摄入的食物。然而，近端胃也具有特征性的紧张性收缩，有助于向下推进胃排空。

在胃的远端，胃体下部和胃窦的高压蠕动收缩将食物研磨并液化成食糜。一旦食物颗粒达到足够小的尺寸，就会通过幽门推入十二指肠。

胃十二指肠运动受内源性和外源性神经及激素信号调控。神经调控来源于肠神经系统，以及通过胃机械感受器的交感神经和副交感神经系统，而某些激素（如胃泌素、CCK）有助于近端胃舒张和远端胃收缩。

十二指肠内的食糜会启动负反馈回路，抑制胃的进一步排空。

消化性溃疡病
定义和流行病学

消化性溃疡是指胃或十二指肠黏膜层发生缺损（直径≥5 mm），且穿透黏膜肌层。直径＜5 mm 或未穿透黏膜肌层的病变被定义为糜烂。男性和女性患消化性溃疡病（PUD）的风险相同。在美国，罹患 PUD 的终生风险为 5%～10%。

胃酸在食物消化中发挥重要作用。PUD 的发生是胃酸和其他胃内有害物质与胃保护功能之间失去平衡的结果。部分 PUD 患者确实分泌过量的胃酸，特别是在十二指肠溃疡中，幽门螺杆菌（*Helicobacter pylori*）引起胃窦分泌生长抑素减少，导致胃泌素和胃酸分泌过多（图 7.3）。然而，大多数 PUD 患者的胃酸分泌正常或偏低，这表明黏膜屏障防御功能缺陷是 PUD 的主要病理生理学原因。

PUD 的两大病因是幽门螺杆菌感染和应用非甾体抗炎药（NSAID）。两者均会损害黏膜防御机制，使患者易患消化性溃疡。当两者同时存在时，可协同增加患 PUD 的风险。随着年龄的增长，PUD 的发生风险增加。此外，由于幽门螺杆菌感染在普通人群中的患病率持续下降，而 NSAID 在老年人中的使用率升高，PUD 在年轻人群（NSAID 使用率和幽门螺杆菌感染率均较低）中的发病率有所下降，而在 65 岁及以上人群中的发病率有所上升。

其他因素也会增加患 PUD 的风险。例如，吸烟会阻碍溃疡愈合，增加复发风险，并与较高的 PUD 相

is an association between PUD development and concomitant use of high-dose corticosteroids with NSAIDs, though there is no evidence that corticosteroids alone cause PUD.

Less common causes of PUD include hypersecretory states such as Zollinger-Ellison syndrome, Crohn's disease, vascular insufficiency, viral infection, radiation therapy, and cancer therapy. Development of PUD may also be influenced by other factors such as stress, personality type, alcohol consumption, occupation, and diet, though these play a relatively minor role compared with the effects of *H. pylori* infection and NSAID usage.

Additionally, certain chronic diseases are positively correlated with PUD. These include chronic obstructive pulmonary disease, systemic mastocytosis, cirrhosis, and uremia.

Given that PUD is a complex disease resulting from diverse pathophysiologic processes, this chapter focuses on the different etiologic agents and mechanisms individually, after considering the shared clinical features.

Clinical Presentation

The clinical presentation of PUD varies depending on the location and severity of the ulcer. Uncomplicated PUD typically presents as sharp, burning, nonradiating epigastric abdominal pain. In duodenal ulcers the pain tends to occur 2 to 3 hours after the ingestion of food or at night, when the stomach is empty. The opposite is often true of gastric ulcers. Patients with duodenal ulcers tend to present with weight gain because the ingestion of food relieves symptoms, whereas patients with gastric ulcers tend to be food averse and are more likely to present with weight loss. Older patients (>60 years) may report no pain at all at the time of presentation and may instead present with nonspecific complaints, such as confusion, restlessness, abdominal distention, and falls. In pregnant patients, symptoms are often fairly mild and might even improve as the pregnancy progresses. They may also present as abnormal patterns of nausea and vomiting of pregnancy, such as nocturnal vomiting or worsening of vomiting in the third trimester. Most patients with PUD present after several weeks or months of symptoms, unless there is a complication that necessitates urgent medical care.

Diagnosis

The diagnosis of PUD requires clinical suspicion in patients with the appropriate clinical presentations. Physical exam may determine focal epigastric tenderness.

Contrast imaging with a barium upper GI series used to be the primary method of diagnosis but is now supplanted by the widespread availability of upper gastrointestinal endoscopy, now considered the "gold standard" for diagnosis because it permits direct visualization of the ulcer or ulcers.

In addition to providing a diagnosis of PUD, endoscopy also enables tissue sampling by biopsy to evaluate for malignancy and *H. pylori* infection. Furthermore, endoscopy can be therapeutic, providing curative hemostasis in patients with acute life-threatening GI bleeding secondary to PUD.

Causes of Peptic Ulcer Disease

There are several conditions associated with the development of ulcer disease; these may be present in isolation or coexist with each other. Identifying specific causes is important to prevent recurrences.

Helicobacter pylori

H. pylori is a flagellated gram-negative bacillus that colonizes the gastric epithelium of half of the world's population. This bacterium is responsible for over 80% of duodenal ulcers and at least half of all cases of gastric ulcers. However, only a fraction of patients with *H. pylori* infection

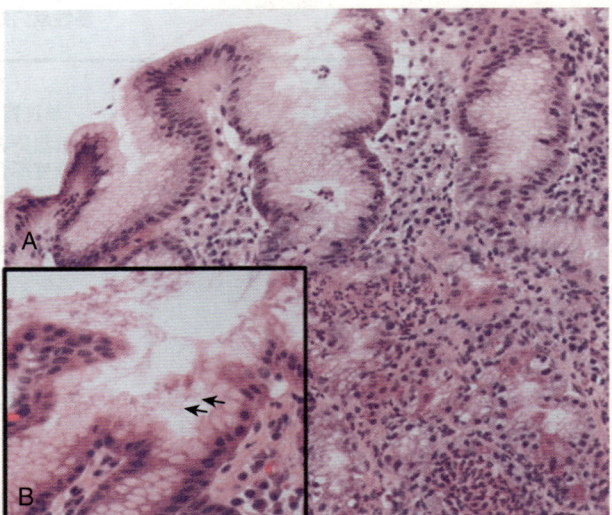

Fig. 7.4 (A) Gastric biopsy (hematoxylin and eosin stain) showing gastric mucosa with intense inflammatory infiltrate including clusters of neutrophils infiltrating gastric pit and surface epithelium and lymphocytes and plasma cells in the lamina propria. At high power (B) *H. pylori* organisms can be seen faintly *(arrows)* adjacent to surface epithelial cells. (Courtesy of Murray Resnick, MD, PhD, Adjunct Professor of Pathology and Laboratory Medicine, Warren Alpert Medical School, Providence, RI.)

develop PUD. *H. pylori* infection is also a strong risk factor for PUD and malignancy (adenocarcinoma and mucosa-associated lymphoid tissue [MALT] lymphoma), as well as a cause of iron deficiency anemia and immune thrombocytopenic purpura (ITP). Infection is transmitted via the fecal-oral route and typically occurs during childhood. *H. pylori* infection tends to persist throughout the lifetime of the host if left untreated, despite a strong gastric inflammatory response and both cell-mediated and humoral immune system recognition.

Rates of *H. pylori* infection differ globally, with highest prevalence in the developing world. In the United States, infection rates are 10% to 15% in persons under 12 years old and 50% to 60% in persons older than 60 years. There is increased prevalence in persons with lower socioeconomic status, increased household crowding and, in the United States, higher prevalence in immigrants from the developing world.

H. pylori has several unique characteristics enabling gastric colonization. *H. pylori* can survive in gastric acid by producing urease, which catalyzes the conversion of urea (which is present in gastric juice) into ammonia, thus neutralizing *H. pylori*'s microenvironment. *H. pylori*'s flagella allow the organism to move fluidly through the stomach's viscous mucous layer toward gastric epithelial cells, where *H. pylori* uses a series of adhesins and receptors to attach and chronically infect its host. At the gastric epithelium, *H. pylori* induces an inflammatory response consisting of neutrophils, leukocytes, plasma cells, and macrophages. Neutrophilic infiltration of the gastric epithelium causing chronic gastritis is a hallmark of *H. pylori* infection, easily recognizable in gastric biopsies (Fig. 7.4).

Determinants of pathogenicity include the location of infection within the stomach, *H. pylori* genomic heterogeneity, and differences in host response. For example, infections that are most predominant in the antrum are more strongly associated with duodenal ulcers and increased acidity due to depletion of antral somatostatin-producing cells leading to uninhibited gastrin secretion. In contrast, *H. pylori* colonization of the corpus is correlated with gastric ulcers, gastric adenomas, and decreased acid production due to inflammation-mediated inhibition of parietal cell secretion and subsequent parietal cell

关死亡率有关。此外，同时使用大剂量皮质类固醇和 NSAID 与 PUD 有关，尽管目前没有证据表明单用皮质类固醇会导致 PUD。

少见的 PUD 病因包括高胃酸分泌状态，如佐林格-埃利森综合征（ZES）、克罗恩病、血管功能不全、病毒感染、放疗和癌症治疗。PUD 的发生还可能受其他因素的影响，如压力、人格类型、饮酒、职业和饮食。与幽门螺杆菌感染和使用 NSAID 的影响相比，这些因素的作用较小。

此外，某些慢性疾病也可能导致 PUD，包括慢性阻塞性肺疾病、系统性肥大细胞增多症、肝硬化和尿毒症。

鉴于 PUD 是一种由多种病理生理学过程引起的复杂疾病，本章在讨论其共同的临床特点后，将逐一重点介绍不同的病因和发病机制。

临床表现

PUD 的临床表现因溃疡的位置和严重程度而异。PUD 的典型表现为尖锐的、烧灼样或非放射性上腹部疼痛。十二指肠溃疡的疼痛通常在进食后 2～3 h 或夜间空腹时发生，而胃溃疡则相反。十二指肠溃疡患者易出现体重增加，因为进食可缓解症状，而胃溃疡患者则易出现厌食，从而导致体重减轻。老年患者（＞60 岁）在就诊时可能没有上腹部疼痛，而是表现为非特异性症状，如意识模糊、不安、腹胀和跌倒。孕妇的症状通常相对较轻，甚至可能随着妊娠进程而有所改善。孕妇患者可能表现为妊娠期呕吐习惯的改变，如夜间呕吐或妊娠晚期呕吐加重。大多数 PUD 患者在出现症状数周或数月后就诊，除非出现需要紧急救治的并发症。

诊断

具有上述临床表现的患者应疑诊 PUD。体格检查可能发现上腹部局部压痛。

上消化道钡剂造影是既往主要的诊断方法，但现在已被广泛应用的上消化道内镜所取代。内镜被认为是诊断 PUD 的"金标准"，因其可直接观察溃疡。

除诊断 PUD 外，内镜可通过活检进行组织取样，以发现恶性肿瘤和幽门螺杆菌感染。此外，内镜检查还可进行治疗，如 PUD 引起危及生命的急性消化道出血时可行内镜下止血治疗。

PUD 的原因

PUD 的多种病因可能单独存在，也可能同时存在。识别特定病因对于预防 PUD 复发很重要。

幽门螺杆菌

幽门螺杆菌是一种带鞭毛的革兰氏阴性杆菌，全球 1/2 的人口存在胃黏膜上皮的幽门螺杆菌定植。80% 以上的十二指肠溃疡和至少 50% 的胃溃疡由幽门螺杆菌感染所致。然而，只有一小部分幽门螺杆菌感染者

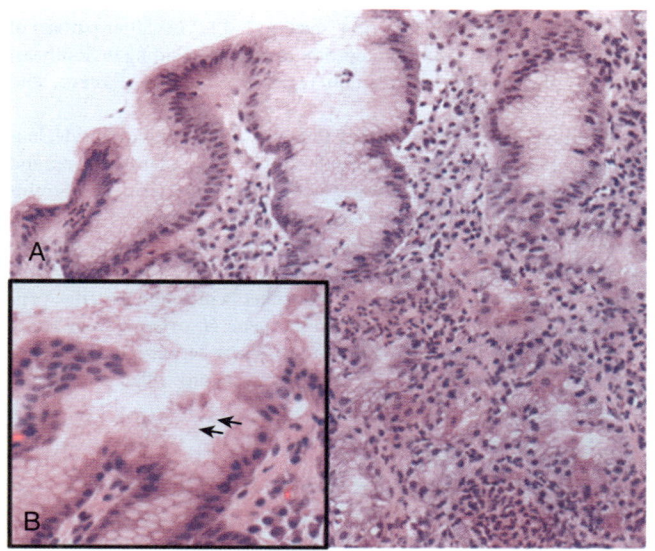

图 7.4　A. 胃活检（苏木精和伊红染色）显示胃黏膜有明显炎症浸润，包括中性粒细胞群浸润胃小凹和表面上皮，固有层中有淋巴细胞和浆细胞浸润。B. 在高倍镜下隐约可见幽门螺杆菌（箭头）与表面上皮细胞相邻（授权自 Murray Resnick，MD，PhD，Adjunct Professor of Pathology and Laboratory Medicine，Warren Alpert Medical School，Providence，RI.）

会发展为 PUD。幽门螺杆菌感染是 PUD 和恶性肿瘤［如胃腺癌和黏膜相关淋巴组织（MALT）淋巴瘤］的高危因素，还可引起缺铁性贫血和免疫性血小板减少性紫癜（ITP）。感染通过粪口途径传播，通常发生在儿童期。尽管可引起强烈的胃黏膜炎症反应且免疫细胞和体液免疫系统能够识别幽门螺杆菌，但如果不进行治疗，感染通常会持续终生。

全球幽门螺杆菌感染的患病率各不相同，在发展中国家最高。在美国，12 岁以下儿童的感染率为 10%～15%，60 岁以上人群的感染率为 50%～60%。社会经济地位较低、共同居住人数较多、来自发展中国家的移民等人群的感染率更高。

幽门螺杆菌具有多种独有的特性，使其能够在胃内定植。幽门螺杆菌通过产生尿素酶，催化胃酸中的尿素分解产生氨，从而中和胃酸，形成适合其生存的微环境。幽门螺杆菌的鞭毛使其能够通过胃的黏液层向胃上皮细胞移动，幽门螺杆菌利用一系列黏附素和受体附着于胃上皮并长期感染宿主。在胃上皮，幽门螺杆菌诱发中性粒细胞、白细胞、浆细胞和巨噬细胞介导的炎症反应。胃上皮中性粒细胞浸润导致的慢性胃炎是幽门螺杆菌感染的标志，在胃活检中易于识别（图 7.4）。

幽门螺杆菌的致病性取决于其在胃内的感染位置、幽门螺杆菌的基因组异质性和宿主反应的差异。例如，发生在胃窦的感染与十二指肠溃疡和胃酸分泌增加相关，这是由于感染导致胃窦分泌生长抑素的细胞数量减少引起胃泌素过度分泌。相比之下，幽门螺杆菌在胃体的定植与胃溃疡、胃腺癌和胃酸分泌减少相关，这是由于炎症介导的壁细胞分泌抑制及壁细胞数量减少引起萎缩性

loss resulting in atrophic gastritis (see Fig. 7.3). This latter pattern of gastric inflammation is most common in persons residing in Southeast Asia, South America, and certain regions of Central, Eastern, and Southern Europe.

Additionally, *H. pylori's* ability to produce lipopolysaccharide, leukocyte-activating factors, specific adhesins and vacuolating toxins, and a type IV bacterial secretory system contribute to its virulence. Strains with more of these pathogenic factors have been associated with more severe disease states. The most important of those pathogenic markers is cytotoxin-associated gene *(cagA)*, a marker of the presence of the type IV secretory system, which is associated with acute gastritis, peptic ulcers, and gastric cancer. This multigene *H. pylori* system serves as a "molecular syringe" functioning to insert certain *H. pylori* proteins directly into host epithelial cells to activate pro-inflammatory and pro-oncogenic signaling pathways.

Diagnosis of *H. pylori*

In persons with clinical manifestations of *H. pylori*, eradication of the infection leads to improved outcomes. Because eradication of *H. pylori* from asymptomatic patients has not yet been shown to significantly prevent disease, *H. pylori* diagnostic testing is generally reserved for those patients with certain *H. pylori*–associated diseases or conditions such as PUD, uninvestigated dyspepsia without alarm symptoms, unexplained iron deficiency anemia, idiopathic thrombocytopenic purpura, early gastric cancer, and low-grade MALT lymphoma. It is remarkable that 80% of patients with low-grade MALT lymphoma and *H. pylori* infection will be cured by *H. pylori* eradication.

There are two categories of diagnostic tests for *H. pylori*: invasive and noninvasive. Noninvasive tests include urea breath test and stool antigen test, and the invasive tests are performed on endoscopic biopsies by histology, rapid urease test, and culture. The sensitivity of these tests, however, is decreased by proton pump inhibitors (PPIs), antibiotics, and bismuth compounds. Blood tests for the presence of *H. pylori* antibodies are relatively inaccurate and no longer recommended. They are particularly poor at monitoring the outcome of treatment because they may remain positive months to years after successful eradication.

For the urea breath test, patients must stop taking PPIs 2 weeks prior to the test. They ingest urea in which the carbon atoms are labeled with either radioactive carbon-14 or nonradioactive carbon-13. If present, *H. pylori* hydrolyzes the urea into ammonia. The presence of a labeled carbon atom in exhaled CO_2 indicates active *H. pylori* infection, and with a 95% specificity and sensitivity, it is the best choice for test of cure.

The stool antigen test detects fecal antigens by immunoassay. Proton pump inhibitors must be stopped 2 weeks prior to the test, but it is a good test for both detection and eradication, though their sensitivity and specificity are slightly lower than the urea breath test.

Invasive tests all require endoscopic biopsies. The *H. pylori* can be visualized histologically (especially if immunohistochemistry or other special stains are used) and the presence of chronic active gastritis, a hallmark of *H. pylori* infection, noted. Additionally, the biopsy can be tested with a rapid urease test, which detects pH changes in the urea-rich test matrix when the *H. pylori* derived urease converts urea to ammonia. Biopsies may also be used to culture *H. pylori*; however, this is a relatively costly and time-consuming process that is currently rarely used. The major advantage of this method is that it allows testing for antibiotic resistance of individual strains. This is an increasingly important focus of research and likely to be important in clinical practice, too, due to the emergence of multiply antibiotic-resistant *H. pylori*.

Given the increasing incidence of antibiotic resistance in *H. pylori*, a test of cure 4 weeks after the end of treatment and 2 weeks after cessation of PPI treatment with a stool antigen or breath tests is recommended to confirm eradication of *H. pylori*.

Treatment of *H. pylori*

Treatment consists of combination therapy with antibiotics and acid inhibitors to guarantee adequate antibiotic coverage and to ensure penetration of the antibiotics into the gastric mucosa (Fig. 7.5). Additionally, the duration of therapy must be long enough to ensure eradication.

The increasing rates of antibiotic resistance, especially to clarithromycin and levofloxacin, make it imperative that providers ask patients about any prior macrolide antibiotic exposures, because prior exposure is associated with likely resistance. They have also spurred efforts to measure local antibiotic resistance rates.

The treatment options are bismuth quadruple therapy, which consists of a PPI, bismuth, tetracycline, and metronidazole for 14 days, and clarithromycin triple therapy, which consists of a PPI, clarithromycin, and amoxicillin or metronidazole for 14 days. Given the increasing rates of clarithromycin resistance, however, clarithromycin triple therapy is falling out of favor and should only be used in regions where it is known that *H. pylori* clarithromycin resistance rates are less than 15% and in patients with no history of macrolide exposure. Otherwise, bismuth quadruple therapy is the current therapy of choice with an expected cure rate of 80% to 90%.

If a patient fails initial treatment, then second-line therapy for that patient should avoid any antibiotics that were previously taken by the patient. If the patient failed first-line bismuth quadruple therapy, salvage therapy should contain either clarithromycin or levofloxacin depending on local antimicrobial resistance patterns and the patient's prior antibiotic exposures. If the patient failed clarithromycin triple therapy, bismuth quadruple therapy should be tried next. Other "salvage" options in cases of recurrent failure include regimens containing rifabutin and dual regimens of high-dose amoxicillin and high-dose PPIs.

H. pylori infection treatment is complete only after eradication has been confirmed with a test of cure, as outlined above.

NSAID-Induced PUD

NSAIDs are a class of drugs that are very useful in the treatment of pain, arthritis, and inflammatory diseases; however, their use can be limited by their side effect profile. Upper GI side effects are dose dependent and include PUD and GI bleeds. Side effects are also more common in patients with certain risk factors, such as age older than 65 years, past history of PUD, heart disease, and concomitant therapy with antiplatelet agents, corticosteroids, and anticoagulants. There is synergism between *H. pylori* infection and chronic NSAID use in terms of PUD risk.

NSAID-induced PUD accounts for approximately 100,000 hospital admissions annually, and about 25% of persons on chronic NSAID therapy will develop PUD. Chronic NSAID users who have the above-mentioned risk factors have a 9% risk of having a serious adverse event, while those who do not have risk factors only have a 0.4% risk. Thus, before starting a patient on chronic NSAIDs, it is important to evaluate their risk factors and consider alternative therapies, if appropriate.

Mechanism of Injury

Half of people taking NSAIDs will develop NSAID-induced gastropathy consisting of superficial mucosal hemorrhages and erosions. These asymptomatic erosions are usually found incidentally during upper endoscopies performed for other reasons and are mainly concentrated in the gastric antrum. Most cases of NSAID gastropathy will not progress to PUD.

胃炎（图 7.3）。后一种胃炎模式在东南亚、南美洲，以及中欧、东欧和南欧的某些地区人群中最为常见。

此外，幽门螺杆菌通过产生脂多糖、白细胞活化因子、特定的黏附素和空泡毒素及Ⅳ型细菌分泌系统来增强其毒力。具有更多致病因子的菌株与更严重的疾病状态相关。这些致病因子中最重要的是细胞毒素相关基因（cagA），它是Ⅳ型细菌分泌系统存在的标志，与急性胃炎、消化性溃疡和胃癌相关。这种多基因幽门螺杆菌系统可作为"分子注射器"直接将某些幽门螺杆菌蛋白插入宿主上皮细胞，激活促炎和促癌的信号通路。

幽门螺杆菌感染的诊断

对于有临床症状的患者，根除幽门螺杆菌感染可以改善预后。由于尚未发现对无症状患者进行根除治疗可以预防患病，通常仅对患有某些幽门螺杆菌相关疾病或状态的患者进行幽门螺杆菌检测，如 PUD、未经检查的无报警症状的消化不良、原因不明的缺铁性贫血、特发性血小板减少性紫癜、早期胃癌和低级别 MALT 淋巴瘤。值得注意的是，80% 合并幽门螺杆菌感染的低级别 MALT 淋巴瘤患者通过根除幽门螺杆菌可以被治愈。

幽门螺杆菌的检测分为侵入性和非侵入性两类。非侵入性检查包括尿素呼气试验和粪便抗原试验，侵入性检查通过内镜活检进行，包括组织学检查、快速尿素酶试验和培养。但是，质子泵抑制剂（PPI）、抗生素和铋剂会降低这些检测的敏感性。幽门螺杆菌抗体血液检测的准确性较低，故不推荐应用。由于在根除治疗成功后数月到数年内抗体可能仍呈阳性，因此抗体检测在监测治疗结果方面的作用较差。

对于尿素呼气试验，患者必须在检查前 2 周停用 PPI。患者摄入放射性 ^{14}C 或非放射性 ^{13}C 标记的尿素，如果胃内存在幽门螺杆菌，尿素将被分解为氨。在呼出的二氧化碳中检测到标记的碳原子提示存在活动性幽门螺杆菌感染，该试验的特异性和敏感性为 95%，是治疗后验证根除的最佳选择。

粪便抗原试验是指通过免疫分析法检测粪便中幽门螺杆菌的抗原。患者必须在检查前 2 周停用 PPI，尽管该试验的敏感性和特异性略低于尿素呼气试验，但它仍然是幽门螺杆菌检测和治疗效果监测的较好选择。

所有侵入性检查都需要内镜活检。组织学检查可以直接观察到幽门螺杆菌（特别是使用免疫组织化学染色或其他特殊染色），并发现幽门螺杆菌感染的标志，即慢性活动性胃炎。此外，可通过快速尿素酶试验检测活检样本，即在幽门螺杆菌产生的尿素酶将尿素分解为氨时检测富含尿素基质中的 pH 值变化。活检样本还可用于培养幽门螺杆菌，但该检查费用较昂贵且过程耗时，目前很少使用。活检标本培养的主要优势是可以检测个别菌株的抗生素耐药性。这已成为日益重要的研究热点，且由于出现了多重抗生素耐药性幽门螺杆菌，这在临床工作中也会变得更加重要。

由于幽门螺杆菌抗生素耐药性的增加，建议在治疗结束后 4 周、停止 PPI 治疗 2 周后，通过粪便抗原或呼气试验确认幽门螺杆菌已根除成功。

幽门螺杆菌感染的治疗

治疗包括抗生素和抑酸剂的联合治疗，以确保足量抗生素覆盖并渗透到胃黏膜内（图 7.5）。此外，治疗时间必须足够长以确保根除。

由于抗生素耐药率不断升高，特别是对克拉霉素和左氧氟沙星的耐药，医生必须提前询问患者既往是否使用过大环内酯类抗生素，因为既往用药情况与耐药性的产生有关。这也促使人们更加积极地评估当地抗生素的耐药率。

治疗方案包括含铋剂的四联治疗（包括 PPI、铋剂、四环素和甲硝唑，共 14 天）和克拉霉素三联治疗（包括 PPI、克拉霉素和阿莫西林或甲硝唑，共 14 天）。然而，由于克拉霉素耐药率的升高，克拉霉素三联治疗不再作为首选，仅在克拉霉素耐药率 < 15% 的地区和无大环内酯类暴露史的患者中使用。此外，铋剂四联治疗是目前的首选治疗，预期治愈率为 80%～90%。

如果患者初次根除失败，则二线治疗应避免既往使用的任何抗生素。如果初次铋剂四联治疗失败，挽救治疗应包含克拉霉素或左氧氟沙星，具体取决于当地的抗生素耐药模式和患者既往的抗生素使用史。如果克拉霉素三联治疗无效，则应尝试铋剂四联治疗。对于复发后根除失败的病例，其他挽救治疗包括含有利福布汀的治疗方案和大剂量阿莫西林联合大剂量 PPI 的双联治疗方案。

如上所述，幽门螺杆菌感染的治疗只有在通过幽门螺杆菌检查确认根除后才算结束。

NSAID 诱导的 PUD

NSAID 是一类对治疗疼痛、关节炎和炎症性疾病非常有效的药物，然而，其使用可能受其副作用的限制。NSAID 的上消化道副作用呈剂量依赖性，副作用包括 PUD 和消化道出血。这些副作用在具有高危因素的患者中更常见，如年龄 > 65 岁、既往有 PUD 病史、心脏病，以及同时使用抗血小板药物、皮质类固醇和抗凝剂的患者。幽门螺杆菌感染和长期使用 NSAID 在 PUD 发生风险方面存在协同作用。

每年约有 10 万例 NSAID 诱导的 PUD 住院病例，约 25% 长期使用 NSAID 的患者将罹患 PUD。具有上述危险因素的长期 NSAID 使用者发生严重不良事件的风险为 9%，而没有危险因素的患者仅为 0.4%。因此，在开始长期使用 NSAID 之前，评估患者的危险因素并考虑是否应用替代治疗非常重要。

损伤机制

服用 NSAID 的患者中有 50% 会出现 NSAID 诱导的胃病，表现为浅表黏膜出血和糜烂。这些无症状的糜烂通常在因其他原因进行上消化道内镜时被偶然发现，主要集中在胃窦。大多数 NSAID 诱导的胃病不会发展为 PUD。

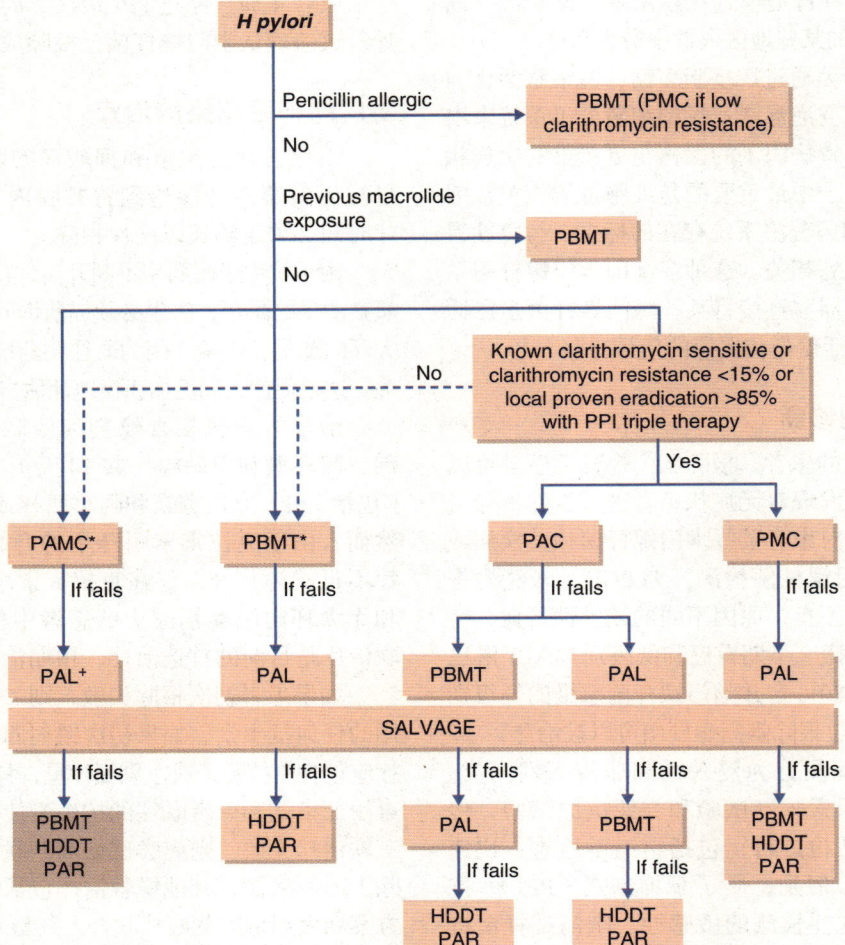

Fig. 7.5 *H. pylori* eradication therapy algorithm. *PAC*, Clarithromycin-based PPI triple therapy with amoxicillin; *PAL*, levofloxacin-based therapy; *PAMC*, concomitant non-bismuth quadruple therapy; *PAR*, rifabutin containing therapy; *PBMT*, PPI/bismuth/metronidazole/tetracycline quadruple therapy; *PMC*, clarithromycin-based PPI triple therapy with metronidazole; *HDDT*, high-dose dual therapy. (From Fallone CA, Moss SF, Malfertheiner P. Reconciliation of recent *Helicobacter pylori* treatment guidelines in a time of increasing resistance to antibiotics. Gastroenterology 2019;157:44-53.)

Once ingested and exposed to gastric acid, NSAIDs become weak acids and are able to cross the lipid bilayer membranes of gastric epithelial cells. There, they lose a hydrogen atom and become trapped intracellularly, disrupting normal cell function. This leads to decreased cellular integrity and increased cellular permeability leaving gastric epithelial cells vulnerable to topical injury, hemorrhages, erosions, and cell death.

Additionally, NSAIDs also inhibit the arachidonic acid pathway, which is crucial for the synthesis of prostaglandins (PGs) that protect gastric epithelial cells, and for mucosal integrity. The synthesis of PGs is catalyzed by cyclooxygenases (COX). The COX-1 isoform is constitutively expressed in the GI tract independent of external factors. In contrast, COX-2 is largely inducible, promoting PG synthesis under the influence of inflammatory mediators that are present in pro-inflammatory states. PGs play a very important role in gastric mucosal protection by increasing mucus and bicarbonate production, increasing blood flow to the gastric mucosa, and promoting epithelial cell repair and turnover after injury. Inhibition of PG synthesis by NSAIDs leaves epithelial cells vulnerable to unopposed injury from gastric acid and pepsin. Aspirin exposes patients to PUD in a similar way. It acetylates COX-1, thus irreversibly inhibiting it.

The more common NSAIDs, such as ibuprofen, naproxen, diclofenac, and aspirin, are nonselective COX inhibitors. Selective COX-2 inhibitors, such as celecoxib and valdecoxib, were developed with the aim of reducing gastric toxicity by primarily acting at sites of inflammation, thus leaving COX-1 function intact. Though the COX-2 inhibitors have fewer GI side effects, they have been associated with increased cardiovascular events such as myocardial infarctions and strokes. The COX-2 inhibitors that are still on the market now carry a black box warning.

Prevention and Therapy of NSAID-Induced PUD

Prevention and treatment of NSAID-induced PUD can be divided into three categories: primary prevention, treatment, and secondary prevention.

Prior to prescribing chronic NSAIDs, providers should assess a patient's risk for NSAID-induced adverse side effects, such as history of ulcers and GI bleeding, age older than 65 years, concomitant *H. pylori* infection, and co-prescription with antiplatelet agents, steroids, and anticoagulants.

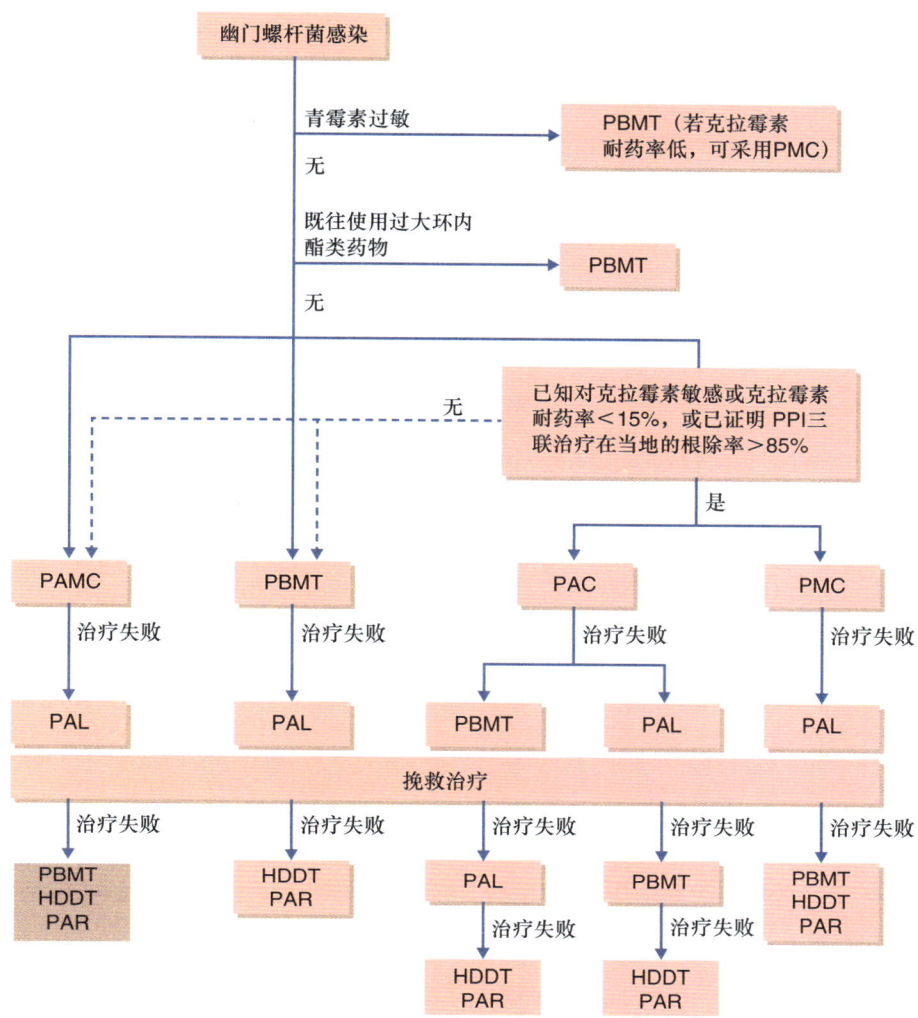

图 7.5 幽门螺杆菌根除治疗流程。PAC，基于克拉霉素的 PPI 三联治疗＋阿莫西林；PAL，基于左氧氟沙星的治疗；PAMC，同时使用非铋剂的四联治疗；PAR，含有利福布汀的治疗；PBMT，PPI/铋剂/甲硝唑/四环素四联治疗；PMC，基于克拉霉素的 PPI 三联治疗＋甲硝唑；HDDT，大剂量双联治疗（引自 Fallone CA，Moss SF，Malfertheiner P. Reconciliation of recent Helicobacter pylori treatment guidelines in a time of increasing resistance to antibiotics. Gastroenterology 2019；157：44-53.）

NSAID 被摄入并接触胃酸后会变成弱酸，能够穿过胃上皮细胞的脂质双层膜，然后丢失 1 个 H^+ 并滞留在细胞内，干扰细胞的正常功能。这会导致细胞完整性下降和通透性增加，使胃上皮细胞更易受到局部损伤、出血、糜烂和细胞死亡的影响。

此外，NSAID 还可抑制花生四烯酸通路，该通路对前列腺素（PG；保护胃上皮细胞和维持胃黏膜完整性）的合成至关重要。PG 的合成由环氧合酶（COX）催化。COX-1 在胃肠道中独立于外界因素而持续表达，而 COX-2 在很大程度上为诱导型，在促炎状态下受炎症介质影响而诱导 PG 合成。PG 可增加黏液和 HCO_3^- 的产生、增加胃黏膜的血流量、促进上皮细胞在损伤后的修复和更新，从而在胃黏膜保护中发挥非常重要的作用。NSAID 可抑制 PG 的合成，使上皮细胞易受胃酸和胃蛋白酶的损伤。阿司匹林通过乙酰化 COX-1 从而产生不可逆地抑制作用，以相同的机制使患者发生 PUD。

常用的 NSAID（如布洛芬、萘普生、双氯芬酸和阿司匹林）均为非选择性 COX 抑制剂。选择性 COX-2 抑制剂（如塞来昔布和伐地考昔）不影响 COX-1 的功能，主要作用于炎症部位，从而减少胃毒性。虽然 COX-2 抑制剂的胃肠道副作用较少，但其与心血管事件（如心肌梗死和卒中）增加有关。目前上市的 COX-2 抑制剂仍然都带有黑框警告。

NSAID 诱导的 PUD 的预防和治疗

NSAID 诱导的 PUD 的预防和治疗可分为三类：一级预防、治疗和二级预防。

在开具长期 NSAID 处方前，医生应评估患者发生 NSAID 诱导的不良反应的风险，如溃疡和胃肠道出血病史、年龄＞65 岁、伴有幽门螺杆菌感染，以及同时使用抗血小板药物、类固醇和抗凝剂。

Those patients with risk factors for developing NSAID-induced PUD should receive co-therapy with a gastroprotective agent. Currently there are several treatment options, including H2 receptor antagonists (H2RAs), synthetic prostaglandins, and PPIs. PPIs remain the co-treatment of choice because they are most efficacious in this regard and generally very well tolerated.

H2RAs work by blocking histamine 2 receptors in parietal cells, thus decreasing acid production. However, in clinical trials their effects on NSAID ulcer prevention have been very limited.

Prostaglandins such as misoprostol work similarly to endogenous prostaglandins in the protection of the stomach and duodenal lining. Unfortunately, prostaglandins are poorly tolerated due to their side effect profile, which includes diarrhea and abdominal pain.

PPIs inhibit the H+/K+-ATPase in parietal cells, hence reducing acid secretion into the gastric lumen. Prescription of PPIs together with NSAIDs significantly reduces GI-related NSAID complications with a 10% to 15% absolute risk reduction in ulcer formation and ulcer-related bleeding in high-risk patients taking nonselective NSAIDs. It must be noted, though, that recent studies have shown that selective COX-2 inhibitors plus a PPI provide better GI protection compared to a nonselective NSAID plus PPI.

With the widespread overuse of chronic PPIs in recent years (principally for GERD and dyspepsia), several likely adverse side effects of PPIs have come to light. These include increased risk of micronutrient deficiencies such as hypomagnesemia, iron and vitamin B_{12} deficiency, and GI-related infections, such as *Clostridioides difficile* infection (CDI) and small intestinal bacterial overgrowth (SIBO). Additionally, PPI use has been associated with increased incidence of osteoporosis and bone fractures and acute interstitial nephritis. More controversially, associations of chronic PPI usage with chronic kidney disease, cerebrovascular disease, upper GI cancers, and dementia have been reported in some studies, though almost entirely from observational cohorts. Better controlled prospective studies are needed to clarify any causal link between PPIs and these side effects. However, given these potential side effects, patients should be evaluated individually for PPI co-prescription with NSAIDs, and the lowest effective doses should be used when prescribing long-term in primary prophylaxis.

H. pylori infection in the setting of chronic NSAID has been shown to increase the risk of PUD, more specifically for duodenal ulceration. The risk for developing ulcers in *H. pylori* positive patients starting chronic NSAID therapy is higher during the first few months after starting therapy. Therefore, *H. pylori* testing, and treatment is recommended prior to starting chronic NSAID use.

Treatment of NSAID-related ulcers is more straightforward. First and foremost, the offending NSAID or aspirin should be discontinued if medically possible in order to allow endogenous protective prostaglandins to be formed. Subsequently, acid secretion should be suppressed with standard doses of PPIs (or H2RAs or misoprostol). In patients who require NSAID therapy but have a history of PUD, risk factors should be assessed, and COX-2 inhibitors should be used preferentially, along with co-therapy with a PPI if there are no cardiovascular contraindications to COX-2 inhibitor therapy.

Patients with cardiovascular risk factors for whom aspirin is required for secondary prevention of myocardial infarction cannot stop aspirin therapy. In this case, cardiovascular protection outweighs the benefit of aspirin cessation for PUD treatment. These patients must be tested for *H. pylori*, if they have not been previously tested, and they should be treated if they test positive. Additionally, these patients must remain on PUD prophylaxis with either a PPI or misoprostol.

Zollinger-Ellison Syndrome

PUD generally occurs in patients with normal or near normal rates of acid secretion. However, a rare cause of PUD is the Zollinger-Ellison syndrome (ZES), in which PUD is the direct result of severe acid hypersecretion due to gastrin-producing G-cell tumors, called gastrinomas. These tumors are generally located in the pancreas or the duodenum, and patients with ZES typically present with recurrent, multiple, refractory ulcers as well as PUD-related complications, esophagitis, and diarrhea. Individuals with ZES generally do not have concomitant *H. pylori* infection or use NSAIDs therapy. This condition will be discussed in further detail later in the chapter.

Stress-Induced Ulcers

Critically ill ICU patients are at increased risk of developing stress ulcers that lead to increased risk of clinically significant GI bleeding. The risk is higher in burn victims, those with significant injury, cranial trauma, shock, and mechanical ventilation. Endoscopically, stress-related mucosal damage is found in 60% to 100% of patients recently admitted to the ICU. Stress ulcers are typically multiple and shallow. They usually present with hematemesis or melena in the ICU patient.

ICU patients are predisposed to stress ulcers due to decreased splanchnic vascular perfusion and impaired microcirculation due to hypovolemia, shock, and low cardiac output leading to gut ischemia and injury. Additionally, they are often subject to pro-inflammatory states, associated with decreased innate mucosal defenses.

Prevention of stress ulcers with acid suppression through prophylactic treatment with PPIs or H2RAs has been common practice for the past four decades. Recently, the side effect profile of these agents has been evaluated against the risk of stress ulcer bleeds. Serious side effects of PPIs and H2RAs in the ICU setting include increased rate of nosocomial infections, such as ventilator-associated pneumonia and CDI. Consequently, stress ulcer prophylaxis should be reserved only for those patients at high risk for life-threatening GI bleeding such as patients with a history of GI bleeding within the past 12 months, greater than 48 hours of mechanical ventilation, spinal or traumatic brain injuries, and patients with coagulopathies.

Idiopathic Ulcers

Ulcers that appear to arise spontaneously with no known cause are called idiopathic ulcers. Idiopathic PUD (IPUD) prevalence varies by geographic location and has a prevalence of about 15% in developed countries as compared to around 80% in developing countries. With the advent of increased *H. pylori* treatment, the incidence of non–*H. pylori* idiopathic ulcers has increased dramatically, mainly in Asian countries. Idiopathic ulcers, similar to *H. pylori* ulcers, have a slightly higher likelihood of being located in the duodenum.

Diagnosis of idiopathic ulcers requires exclusion of all known causes of PUD such as missed *H. pylori* infection, surreptitious use of ulcerogenic medications, certain systemic diseases such as Crohn's disease, eosinophilic gastroenteritis, vasculitis, ZES, and other infections besides *H. pylori* that may lead to ulcers such as cytomegalovirus (CMV), herpes simplex virus (HSV), tuberculosis (TB), and syphilis.

IPUD carries an increased risk of ulcer recurrence when compared with other etiologies. One study concluded that recurrence rates for *H. pylori*–positive, NSAID-induced, and IPUD-related ulcers were 4.1%, 11.7%, and 23.2%, respectively.

Treatment consists of PPI administration for 4 to 8 weeks, or longer in the case of complicated disease. After PPI administration, it is important to monitor patients clinically. If there is recurrence, maintenance therapy is reasonable.

General PUD Treatment

As highlighted above, the single most important treatment option for PUD is to tailor therapy based on ulcer etiology. Generally, ulcers will heal with antisecretory treatment with a PPI. Uncomplicated duodenal

对于存在危险因素的患者，应同时使用胃黏膜保护剂。目前的治疗方案包括 H_2 受体拮抗剂（H_2RA）、合成前列腺素和 PPI。PPI 仍是首选的联合治疗药物，因其最有效且耐受性较好。

H_2RA 可通过阻断壁细胞的 H_2 受体来减少胃酸的产生。然而，在临床试验中，它们对 NSAID 诱导的溃疡的预防作用非常有限。

前列腺素（如米索前列醇）类似于内源性前列腺素，能保护胃和十二指肠。然而，由于其副作用（包括腹泻和腹痛），前列腺素的耐受性较差。

PPI 通过抑制壁细胞的 H^+-K^+ ATP 酶，从而减少胃酸分泌。PPI 与 NSAID 联用可显著减少 NSAID 的胃肠道并发症，在使用非选择性 NSAID 的高危患者中，溃疡形成和溃疡相关出血的绝对风险降低了 10%～15%。需要注意的是，近期研究表明，选择性 COX-2 抑制剂联合 PPI 比非选择性 NSAID 联合 PPI 具有更好的胃肠道保护作用。

近年来，随着广泛的长期过度使用 PPI（主要用于治疗 GERD 和消化不良），PPI 的一些潜在不良反应也逐渐显现，包括微量营养素缺乏（如低镁血症、铁和维生素 B_{12} 缺乏）和胃肠道相关感染［如艰难梭菌感染（CDI）和小肠细菌过度生长（SIBO）］。此外，PPI 的使用与骨质疏松症、骨折和急性间质性肾炎的发生率升高有关。更具争议的是，部分研究显示，长期使用 PPI 与慢性肾脏病、脑血管疾病、上消化道癌症和痴呆有关，尽管这些研究几乎全部来自观察性队列。未来需要试验设计更合理的前瞻性研究来阐明 PPI 与这些副作用之间的因果关系。然而，鉴于这些潜在的副作用，应进行患者个体化评估来确定 NSAID 联用 PPI 的必要性，长期处方应使用最低有效剂量进行一级预防。

研究表明，在长期使用 NSAID 的情况下，幽门螺杆菌感染会增加 PUD 的风险，特别是十二指肠溃疡。幽门螺杆菌阳性患者在开始长期 NSAID 治疗的最初几个月内发生溃疡的风险更高。因此，在开始长期使用 NSAID 前，建议行幽门螺杆菌检测和治疗。

NSAID 相关溃疡的治疗较为简单。首先，应在医生指导下停用引起溃疡的 NSAID（如阿司匹林），以便生成内源性保护性前列腺素。随后，应使用标准剂量的 PPI（或 H_2RA、米索前列醇）抑制胃酸分泌。在需要 NSAID 治疗但有 PUD 病史的患者中，应评估危险因素，若无心血管疾病禁忌证，首选 COX-2 抑制剂联用 PPI 进行治疗。

对于有心血管疾病风险且需要使用阿司匹林进行心肌梗死二级预防的患者，不能停用阿司匹林。在这种情况下，心血管保护比停用阿司匹林对 PUD 的获益更重要。这些患者必须进行幽门螺杆菌检测（如果从未检测过），如果检测结果为阳性，应进行治疗。此外，这些患者必须继续使用 PPI 或米索前列醇进行 PUD 预防。

佐林格-埃利森综合征（ZES）

PUD 通常发生在胃酸分泌正常或接近正常的患者中。ZES 是导致 PUD 的一种罕见病因，在这种情况下，分泌胃泌素的 G 细胞肿瘤（即胃泌素瘤）引起严重的高胃酸分泌，直接导致 PUD。这些肿瘤通常位于胰腺或十二指肠，ZES 患者通常表现为反复发作的多发性难治性溃疡，以及与 PUD 相关的并发症、食管炎和腹泻。ZES 患者通常没有幽门螺杆菌感染或 NSAID 治疗史（见下文）。

应激性溃疡

重症监护病房（ICU）的危重患者发生应激性溃疡的风险增加，进而导致具有临床意义的消化道出血风险增加。烧伤、重伤、颅脑创伤、休克和接受机械通气的患者风险更高。60%～100% 新入住 ICU 的患者内镜下可见应激相关黏膜损伤。应激性溃疡通常为多发和浅表溃疡。ICU 患者的应激性溃疡通常表现为呕血或黑便。

ICU 患者易患应激性溃疡是由于低血容量、休克和低心输出量导致的脏器血流灌注减少和微循环障碍，从而导致肠道缺血和损伤。此外，患者通常处于促炎状态，与黏膜防御功能减弱有关。

近 40 年来，使用 PPI 或 H_2RA 进行抑酸治疗从而预防应激性溃疡已成为常规做法。近期，这些药物的副作用与应激性溃疡出血的风险得到了评估。PPI 和 H_2RA 在 ICU 环境中的严重副作用包括院内感染率升高，如呼吸机相关性肺炎和 CDI。因此，应激性溃疡的预防应仅限于危及生命的消化道出血高危患者，如过去 12 个月内有消化道出血史、机械通气超过 48 h、脊柱或创伤性脑损伤及凝血障碍患者。

特发性溃疡

病因不明的溃疡被称为特发性溃疡。特发性消化性溃疡病（IPUD）的患病率因不同地区而异，发达国家的患病率约为 15%，发展中国家则约为 80%。随着幽门螺杆菌根除治疗的普及，非幽门螺杆菌特发性溃疡的发病率显著升高，主要见于亚洲国家。特发性溃疡与幽门螺杆菌溃疡类似，发生于十二指肠的可能性略大。

IPUD 的诊断需要排除所有已知的 PUD 病因，如漏诊的幽门螺杆菌感染、隐秘使用致溃疡药物、某些系统性疾病（如克罗恩病、嗜酸细胞性胃肠炎、血管炎、ZES），以及除幽门螺杆菌外可能导致溃疡的其他病原体感染，包括巨细胞病毒（CMV）感染、单纯疱疹病毒（HSV）感染、结核（TB）和梅毒。

与其他病因相比，IPUD 的溃疡复发风险更高。一项研究显示，幽门螺杆菌阳性、NSAID 诱导的 PUD 和 IPUD 相关的溃疡的复发率分别为 4.1%、11.7% 和 23.2%。

治疗 IPUD 需使用 4～8 周的 PPI，复杂疾病则需要更长时间的用药。在 PPI 治疗后，应对患者进行临床监测。如果复发，则需要进行维持治疗。

PUD 的一般治疗

如上所述，PUD 最重要的治疗是针对溃疡病因的治疗。一般来说，用 PPI 抑制胃酸分泌可以治愈溃疡。无并发症的十二指肠溃疡经 PPI 治疗 14 天可愈合，特别

ulcers, specifically those associated with *H. pylori* infection, will heal with 14 days of PPI treatment, which is part of *H. pylori* treatment itself. Complicated ulcers, however, necessitate a longer treatment of 8 to 12 weeks. NSAID-induced ulcers should be treated for a minimum of 8 weeks if the NSAID is stopped. Idiopathic ulcers must be evaluated as previously mentioned. Patients with ZES will need treatment as outlined later.

Maintenance Treatment
In addition to detailed evaluation of the etiology of ulceration for each individual patient and treatment according to the root cause of PUD (i.e., *H. pylori* infection, NSAIDs, ZES), some patients will require maintenance therapy to prevent ulcer recurrence.

After eliminating risk factors for PUD, patients with the following high-risk characteristics may benefit from antisecretory therapy with a PPI: (1) giant ulcer (>2 cm) and age older than 50 or multiple comorbidities, (2) *H. pylori*–negative ulcer disease, (3) non-NSAID disease, (4) refractory peptic ulcers defined as ulcers that do not heal after 12 weeks of PPI treatment, (5) *H. pylori* eradication failure, (6) recurrent peptic ulcer, (7) continued NSAID use. Maintenance therapy regimens include either an H2RA or a PPI at the lowest possible therapeutic dose. The risks of chronic PPIs versus the likelihood of developing PUD should be reviewed periodically.

Special Considerations
Patients that require dual antiplatelet therapy, specifically aspirin and clopidogrel, for treatment after cardiac catheterization, unstable angina, NSTEMI or stroke tend to be co-treated with PPIs to reduce GI side effects. Both PPIs and clopidogrel are metabolized by CYP2C19, leading to concerns that PPIs may decrease the efficacy of clopidogrel and lead to catastrophic events. This risk, however, has been assessed by various systematic reviews and, although the research obviously shows that PPIs decrease the risk of GI events, it has not demonstrated a clear adverse effect on patients on clopidogrel.

Additionally, new anticoagulants, such as dabigatran, rivaroxaban, apixaban, and edoxaban, are becoming more commonly used in patients who need long-term anticoagulation. Though research on these drugs and GI bleeding as it relates specifically to PUD is lacking, these drugs are linked to increased risk of GI bleeding overall and likely lead to increased bleeding in patients with PUD.

Surgery
The efficacy of nonsurgical ulcer treatment has increased dramatically with the discovery of *H. pylori* eradication treatment and antisecretory therapy. As a result, surgery is rarely used to treat PUD. It is an important therapeutic option, however, for patients with complications, such as gastric outlet obstruction, bleeding and perforation.

Complications of PUD
The most common complications of PUD include bleeding, perforation, and obstruction, with bleeding being the most common and obstruction being the least common.

Bleeding
GI bleeding accounts for half a million hospitalizations per year and about $5 billion in annual costs in the United States. Upper GI bleeds (UGIBs) make up half of those hospitalizations and carry a significant mortality rate of up to 7.4%. Peptic ulcers are the most frequent cause of UGIBs, making up about a third of all cases.

Bleeding ulcers present with the classic symptoms of an UGIB and vary depending on the severity of the bleed. In chronically bleeding UGIB, patients present with occult blood in the stool and possibly iron deficiency anemia. When the bleed is acute, patients will have coffee-ground emesis and melena (black and tarry stool); however, a patient with a brisk UGIB may present with hematemesis and, possibly, hematochezia with hypotension. Treatment of bleeding ulcers includes fluid resuscitation, blood transfusions when hemoglobin levels fall below 7 g/dL or below 8 g/dL in patients with existing cardiovascular disease or who are symptomatic, intravenous PPI therapy (which should be switched to oral therapy as soon as the patient tolerates oral medications), and an esophagogastroduodenoscopy (EGD) within 24 hours of admission. If the patient has high-risk clinical features, such as hemodynamic instability or hematemesis, EGD should be performed within 12 hours of admission. Endoscopic intervention is dictated by the features of the bleeding ulcer. Typically, endoscopic interventions, such as injections, sclerotherapy, or clips, are employed if there is active bleeding from the ulcer, or if there is a clot adherent to the ulcer. In active bleeding, combination therapy such as injected epinephrine followed by the application of clips produces improved outcomes over a single modality. Hospital discharge is dependent on the patient's clinical status, but it is typically after 3 days of hospitalization for patients with high-risk bleeds.

Perforation
Perforation of a peptic ulcer accounts for 2% to 10% of ulcer complications. Perforation happens when an ulcer penetrates the full thickness of the stomach or duodenal wall. It should be suspected if a patient develops sudden, severe abdominal pain. On physical examination, the patient will have exquisite abdominal pain and tenderness, guarding, and, potentially, signs of peritonitis such as rebound tenderness. Upright chest and abdominal radiographs will show free peritoneal air under the diaphragm; however, if they do not, and the clinical suspicion for perforation is high, the next most useful imaging modality, if the perforation happened within the previous 6 hours, is ultrasound. After 6 hours have elapsed, CT may provide diagnostic value.

Patients with an abdominal perforation need to be treated for hemodynamic instability and receive antibiotics targeting enteric bacteria. Additionally, they should undergo an emergent surgical evaluation. Risks of surgery must be weighed against the individual patient's risk of perforation-related mortality. However, nonoperative management is appropriate only for a small number of patients, and the most effective treatment remains surgical repair of the perforation.

Gastric Outlet Obstruction
Though much less common than UGIB and perforation, gastric outlet obstruction (GOO) is a serious complication of a peptic ulcer located at the pylorus. Though PUD historically accounted for the majority of cases of obstruction, the incidence of GOO in PUD has declined as treatment for PUD has steadily improved. Currently, the leading cause of GOO is malignancy, therefore malignancy must be ruled out by endoscopy in all cases.

The precise etiology of GOO is unknown; however, it is more prevalent in patients with duodenal or pyloric ulceration. Causes of GOO secondary to PUD are likely multifactorial, from inflammatory-related causes such as spasm, edema, and pyloric dysmotility in the acute setting to more chronic causes such as scarring and fibrosis as the ulcer heals.

Patients with GOO present with early satiety, nausea, bloating, vomiting, and weight loss. On physical exam, patients will have stigmata of dehydration, abdominal distention, and a succussion splash. At presentation, patients should undergo gastric decompression to clear the gastric contents, and electrolyte abnormalities must be evaluated and treated along with IV rehydration.

是与幽门螺杆菌感染相关的溃疡，这也是幽门螺杆菌治疗的一部分。然而，复杂溃疡需要长达 8～12 周的治疗。NSAID 诱导的溃疡应在停药后至少治疗 8 周。特发性溃疡必须进行评估。ZES 患者需要进行治疗（见下文）。

维持治疗

除了根据每位患者的溃疡病因（如幽门螺杆菌感染、NSAID、ZES）进行详细评估和治疗外，部分患者还需要维持治疗以防止溃疡复发。

在消除 PUD 的危险因素后，具有以下高危特征的患者可能会受益于使用 PPI 的抑酸治疗：①巨大溃疡（＞2 cm）且年龄＞50 岁或有多种合并症；②幽门螺杆菌阴性的溃疡病；③非 NSAID 相关疾病；④难治性消化性溃疡，即经 PPI 治疗 12 周后未愈合的溃疡；⑤幽门螺杆菌根除失败；⑥复发性消化性溃疡；⑦持续使用 NSAID。维持治疗方案包括使用最低有效剂量的 H_2RA 或 PPI。应定期评估长期使用 PPI 的风险与 PUD 发生的可能性。

特殊注意事项

因心脏导管术后、不稳定型心绞痛、非 ST 段抬高型心肌梗死或卒中而需要接受双联抗血小板治疗（特别是阿司匹林和氯吡格雷）的患者，常联用 PPI 以减少胃肠道副作用。由于 PPI 和氯吡格雷均通过 CYP2C19 代谢，PPI 可能降低氯吡格雷的疗效并引发严重不良事件。多项系统综述评估了这种风险，研究表明，PPI 可降低胃肠道事件的风险，但并未显示对使用氯吡格雷的患者有明显的不良影响。

此外，新型抗凝剂（如达比加群、利伐沙班、阿哌沙班和艾多沙班）已越来越多地被用于需要长期抗凝治疗的患者。尽管关于这些药物与 PUD 相关的胃肠道出血的研究尚少，但其总体上与胃肠道出血风险增加有关，可能会导致 PUD 患者出血率升高。

手术

随着幽门螺杆菌根除治疗和抑酸治疗的应用，非手术治疗溃疡的效果显著提升。因此，手术治疗 PUD 的情况较少。然而，对于有并发症的患者，如胃出口梗阻、出血和穿孔，手术仍然是重要的治疗选择。

PUD 的并发症

PUD 最常见的并发症包括出血、穿孔和梗阻，其中出血最常见，梗阻最少见。

出血

在美国，消化道出血每年导致约 50 万次住院，每年花费约 50 亿美元。上消化道出血（UGIB）占总住院人次的 1/2，死亡率高达 7.4%。消化性溃疡是 UGIB 最常见的原因，约占所有病例的 1/3。

出血性溃疡可表现为 UGIB 的典型症状，其严重程度因出血情况而异。慢性 UGIB 的患者可能出现大便隐血和缺铁性贫血。急性出血时，患者可表现为呕吐咖啡渣样物和黑便（黑色柏油样便）；然而，快速大量的 UGIB 患者可能表现为呕血、血便和低血压。溃疡出血的治疗包括液体复苏、输血（当血红蛋白＜7 g/dl，或血红蛋白＜8 g/dl 且伴有心血管疾病，或有症状时）、静脉使用 PPI（可耐受口服的患者尽早更换为口服治疗），入院 24 h 内进行食管胃十二指肠镜（EGD）检查。如果患者有高危临床特征，如血流动力学不稳定或呕血，应在入院 12 h 内进行 EGD。内镜干预措施取决于出血性溃疡的特征。通常情况下，如果溃疡有活动性出血或有血块附着，可采用注射（血管收缩药或凝血酶）、硬化治疗或夹子等内镜干预措施。在出现活动性出血的情况下，组合治疗（如注射肾上腺素后应用夹子）的效果优于单一治疗。出血性溃疡患者的出院时间取决于其临床状态，通常可在住院 3 天后出院。

穿孔

消化性溃疡穿孔占溃疡并发症的 2%～10%。当溃疡穿透胃或十二指肠壁全层时，即会发生穿孔。如果患者突然出现剧烈腹痛，应考虑溃疡穿孔。体格检查时，患者可有剧烈腹痛和压痛、拒按及可能的腹膜炎征象（反跳痛）。立位胸腹部 X 线片可显示膈下游离气体；但是，如果未显示，且临床上高度怀疑穿孔，在穿孔发生后 6 h 内进一步行超声检查有助于诊断。超过 6 h 后，CT 可能具有诊断价值。

腹部穿孔患者需要纠正血流动力学并接受针对肠道细菌的抗生素治疗。此外，应进行紧急手术评估。必须权衡患者的手术风险与穿孔相关死亡风险。然而，非手术管理仅适用于少数患者，最有效的治疗仍然是穿孔修复手术。

胃出口梗阻

虽然远不如 UGIB 和穿孔常见，但胃出口梗阻（GOO）是幽门溃疡的严重并发症。虽然 PUD 既往是梗阻的主要原因，但随着 PUD 治疗的不断改进，GOO 的发生率已经下降。目前，GOO 的主要原因是恶性肿瘤，因此在所有病例中必须通过内镜排除恶性肿瘤。

GOO 的确切病因尚不清楚；但在十二指肠或幽门溃疡患者中更为常见。PUD 引起的 GOO 的原因可能是多因素的，包括急性期的炎症相关原因（如痉挛、水肿和幽门动力障碍）、溃疡愈合时的慢性原因（如瘢痕和纤维化）等。

GOO 患者可表现为早饱、恶心、腹胀、呕吐和体重减轻。体格检查时，患者会有脱水的体征、腹部膨隆和振水音。患者入院时应进行胃减压，以清除胃内容物，并在静脉补液的同时评估和治疗电解质紊乱。

Radiographic imaging will demonstrate an enlarged gastric bubble and dilated proximal duodenum on abdominal radiographs. Computed tomography of the abdomen will generally show gastric distention and retained chyme in the gastric cavity with an associated fluid level (Fig. 7.6).

Ultimately, patients must undergo EGD for diagnostic and possible therapeutic purposes (Fig. 7.7). Endoscopic biopsies must be obtained from the site of obstruction to evaluate for malignancy and from the antrum and body to determine if there is underlying *H. pylori* infection. If PUD is suspected, antisecretory IV treatment with a PPI must be initiated to promote healing of the ulcer and alleviation of the obstruction. Oral alimentation must be introduced slowly, as tolerated by the patient. Patients with refractory obstruction who fail conservative treatment may be treated endoscopically with balloon dilation, endoscopic stent placement, or even surgery. Additionally, patients should receive treatment for *H. pylori* and other causes of PUD, if indicated.

ZOLLINGER-ELLISON SYNDROME

Definition and Epidemiology

ZES is a rare condition that results from ectopic gastrin secretion due to a neuroendocrine tumor, called a *gastrinoma*. This leads to elevated levels of basal acid secretion in the stomach. Symptoms such as multiple or *H. pylori*–negative duodenal ulcers, recurrent ulcers, refractory ulcers, esophagitis, and unexplained diarrhea should raise clinical suspicion of ZES. Gastrinomas are primarily located in the duodenum (60% to 80%) or pancreas (10% to 14%) in an area known as the "gastrinoma triangle." They are also rarely found in other areas such as the stomach, liver, bile duct, and ovary. ZES tends to present in patients between 45 and 50 years old, and there is a slight male predominance with an estimated male to female ratio of 2:1 to 3:2. The diagnosis is often delayed due to low clinical suspicion.

Although the majority of ZES cases develop sporadically, 10% to 54% of ZES cases are found in patients with multiple endocrine neoplasia type 1 (MEN1). Multiple endocrine neoplasia type 1 is an autosomal dominant genetic disorder, usually of the *menin* gene located on chromosome 11q13. In addition to gastrinomas, patients with MEN1 also have increased incidence of parathyroid hyperplasia, pancreatic endocrine tumors, pituitary adenomas, and adrenal adenomas. Therefore, patients diagnosed with ZES must be screened for MEN1.

Pathophysiology of ZES

The main pathologic characteristic of ZES is excessively elevated levels of circulating gastrin, secreted autonomously from gastrinomas. Unlike physiologic gastrin production, gastrin release from gastrinomas is not subject to regular inhibitory feedback loops. This unregulated acid secretion causes excessive acid secretion that eventually leads to peptic ulceration in 90% of people with ZES. Exaggerated gastrin levels also act as trophic factors for ECL and parietal cells resulting in hypertrophic gastric rugae that are visible on endoscopy.

Clinical Presentation

In addition to an elevated risk of PUD, as detailed above, a third of patients may present with unexplained diarrhea, which can sometimes lead to electrolyte imbalances such as hypokalemia, steatorrhea, and weight loss. Diarrhea may be the sole clinical manifestation in about 20% of patients. Diarrhea occurs when the high acid load reaches the small intestine causing direct enterocyte damage, inactivation of pancreatic lipase, and precipitation of bile acids, which interferes with micelle formation.

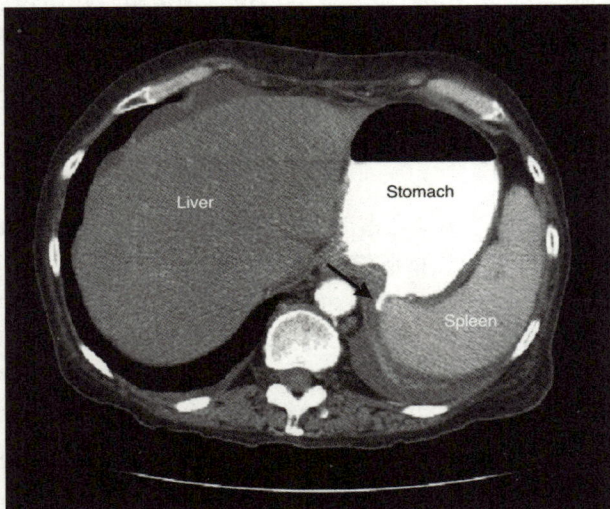

Fig. 7.6 Transverse view of an abdominal CT demonstrating a gastric outlet obstruction with significant narrowing at the distal stomach *(arrow)*. This has caused gastric distention with retained fluid in the stomach and a visible fluid level. (From Mönkemüller, et al. Gastrointestinal Endoscopy 2012;75:463-465.)

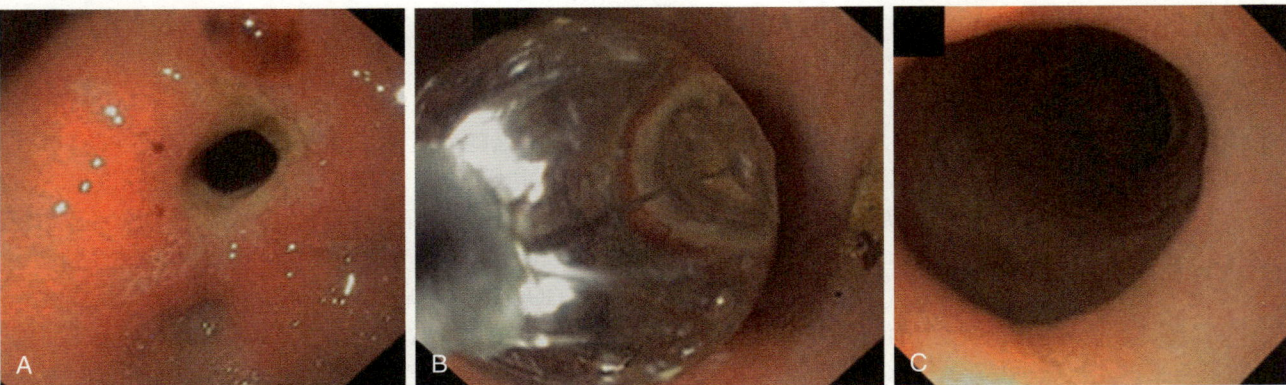

Fig. 7.7 Endoscopic appearance of gastric outlet obstruction due to a pyloric channel stricture. (A) Pyloric channel stricture. (B) Endoscopic view of balloon dilation of the pyloric stricture. (C) Post-procedure view of the pylorus after successful balloon dilation. (From Kochhar et al. Gastrointestinal Endoscopy 2018;8:899-908.)

腹部X线平片可见胃泡增大和近端十二指肠扩张的征象。腹部CT通常会显示胃腔扩张和胃内食糜潴留伴有液平（图7.6）。

最终，GOO患者必须接受胃镜检查，以进行诊断和可能的治疗（图7.7）。必须从梗阻部位进行内镜活检以排除恶性肿瘤，并从胃窦和胃体进行活检以确定是否存在幽门螺杆菌感染。如果疑诊PUD，必须开始静脉使用PPI治疗，以促进溃疡愈合和解除梗阻。经口饮食应根据患者的耐受情况逐步恢复。对于保守治疗失败的顽固性梗阻患者，可通过内镜下气囊扩张、内镜支架置入甚至手术进行治疗。此外，若有指征，应对患者进行幽门螺杆菌和其他PUD病因的治疗。

佐林格-埃利森综合征（ZES）

定义和流行病学

ZES是一种罕见疾病，由神经内分泌肿瘤（即胃泌素瘤）引起异位胃泌素分泌增加所致。这导致胃内基础胃酸分泌水平升高。当患者症状类似于多发性或幽门螺杆菌阴性的十二指肠溃疡、复发性溃疡、难治性溃疡、食管炎和不明原因的腹泻时，应临床疑诊ZES。胃泌素瘤主要发生于十二指肠（60%～80%）或胰腺（10%～14%）的"胃泌素瘤三角区"。极少数情况下可见于胃、肝、胆管和卵巢等其他区域。ZES多发生于45～50岁的患者，男性略多于女性，男女性比例估计为2:1～3:2。由于临床认识程度低，诊断常延误。

尽管绝大多数ZES病例呈散发性，但10%～54%的ZES病例见于多发性内分泌肿瘤1型（MEN1）患者。MEN1是一种常染色体显性遗传病，通常与位于染色体11q13上的*menin*基因有关。除胃泌素瘤外，MEN1患者合并甲状旁腺增生、胰腺内分泌肿瘤、垂体腺瘤和肾上腺腺瘤的发生率也升高。因此，诊断为ZES的患者必须筛查MEN1。

ZES的病理生理学

ZES的主要病理学特征是胃泌素瘤自主分泌过量的胃泌素进入循环。与生理性胃泌素分泌不同，胃泌素瘤的胃泌素释放不受正常的抑制反馈机制调控。这种不受控制的酸分泌会使酸分泌过量，最终导致90%的ZES患者出现消化性溃疡。过量的胃泌素水平还可作为ECL和壁细胞的营养因子，导致在内镜中可见胃皱襞肥大。

临床表现

除上文所述的增加PUD发生风险外，约1/3的ZES患者可能出现不明原因的腹泻，有时会导致电解质失衡（如低钾血症）、脂肪泻和体重减轻。腹泻可能是约20%患者的唯一临床表现。当高酸负荷到达小肠时，会导致肠上皮细胞直接损伤、胰脂肪酶失活和胆酸沉淀，干扰微胶粒形成，导致腹泻。

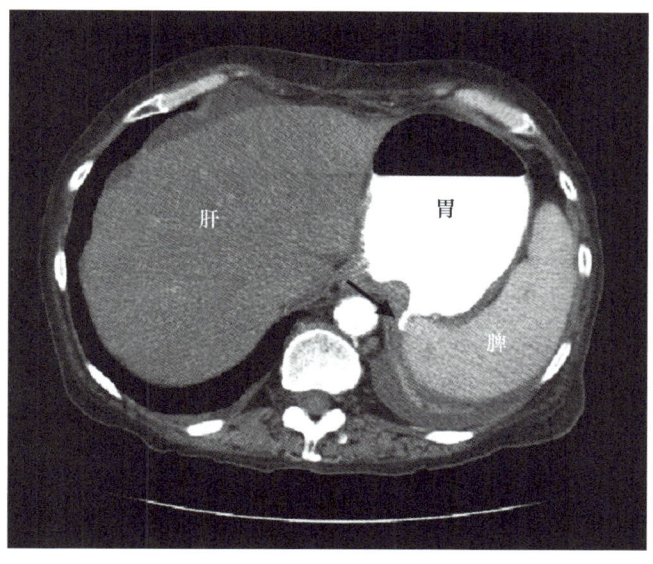

图7.6 腹部CT横断面显示胃出口梗阻伴胃远端明显狭窄（箭头）。这导致胃胀气，胃内有液体潴留，可见液平（引自Mönkemüller, et al. Gastrointestinal Endoscopy 2012; 75: 463-465.）

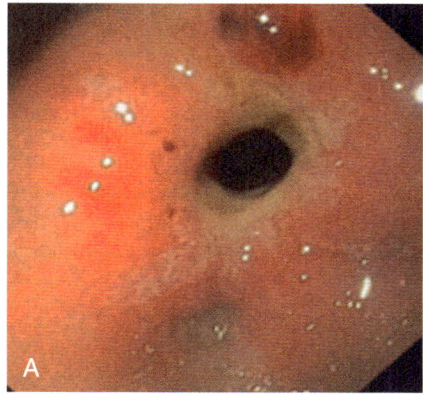 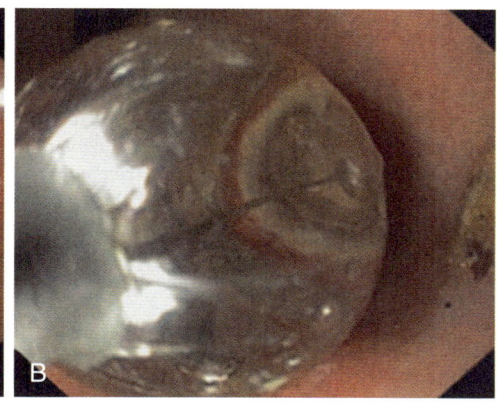 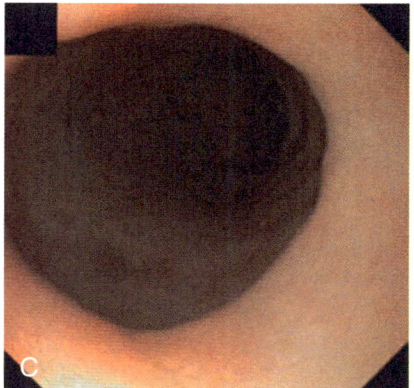

图7.7 幽门狭窄导致的胃出口梗阻的内镜下表现。**A**.幽门狭窄。**B**.气囊扩张治疗幽门狭窄的内镜视图。**C**.气囊扩张成功后的幽门术后视图（引自Kochhar et al. Gastrointestinal Endoscopy 2018; 8: 899-908.）

Other manifestation of ZES include esophageal syndromes from gastric acid hypersecretion, such as dysphagia, esophagitis, esophageal ulceration, strictures, or even perforation. In fact, reflux esophagitis may occur in up to 40% of patients with ZES.

Diagnosis

As in the diagnosis of other rare diseases, the most important factor in diagnosing ZES is having a high index of suspicion for ZES in patients that present with classic symptoms, as detailed above. These classic symptoms, however, may be hard to discern in the age of ubiquitous PPI use because these antisecretory agents may mask ZES symptoms. Diagnosis of ZES requires the presence of hypergastrinemia and hyperchlorhydria.

Initially, patients with suspected ZES should be evaluated by obtaining a fasting gastrin level and obtaining a gastric pH. A low gastric pH in conjunction with high gastrin levels is characteristic because, in achlorhydric states, gastrin will be appropriately elevated but so will pH. Because PPIs also affect the gastric pH, PPIs must be discontinued for at least 1 week prior to testing. PPI discontinuation in patients with ZES incurs serious risks and should be done only after careful evaluation of the risks and benefits of PPI withdrawal for diagnostic purposes under the supervision of experienced practitioners. Some case reports have described serious health complications of ZES that developed just 48 hours after PPI withdrawal.

Gastrin levels greater than ten times the upper limit of normal (ULN) with a gastric pH less than 2 establishes the diagnosis of ZES. However, most patients with ZES will have equivocal gastrin levels. A secretin stimulation test can help make the diagnosis in this case.

The secretin stimulation test takes advantage of the paradoxical increase in gastrin secretion after the administration of secretin in patients with gastrinomas. Similar to gastrin and gastrin pH levels, the secretin test must be obtained while the patient is not under antisecretory therapy. Gastrin levels are obtained before and after the administration of 2 U/kg of secretin. The test is positive if gastrin levels increase at least 120 pg/mL with secretin administration.

After the diagnosis of ZES is made, all patients must be screened for MEN1 by measuring calcium, parathyroid hormone (PTH), and MEN1 germline mutation testing. In addition, first-degree relatives of patients with MEN1 also must be screened. Because a majority of gastrinomas are malignant, it is critical to attempt to localize the gastrinoma with the purpose of tumor resection.

A useful imaging modality for localizing gastrinomas is a somatostatin-receptor scintigraphy (SRS) scan combined with CT scan, but other modalities such as CT, MRI, and ultrasonography may also be used. In experienced hands, upper endoscopy with endoscopic ultrasound (EUS) has similar sensitivity to SRS (74% and 75% respectively) and can be helpful in determining the location of the gastrinoma.

Treatment of ZES

After ruling out other causes of hypergastrinemia (such as pernicious anemia or PPI-induced hypergastrinemia, in which the high gastrin occurs secondary to *low* acid secretion), the most important treatment goal for ZES is reduction and normalization of acid secretion, which can be achieved through PPI therapy. To control acid secretion in ZES, PPIs typically need to be taken at elevated doses, sometimes double the standard dose or higher. PPI treatment must be titrated to achieve a basal acid output (BAO) that is less than 10 mmol/hour the hour preceding the next scheduled dose. When patients are unable to take oral medications, IV PPI therapy must be administered to control acid secretion. In extreme cases, vagotomy may be performed to decease acid secretion.

Surgery can sometimes uncover a hitherto unrecognized primary tumor. Additionally, it allows for evaluation of tumor grade and stage and removes the source of the ectopic gastrin production. Regardless, surgery significantly improves survival rates in patients with ZES. Gastrinomas tend to metastasize via a hematogenous route primarily to the lymph nodes, followed by the liver. Up to 50% of patients will have liver metastases at presentation.

GASTRITIS

Gastritis is a general term that is used to describe inflammation in the gastric mucosa. Gastric inflammation can be caused by a variety of conditions, most commonly *H. pylori* infection and NSAID gastritis (more strictly in the latter case termed *gastropathy*, because inflammation is rather mild). Gastritis can be acute or chronic and may be secondary to other infectious causes, autoimmune disorders, drugs, and ischemia. Every effort should be made to identify the cause of gastritis, though many times a specific diagnosis may not be identifiable.

Atrophic gastritis is a histopathologic entity of glandular loss that results from chronic inflammation. It can be divided into two major types: multifocal (secondary to environmental factors, *H. pylori*, specific diets) or corpus predominant (autoimmune) gastritis. This section will focus on the corpus predominant subtype, autoimmune metaplastic atrophic gastritis (AMAG).

AMAG is a chronic inflammatory gastritis caused by autoantibodies against intrinsic factor and the parietal cells in the fundus and body. It has a prevalence of 2% with a female to male ration of 3:1, and it is more common in persons with other autoimmune diseases, specifically diabetes mellitus and autoimmune thyroid disease. AMAG increases the risk of intestinal-type gastric adenocarcinoma and gastric carcinoid tumors. Patients typically present with nonspecific GI symptoms and are generally diagnosed relatively late in their disease, once they have hematologic manifestations, such as macrocytic anemia due to vitamin B_{12} deficiency (pernicious anemia). Due to the inability to absorb vitamin B_{12}, these patients may present with concomitant neurologic and psychiatric symptoms, though this happens in less than 10% of cases. On biopsy, patients will have gastric body mucosal atrophy as well as ECL hyperplasia in the setting of hypochlorhydria (and resultant hypergastrinemia). Treatment consists of vitamin B_{12} supplementation and surveillance for associated diseases.

Infectious gastritis may be caused by infections other than *H. pylori*, such as CMV, *Mycobacterium avium-intracellulare*, enterococcal infections, HSV, as well as parasitic and fungal infections. Treatment for infectious gastritis involves treatment of the specific microbe causing damage to the gastric mucosa.

Eosinophilic gastritis (EG) is a part of a continuum of eosinophil-associated gastrointestinal disorders (EGIDs). It is associated with systemic eosinophilia in about 75% of patients with EGID. In EG, there is an eosinophilic infiltration, which rarely includes all layers of the gastric wall. There is mucosal involvement in 60% of cases, muscular involvement in 30% of cases, and subserosal involvement in 10% of cases. Diagnosis is difficult, given the varying locations of infiltration, and the nonspecific appearance of the stomach on EGD. Eosinophilic gastritis may be a cause of GOO. Treatment includes systemic steroids; however, there has been some success treating patients with elemental diets free of allergenic foods.

Ménétrier's disease is a very rare condition associated with hypertrophy of the gastric mucosa primarily in the body of the stomach. Histologically, there is proliferation of the gastric glands with cystic dilation of the basilar portion. The etiology of the disease is unknown, and the diagnosis is difficult to make. Diagnosis generally necessitates

ZES 的其他表现包括胃酸分泌过多导致的食管综合征，如吞咽困难、食管炎、食管溃疡、狭窄，甚至穿孔。事实上，高达 40% 的 ZES 患者可能出现反流性食管炎。

诊断

与其他罕见疾病的诊断一样，诊断 ZES 最重要的是高度怀疑出现上述临床表现的患者。然而，在普遍使用 PPI 的时代，这些典型症状可能难以辨别，因为这些抑酸剂可能会掩盖 ZES 的症状。诊断 ZES 需要存在高胃泌素血症和高胃酸分泌。

首先，疑诊 ZES 的患者应通过检测空腹胃泌素水平和胃液 pH 值。由于在胃酸缺乏的状态下，胃泌素也会适当升高，但 pH 值同样会升高，因此胃液 pH 值低且胃泌素水平高是 ZES 的特征。由于 PPI 会影响胃液 pH 值，因此必须在检测前停用 PPI 至少 1 周。ZES 患者停用 PPI 会带来严重风险，因此必须在经验丰富的医生指导下仔细评估 PPI 停药的风险和获益后停药。一些病例报告描述了 ZES 患者在停用 PPI 后仅 48 h 内发生严重并发症。

当胃泌素水平＞正常值上限（ULN）10 倍且胃液 pH 值＜2 时，可诊断 ZES。然而，大多数 ZES 患者的胃泌素水平不稳定。在这种情况下，可通过促胰液素刺激试验帮助诊断。

促胰液素刺激试验是给予胃泌素瘤患者注射促胰液素，随后胃泌素分泌会反常性增加。类似于检测胃泌素和胃液 pH 值水平，促胰液素检测必须在患者未接受抑酸治疗时进行。分别在检查前和注射 2 U/kg 促胰液素后检测胃泌素水平。如果注射促胰液素后胃泌素增加≥ 120 pg/ml，则试验结果为阳性。

确诊 ZES 后，所有患者必须通过检测钙、甲状旁腺激素（PTH）和 MEN1 种系突变检测，以筛查 MEN1。此外，MEN1 患者的一级亲属也必须接受筛查。由于绝大多数胃泌素瘤为恶性，因此为了达到肿瘤切除的目的，对其进行定位至关重要。

一种用于胃泌素瘤定位的有效成像方式是将生长抑素受体显像（SRS）与 CT 结合，也可使用其他方式（如 CT、MRI 和超声）进行定位。对于经验丰富的医生，上消化道超声内镜（EUS）与 SRS 具有相似的敏感性（分别为 74% 和 75%），有助于确定胃泌素瘤的位置。

ZES 的治疗

在排除其他高胃泌素血症的原因（如恶性贫血或 PPI 引起的高胃泌素血症，高胃泌素继发于低胃酸分泌）后，ZES 最重要的治疗目标是减少酸分泌并使之正常化，这可以通过 PPI 治疗来实现。为了控制 ZES 患者的酸分泌，通常需要服用较高剂量的 PPI，有时是标准剂量的 2 倍甚至更高。PPI 治疗必须调整剂量，以达到下次计划用药前 1 h 的基础酸分泌（BAO）＜ 10 mmol/h 的目标。当患者无法口服药物时，必须通过静脉使用 PPI 来控制酸分泌。在严重病例中，可通过迷走神经切断术减少酸分泌。

手术有时可以发现既往未被发现的原发性肿瘤。此外，手术还可评估肿瘤的分级和分期，并消除异位胃泌素分泌的来源。手术可显著提高 ZES 患者的生存率。胃泌素瘤倾向于血行转移，主要转移至淋巴结，其次是肝。多达 50% 的患者在确诊时已出现肝转移。

胃炎

胃炎是胃黏膜炎症的总称。胃炎可由多种原因引起，最常见的是幽门螺杆菌感染和使用 NSAID（后一种情况应更严格地被称为胃病，因为炎症相对较轻）。胃炎可为急性或慢性，并可能继发于其他感染性原因、自身免疫病、药物和缺血。应尽一切努力明确胃炎的病因，尽管很多时候可能无法确定其具体的诊断。

萎缩性胃炎是慢性炎症导致腺体减少的一种组织病理学形式。它可分为两大类：多灶性萎缩性胃炎（继发于环境因素、幽门螺杆菌、特定饮食）和胃体为主型（自身免疫性）萎缩性胃炎。此处重点介绍胃体为主的亚型，即自身免疫性化生性萎缩性胃炎（AMAG）。

AMAG 是一种由针对内因子和胃底及胃体壁细胞的自身抗体引起的慢性炎症性胃炎。其患病率为 2%，女性与男性的比例为 3 : 1，在合并其他自身免疫病的患者中更常见，尤其是糖尿病和自身免疫性甲状腺疾病。AMAG 会增加肠型胃腺癌和胃类癌的风险。患者通常表现出非特异性胃肠道症状，且诊断滞后，常由维生素 B_{12} 缺乏导致巨幼细胞贫血（恶性贫血）出现血液系统表现时才被诊断。虽然仅见于不足 10% 的患者，但由于无法吸收维生素 B_{12}，这些患者可能出现神经和精神症状。活检可见胃体黏膜萎缩及在低胃酸分泌（以及继发的高胃泌素血症）背景下的 ECL 增生。治疗包括维生素 B_{12} 补充和对相关疾病的监测。

感染性胃炎可能由幽门螺杆菌以外的病原体感染引起，如 CMV、鸟-胞内分枝杆菌复合菌、肠球菌、单纯疱疹病毒（HSV），以及寄生虫和真菌感染。感染性胃炎的治疗应针对引起胃黏膜损伤的特定微生物。

嗜酸细胞性胃炎（EG） 是嗜酸性粒细胞相关性胃肠疾病（EGID）的一部分。约 75% 的 EGID 患者伴有系统性嗜酸性粒细胞增多症。在 EG 中，存在嗜酸性粒细胞浸润，但很少浸润胃壁全层。60% 的患者有黏膜受累，30% 的患者有肌层受累，10% 的患者有浆膜下层受累。鉴于浸润部位的不同且胃在食管胃十二指肠镜下的表现无特异性，故诊断较为困难。EG 可能是胃出口梗阻的原因。治疗包括使用全身性类固醇；此外，使用不含过敏原的元素饮食治疗已取得一定成功。

梅内特里耶病（Ménétrier 病） 是一种非常罕见的疾病，主要发生在胃体，与黏膜增生相关。组织学表现为胃腺体增生伴有基底部囊性扩张。该病的病因未知，诊断困难。诊断通常需要评估胃黏膜在内镜下的外观及一系列特征性症状。临床常见的症状包括恶心、

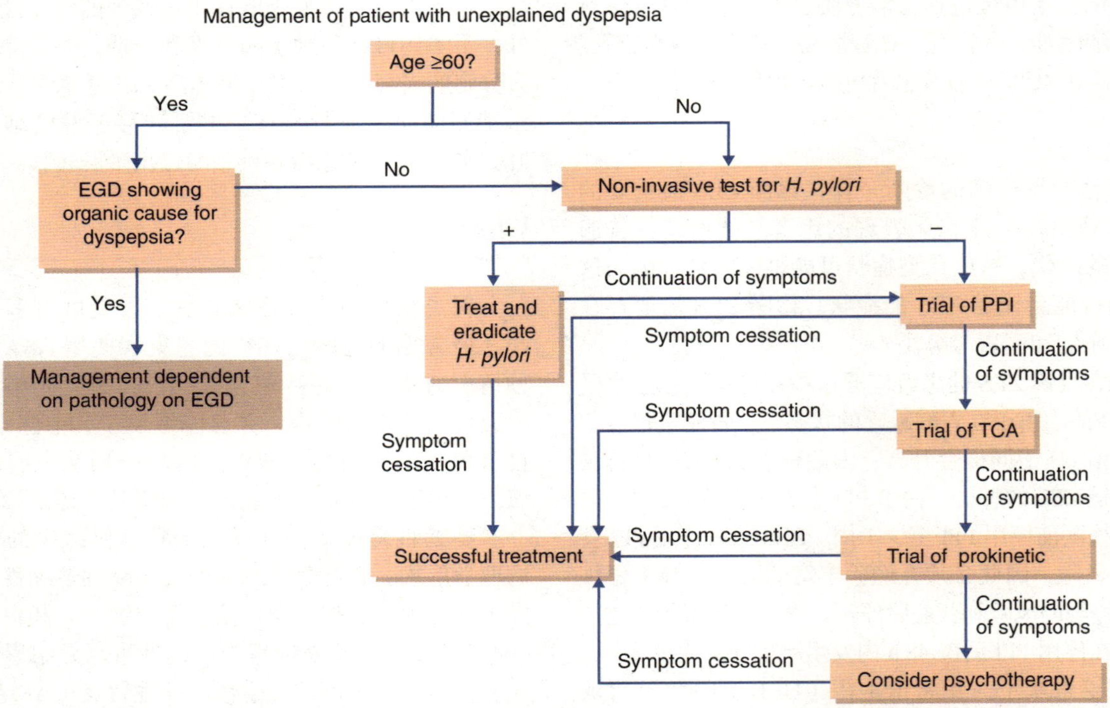

Fig. 7.8 Guideline for management of patients with dyspepsia. *EGD*, Esophagogastroduodenoscopy; *TCA*, tricyclic antidepressant. (Adapted from Moayyedi PM, Lacy BE, Andrews CN, Enns RA, Howden CW, Vakil N. ACG and CAG Clinical Guideline: Management of Dyspepsia. Am J Gastroenterol. 2017;112:988-1013.)

evaluation of the gross appearance of the gastric mucosa during endoscopy along with the characteristic constellation of symptoms. Clinically, there is associated nausea, vomiting, anemia, hypochlorhydria, and peripheral edema secondary to hypoalbuminemia.

Lymphocytic gastritis is another rare disorder characterized by mucous and gastric epithelium infiltration by T cells. It is associated with celiac disease, *H. pylori* gastritis, collagenous colitis, and Ménétrier's disease.

FUNCTIONAL (NONULCER) DYSPEPSIA

When a patient presents with a constellation of symptoms similar to that of PUD or gastritis without evidence of ulceration on EGD, they are said to have *nonulcer dyspepsia (NUD)*. Nonulcer dyspepsia is a diagnosis of exclusion. The etiology of NUD is not well understood; however, patients with NUD may have impaired gastric mucosal integrity, dysmotility, dysregulation of the gut-brain axis, or sensory dysfunction. Psychosocial factors and psychiatric disorders such as depression and anxiety, however, are very strongly associated with NUD. NUD affects 10% to 30% of the world's population.

Specific diagnostic criteria include bothersome postprandial fullness, early satiety, epigastric pain, or epigastric burning, in addition to a lack of evidence of an organic or structural explanation of the symptoms on EGD, imaging, or laboratory studies. Patients older than 60 years of age should have an EGD to evaluate for possible malignancy. Depending on individual clinical symptoms, some patients may benefit from motility studies to evaluate for dysmotility and gastroparesis (Fig. 7.8).

Unfortunately, treatment for NUD is limited and therapeutic modalities have not been well studied. Some (about 1 in 10) dyspeptic patients with NUD who test positive for *H. pylori* may respond to *H. pylori* eradication even if they do not have evidence of PUD on endoscopy. Antisecretory therapy with a PPI or H2RA is recommended for *H. pylori*–negative patients and those that have been successfully treated for *H. pylori* who continue to have symptoms. Tricyclic antidepressants are recommended for patients that continue to be symptomatic despite *H. pylori* eradication and antisecretory therapy. Further treatment options include prokinetics, such as cisapride and domperidone, though these are not available in the United States. Patients who do not respond to therapy and have ongoing, bothersome symptoms may benefit from psychological therapies, the most common being cognitive behavioral therapy.

CYCLIC VOMITING SYNDROME

Cyclic vomiting syndrome (CVS) is an idiopathic condition that presents both in children and adults with the mean age of presentation of 37 years in the adult population. The etiology of CVS is largely unknown, but it has been observed to be triggered in patients with chronic cannabis use, migraine headaches, and by certain foods (which typically also trigger migraine headaches). Characteristically, patients present with bouts of vomiting lasting hours to days with absence of vomiting between episodes. Adult patients will commonly report alleviation of symptoms while taking hot showers or baths.

Diagnosing CVS is difficult, and many years may elapse before a clear diagnosis is made. Clinicians may often misdiagnose patients with recurrent infectious gastroenteritis or other self-limiting causes of vomiting. Specific criteria for diagnosis include (1) stereotypical bouts of acute vomiting lasting less than 1 week, (2) three or more episodes in the prior year and two in the past 6 months, occurring at least 1 week apart, (3) absence of vomiting between episodes. The diagnosis of CVS must be made only after excluding other possible diagnoses.

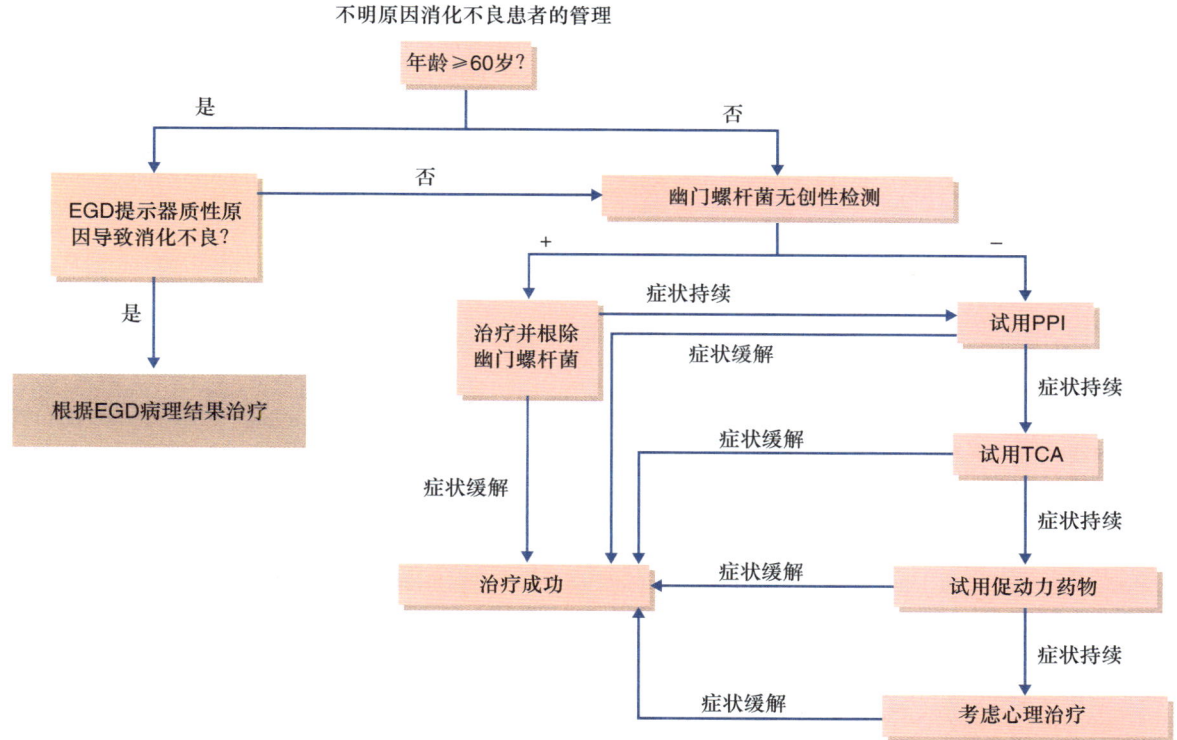

图7.8 消化不良患者的管理指南。EGD，食管胃十二指肠镜；TCA，三环类抗抑郁药（改编自 Moayyedi PM，Lacy BE，Andrews CN，Enns RA，Howden CW，Vakil N. ACG and CAG Clinical Guideline: Management of Dyspepsia. Am J Gastroenterol. 2017; 112: 988-1013.）

呕吐、贫血、低胃酸分泌，以及由低白蛋白血症引起的外周水肿。

淋巴细胞性胃炎是一种罕见疾病，其特征是T淋巴细胞浸润黏膜和胃上皮。它与乳糜泻、幽门螺杆菌胃炎、胶原性结肠炎和梅内特里耶病有关。

功能性（非溃疡性）消化不良

当患者表现出与PUD或胃炎相似的一系列症状，但在食管胃十二指肠镜中没有溃疡证据时，被称为非溃疡性消化不良（NUD）。NUD是一种排除性诊断。其病因尚不完全清楚；然而，NUD患者可能存在胃黏膜完整性受损、胃肠动力障碍、脑-肠轴失调或感觉功能障碍。此外，心理社会因素和精神疾病（如抑郁症和焦虑症）与NUD的相关性较强。NUD的全球患病率为10%～30%。

NUD的具体诊断标准包括：令人困扰的餐后饱胀、早饱、上腹痛或上腹灼热感，以及在食管胃十二指肠镜、影像学检查或实验室检查中未发现可解释症状的器质性或结构性病变。60岁以上患者应进行食管胃十二指肠镜，以评估可能的恶性肿瘤。根据个体的临床症状，部分患者可能会获益于动力学检查，以评估胃肠动力障碍和胃轻瘫（图7.8）。

然而，目前NUD的治疗方法有限，针对治疗方法的研究尚不充分。幽门螺杆菌根除治疗对约10%的幽门螺杆菌阳性的NUD患者可能有效，即使这些患者在内镜检查中没有发现PUD的证据。对于幽门螺杆菌阴性及幽门螺杆菌根除成功后仍有症状的患者，推荐使用PPI或H_2RA进行抑酸治疗。对于进行幽门螺杆菌根除和抑酸治疗后仍有症状的患者，建议使用三环类抗抑郁药。进一步的治疗选择包括促动力药物，如西沙必利和多潘立酮，但这些药物在美国未上市。对于无治疗反应且持续有令人困扰的症状的患者，心理治疗可能有帮助，最常见的是认知行为疗法。

周期性呕吐综合征

周期性呕吐综合征（CVS）是一种特发性疾病，儿童和成人均可发病，成人的平均发病年龄为37岁。CVS的病因尚不完全清楚，但据观察，长期使用大麻、偏头痛和某些食物（通常也会引发偏头痛）会引发CVS。患者的典型临床表现为持续数小时到数天的发作性呕吐，发作间期无呕吐症状。成人患者的症状通常在泡热水澡或淋浴时缓解。

诊断CVS较为困难，明确诊断可能需要数年时间。临床医生常误诊为复发性感染性胃肠炎或呕吐的其他自限性病因。诊断标准包括：①固定模式的发作性呕吐，呈急性发作，持续时间<1周；②近1年内发作≥3次，近6个月发作≥2次，且间隔至少1周；③发作间期无呕吐。CVS的诊断必须在排除其他可能的诊断后才能做出。

In the acute setting, therapy is supported with IV fluids, antiemetics, and slow reintroduction of food as tolerated by the patient. Antiemetics taken prior to the attack during the prodromal period may prevent or reduce the longevity of symptoms. Maintenance therapy consists of avoidance of triggers and, if appropriate, psychosocial treatment. When a patient presents with CVS in the setting of cannabis use, cannabis use must be stopped.

RAPID GASTRIC EMPTYING

Rapid gastric emptying, also known as *dumping syndrome*, is a debilitating condition manifesting in postprandial gastrointestinal and vasomotor symptoms that occur following esophageal, gastric, or bariatric surgery. It is due to premature delivery of food into the small intestine. Postsurgical rapid gastric emptying occurs in 25% to 50% of cases with 5% to 10% of patients experiencing debilitating symptoms; however, this diagnosis is also correlated with diabetes mellitus, and idiopathic cases have also been reported. Rapid gastric emptying can be divided into two categories, early and late dumping syndrome, of which the early variation is most common. It is defined as less than 30% retention of gastric contents within 1 hour of solid meal ingestion.

In early rapid gastric emptying, hyperosmolar food is delivered to the small intestine triggering the release of vasoactive substances such as neurostatin, vasoactive intestinal peptide (VIP), and glucose modulators such as incretins, insulin, and glucagon. This results in gastrointestinal symptoms such as early satiety, pain, diarrhea, nausea, cramps, and bloating, vasomotor symptoms such as hypotension, and sympathetic nervous system response such as facial flushing, palpitations, and diaphoresis within 30 minutes of meal ingestion.

The symptoms of late gastric emptying are a result of hyperinsulinemia and subsequent reactive hypoglycemia. Hyperinsulinemia occurs secondary to an increased release of incretins in response to undigested carbohydrates in the small intestine. Symptoms, including diaphoresis, tremulousness, decreased concentration, and altered levels of consciousness, occur 1 to 3 hours postprandially. Early and late gastric emptying may be present in isolation, but they frequently coexist.

Diagnosis of rapid gastric emptying primarily relies on a high clinical suspicion in patients with typical clinical symptoms of rapid gastric emptying. Other diagnostic modalities include oral glucose tolerance test and radionuclide scintigraphy.

First-line treatment includes lifestyle modifications to reduce the amount of food taken per meal, eating at more frequent intervals, and separating solid from liquid food ingestion. Additionally, it can be helpful to lie down after meals and decrease carbohydrate and lactose ingestion. Early consultation with a dietitian is important to ensure that an adequate nutritional status is maintained. When lifestyle modification methods fail to alleviate symptoms, pharmacologic options include acarbose, guar gum, or symptomatic treatment with loperamide, tincture of opium, and other methods of pain control. Octreotide, which inhibits the secretion of vasoactive agents, may also be helpful.

GASTROPARESIS

Gastroparesis occurs when there is delayed gastric emptying into the small intestine, causing a characteristic constellation of symptoms. It is most commonly seen in diabetics, postsurgical patients, and those on chronic scheduled opioid therapy. A third of cases are idiopathic, and women are more likely than men to develop this disorder. Up to 30% to 50% of patients with type 1 diabetes have delayed gastric emptying, as do 15% to 30% of patients with type 2 diabetes.

Diabetic gastroparesis is better understood than idiopathic gastroparesis. The etiology of diabetic gastroparesis is similar to that of diabetic neuropathy with possible denervation of the vagus nerve causing a delay in gastric emptying. Additionally, patients with diabetes-related gastroparesis have been found to have decreased numbers of interstitial cells of Cajal (ICCs), the pacemaker cells of the GI tract, as well as decreased levels of nitric oxide release from enteric neural cells. Although patients with idiopathic gastroparesis also have decreased numbers of ICCs, the cause of idiopathic gastroparesis is less well understood, though enterovirus infections have been implicated.

Clinically, patients experience early satiety, abdominal distension, nausea, vomiting, anorexia, and malnutrition. Though all patients with gastroparesis experience nausea, patients with diabetes tend to have more severe and more frequent episodes of vomiting when compared to those with idiopathic gastroparesis. Patients with idiopathic gastroparesis are more likely to have severe postprandial fullness and early satiety.

Some patients with idiopathic gastroparesis are misdiagnosed as having nonulcer dyspepsia, therefore a high index of suspicion is key to the diagnosis. After gastric outlet obstruction has been ruled out, the timing of gastric emptying may be evaluated with gastric emptying scintigraphy, breath testing, or a wireless motility capsule. It is very important that patients refrain from taking prokinetic or gastroparetic agents prior to these studies.

Treatment takes a stepwise approach beginning with dietary modifications (small, spaced out meals), improving glucose control in diabetic patients, and adding prokinetic agents. More invasive procedures such as gastric pacemakers may be tried in severe cases.

GASTRIC VOLVULUS

Gastric volvulus is a rare condition that affects both adult and pediatric patients, where the stomach rotates at least 180 degrees along its transverse or longitudinal axis causing gastric inlet or outlet obstruction. In extreme cases, gastric volvulus may cause strangulation, necrosis, and perforation; therefore it is considered a surgical emergency. The mortality rate for acute gastric volvulus ranges between 15% to 20%, whereas it is 0% to 13% for chronic cases. Rotation of the stomach is generally caused by paraesophageal hernias, structural abnormalities (such as neoplasms), adhesions, and gastric ligamentous laxity (Fig. 7.9).

Clinically, presentation varies depending on acuity and degree of obstruction. Borchardt triad of acute abdominal pain, severe retching without vomiting, and inability to place a gastric tube is present in 70% of cases with acute gastric volvulus. If the volvulus is severe enough to cause strangulation and necrosis, hematemesis may be seen. Patients with chronic gastric volvulus may present with vague symptoms such as abdominal pain, dysphagia, and bloating. These may be misdiagnosed as other upper GI disorders.

Given the rarity and nonspecific presentation of gastric volvulus, diagnosis is often done while investigating other causes for the patient's symptoms. Evidence of gastric outlet obstruction with an interruption, such as two pockets of air-fluid levels, is seen on radiographs. Additionally, given the correlation with esophageal hernias, these can also be seen on radiographs and should increase index of suspicion for gastric volvulus. These patients typically have subsequent abdominal CT scans that show abnormal location of the antrum and evidence of GOO.

Treatment can be divided into three categories: conservative, endoscopic, or surgical. In the acute setting, patients must be treated and

在急性发作时，治疗包括静脉输液、止吐药及在患者耐受时缓慢恢复进食。在发作前驱期服用止吐药可预防症状或缩短持续时间。维持治疗包括避免诱因，条件允许时可进行社会心理治疗。当患者在使用大麻的背景下出现 CVS 时，必须停止使用大麻。

胃排空加快

胃排空加快又称倾倒综合征，是食管手术、胃部手术或减重术后出现的一种表现为餐后胃肠道症状和血管运动症状的疾病。其由食物过早进入小肠引起。术后快速胃排空发生于 25%～50% 的病例，其中 5%～10% 的患者有虚弱的症状；但是，该诊断也与糖尿病相关，且也有特发性病例的报道。胃排空加快可分为早期和晚期，其中早期胃排空加快最为常见。其定义为固体餐摄入后 1 h 内胃内容物保留 < 30%。

在早期胃排空加快时，高渗食物进入小肠会刺激血管活性物质［如神经肽、血管活性肠肽（VIP）］和葡萄糖调节物质［如肠促胰岛素、胰岛素和胰高血糖素］的释放，导致在进餐后 30 min 内出现胃肠症状（如早饱、疼痛、腹泻、恶心、痉挛痛和腹胀）、血管运动症状（如低血压）和交感神经系统反应（如面部潮红、心悸和出汗）。

晚期胃排空加快的症状由高胰岛素血症和随后的反应性低血糖引起。小肠中未消化的碳水化合物引起肠促胰岛素释放增加，可导致高胰岛素血症。症状包括出汗、震颤、注意力减退和意识水平改变，通常在进餐后 1～3 h 发生。早期和晚期胃排空加快可单独存在，但通常共存。

胃排空加快的诊断主要依赖于对具有典型临床症状的患者持有高度临床怀疑。其他诊断方法包括口服葡萄糖耐量试验和放射性核素显像。

首选治疗方法包括生活方式改变，减少每餐的进食量，增加进餐频率，分开摄入固体和液体食物。此外，餐后平卧并减少碳水化合物和乳糖摄入可能有帮助。尽早咨询营养师对确保维持适当的营养状况很重要。当生活方式改变无法缓解症状时，药物治疗包括阿卡波糖、瓜尔胶或对症治疗药物（洛哌丁胺、鸦片酊和其他疼痛控制方法）。奥曲肽（抑制血管活性物质分泌）也可能有所帮助。

胃轻瘫

胃轻瘫是指胃排空至小肠的时间延迟，引起一系列特征性症状。这种情况最常见于糖尿病、术后及长期服用阿片类药物的患者。约 1/3 的病例属于特发性胃轻瘫，多见于女性。30%～50% 的 1 型糖尿病患者和 15%～30% 的 2 型糖尿病患者存在胃排空延迟。

相比于特发性胃轻瘫，目前对糖尿病性胃轻瘫的认识更深入。糖尿病性胃轻瘫的病因类似于糖尿病神经病变，可能是由于迷走神经的去神经作用导致胃排空延迟。此外，糖尿病性胃轻瘫患者的肠间质卡哈尔（Cajal）细胞（ICC；即消化道的起搏细胞）数量减少，以及肠神经细胞中一氧化氮释放水平降低。虽然特发性胃轻瘫患者的 ICC 数量也会减少，但其病因尚不清楚，可能与肠道病毒感染有关。

临床上，患者表现为早饱、腹胀、恶心、呕吐、厌食和营养不良。虽然所有胃轻瘫的患者都会出现恶心，但与特发性胃轻瘫患者相比，糖尿病性胃轻瘫患者的呕吐发作更严重且频繁。特发性胃轻瘫患者更可能出现严重的餐后饱胀和早饱。

一些特发性胃轻瘫患者可能会被误诊为非溃疡性消化不良，因此高度怀疑是诊断的关键。在排除胃出口梗阻后，可通过胃排空显像、呼气试验或无线动力胶囊来评估胃排空时间。在进行这些检查之前，患者应避免服用促动力或促胃轻瘫的药物。

治疗应采取循序渐进的方法，先进行饮食调整（少量多餐），改善糖尿病患者的血糖控制，并添加促动力药物。严重患者可以尝试更具侵入性的治疗方法，如胃起搏器。

胃扭转

胃扭转是一种罕见疾病，即胃在其横轴或纵轴上至少旋转 180°，导致胃入口或出口梗阻，成人和儿童均可患病。在极端情况下，胃扭转可能导致绞窄、坏死和穿孔，因此被视为外科急症。急性胃扭转的死亡率为 15%～20%，而慢性胃扭转的死亡率为 0%～13%。胃的扭转通常由食管旁疝、结构异常（如肿瘤）、粘连和胃韧带松弛引起（图 7.9）。

临床上，患者的表现因急性程度和梗阻程度而异。70% 的急性胃扭转患者会出现 Borchardt 三联征（急性腹痛、严重干呕但不呕吐、胃管放置困难）。如果严重扭转引起绞窄和坏死，可能会出现呕血。慢性胃扭转患者的临床症状可能不明显，如腹痛、吞咽困难和腹胀。这些症状可能会被误诊为其他上消化道疾病。

由于胃扭转的罕见性和非特异性表现，诊断通常在排除其他原因后做出。患者 X 线检查可有胃出口梗阻的证据，如两个气液平的中断。此外，由于与食管疝的相关性，X 线检查观察到食管疝时应警惕胃扭转。这些患者通常会在随后进行的腹部 CT 中发现胃窦位置异常和胃出口梗阻的证据。

治疗可分为三类：保守治疗、内镜治疗或手术治疗。急性胃扭转时，必须稳定患者病情并进行治疗。

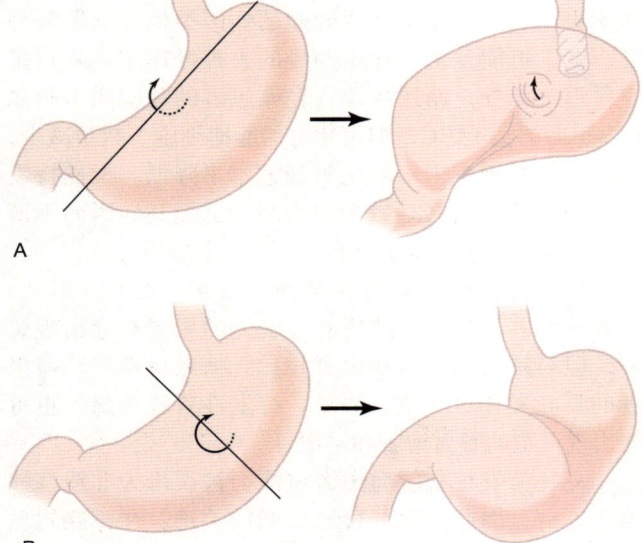

Fig. 7.9 The two major types of gastric volvulus. (A) Organoaxial volvulus, in which there is anterior rotation about the cardiopyloric axis, resulting in an upside-down stomach with the greater curve on top and the lesser curve on the bottom. Obstruction may occur at the gastroesophageal junction and the pyloroantral area. (B) Mesenteroaxial volvulus, in which there is anterior rotation about an axis perpendicular to the cardiopyloric axis. The greater curve remains on the bottom. (From Tsang, Tat-Kin et al. Endoscopic reduction of gastric volvulus: The alpha-loop maneuver Gastrointestinal Endoscopy 1995; 42: 244-248.)

stabilized. Conservative therapy consists of placing a gastric tube and laying patients in the prone position. It is generally reserved for stable patients with viable stomach tissue at the time of presentation. An endoscopic approach affords therapeutic and diagnostic value because it can assess the condition of the gastric mucosa and may sometimes lead to resolution of the volvulus with insufflation. Critically ill patients with evidence of tissue compromise generally must undergo surgery to relieve the volvulus and resect damaged tissue. Surgery also repairs gastric perforations and hiatal hernias. Patients generally undergo a gastropexy (fixation of the stomach to the anterior abdominal wall) to prevent future episodes.

SUGGESTED READINGS

Cook D, Guyatt G: Prophylaxis against gastrointestinal bleeding in hospitalized patients, N Engl J Med 378:2500–2516, 2018.
Crowe SE: Helicobacter pylori Infection, N Engl J Med 380:1158–1165, 2019.
Laine L, Jensen DM: Management of patients with ulcer bleeding, Am J Gastroenterol 107:345–360, 2012.
Lanas A, Chan FKL: Peptic ulcer disease, Lancet 530:613–624, 2017.
Moayyedi PM, Lacy BE, Andrews CN, Enns RA, Howden CW, Vakil N: ACG and CAG clinical guideline: management of dyspepsia, Am J Gastroenterol 112:988–1013, 2017.
Murugesan SV, Varro A, Pritchard DM: Review article: Strategies to determine whether hypergastrinemia is due to Zollinger-Ellison syndrome rather than a more common benign cause, Aliment Pharmacol Ther 29:1055–1068, 2009.
Siddique O, Ovalle A, Siddique AS, Moss SF: Helicobacter pylori infection: an update for the internist in the age of increasing global antibiotic resistance, Am J Med 131:473–479, 2018.

保守治疗包括放置胃管和让患者取俯卧位。这种治疗通常仅适用于病情稳定、胃部组织仍存活的患者。内镜治疗具有诊断和治疗价值，可评估胃黏膜情况，且有时可通过注气来缓解胃扭转。有组织损伤证据的危重患者通常必须接受手术，以解除扭转并切除受损组织。手术还可修复胃穿孔和食管裂孔疝。患者通常需要接受胃固定术（将胃固定在前腹壁上），以防止复发。

推荐阅读

Cook D, Guyatt G: Prophylaxis against gastrointestinal bleeding in hospitalized patients, N Engl J Med 378:2500–2516, 2018.

Crowe SE: Helicobacter pylori Infection, N Engl J Med 380:1158–1165, 2019.

Laine L, Jensen DM: Management of patients with ulcer bleeding, Am J Gastroenterol 107:345–360, 2012.

Lanas A, Chan FKL: Peptic ulcer disease, Lancet 530:613–624, 2017.

Moayyedi PM, Lacy BE, Andrews CN, Enns RA, Howden CW, Vakil N: ACG and CAG clinical guideline: management of dyspepsia, Am J Gastroenterol 112:988–1013, 2017.

Murugesan SV, Varro A, Pritchard DM: Review article: Strategies to determine whether hypergastrinemia is due to Zollinger-Ellison syndrome rather than a more common benign cause, Aliment Pharmacol Ther 29:1055–1068, 2009.

Siddique O, Ovalle A, Siddique AS, Moss SF: Helicobacter pylori infection: an update for the internist in the age of increasing global antibiotic resistance, Am J Med 131:473–479, 2018.

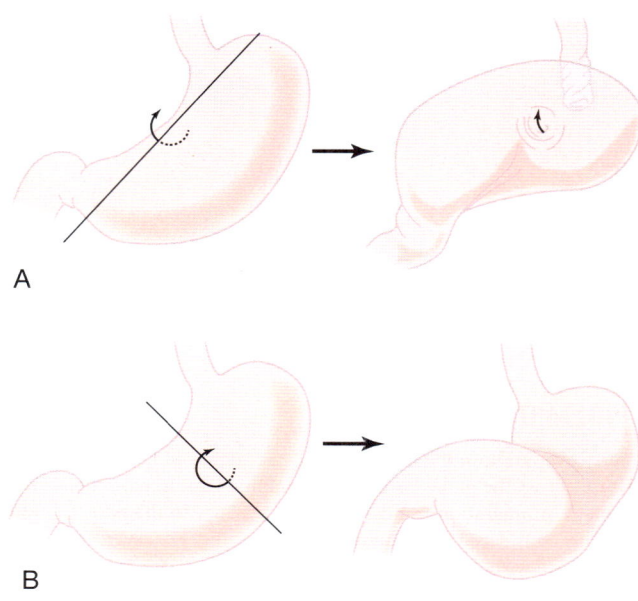

图 7.9　胃扭转的两种主要类型。**A**. 器官轴性胃扭转，胃围绕贲门-幽门轴进行前向旋转，导致胃上下颠倒，大弯位于顶部，小弯位于底部。梗阻可发生于胃食管连接处和幽门前区。**B**. 肠系膜轴性胃扭转，胃围绕垂直于贲门-幽门轴的轴线进行前向旋转。大弯保持在底部（引自 Tsang，Tat-Kin et al. Endoscopic reduction of gastric volvulus：The alphaloop maneuver Gastrointestinal Endoscopy 1995；42：244-248.）

Inflammatory Bowel Disease

Talha A. Malik, Michael F. Picco, Francis A. Farraye

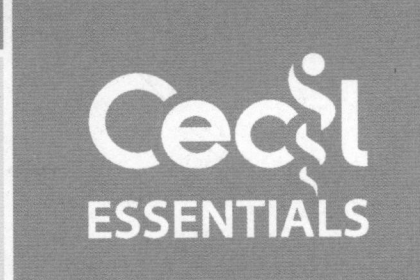

INTRODUCTION

Inflammatory bowel disease (IBD) comprises two chronic disorders: ulcerative colitis (UC) and Crohn's disease. The diagnosis of IBD is based on review of clinical, endoscopic, radiologic, and histologic data. Although the cause of these two diseases has yet to be defined, new and emerging targeted anti-inflammatory treatments hold great promise in helping to reduce morbidity and improve the quality of life of individuals with IBD.

UC is characterized by chronic inflammatory changes that involve the colonic mucosa in a continuous superficial fashion, typically starting in the rectum and extending proximally. Depending on the extent of the disease, UC can be divided into proctitis (rectum only), proctosigmoiditis (rectum and sigmoid), left-sided colitis (extending to the splenic flexure), and pancolitis (inflammation extends proximal to the splenic flexure). This classification is significant for both prognosis and therapy. Unlike UC, Crohn's disease can involve any segment of the gastrointestinal tract from the mouth to the anus, often in a discontinuous fashion. It is characterized by transmural chronic inflammation, which results in complications such as abscesses, fistulas, and strictures.

Historical Perspective

Ulcerative colitis was first described in ancient Greece by Hippocrates as a condition characterized by chronic diarrhea and bloody stools. In 1859, Samuel Wilks, a British physician, described "ulcerative colitis" as a discrete disease entity.

In 1913, the British physician Kennedy Dalziel first described patients with transmural inflammation of the small and large intestines. Subsequently, in 1932, Dr. Burrill Crohn, Dr. Leon Ginzburg, and Dr. Gordon Oppenheimer published papers describing a condition that caused inflammation of the terminal ileum and which they called regional or terminal ileitis. This disease entity later began to be referred as Crohn's disease.

The first breakthrough that established IBD as the major intestinal autoimmune disease occurred in the 1950s when it was demonstrated that symptoms in patients with both UC and Crohn's disease responded to corticosteroids. In the 1980s, traditional immune modulators, mainly thiopurines, were used as first-line steroid sparing agents. In 1997, Targan and colleagues published findings from the "Crohn's Disease cA2 Study" that looked at the efficacy of infliximab, a biologic antibody against tumor necrosis factor (TNF) cA2 in the induction of remission in luminal Crohn's. This began the era of biologics. During the first decade of the 21st century, biologics given intravenously or as subcutaneous injections emerged as the most effective therapeutic agents used to induce and maintain remission in moderate to severe UC and Crohn's disease. Since then, new oral agents are now available and effective in the treatment of patients with IBD.

EPIDEMIOLOGY

There is variation in the incidence and prevalence of UC and Crohn's disease across the globe based on geographic region, particular environment, immigration trends, and ethnic group. In the past, UC was generally considered to be slightly more common. However, this trend has changed with the rising incidence of Crohn's disease. It is estimated that there are more than 2 million people with IBD in North America. The annual incidence in North America of both UC and Crohn's disease is estimated to be between 0 to 20 per 100,000 persons. The estimates for prevalence of UC and Crohn's disease in North America are 35 to 250 per 100,000 and 25 to 300 per 100,000, respectively. The incidence and prevalence of IBD reflect the interplay of complex genetic and environmental factors that contribute to these disorders. For example, both diseases are more common in northern climates and among white individuals, particularly among populations of European descent living in North America, South Africa, and Australia. Although incidence rates of IBD are lowest among Hispanic and Asian populations, IBD can occur in any ethnic or racial group from anywhere in the world. The cause of IBD remains unknown, but it is believed to result from a combination of genetic, immunologic, infectious, and environmental factors. In addition, research points toward a relationship between the human microbiome and dysfunction of the immune system in patients with IBD.

UC and Crohn's disease can occur at any age, but the peak age of onset for UC is between 30 and 40 years of age and for Crohn's disease it is between 20 and 30 years. There is another peak, especially for UC, between 60 and 70 years of age based on studies in several European cohorts. The incidence and prevalence of UC and Crohn's disease appear to be similar in North American men and women.

RISK FACTORS AND PATHOPHYSIOLOGY

IBD is likely a result of an uncontrolled immune-mediated inflammatory response in genetically predisposed individuals to an environmental trigger that interacts with the intestinal flora and primarily affects the alimentary tract.

Approximately 5% to 20% of patients with IBD have a first-degree relative with the disease, and first-degree relatives of IBD patients have about a 10- to 15-fold increased risk for developing IBD, predominantly with the same disease as the proband. A positive family history is more frequently observed in patients with Crohn's disease compared with UC, suggesting that genetic factors are more important in the etiology of Crohn's disease. The lifetime risk of developing IBD in first-degree relatives has been estimated at 5% in Crohn's disease and about 2% in UC among non-Ashkenazi Jewish populations and 8% and 5% within Ashkenazi Jewish populations, respectively.

炎症性肠病

王吉林　译　左秀丽　刘苶　审校　房静远　通审

引言

炎症性肠病（IBD）包括两种慢性疾病：溃疡性结肠炎（UC）和克罗恩病（CD）。IBD 的诊断需依据临床表现、内镜检查、影像学检查和病理结果来综合判断。尽管这两种慢性疾病的病因尚未完全明确，但新型靶向抗炎药物在降低疾病严重程度和改善 IBD 患者生活质量方面具有巨大潜力。

UC 是结直肠黏膜的慢性炎症性疾病，病变表浅，呈连续性分布，通常起始于直肠并向近端肠段延伸。根据病变累及的范围，UC 可分为直肠炎（局限于直肠）、直乙结肠炎（直肠和乙状结肠）、左半结肠炎（延伸至脾曲）和全结肠炎（炎症延伸至脾曲以上）。这种分型对于治疗和预后具有重要意义。与 UC 不同，CD 可累及从口腔到肛门的任何消化道部分，通常呈节段性分布。其特征是肠壁全层慢性炎症，可导致脓肿、瘘管和狭窄等并发症。

诊疗的历史回顾

UC 最早由古希腊的希波克拉底描述，他将其定义为一种以慢性腹泻和血便为特征的病症。1859 年，英国医生塞缪尔·威尔克斯将"溃疡性结肠炎"描述为一种独立的疾病。

1913 年，英国医生肯尼迪·达齐尔首次报道了患有小肠和结肠全层炎症的患者。1932 年，伯里尔·克罗恩医生、莱昂·金兹堡医生和戈登·奥本海默医生在论文中描述了一种引起末端回肠炎症的疾病，他们将其称为区域性回肠炎或末端回肠炎。这种疾病后来被称为 CD。

20 世纪 50 年代，IBD 首次被确立为主要的肠道自身免疫病，因为当时发现皮质类固醇能改善 UC 和 CD 患者的症状。20 世纪 80 年代，传统免疫调节剂（主要是硫嘌呤类药物）被用作一线类固醇减停剂。1997 年，塔尔甘等发表了"Crohn's Disease cA2 Study"的研究结果，该研究主要探讨了针对肿瘤坏死因子（TNF）cA2 的生物抗体英夫利昔单抗在诱导 CD 缓解方面的有效性，这标志着生物制剂时代的开始。在 21 世纪的最初 10 年，通过静脉注射或皮下注射生物制剂成为诱导和维持中重度 UC 和 CD 缓解最有效的治疗。此后，新型口服小分子药物陆续进入临床使用，且被证实有效。

流行病学

在全球范围内，UC 和 CD 的发病率和患病率因地理区域、特定环境、移民趋势和种族而异。过去通常认为 UC 更为常见。然而，随着 CD 发病率的上升，这一趋势已经发生改变。据估计，北美地区的 IBD 患者超过 200 万人。在北美地区，估计 UC 和 CD 的年发病率均为（0~20）/100 000，估计 UC 和 CD 的患病率分别为（35~250）/100 000 和（25~300）/100 000。IBD 发病率和患病率的差异也反映了复杂的遗传因素和环境因素相互作用对 IBD 发病的影响，例如，UC 和 CD 在北方气候地区和白种人中更常见，特别是北美、南非和澳大利亚的欧裔人群。西班牙裔和亚洲人群的 IBD 发病率最低，但 IBD 可以发生于世界上任何地区、人群和种族。IBD 的病因仍未完全明确，但通常认为是由遗传、免疫、感染和环境因素的共同作用所致。此外，近期研究显示肠道微生态和免疫系统功能紊乱也与 IBD 的发生有关。

UC 和 CD 可在任何年龄发病，但 UC 的发病高峰年龄为 30~40 岁，而 CD 的发病高峰年龄为 20~30 岁。欧洲队列研究发现，UC 的另一发病高峰年龄为 60~70 岁。在北美地区，UC 和 CD 的发病率和患病率无明显性别差异。

危险因素和病理生理学

IBD 可能是遗传易感个体因环境诱因与肠道菌群的相互作用导致免疫介导的炎症反应失控而发病，主要累及消化道。

5%~20% 的 IBD 患者的一级亲属罹患 IBD，IBD 患者一级亲属的发病风险是普通人群的 10~15 倍，且大多与先证者疾病类型相同。与 UC 相比，CD 的阳性家族史更常见，表明遗传因素在 CD 的发病中占有更重要的地位。在非阿什肯纳兹犹太人群中，估计 IBD 患者的一级亲属罹患 CD 和 UC 的终身风险分别为 5% 和 2%，在阿什肯纳兹犹太人群中分别为 8% 和 5%。

Through genome-wide association studies (GWAS), over 200 genetic loci have been identified as being associated with IBD. However, there is little diagnostic utility in clinical practice of these genetic variants due to their overall low incidence in IBD populations. With increasingly diverse populations being studied, this may change. Examples of single nucleotide polymorphisms (SNPs) associated with Crohn's include sequences in the *NOD2*, IL23-receptor and the *ATG16L1* genes. It is thought that *NOD2* variants may predict more complicated disease, mainly in European patients with stricturing ileal and penetrating disease. IL-12 variants may be associated with risk for early surgery.

Additionally, other genes associated with IBD that have been identified through GWAS include *IRGM*, *LRRK*, *FUT2*, *CARD9*, *TNFSF15*, *FCG2RA*, *NKX2-3*, *PTPN2*, *ZNF365*, *ECM1*, *STAT3*, and *IL10R* among others. As mentioned, these variants have little diagnostic or therapeutic utility in clinical practice at this time due to lack of replication of associations noted in small studies.

Profound alterations in mucosal immunology have been demonstrated in patients with IBD. In the normal immunologic state of the intestine, activated lymphoid tissue is abundant within the mucosal compartment. This state has been described as controlled or physiologic inflammation, and it likely develops in response to constant encounters with antigenic substances (derived from host microbial flora or dietary and environmental sources) that have crossed the epithelial barrier from the luminal environment. Indeed, one of the main functions of the intestinal immune system is to discriminate noxious or harmful substances and organisms from nonharmful ones. As a result, a large and well-maintained network of many different mucosal immune cells exists, including cells involved in reducing immune responses (regulatory cells) and those involved in activating immune responses. In IBD, this homeostatic balance, or immune tolerance, is dysregulated, resulting in overactivation of the immune system.

In the past, it was thought that inflammation in Crohn's was predominantly mediated by T_H1 cells and in UC it was primarily mediated by T_H2 cells; there is now considerable evidence that each of their pathogeneses is more complex and nuanced, whereby both types of T helper cells appear to play a role. Furthermore, there is recent evidence that T_H17 cells produce pro-inflammatory cytokines that facilitate inflammation in IBD, the most notable of which appear to be IL-6 and IL-17. Moreover, IL-23R is expressed in high numbers on T_H17 cells and has been postulated to play a key role in propagation of inflammation in both UC and Crohn's disease.

Overall, the immune mechanisms mediating inflammation in IBD are complex and work through significant interactions with environmental triggers, the genome, and the gut microbiome to produce active disease necessitating the need for a personalized approach to management.

As alluded to, environmental factors also are believed to play a role in the pathogenesis of IBD because the disease is more common in industrialized countries. Moreover, the frequency has increased in countries as they become more industrialized. It has been postulated that poor sanitation, food contamination, and crowded living conditions are associated with helminthic infection, which leads to regulatory T-cell conditioning and stimulation of IL-10 and transforming growth factor-β production by mononuclear cells, thereby preventing intestinal inflammation.

The only environmental factor clearly associated with IBD is tobacco smoking. Tobacco seems to be protective against UC, with an older age of onset in former smokers. Among UC patients, smoking cessation may cause an exacerbation. Moreover, studies have shown that tobacco smokers with UC may have a milder disease course, require less immune suppression, and have a reduced need for surgery.

Conversely, Crohn's disease is associated with a more aggressive disease course. Tobacco consumption is associated with a 2-fold increase in the risk of development of Crohn's disease and an earlier age of onset. Passive smoking may also increase the risk. Smoking leads to more frequent exacerbations of Crohn's disease, an increased need for immunosuppression and surgery, as well as a higher risk of post-resection recurrence. Not all studies demonstrate these associations, suggesting a gene-environment interaction of tobacco and IBD with the divergent effects on UC and Crohn's disease not well understood.

Diet may also play a role. There is observational evidence that patients with Crohn's disease consumed a much higher quantity of refined sugars represented by sugar, candy, and sweetened foods like cakes and cookies prior to their diagnosis. Subsequently, it was suggested that high sugar intake itself could also interact with intestinal flora and produce pro-inflammatory intestinal agents. In addition to increased intake of refined sugars, newly diagnosed patients with IBD consumed less dietary fiber, raw fruit, and vegetables when compared to healthy controls. A systematic review of past epidemiologic surveys and case control studies performed in Japanese patients suggested an association between increased consumption of animal meat in addition to carbohydrates as potential risk for development of Crohn's disease. The researchers hypothesized that Western dietary patterns may be responsible for the increased occurrence of IBD in Japan.

Study of the relationship between obesity and IBD is especially important because of credible molecular evidence that links adipose tissue physiology to intestinal inflammation. However, it is still not entirely clear whether this link translates into a causal or clinically meaningful association between obesity and Crohn's disease.

Recently, there has been interest in understanding the association between cannabis and IBD. There are no credible epidemiologic data suggesting that cannabis plays a role in the development of IBD or its management. However, studies are ongoing.

Medications suggested to be potential risk factors for the development of IBD include, most importantly, nonsteroidal anti-inflammatory drugs (NSAIDs). NSAIDs have also been implicated in exacerbating existing disease. Other medications potentially linked to development of IBD include oral contraceptives, hormone replacement therapy, and antibiotics, but evidence for these is not as strong as with NSAIDs.

Mycobacterium avium subspecies *paratuberculosis* has been linked to Crohn's disease but this association has not been confirmed. Similarly, associations between *Salmonella*, *Campylobacter*, and measles virus have been reported to increase the risk of IBD, but not proven.

Poor hygiene (lack of sanitation), especially early in life, may protect against the development of IBD. Other potential associations include stress, anxiety, depression, disruptive sleep pattern, and sedentary lifestyle. Although provocative, these associations have not been confirmed in well-designed prospective studies.

CLINICAL PRESENTATION

Intestinal Manifestations
Ulcerative Colitis
UC is characterized by chronic inflammation of the mucosal surface that involves the rectum and extends proximally through the colon in a continuous manner. The extent and severity of colonic inflammation determine prognosis and presentation (insidious vs. acute onset). Most patients initially exhibit diarrhea, abdominal pain, urgency to defecate, rectal bleeding, and the passage of mucus per rectum. At presentation, approximately 40% to 50% of patients have proctitis or proctosigmoiditis, 30% to 40% have left-sided colitis (disease extending to the splenic flexure), and the remaining 20% to 25% have pancolitis. Though data

全基因组关联分析（GWAS）已鉴定出 200 多个与 IBD 相关的遗传位点。然而，这些遗传变异在 IBD 患者中的总体发生率较低，因此其临床诊断价值有限。随着研究人群的多样化，这种情况正在发生改变。与 CD 相关的单核苷酸多态性（SNP）包括 NOD2、IL23 受体和 ATG16L1 基因等。研究显示，NOD2 基因变异能预测更复杂的疾病状态，特别是对欧洲 IBD 患者发生回肠狭窄和穿透性病变有较高的预测价值，而 IL-12 的遗传变异可能与早期手术风险相关。

此外，GWAS 鉴定出的与 IBD 相关的其他基因包括 IRGM、LRRK、FUT2、CARD9、TNFSF15、FCG2RA、NKX2-3、PTPN2、ZNF365、ECM1、STAT3 和 IL10R 等。如前所述，由于研究较少及重复性欠佳，这些遗传变异位点在临床实践中几乎没有诊断或治疗价值。

IBD 患者的黏膜免疫功能会发生显著改变。在肠道的正常免疫状态下，由于不断遇到从管腔环境穿过上皮屏障的抗原物质（包括来源于宿主自身的微生物菌群、饮食和环境因素），黏膜层丰富的淋巴组织处于活化状态，这种状态被称为可控性或生理性炎症。事实上，肠道免疫系统的主要功能之一就是区分来源物质对机体是否有害。因此，机体存在很多不同的黏膜免疫细胞，包括参与抑制免疫应答的细胞（调节细胞）和参与激活免疫应答的细胞，这些免疫细胞构成了数量庞大且稳定有序的免疫调节网络。在 IBD 患者中，这种稳态失衡或免疫耐受失调，导致免疫系统的过度激活。

既往通常认为 CD 中的炎症主要由 T_H1 细胞介导，而 UC 主要由 T_H2 细胞介导；目前已有大量证据表明，它们的发生机制更为复杂和微妙，两种类型的辅助性 T 细胞似乎都发挥了作用。此外，新证据表明 T_H17 细胞可产生促炎症细胞因子，从而促进 IBD 中炎症的发生，其中作用最显著的是 IL-6 和 IL-17。此外，IL-23R 在 T_H17 细胞上大量表达，这可能在 UC 和 CD 的炎症进展中发挥关键作用。

总的来说，介导 IBD 炎症的免疫机制非常复杂，与环境因素、基因和肠道菌群之间存在显著的相互作用，因此 IBD 患者需采取个性化管理方法。

如前所述，由于 IBD 在工业化国家中更常见，故环境因素被认为发挥一定作用。随着各国的工业化程度不断提高，IBD 的发病率也随之升高。据推测，卫生条件差、食物污染和居住条件拥挤均与寄生虫感染有关，这可导致调节性 T 细胞的表达，并刺激单核细胞产生 IL-10 和转化生长因子 β（TGF-β），从而防止肠道发生炎症。

目前，吸烟是唯一明确与 IBD 有关的环境因素，吸烟似乎对 UC 有保护作用，吸烟者 UC 的发病年龄较大。在 UC 患者中，戒烟可能会导致病情恶化。此外，研究表明，吸烟的 UC 患者可能病情较轻，更少需要免疫抑制治疗，需要手术的概率也较低。

相反，吸烟与 CD 病情更严重有关。吸烟使 CD 的发生风险增加 2 倍，且发病年龄更小。被动吸烟也会增加 CD 的发生风险。吸烟会导致 CD 发作更频繁，对免疫抑制剂和手术的需求增加，术后的复发风险增加。并非所有研究结果都表明存在这种相关性，这提示吸烟和 IBD 之间存在基因-环境交互作用，且吸烟对 UC 和 CD 的不同影响的机制尚不明确。

饮食也在 IBD 的发生中发挥一定作用。观察性研究发现，在诊断 CD 前，患者摄入的精制糖（糖、糖果，以及蛋糕和饼干等甜点）更多。后续研究指出，摄入的高糖可与肠道菌群相互作用，产生肠道促炎症因子。与健康对照组相比，新发 IBD 患者除精制糖的摄入增加外，还存在膳食纤维、新鲜蔬菜和水果的摄入减少。一项对日本患者进行的流行病学调查和病例对照研究的系统综述表明，除碳水化合物外，动物肉类的摄入量增加是 CD 发生的潜在风险。研究人员推测，西方化的饮食模式可能是导致日本 IBD 发病率升高的原因。

研究肥胖与 IBD 之间的关系具有非常重要的意义，因为脂肪组织与肠道炎症相关存在确切的分子证据。但是，肥胖与 CD 之间是否存在因果关系，或两者的关联是否具有临床意义，目前尚不清楚。

近期有关大麻和 IBD 相关性的研究引起了人们的关注，目前尚无可靠的流行病学证据表明大麻在 IBD 的发生及疾病控制中发挥作用，相关研究仍在进行中。

药物也可能是 IBD 的潜在危险因素，其中最主要的是非甾体抗炎药（NSAID），NSAID 会加重 IBD 的病情。其他可能与 IBD 相关的药物包括口服避孕药、激素替代治疗药物和抗生素等，但这些药物与 IBD 的相关性没有 NSAID 那么确切。

鸟分枝杆菌的副结核亚种与 CD 发病有关，但尚未得到证实。同样，也有报道显示沙门菌、空肠弯曲菌和麻疹病毒会增加 IBD 的发生风险，但也未得到证实。

不良卫生条件（缺乏卫生设施），尤其是在生命早期阶段，可能会防止 IBD 的发生。其他潜在的关联因素包括应激、焦虑、抑郁、睡眠紊乱和久坐的生活方式等。尽管这些关联引人关注，但它们尚未在设计良好的前瞻性研究中得到确认。

临床表现

肠道表现

溃疡性结肠炎

UC 是累及结直肠黏膜的慢性炎症性疾病，病变常从直肠开始，呈连续性分布而向近端蔓延，可累及全结肠。患者的预后和临床表现（隐匿性 vs. 急性发作）取决于结肠炎症的范围和严重程度。大多数患者的初发表现为腹泻、腹痛、排便急迫、血便和黏液便。初次就诊时，40%～50% 的患者为直肠炎或直乙结肠炎，30%～40% 为左半结肠炎（病变延伸至脾曲），其余 20%～25% 为全结肠炎。尽管数据因队列研究人群不

are variable, depending on the cohort, it has been observed that up to 50% of patients diagnosed with proctitis or proctosigmoiditis will progress to more extensive disease by 25 years of follow-up.

The typical clinical course of UC is one of chronic intermittent exacerbations followed by periods of remission. A disease flare may be suggested by the development of diarrhea, hematochezia, and abdominal pain, with dehydration, fever, and tachycardia suggesting more severe disease. Elevated fecal calprotectin, erythrocyte sedimentation rate (ESR) or C-reactive protein (CRP) level may also indicate a flare. Anemia commonly occurs and is caused by chronic blood loss from the involved colonic mucosa as well as bone marrow suppression from the systemic inflammatory process. Perforation can occur in patients with severe or fulminant colitis, especially those taking corticosteroids, and in the setting of toxic megacolon. Toxic megacolon is characterized by gross dilation of the large bowel associated with fever, abdominal pain, dehydration, tachycardia, and bloody diarrhea.

Crohn's Disease

The clinical presentation of Crohn's disease depends on the section of gastrointestinal tract involved and the type of inflammation. Crohn's disease can involve any portion of the gastrointestinal tract; the most common site is ileocecal/ileocolonic (40% of patients), followed by isolated small bowel disease mostly affecting the terminal ileum (30%), and isolated colonic involvement (25%). The remaining sites of Crohn's disease are rarely (5%) affected in isolation and include the esophagus, stomach, and duodenum.

Symptoms in Crohn's disease often include right lower quadrant abdominal pain, fever, weight loss, diarrhea, and sometimes a palpable inflammatory mass on physical exam. Hematochezia may be present with colonic involvement but is less common than in UC. The symptoms can often be present for months or years before a diagnosis is made, and in children, growth retardation may be the sole presenting sign. In contrast to UC, the inflammation in Crohn's disease is transmural and can result in deep ulcerations and the formation of fistulous tracts. Fistulas may form between different segments of bowel (e.g., enteroenteric, enterocolonic) or between bowel and skin (enterocutaneous), bowel and bladder (enterovesicular), or rectum and vagina (rectovaginal). Over time, as many as 30% to 40% of patients will develop perianal involvement with fissures, fistulas or abscesses.

Chronic inflammation can cause fibrosis and stricture formation, which in turn may result in partial or complete intestinal obstruction with the patient complaining of abdominal pain, distention, nausea, and vomiting. Strictures can also lead to stasis with subsequent small intestinal bacterial overgrowth. Small bowel disease may lead to vitamin D deficiency. Extensive ileal mucosal disease may lead to malabsorption of vitamin B_{12} (resulting in a megaloblastic anemia and neurologic side effects if not corrected) and malabsorption of bile salts (resulting in diarrhea induced by unabsorbed bile salts and potential fat-soluble vitamin deficiency). Depletion of the bile salt pool can lead to the formation of gallstones. Weight loss may result from generalized malabsorption caused by loss of absorptive surfaces. Chronic fat malabsorption leads to luminal binding of free fatty acids to calcium; this allows oxalate, which normally is poorly absorbed because it complexes to calcium in the gut lumen, to be absorbed in the colon. The increase in oxalate absorption increases the risk for urinary calcium oxalate stone formation. Patients with an ileostomy or chronic volume loss from diarrhea are also at increased risk for uric acid stones.

Extraintestinal Manifestations

Although both UC and Crohn's disease primarily involve the bowel, they are also associated with inflammatory manifestations in other organ systems. This reflects the systemic nature of these disorders

TABLE 8.1 Extraintestinal Manifestations of Inflammatory Bowel Disease

Skin
Pyoderma gangrenosum
Erythema nodosum
Sweet syndrome

Hepatobiliary
Primary sclerosing cholangitis
Cholelithiasis
Autoimmune hepatitis

Musculoskeletal
Seronegative arthritis
Ankylosing spondylitis
Sacroiliitis

Ocular
Uveitis
Episcleritis

Miscellaneous
Hypercoagulable state
Autoimmune hemolytic anemia
Amyloidosis

(Table 8.1). Extraintestinal manifestations can occur in parallel or independently of disease activity and they can become more difficult to treat than the bowel disease itself.

The most common extraintestinal manifestation is arthritis, which is seen in about 9% to 50% of patients and is divided into two major types: axial and peripheral. Axial arthropathy consists of sacroiliitis or ankylosing spondylitis and does *not* parallel activity of bowel disease. Ankylosing spondylitis occurs in 5% to 10% of IBD patients and manifests with low back pain and stiffness that is usually worse during the night, in the morning, or after inactivity. Sacroiliitis alone (without ankylosing spondylitis) is common in IBD (up to 20% of patients) but in many cases is asymptomatic. Peripheral arthropathy is divided into type 1 and type 2. Type 1 peripheral arthropathy affects peripheral large joints. It is an asymmetric, seronegative, oligoarticular, nondeforming arthritis that may involve the knees, hips, wrists, elbows, and ankles. This peripheral arthropathy usually parallels disease activity. Peripheral arthropathy type 2 involves typically metacarpal phalangeal (MCP) joints, is typically symmetrical, and does *not* parallel disease activity.

Liver complications of IBD include both parenchymal and biliary tract diseases. Parenchymal diseases include fatty liver, pericholangitis, and chronic active hepatitis. Pericholangitis, also known as small-duct sclerosing cholangitis, is the most common of these diseases. It usually is asymptomatic, identified only by abnormalities in alkaline phosphatase and γ-glutamyl transpeptidase (GGT) on laboratory tests and histologically by portal tract inflammation and bile ductule degeneration. Small-duct sclerosing cholangitis may progress to cirrhosis.

Biliary tract disease includes an increased incidence of gallstones and primary sclerosing cholangitis (PSC). PSC is a chronic cholestatic liver disease marked by fibrosis of the intrahepatic and extrahepatic bile ducts. It occurs in 1% to 4% of patients with UC and less often in those with Crohn's disease. Overall, about 70% of patients with PSC have UC. Fibrosis leads to strictures of the bile ducts, which in turn may lead to recurrent cholangitis (with fever, right upper quadrant pain, and jaundice) and progression to cirrhosis. In addition, about 10% of patients develop cholangiocarcinoma. Medical or surgical

同而有差异，但研究发现，在长达 25 年的随访中，约 50% 最初表现为直肠炎或直乙结肠炎的 UC 患者，其病变范围会进一步进展。

UC 的典型临床病程呈慢性间歇性加重，随后是缓解期。腹泻、便血和腹痛提示疾病发作，而脱水、发热和心动过速提示病情严重。粪便钙卫蛋白、红细胞沉降率（ESR）或 C 反应蛋白（CRP）水平升高也可提示疾病发作。UC 患者常出现贫血，主要原因包括受累结肠黏膜慢性失血和全身炎症导致的骨髓抑制。重度或爆发型 UC 患者可能会发生肠穿孔，尤其是正在使用皮质类固醇或中毒性巨结肠的患者。中毒性巨结肠表现为结肠显著扩张，伴有发热、腹痛、脱水、心动过速和血性腹泻。

克罗恩病

CD 的临床表现取决于受累消化道的部位和炎症类型。病变可累及胃肠道的任何部位，最常见的受累部位是回盲肠 / 回结肠（40%），其次是末段回肠（30%）和结肠（25%）。其他部位（如食管、胃、十二指肠）较少见（5%），且很少单独受累。

CD 的常见症状包括右下腹痛、发热、体重减轻和腹泻，体格检查有时可触及炎性包块。结肠受累时可出现便血，但比 UC 少见。这些症状通常在确诊 CD 前已经存在数月甚至数年，在儿童患者中，生长发育迟缓可能是唯一的临床表现。与 UC 不同，CD 是透壁性炎症，因此可导致深溃疡和瘘管形成。瘘管形成可发生在不同肠段之间（如小肠-小肠瘘、小肠-结肠瘘），肠道与皮肤之间（肠-皮瘘），肠道与膀胱之间（肠-膀胱瘘），以及直肠与阴道之间（直肠-阴道瘘）。随着时间推移，30% ~ 40% 的 CD 患者会出现肛周病变，包括肛裂、肛瘘和肛周脓肿等。

慢性炎症可引起纤维化和肠腔狭窄，进而导致不完全性或完全性肠梗阻，患者常表现为腹痛、腹胀、恶心和呕吐。肠腔狭窄也可导致肠内容物潴留，并引发小肠细菌过度生长。小肠病变可引起维生素 D 缺乏。广泛的回肠黏膜病变可引起维生素 B_{12} 和胆盐吸收不良，前者可导致巨幼细胞贫血和神经系统症状，后者可导致因胆盐未被吸收而引起的腹泻和潜在的脂溶性维生素缺乏。胆汁中胆盐不足可导致胆结石。肠道吸收面积减小导致的吸收不良可引起体重减轻。慢性脂肪吸收不良可导致肠腔内游离脂肪酸和钙结合，使得本来与钙结合的草酸盐游离并被结肠吸收。草酸盐吸收过多、回肠造瘘术和腹泻导致的慢性循环容量不足可增加尿路草酸钙结石形成的风险。

肠外表现

尽管 UC 和 CD 主要累及肠道，但炎症也可累及多器官，这反映出两种疾病在本质上是系统性疾病（表

表 8.1　IBD 的肠外表现

皮肤
坏疽性脓皮病
结节性红斑
Sweet 综合征

肝胆系统
原发性硬化性胆管炎
胆石症
自身免疫性肝炎

肌肉骨骼系统
血清阴性关节炎
强直性脊柱炎
骶髂关节炎

眼部
葡萄膜炎
巩膜外层炎

其他
高凝状态
自身免疫性溶血性贫血
淀粉样变性

8.1）。肠外表现与疾病活动性平行或独立发生，且比肠道病变更难处理。

最常见的肠外表现是关节炎，可见于 9% ~ 50% 的 IBD 患者，分为两种类型：中轴型和外周型。中轴型关节病包括骶髂关节炎和强直性脊柱炎，其与肠道炎症活动性不平行。强直性脊柱炎发生于 5% ~ 10% 的 IBD 患者，表现为腰痛和僵硬感，通常在夜间及晨起时明显，活动后减轻。单纯骶髂关节炎（不伴有强直性脊柱炎）在 IBD 中很常见（发病率高达 20%），但多数患者无症状。外周型关节病可分为 1 型和 2 型。1 型外周型关节病主要影响外周大关节，表现为不对称性、血清阴性、不变形的寡关节炎，可累及膝关节、髋关节、腕关节、肘关节和踝关节，病变通常与肠道疾病活动性平行。2 型外周型关节病通常影响掌指关节（MCP），呈对称性，且与疾病活动性不平行。

IBD 的肝并发症包括肝实质病变和胆道疾病。肝实质病变包括脂肪肝、胆管周围炎和慢性活动性肝炎。胆管周围炎（又称小胆管硬化性胆管炎）最常见，通常无症状，仅能通过实验室检测碱性磷酸酶和 γ-谷氨酰转移酶（GGT）水平异常，以及组织学检查见汇管区炎症和胆小管退化来诊断。胆管周围炎可进展为肝硬化。

胆道疾病包括发病率升高的胆石症和原发性硬化性胆管炎（PSC）。PSC 是一种慢性胆汁淤积性肝病，特征性表现是肝内和肝外胆管纤维化，见于 1% ~ 4% 的 UC 患者，但在 CD 患者中少见。约 70% 的 PSC 患者合并 UC。胆管纤维化可导致胆管狭窄，继而引起反复发作的胆管炎，表现为发热、右上腹痛和黄疸，可进一步发展为肝硬化。此外，约 10% 的患者会发生胆

TABLE 8.2 Differentiating Features of UC and Crohn's Disease

	Ulcerative Colitis	Crohn's Disease
Site of involvement	Involves colon only	Any area of the gastrointestinal tract
	Rectum almost always involved	Rectum usually spared
Pattern of involvement	Continuous	Skip lesions
Diarrhea	Bloody	Usually nonbloody
Severe abdominal pain	Rare	Frequent
Perianal disease	No	In 30% of patients
Fistula	No	Yes
Endoscopic findings	Erythematous and friable	Aphthoid and deep ulcers
	Superficial ulceration	Cobblestoning
Radiologic findings	Tubular appearance resulting from loss of haustral folds	String sign of terminal ileum
		RLQ mass, fistulas, abscesses
Histologic features	Mucosal involvement only	Transmural
	Crypt abscesses	Crypt abscesses, granulomas (about 30%)
Smoking	Protective	Worsens course
Serology	pANCA more common	ASCA more common

ASCA, Anti–*Saccharomyces cerevisiae* antibodies; *pANCA*, perinuclear antineutrophil cytoplasmic antibody; *RLQ*, right lower quadrant.

therapy for IBD does not modify the course of PSC and most patients progress to cirrhosis and may require liver transplantation.

The two classic dermatologic manifestations that can be associated with IBD are pyoderma gangrenosum and erythema nodosum. Pyoderma gangrenosum occurs in about 5% of patients and is characterized by a discrete ulcer with a necrotic base, usually on the legs. The ulcer may spread and become large and deep, destroying soft tissues. Pyoderma is unrelated to disease activity. Treatment is usually with systemic or intralesional steroids, or both. Other treatment options include dapsone, cyclosporine, and anti-TNF agents. Erythema nodosum occurs in 10% of IBD patients, usually with peripheral arthropathy, and produces raised, tender nodules, usually over the anterior surface of the legs. Erythema nodosum responds to treatment for the underlying bowel disease. A less common dermatologic manifestation of IBD is Sweet syndrome or acute febrile neutrophilic dermatosis. This condition is characterized by the sudden onset of fever, leukocytosis, and tender, erythematous, well-demarcated papules and plaques that show dense neutrophilic infiltrates on histologic examination.

Ocular manifestations of IBD include uveitis and episcleritis. They occur in 1% to 5% of patients. Uveitis (or iritis) is an inflammatory condition of the anterior chamber that produces blurred vision, photophobia, headache, and conjunctival injection that may not parallel disease activity. Local therapy includes corticosteroids and atropine. Episcleritis is typically associated with disease activity. It produces burning eyes and scleral injection without vision deficits and is treated with topical corticosteroids.

DIAGNOSIS AND DIFFERENTIAL DIAGNOSIS

The diagnosis of IBD is based on a constellation of clinical features and endoscopic, radiographic, and histologic findings. Laboratory tests are not specific and usually demonstrate inflammation (leukocytosis) and anemia when the disease is active. Perinuclear antineutrophil cytoplasmic antibody (pANCA) is positive in up to 70% of patients with UC but is uncommon in patients with Crohn's disease, whereas anti–*Saccharomyces cerevisiae* antibodies (ASCA) are common (up to 60%) in Crohn's disease but not typically found in UC (Table 8.2). Additional markers, mainly for Crohn's disease, have improved the sensitivity and specificity of serologic testing, including antibodies to OmpC (*Escherichia coli* outer membrane porin C) and antibodies to bacterial flagellins CBir1, FlaX, and A4-Fla2. Due to lack of sensitivity and specificity, laboratory testing is of limited value and should not be used to make a diagnosis of IBD.

Colonoscopy findings in patients with UC are nonspecific, typically revealing granular mucosa, decreased vascular markings, exudate, and superficial ulcerations (Fig. 8.1) typically beginning in the rectum. In more severe cases, the mucosa is friable, with deeper ulcerations. Patients with long-standing severe disease can develop pseudopolyps, which represent islands of normal tissue in regions of previous ulceration. In Crohn's disease (Fig. 8.2), endoscopic examination may show aphthoid erosions, deep linear or stellate ulcers, edema, erythema, exudate, and friability with intervening areas of normal mucosa (skip lesions). However, a diagnosis of indeterminate colitis is made in 10% to 15% of patients because of an overlap of findings. For example, colonic Crohn's disease may produce superficial continuous rectal involvement similar to that seen in UC. Similarly, chronic UC

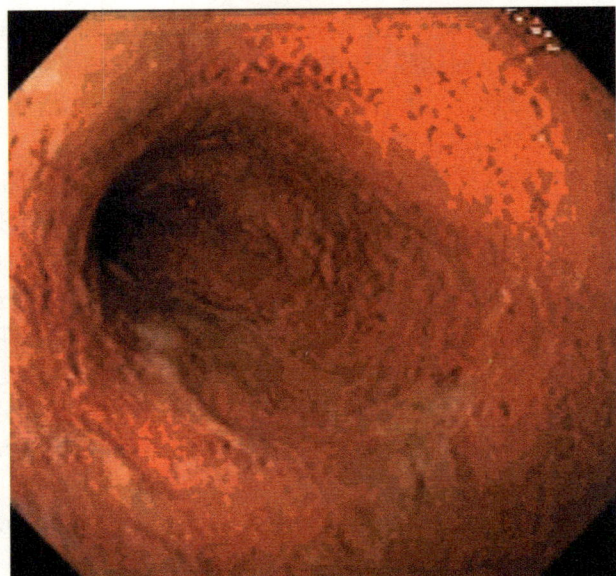

Fig. 8.1 Endoscopic image of ulcerative colitis demonstrates diffuse inflammation characterized by erythema, edema, friability, and hemorrhage.

表 8.2 UC 和 CD 的鉴别诊断要点

	UC	CD
病变累及范围	仅累及结肠 直肠普遍受累	可累及消化道的任何部位 直肠很少受累
病变形式	连续性病变	跳跃性病变
腹泻	血便	通常无血便
剧烈腹痛	少见	常见
肛周病变	无	见于 30% 的患者
瘘管形成	无	有
内镜表现	黏膜红斑、质脆 浅溃疡	口疮样溃疡和深大溃疡 铺路石样改变
影像学表现	结肠袋减少或消失，铅管征	末端回肠线样征 右下腹包块、瘘管、脓肿
组织学特点	局限于黏膜层 隐窝脓肿	透壁炎症 隐窝脓肿、肉芽肿（见于 30% 的患者）
吸烟	保护因素	危险因素
血清学标志物	pANCA 较常见	ASCA 较常见

pANCA，核周中性粒细胞胞质抗体；ASCA，抗酿酒酵母菌抗体。

管癌。内科或外科治疗均不能改变 PSC 的病程，大多数患者会进展为肝硬化，可能需要肝移植。

IBD 的两种典型皮肤表现是坏疽性脓皮病和结节性红斑。坏疽性脓皮病可见于约 5% 的患者，特征性表现是伴有坏死基底的孤立性溃疡，常发生于下肢。溃疡可蔓延、加深变大，并破坏软组织。坏疽性脓皮病与 IBD 活动性无关。治疗上通常需全身使用和（或）局部使用类固醇。其他治疗药物包括氨苯砜、环孢素和抗 TNF 制剂。结节性红斑可发生于 10% 的 IBD 患者，常伴有外周型关节病，可出现隆起的痛性结节，常见于胫前。治疗肠道病变有利于控制结节性红斑。IBD 患者较少见的皮肤表现是 Sweet 综合征（又称急性发热性嗜中性细胞皮肤病）。Sweet 综合征的临床特点为起病急，突然出现发热、白细胞增多、皮肤出现界限清晰的痛性丘疹或红斑，组织学检查可见大量中性粒细胞浸润。

IBD 的眼部病变包括葡萄膜炎和巩膜外层炎，可发生于 1%～5% 的患者。葡萄膜炎（或虹膜炎）是发生于前房的炎症性疾病，可导致视物模糊、畏光、头痛和结膜充血，这些症状与 IBD 活动性不平行。局部治疗可使用皮质类固醇和阿托品。巩膜外层炎通常与 IBD 活动性相关，表现为眼部灼热感和巩膜充血，不伴有视力缺陷，治疗选择局部使用皮质类固醇。

诊断和鉴别诊断

IBD 的诊断主要基于临床表现、内镜检查、影像学检查和病理组织学检查结果。实验室检查无特异性，仅在活动期提示炎症（白细胞增多）和贫血。核周抗中性粒细胞胞质抗体（pANCA）在高达 70% 的 UC 患者中呈阳性，但在 CD 患者中不常见，而抗酿酒酵母菌抗体（ASCA）在 CD 患者中很常见（高达 60%），但在 UC 患者中少见（表 8.2）。其他血清学标志物包括针对大肠杆菌外膜孔蛋白 C（OmpC）的抗体和针对细

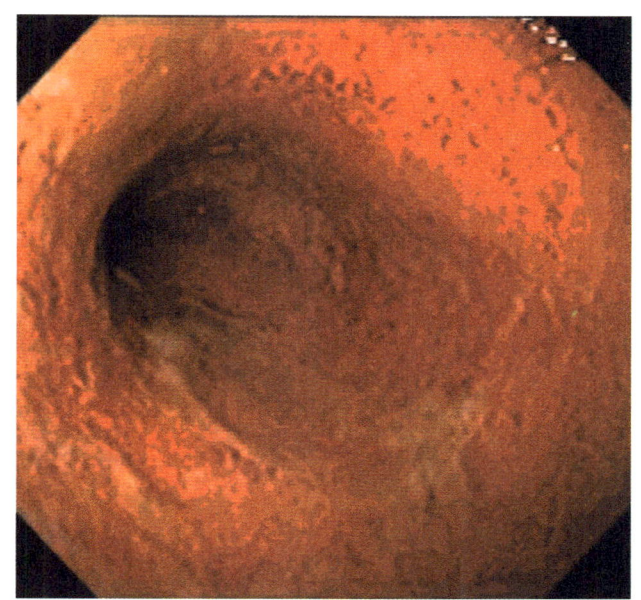

图 8.1 UC 的内镜图像显示黏膜弥漫性炎症，特征为黏膜红斑、水肿、质脆和出血

菌鞭毛蛋白（CBir1、FlaX 和 A4-Fla2）的抗体，这些标志物可以提高 CD 血清学诊断的敏感性和特异性。然而，目前实验室检查在诊断 IBD 方面仍缺乏足够的敏感性和特异性，尚不能用于 IBD 的诊断。

UC 的结肠镜表现无特异性，典型表现包括肠黏膜呈细颗粒状改变、血管纹理减少、黏膜表面可见渗出物和浅溃疡形成（图 8.1），通常起自直肠。严重者可出现黏膜变脆和深溃疡，病程长者可出现假息肉，由既往溃疡区域与残存的岛状黏膜构成。CD（图 8.2）内镜下可表现为口疮样糜烂、深的纵行溃疡或星状溃疡、黏膜充血水肿、渗出明显、脆性增加，其间有正常黏膜（呈跳跃性病变）。由于病变表现重叠，10%～15% 的患者会被诊断为未定型结肠炎，如结肠型 CD 可出现与 UC 类似的累及直肠的连续性浅表炎症。同样，慢性 UC 偶可引起末端回肠的炎症性改变，被称为倒灌性回

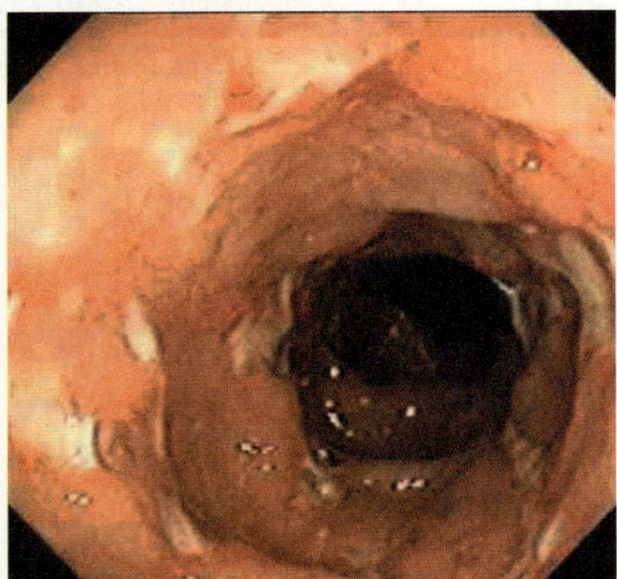

Fig. 8.2 Endoscopic image of Crohn's disease demonstrates linear ulcers in areas of otherwise normal mucosa.

can infrequently result in inflammation of the terminal ileum, called backwash ileitis, usually when severe disease of the cecum or ascending colon is present. In many patients with indeterminate colitis, repeated examination is necessary, or complications may develop that help identify the disease form.

Several types of radiologic studies can be used to diagnose IBD. In Crohn's disease, the most sensitive radiographic test to diagnose small bowel disease is CT or MR enterography. On traditional small bowel radiography, segments of edematous bowel appear thickened next to uninvolved mucosa, a characteristic pattern referred to as *cobblestoning*. Tight, long strictures in the small bowel can be identified and are called a *string sign*. Cross-sectional imaging with computed tomographic (CT) enterography and magnetic resonance enterography (MRE) has replaced traditional small bowel radiography. Cross-sectional imaging can identify bowel wall thickening with surrounding inflammation, as well as intra-abdominal abscesses and fistulas (Figs. 8.3 and 8.4). A characteristic finding on cross-sectional imaging in Crohn's disease is infiltration of the mesentery with fat, commonly known as *creeping fat*.

Video capsule endoscopy allows for direct visualization of the small bowel mucosa where erosions or ulcerations of the small bowel may be found (Fig. 8.5). Patients with known or suspected strictures should be evaluated for risk of capsule retention before undergoing capsule endoscopy.

Mucosal biopsies in IBD reveal acute and chronic inflammation with infiltration by plasma cells, neutrophils, lymphocytes, and eosinophils; focal ulcerations; crypt architectural distortion; and crypt abscesses (Figs. 8.6 and 8.7). The presence of chronic inflammation distinguishes IBD from other types of acute self-limited colitis like enteric infection. In Crohn's disease, the inflammation is transmural and more commonly focal. Granulomas are found in 25% to 30% of histologic specimens in Crohn's disease. The presence of granulomas is not required but can assist in making the diagnosis of Crohn's disease in the right clinical setting (Fig. 8.8). Granulomas are not diagnostic because they can be found in many other diseases, such as Behçet's disease, tuberculosis, *Yersinia* infection, gastrointestinal and hepatic sarcoidosis, and lymphoma.

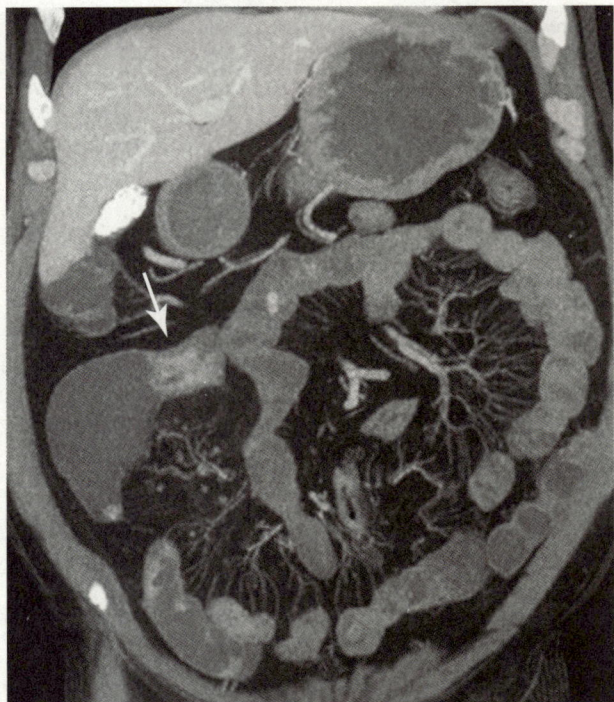

Fig. 8.3 Computed tomographic enterography shows inflammatory stricture *(arrow)* and small bowel wall thickening in a patient with Crohn's disease.

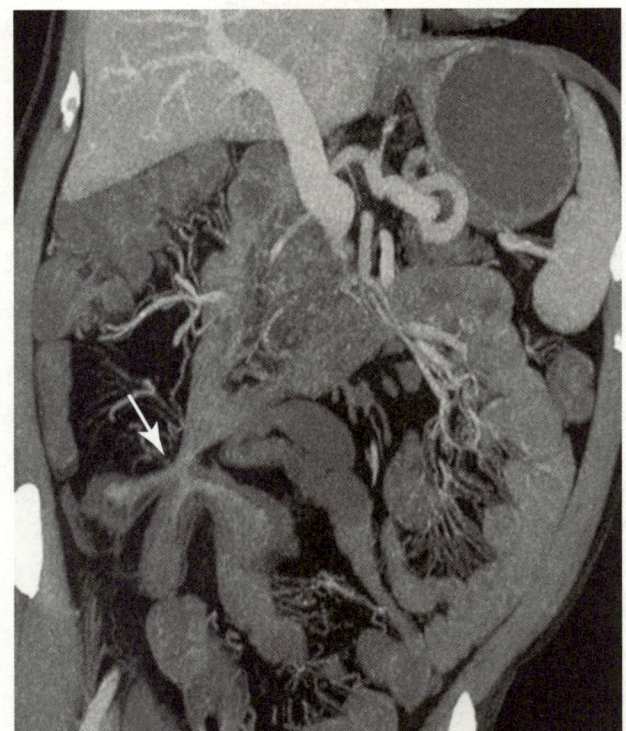

Fig. 8.4 Computed tomographic enterography shows extensive Crohn's disease with fistula *(arrow)*.

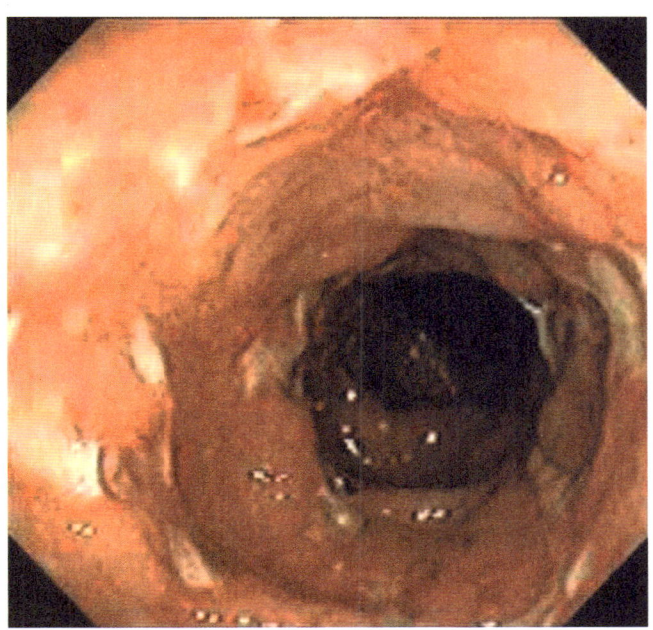

图 8.2 CD 的内镜图像显示在正常黏膜间的纵行溃疡

肠炎，通常见于盲肠和升结肠病变较严重的患者。对于未定型结肠炎患者，有必要进行复查，而并发症的出现也有助于明确疾病类型。

多种影像学检查方法可用于 IBD 的诊断。对于 CD，诊断小肠病变最敏感的影像学检查是 CT 或磁共振小肠成像（MRE）。在传统的小肠影像学检查中，病变肠管水肿增厚与邻近正常黏膜形成特征性的鹅卵石征。影像学检查还可识别出小肠较长的狭窄病变，即线样征。目前，CT 和 MRE 的断层成像已经取代了传统的小肠影像学检查。断层成像检查可发现肠壁增厚和肠壁周围炎症，以及腹腔脓肿和瘘管等病变（图 8.3 和图 8.4）。CD 在断层成像检查中的特征性改变是肠系膜脂肪浸润，被称为"爬行脂肪"。

胶囊内镜可以直接观察小肠黏膜，发现可能存在的糜烂和溃疡性病变（图 8.5）。已知或疑似狭窄的患者在接受胶囊内镜检查前应评估胶囊滞留的风险。

IBD 的黏膜组织学活检可见黏膜的急慢性炎症，伴有浆细胞、中性粒细胞、淋巴细胞和嗜酸性粒细胞浸润，以及局部溃疡、隐窝结构改变和隐窝脓肿（图 8.6 和图 8.7）。慢性炎症的存在有助于将 IBD 与其他类型的急性自限性结肠炎（如肠道感染）区分开来。CD 的炎症常呈透壁性和局灶性。25%～30% 的 CD 活检标本可见肉芽肿，发现肉芽肿有助于 CD 的正确诊断（图 8.8）。但是，肉芽肿不能作为诊断依据，因其还可见于其他疾病，如白塞病、结核病、耶尔森菌感染、胃肠道结节病及肝结节病、淋巴瘤。

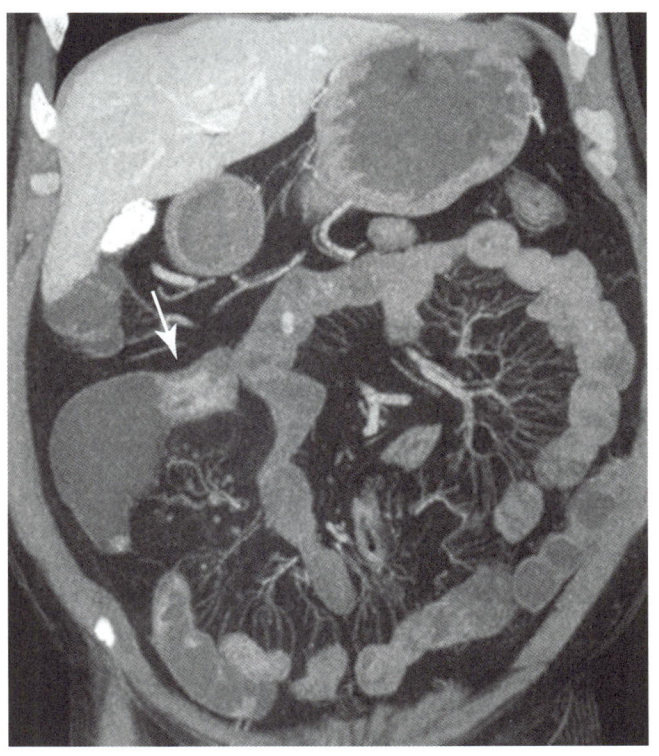

图 8.3 小肠 CT 造影显示 CD 患者的炎症性狭窄（箭头）伴肠壁增厚

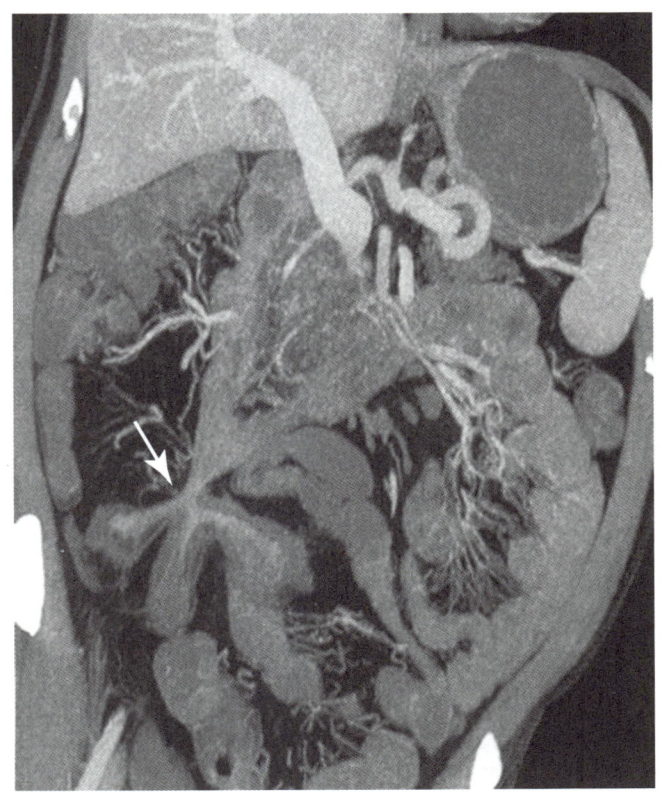

图 8.4 小肠 CT 造影显示 CD 合并瘘管（箭头）

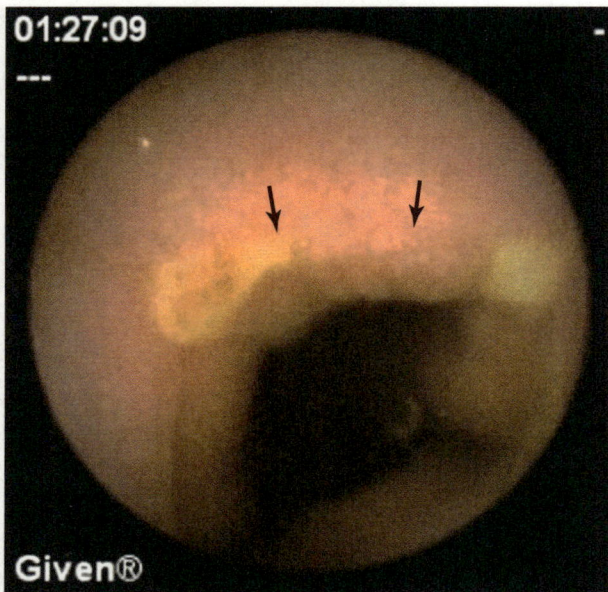

Fig. 8.5 Video capsule endoscopic image shows ulcerated stenosis in a patient with Crohn's disease *(arrows)*.

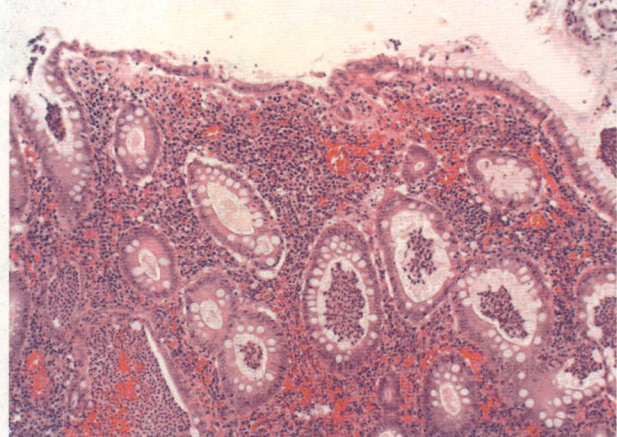

Fig. 8.7 Mucosal biopsy specimen demonstrates crypt branching and a crypt abscess characteristic of ulcerative colitis (hematoxylin and eosin stain).

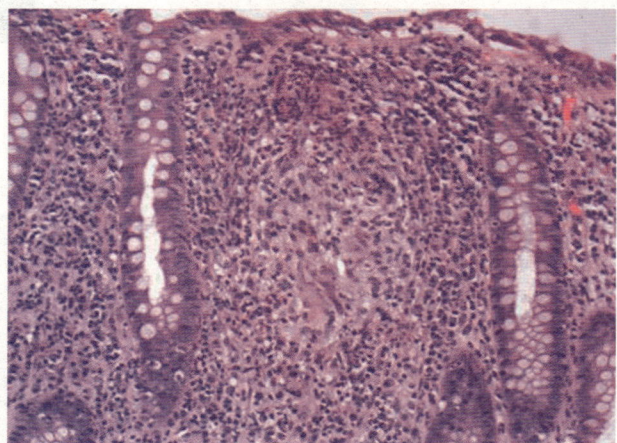

Fig. 8.8 Colonic biopsy specimen demonstrates a chronic inflammatory infiltrate with a granuloma in a patient with Crohn's colitis (hematoxylin and eosin stain).

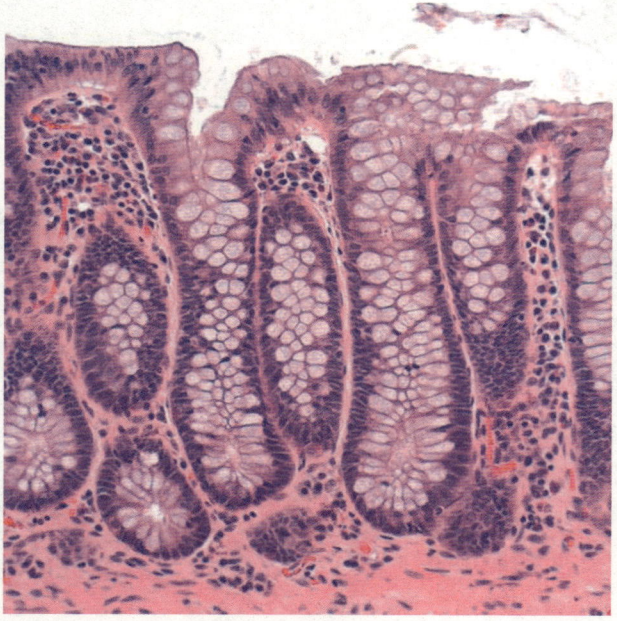

Fig. 8.6 Normal colonic mucosa (hematoxylin and eosin stain).

The differential diagnosis of IBD includes infectious colitis, ischemic colitis, radiation enteritis, enterocolitis induced by nonsteroidal anti-inflammatory drugs, diverticulitis, appendicitis, gastrointestinal malignancies, and irritable bowel syndrome. In patients with acute onset of bloody diarrhea, infectious causes that must be excluded with stool testing include *Salmonella enteritidis*, *Shigella* species, *Campylobacter jejuni*, *Escherichia coli* O157, and *Clostridioides difficile*. *Clostridioides difficile* is more common among patients with IBD. Among the infectious causes, *Yersinia enterocolitica* can mimic Crohn's disease because the pathogen causes ileitis, mesenteric adenitis, fever, diarrhea, and right lower quadrant abdominal pain. *Mycobacterium tuberculosis* infection, strongyloidiasis, and amebiasis must be excluded in high-risk populations, because these infections can mimic IBD, and treatment with corticosteroids can lead to disseminated infection and death.

TREATMENT

Treatment of IBD follows a systematic, standardized, and evidence-based approach. It relies on first identifying the type of IBD, then categorizing severity of disease, and then identifying a management goal, which now encourages a "treat to target" approach and focuses on endoscopic improvement and healing. Next, a therapeutic agent is selected incorporating data from well-designed clinical studies and also patient tolerability and overall safety, convenience, and preference. Furthermore, the treatment of IBD includes a focus on employing more aggressive and effective "top down" strategies by using biologic and newer oral agents earlier in the course in selected patients with moderate to severe disease. Maximizing the efficacy of current therapies now includes achieving therapeutic levels of these drugs when possible in the attempt to achieve endoscopic healing rapidly and thus improve long-term outcomes.

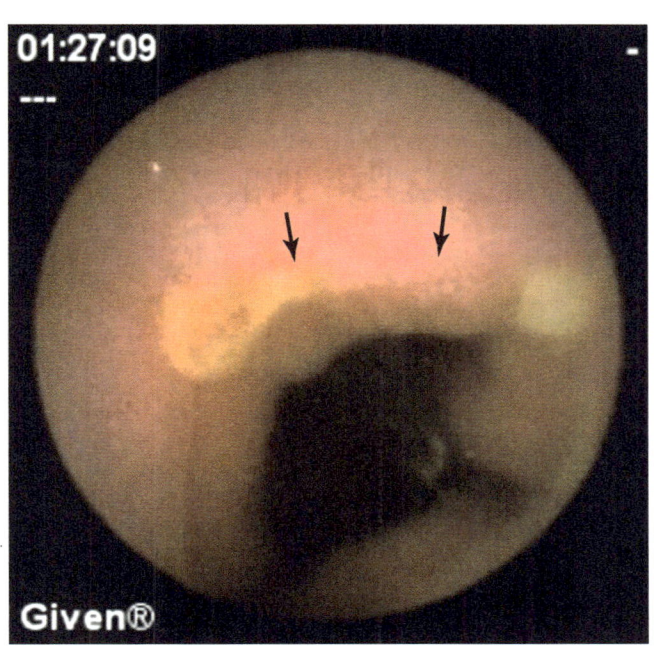

图 8.5　胶囊内镜显示 CD 患者的溃疡性狭窄（箭头）

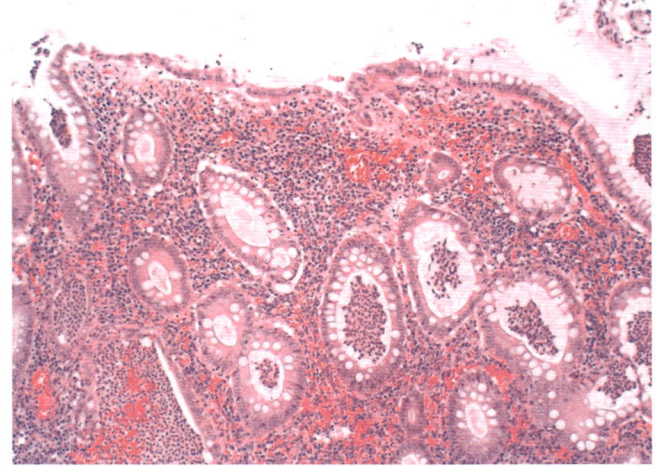

图 8.7　黏膜活检标本显示 UC 患者特征性的隐窝分支和隐窝脓肿（HE 染色）

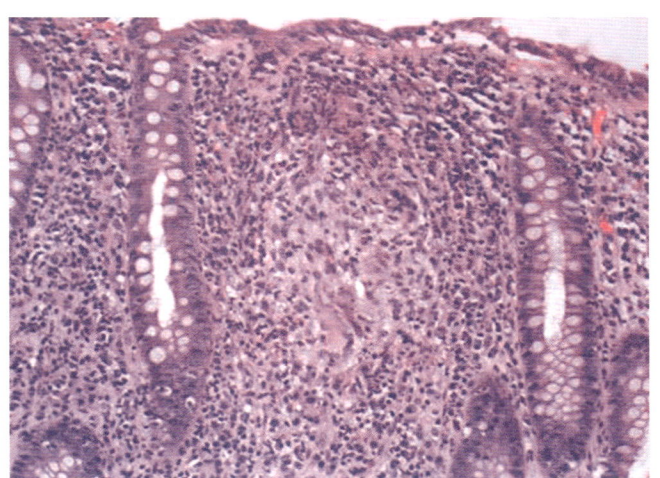

图 8.8　结肠活检标本显示 CD 患者的慢性炎症浸润伴肉芽肿（HE 染色）

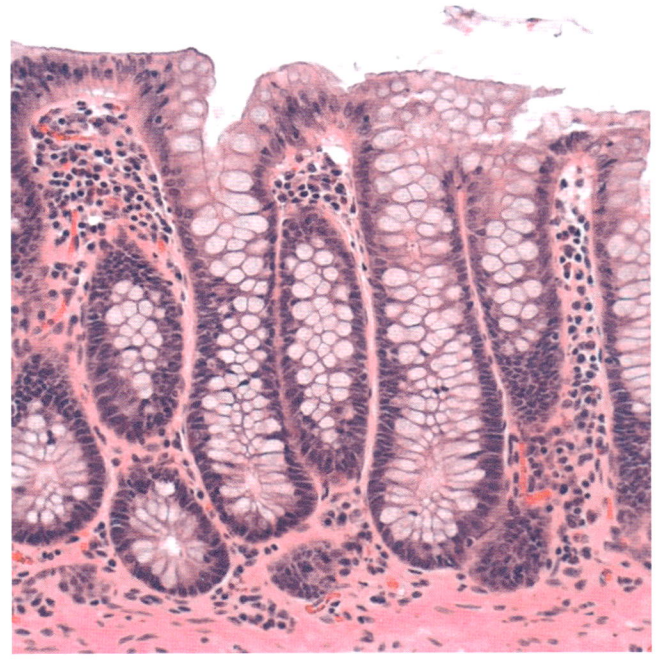

图 8.6　正常结肠黏膜（HE 染色）

　　IBD 的鉴别诊断包括感染性结肠炎、缺血性结肠炎、放射性肠炎、NSAID 引起的结肠炎、憩室炎、阑尾炎、胃肠道恶性肿瘤和肠易激综合征。对于急性起病的血性腹泻患者，必须行粪便检查排除感染性肠炎，致病菌包括沙门菌、志贺菌、空肠弯曲菌、大肠埃希菌 O157 和艰难梭菌。艰难梭菌更常见于 IBD 患者。在感染性病因中，小肠结肠炎耶尔森菌感染可类似于 CD，因为这种病原体可引起回肠炎、肠系膜淋巴结炎、发热、腹泻和右下腹痛。在高危人群中必须排除结核分枝杆菌感染、类圆线虫病和阿米巴病，其临床表现与 IBD 类似，应用皮质类固醇治疗可导致感染播散，甚至造成死亡。

治疗

　　IBD 的治疗应遵循系统化、标准化原则，并基于循证证据。应首先确定 IBD 的类型并划分疾病严重程度，据此制订相应的治疗目标。目前提倡"达标治疗"，侧重于内镜改善和黏膜愈合。随后，选择治疗药物时应依据设计良好的临床研究数据、患者耐受性、整体安全性、便利性和患者偏好。此外，对于部分中重度 IBD 患者，应采用更积极的"降阶梯"治疗策略，即早期使用生物制剂和新型口服小分子药物，从而最大限度地提高现有治疗的疗效，尽可能使这些药物达到治疗水平，以尽快实现黏膜愈合，改善长期预后。

TABLE 8.3 Treatment Options

Disease Severity	Ulcerative Colitis	Crohn's Disease
Mild	Oral and topical 5-ASA compounds Budesonide MMX	Budesonide EC Elemental diet
Moderate	Oral and topical 5-ASA compounds Oral steroids or budesonide MMX Azathioprine, 6-MP Infliximab, adalimumab, golimumab Vedolizumab Tofacitinib Ustekinumab	Oral steroids or budesonide EC Azathioprine, 6-MP Methotrexate Infliximab, adalimumab, certolizumab pegol Vedolizumab Ustekinumab
Severe	Intravenous steroids Cyclosporine Infliximab, adalimumab, golimumab Vedolizumab Tofacitinib Ustekinumab Surgery	Intravenous steroids Methotrexate Infliximab, adalimumab, certolizumab vedolizumab Ustekinumab Surgery

5-ASA, 5-Aminosalicylic acid; *6-MP*, 6-mercaptopurine.

Patients with mild or moderate disease can be managed as outpatients. Patients with severe or fulminant disease—with abdominal pain, fever, tachycardia, anemia, and leukocytosis—require hospital admission and multidisciplinary team management. Because IBD is a chronic recurrent illness, treatment is centered on controlling the acute attack with induction of remission, followed by maintenance of remission. Treatment options for UC and Crohn's disease are summarized in Table 8.3.

In brief, treatment agents for IBD broadly include nontargeted immune suppressants such as corticosteroids, topical anti-inflammatories including 5-aminosalicylic acid (mesalamine) and related agents, antibiotics, and traditional immunomodulators including thiopurine analogs (azathioprine, 6-MP) that inhibit replication of inflammatory cells by inducing cell death or apoptosis and methotrexate, which inhibits replication of inflammatory cells by inhibiting cell division or mitosis.

Newer approved biologic and oral agents work variably by targeting effector pro-inflammatory cytokines such as TNF-alpha and IL-12/23, targeting immune cell function such as the JAK-STAT enzyme pathway or inhibiting cell trafficking such as the alpha-4/beta7 adhesion inhibition.

5-Aminosalicylic Acid (Mesalamine)

The 5-aminosalicylates are given either orally or topically (suppository/enema) or as a combined regimen. They are safe and effective for treatment (i.e., induction of remission) of mild to moderate UC and for maintenance of remission. The efficacy of the 5-aminosalicylic acid (5-ASA) agents in induction or maintenance of remission in Crohn's disease has not been demonstrated. This class of anti-inflammatory medications includes sulfasalazine (Azulfidine) at a dose of 4 to 6 g/day in divided doses. This drug consists of 5-ASA linked to a sulfapyridine moiety; the 5-ASA is released after bacterial lysis of the azo bond in the distal small bowel and colon. Side effects, including headache, nausea, and skin reactions, require discontinuation of sulfasalazine in about 30% of patients. Reversible oligospermia may occur with sulfasalazine. Rare serious side effects include pleuropericarditis, pancreatitis, agranulocytosis, interstitial nephritis, and hemolytic anemia may occur with sulfasalazine and 5-ASA. Patients who take sulfasalazine need folic acid supplementation.

Derivatives of oral 5-ASA compounds include mesalamine (Pentasa, 4 g/day in divided doses; Delzicol, 2.4 g/day in divided doses; Asacol HD, 2.4 to 4.8 g/day in divided doses; Lialda, 2.4 to 4.8 g once daily; Apriso, 1.5 g once a day), olsalazine (Dipentum, 1 to 2 g/day in divided doses), and balsalazide (Colazal, 6.75 g/day in divided doses; Giazo 3.3 g/day in divided doses). Topical forms of mesalamine (Canasa suppositories, 1000 mg once daily; Rowasa enemas, 4 g once nightly) are commonly used because of a more favorable side effect profile.

Corticosteroids

Corticosteroids may be used topically, orally, or intravenously. They are effective for controlling active inflammatory disease but not for maintaining remission and should act as a bridge to maintenance therapy. They are not indicated for maintenance therapy. They are indicated for moderate or severe disease in patients with UC for whom treatment with 5-ASA has failed. The most commonly used agents are parenteral methylprednisolone for severe/fulminant disease requiring hospitalization at doses of 45 to 60 mg intravenously daily and for outpatients, oral prednisone, started in doses between 40 and 60 mg/day. Patients typically improve rapidly, and the medication is usually tapered down slowly (i.e., by 5 to 10 mg/week) until discontinuation. Patients who do not improve after 1 week of oral treatment and those with more severe disease are best treated in the hospital with intravenous corticosteroids.

Controlled trials have shown that budesonide EC (Entocort EC) is more effective than placebo or oral 5-ASA and has similar efficacy to prednisolone for the induction of remission in Crohn's disease of the terminal ileum (level of evidence I, A). Entocort EC (9 mg given once daily as three 3-mg pills) undergoes extensive first-pass hepatic metabolism and is approved for inducing and maintaining remission of ileal and ileocolonic Crohn's disease (level of evidence III, A) with decreased corticosteroid side effects. Budesonide MMX (Uceris 9 mg given once daily) has an extended release that targets the colon and is approved for the treatment of mild to moderate UC but should not be used as maintenance therapy. Corticosteroids have numerous side effects with long-term use.

Traditional Immunomodulators

The traditional immunomodulators used in IBD include azathioprine (Imuran) and its active metabolite, 6-mercaptopurine (6-MP) (Purinethol), as well as methotrexate and cyclosporine. Metabolism of azathioprine and 6-mercaptopurine is based on the enzyme thiopurine methyl transferase (TPMT). TPMT should be measured in each patient before starting therapy to determine starting dose to minimize toxicity and maximize efficacy. Hematologic monitoring for drug toxicity on therapy is essential. Azathioprine and 6-MP are effective therapies for maintaining remission in both Crohn's disease and UC and are used primarily as corticosteroid-sparing agents. They have a slow onset of action (weeks to months) and consequently are not used to induce remission. Side effects include pancreatitis, nausea, abnormal liver enzymes, bone marrow suppression, opportunistic infections, and an increased risk of lymphoma and nonmelanoma skin cancer.

Methotrexate can be used for induction (25 mg subcutaneously once weekly) and maintenance of remission (15 to 25 mg subcutaneously once weekly) in active Crohn's disease; the side effect profile includes bone marrow suppression, mucositis, interstitial pneumonitis, and with long-term use, cirrhosis. Folic acid should be given with methotrexate to reduce the risk of mucositis. Methotrexate has been

表 8.3 IBD 的治疗选择

疾病严重程度	UC	CD
轻度	口服或局部使用 5-ASA 布地奈德缓释片	布地奈德缓释胶囊 要素饮食
中度	口服或局部使用 5-ASA 口服类固醇或布地奈德缓释片 硫唑嘌呤、6-MP 英夫利昔单抗、阿达木单抗、戈利木单抗 维多珠单抗 托法替尼 乌司奴单抗	口服类固醇或布地奈德缓释胶囊 硫唑嘌呤、6-MP 甲氨蝶呤 英夫利昔单抗、阿达木单抗、赛妥珠单抗 维多珠单抗 乌司奴单抗
重度	静脉注射类固醇 环孢素 英夫利昔单抗、阿达木单抗、戈利木单抗 维多珠单抗 托法替尼 乌司奴单抗 手术	静脉注射类固醇 甲氨蝶呤 英夫利昔单抗、阿达木单抗、赛妥珠单抗 维多珠单抗 乌司奴单抗 手术

5-ASA，5-氨基水杨酸；6-MP，6-巯基嘌呤。

轻中度 IBD 患者可在门诊治疗，但重度或暴发性 IBD 患者（如出现腹痛、发热、心动过速、贫血和白细胞增多）需要入院和多学科联合诊疗。由于 IBD 是一种慢性复发性疾病，治疗的重点是控制急性发作，诱导并维持缓解。表 8.3 总结了 UC 和 CD 的治疗方法。

简而言之，IBD 的治疗药物主要包括非靶向免疫抑制剂（如皮质类固醇）、局部抗炎药 [如 5- 氨基水杨酸（美沙拉嗪）及其相关药物]、抗生素、传统免疫抑制剂 [如硫嘌呤类似物（硫唑嘌呤、6- 巯基嘌呤）] 和甲氨蝶呤。硫嘌呤类似物主要通过诱导细胞死亡或凋亡来抑制炎症细胞复制，甲氨蝶呤通过抑制细胞分裂或有丝分裂来抑制炎症细胞复制。

新型生物制剂和小分子药物通过靶向效应分子促炎症细胞因子（如 TNF-α 和 IL-12/23）、靶向免疫细胞功能（如 JAK-STAT 酶通路）或抑制炎症细胞迁移（如 $\alpha_4\beta_7$ 黏附分子）而发挥相应的作用。

5- 氨基水杨酸（美沙拉嗪）

5- 氨基水杨酸类药物可以口服、局部给药（栓剂/灌肠）或联合用药。对于轻中度 UC 的诱导缓解和维持缓解是安全、有效的，但在诱导和维持 CD 缓解方面的疗效尚未得到证实。这类药物包括柳氮磺吡啶，剂量为 4~6 g/d，分次给药。柳氮磺吡啶是 5- 氨基水杨酸（5-ASA）和磺胺吡啶的结合产物，在远端小肠和结肠的细菌作用下裂解偶氮键并释放 5-ASA。柳氮磺吡啶的副作用包括头痛、恶心和皮肤反应，约 30% 的患者需要停药。使用柳氮磺吡啶可能会出现可逆性少精子症。其他罕见的严重副作用包括浆膜炎、胰腺炎、粒细胞缺乏症、间质性肾炎和溶血性贫血。使用柳氮磺吡啶的患者需补充叶酸。

口服 5-ASA 的衍生物包括美沙拉嗪、奥沙拉嗪和巴柳氮。因副作用相对较少，美沙拉嗪局部制剂（如栓剂和灌肠剂）的使用较为普遍。

皮质类固醇

皮质类固醇可以局部、口服或静脉给药，对于控制疾病活动有效，但不能用于维持缓解，适用于 5-ASA 治疗无效的中重度 UC 患者。最常用的皮质类固醇是静脉注射甲泼尼龙，用于需要住院治疗的重度/暴发性 UC 患者，剂量为 40~60 mg/d。门诊患者通常口服泼尼松，起始剂量为 40~60 mg/d。患者病情通常可迅速改善，然后缓慢减量，每周减少 5~10 mg，直至停药。口服治疗 1 周无效的患者或重度 UC 患者，建议住院静脉使用皮质类固醇治疗。

对于回肠末端 CD 患者的诱导缓解，临床对照试验显示布地奈德缓释胶囊的疗效优于安慰剂和口服 5-ASA，与泼尼松疗效相当（推荐类别 I 类，证据等级 A 级）。布地奈德缓释胶囊（9 mg/d，1 次/日）经肝首过效应代谢，已被批准用于回肠和回结肠 CD 的诱导缓解和维持缓解（推荐类别 III 类，证据等级 A 级），副作用较少。布地奈德缓释片（9 mg/d，1 次/日）缓慢释放，作用于结肠，被批准用于轻中度 UC 的治疗，但不能用于维持治疗。应注意长期使用皮质类固醇的副作用。

传统免疫调节剂

用于 IBD 治疗的传统免疫调节剂包括硫唑嘌呤及其活性代谢产物 6- 巯基嘌呤（6-MP）、甲氨蝶呤和环孢素。硫唑嘌呤和 6-MP 的代谢依赖于硫嘌呤甲基转移酶（TPMT）。在开始治疗前，应检测患者 TPMT 水平以确定起始剂量，争取达到疗效最大化和副作用最小化。治疗期间应进行血液学检查，以监测药物毒副作用。硫唑嘌呤和 6-MP 可用于 UC 和 CD 的维持缓解，且通常是为了降低皮质类固醇的使用剂量。此类药物起效缓慢，需数周甚至数月，因此不能用于诱导缓解。副作用包括胰腺炎、恶心、肝功能异常、骨髓抑制、机会性感染，以及患淋巴瘤和非黑色素皮肤癌的风险增加。

甲氨蝶呤可用于活动性 CD 的诱导缓解（25 mg，皮下注射，每周 1 次）和维持缓解（15~25 mg，皮下注射，每周 1 次）；副作用包括骨髓抑制、黏膜炎、间质性肺炎，长期使用还可能导致肝硬化。为了减少黏膜炎的发生，甲氨蝶呤通常与叶酸一起使用。既往有研究探讨了甲氨蝶呤用于 UC 的一线治疗，但结果显

studied as a primary treatment for UC and was not found to be effective. Intravenous cyclosporine (2 mg/kg/day given over 24 hours) is used as a rescue medicine and, in severe UC refractory to intravenous steroids, as a *bridge* treatment to one of the above immunomodulators or biologic agents. Given the potential for both short-term and long-term side effects, as well as the need for close follow-up, patients needing these medications are best managed by gastroenterologists.

Previously used as primary therapy for IBD, azathioprine/6-mercaptopurine and methotrexate are now more commonly used in combination with newer more effective biologic therapies, especially anti-TNF agents.

Biologic Agents

Biologics are a class of medications that target specific aspects of the immune system. The first such agent to be used in IBD was infliximab (Remicade), a chimeric monoclonal antibody to TNF-α, which has been shown to be effective in the treatment of both moderate to severe Crohn's disease, including fistulizing disease, and UC (level of evidence I, A). Anti-TNF agents that are administered subcutaneously include adalimumab (Humira) and golimumab (Simponi), which are fully human monoclonal antibodies, and certolizumab pegol (Cimzia), which is a humanized anti-TNF antibody Fab fragment. Adalimumab, certolizumab pegol, and infliximab are indicated for the treatment of patients with moderate to severe Crohn's disease. Adalimumab, infliximab, and golimumab are approved to treat moderate to severe UC. These agents can be associated with adverse reactions including infusion reactions (infliximab), delayed-type hypersensitivity reaction, and with development of anti-drug antibodies resulting in reduced effectiveness.

Natalizumab (Tysabri), a humanized anti–$α_4$-integrin antibody, blocks inflammatory cell migration and adhesion and is approved for the treatment of moderate to severe Crohn's disease in patients who have had an inadequate response to, or are unable to tolerate, conventional Crohn's disease therapies including inhibitors of TNF-α. Due to its link with progressive multifocal leukoencephalopathy (PML) and approval of a more gut selective agent, vedolizumab, it is now rarely used. Vedolizumab (Entyvio), a humanized monoclonal antibody to α4β7 integrin, is approved for the treatment and maintenance of both Crohn's and UC.

Ustekinumab, a monoclonal antibody against the P40 subunit of IL-12 and IL-23, is approved for the induction and maintenance of remission in moderate to severe Crohn's and UC.

Tofacitinib, an oral small molecule that inhibits Janus kinase (JAK) enzymes, is approved for treatment of moderate to severe UC in patients intolerant of or who have not responded to anti-TNFs. Because of the potent effects these biological drugs and oral agents have on the immune system, careful patient selection and monitoring for complications are necessary. Reactivation of latent tuberculosis and other serious infections have been reported with the anti-TNF agents. Other rare but serious complications include non-Hodgkin's lymphoma, exacerbation of congestive heart failure, abnormal complete blood count (CBC) and liver function test results, venous thrombosis, and demyelinating disease. Natalizumab is associated with rare cases of progressive multifocal leukoencephalopathy caused by the human JC virus.

Future biologic agents with alternative mechanisms of action are being developed. These include several selective IL-23 inhibitors such as risankizumab, mirikizumab, guselkumab, and brazikumab. These biologics selectively target the P19 subunit of the interleukin-23 (IL-23) cytokine, thus being more selective than ustekinumab (Stelara), which inhibits the P40 components of both IL-12 and IL-23. A theoretical advantage of IL-23 selectivity is thought to be reduced potential side effects related to targeting of IL-12, including risk of carcinogenesis suggested in some animal studies.

Additional JAK inhibitors (filgotinib, upadacitinib) are being examined for their role in treatment of IBD. Etrolizumab, a beta7 inhibitor, and ontamalimab, a MadCAM-1 ligand inhibitor, are inhibitors of cell trafficking that are in clinical trials. Ozanimod (RPC1063), an oral agent that acts as a selective agonist and modulator of sphingosine phosphate receptor subtypes 1 and 5, thus inhibiting lymphocyte trafficking to sites of inflammation, is also being tested for its efficacy in UC and Crohn's disease.

The availability of these biologic agents has changed the approach to the management of IBD. The emphasis now has shifted from treating symptoms alone and maintaining clinical remission to treating to a target of endoscopic remission. Endoscopic remission or mucosal healing (as it is typically referred to) is defined as the absence of mucosal ulceration or erosion. The finding of ulceration in the lining of the bowel is associated with higher likelihood of disease flare in asymptomatic patients. Achieving endoscopic remission has been associated with better long-term patient outcomes including longer sustained clinical remissions, lower rates of hospitalization and, in some studies, lower rates of surgery. In this paradigm, after a therapy has been started, an asymptomatic patient will undergo an evaluation 6 to 9 months later to look for evidence of endoscopic remission or ongoing intestinal inflammation. If persistent or significant disease is present, then treatment is typically optimized or changed to try to achieve endoscopic remission. This treat to target approach continues to undergo further study.

Other Agents

Other agents for the treatment of IBD include antibiotics, probiotics, antidiarrheal agents, bile salt resin binders, and nutritional support.

Although used widely in the past for luminal Crohn's, antibiotics are now less commonly employed in routine treatment of patients with luminal Crohn's disease. Current use of antibiotics in active Crohn's is largely limited to treatment of pyogenic complications and in perianal disease. Metronidazole may prevent postoperative recurrence in some patients with luminal Crohn's but adverse effects typically limit its usefulness. There is some evidence for the efficacy of a novel enteric form of rifaximin in mild to moderately active luminal Crohn's disease. The role of antibiotics in UC is unclear, and further studies are required. However, intravenous antibiotics may be used in the initial treatment of severe, toxic, or fulminant colitis when infection is a concern. Antibiotics are useful to treat bacterial overgrowth that can be associated with Crohn's disease.

Probiotics are viable nonpathogenic organisms considered to be food products that after ingestion may prevent or treat intestinal diseases and have been explored in the treatment of IBD. There is some evidence for their efficacy in pouchitis (see later) and UC but no clear benefit in Crohn's disease has been noted thus far. Additional studies are ongoing.

Antidiarrheal agents and bile salt resin binders have no effect on IBD inflammation but can be used as adjuncts for management of diarrhea in patients with IBD, but antidiarrheal agents should be used cautiously during exacerbations of colitis because they may precipitate toxic megacolon. The main role of antidiarrheal medications involves controlling diarrhea in patients who have undergone previous resections. Patients with Crohn's disease who have had less than 100 cm of terminal ileum removed can develop a bile salt malabsorptive state, during which bile salts enter the colon and cause a secretory diarrhea. Bile salt resin binders such as cholestyramine are an effective treatment in these cases. When patients have undergone one or more extensive resections amounting to more than 100 cm of ileum, the bile salt

示效果不佳。静脉用环孢素 [2 mg/(kg·d)，24 h 持续给药] 可用于补救治疗，用于皮质类固醇抵抗的重度 UC 患者，作为上述免疫调节剂或生物制剂的桥接治疗。考虑到潜在的短期和长期副作用及需要密切随访，应在消化科医生的指导下使用这些药物。

硫唑嘌呤 /6-MP 和甲氨蝶呤曾是 IBD 的一线治疗药物，现在常与更有效的生物制剂（尤其是抗 TNF 药物）联合使用。

生物制剂

生物制剂是一类针对机体免疫系统特定靶点的药物。用于 IBD 治疗的首个生物制剂是英夫利昔单抗，它是一种针对肿瘤坏死因子 α（TNF-α）的嵌合型单克隆抗体，对治疗中重度 CD（包括瘘管性病变）和 UC 均有效（推荐类别 I 类，证据等级 A 级）。皮下注射的抗 TNF 药物包括阿达木单抗和戈利木单抗（均为完全人源化单克隆抗体），以及赛妥珠单抗（人源化抗 TNF Fab 片段）。阿达木单抗、赛妥珠单抗和英夫利昔单抗已被批准用于治疗中重度 CD。阿达木单抗、英夫利昔单抗和戈利木单抗被批准用于治疗中重度 UC。这些药物的不良反应包括输液反应（英夫利昔单抗多见）、迟发型超敏反应和产生抗药性抗体，从而导致疗效降低。

那他珠单抗是一种人源化抗 $α_4$ 整合素抗体，能够阻断炎症细胞的迁移和黏附，已被批准用于常规治疗（包括抗 TNF-α 制剂）效果不佳或无法耐受的中重度 CD 患者。由于那他珠单抗与进行性多灶性白质脑病（PML）相关，且更具肠道特异性的维多珠单抗已被批准用于临床，因此那他珠单抗目前已很少使用。维多珠单抗是一种针对 $α_4β_7$ 整合素的人源化单克隆抗体，已被批准用于 CD 和 UC 的诱导缓解和维持治疗。

乌司奴单抗是一种针对 IL-12 和 IL-23 P40 亚基的单克隆抗体，已被批准用于中重度 CD 和 UC 的诱导缓解和维持治疗。

托法替尼是一种口服小分子药物，为 Janus 激酶（JAK）酶抑制剂，已被批准用于治疗抗 TNF-α 制剂不耐受或无效的中重度 UC 患者。由于生物制剂和口服小分子药物对免疫系统的抑制作用较强，因此需严格掌握适应证并密切监测并发症的发生。已有使用抗 TNF-α 制剂引起潜伏结核的再次活动和其他严重感染的报道。其他罕见的严重不良反应包括非霍奇金淋巴瘤、充血性心力衰竭加重、血常规和肝功能异常、静脉血栓形成和脱髓鞘病变。那他珠单抗还与由人类 JC 病毒引起的罕见的 PML 有关。

目前正在开发具有其他作用机制的生物制剂，包括多种选择性 IL-23 抑制剂，如瑞莎珠单抗、米吉珠单抗、古塞库单抗和布雷库单抗。这些生物制剂选择性作用于 IL-23 的 P19 亚基，因此比同时抑制 IL-12 和 IL-23 的 P40 亚基的乌司奴单抗更具选择性。选择性靶向 IL-23 抑制剂的一个理论优势是减少了抑制 IL-12 相关的潜在副作用，包括动物实验中提示的致癌风险。

其他 JAK 酶抑制剂（如非戈替尼和乌帕替尼）在治疗 IBD 中的作用正在研究中。依曲利组单抗（一种 $β_7$ 抑制剂）和昂塔利单抗（一种 MadCAM-1 配体抑制剂）在临床试验中均显示可以抑制炎症细胞的迁移。奥扎莫德（RPC1063）是一种口服鞘氨醇磷酸受体亚型 1 和 5 的选择性激动剂和调节剂，可以抑制淋巴细胞迁移到炎症部位，目前正在研究其对 UC 和 CD 的疗效。

生物制剂的使用已经改变了 IBD 的治疗策略。目前的治疗重点已从单纯的控制症状和维持临床缓解转变为以实现内镜下缓解为目标。内镜下缓解（通常被称为黏膜愈合）是指肠道黏膜无溃疡或糜烂。无症状患者存在肠道溃疡提示其复发风险更高。达到黏膜愈合的患者长期临床预后更好，包括临床缓解的持续时间更长、住院率和手术率更低。在目前的治疗模式下，症状缓解的患者需要在开始治疗后 6～9 个月时评估是否达到黏膜愈合或持续存在肠道炎症。如果持续存在肠道炎症，需优化治疗或更换治疗方法，以期达到黏膜愈合。这种达标治疗策略仍在持续研究中。

其他治疗药物

IBD 的其他治疗药物包括抗生素、益生菌、止泻药、胆盐树脂螯合剂和营养支持治疗。

抗生素既往被广泛用于 CD 的治疗，但目前已很少常规使用。目前抗生素一般仅用于伴有化脓性病变或肛周病变的 CD 患者。甲硝唑可预防部分 CD 患者的术后复发，但副作用限制了其使用。利福昔明是一种新型肠道抗生素，有证据表明其在治疗轻中度 CD 患者中具有一定疗效。抗生素在治疗 UC 中的作用尚不明确，仍需进一步研究，但重度、中毒性或暴发性 UC 患者考虑感染风险时可静脉使用抗生素。抗生素可用于治疗 CD 相关的细菌过度生长。

益生菌是存活的非致病性微生物，被认为是食品级别，摄入后可用于预防和治疗肠道疾病，已被尝试用于 IBD 的治疗。研究发现，益生菌在治疗储袋炎（见下文）和 UC 中有一定疗效，但治疗 CD 的作用不确切。目前更多的研究正在进行中。

止泻药和胆盐树脂螯合剂对 IBD 的肠道炎症无效，但可用于 IBD 伴腹泻患者的辅助治疗。在结肠炎症状加重期间，应谨慎使用止泻药，以免诱发中毒性巨结肠。止泻药主要用于控制肠切除术后患者的腹泻。末端回肠切除 < 100 cm 的 CD 患者可能发生胆盐吸收不良，胆盐进入结肠可能引起分泌性腹泻。胆盐树脂螯合剂（如考来烯胺）可有效治疗此类患者。当经历一次或多次广泛肠切除术且累计切除回肠 > 100 cm 时，

pool is depleted and fat malabsorption develops. These patients may require a low-fat diet supplemented with medium-chain triglycerides and antidiarrheal agents, but bile salt resin binders should not be used.

Nutritional support is an important adjunctive aspect in the management of IBD. However, the role of nutrition as a primary treatment has been limited to patients with small bowel Crohn's disease, especially in children. These patients may achieve and maintain remission with total parenteral nutrition or elemental diets after prolonged periods (at least 4 weeks) and potentially avoid the need for corticosteroids. Many patients with Crohn's disease or UC experience weight loss during exacerbations of their illness and need caloric supplements. Vitamins and minerals can be given orally as a multivitamin with folic acid. Vitamin B_{12} should be supplemented parenterally in patients who have extensive ileal disease or an ileal resection. Patients taking corticosteroids require supplemental calcium and vitamin D, and individuals with extensive small bowel involvement can also develop malabsorption of fat-soluble vitamins (A, D, E, and K), iron, and, rarely, trace minerals. A low-fiber diet may be necessary in patients with active disease or strictures. There is some observational evidence to suggest effectiveness of the specific carbohydrate diet (SCD) in patients with IBD but it is very restrictive in nature; therefore, it is not being widely recommended until further research becomes available.

More studies on diet as a treatment for IBD are needed. Complementary and alternative medicines are used frequently by patients with IBD and it is important that treating clinicians ask about their use.

Surgical Management

Surgical intervention is indicated for patients with complications such as obstruction, perforation, fibrotic stricture, massive gastrointestinal hemorrhage, or toxic megacolon or who are not responsive to medical treatment. The other main indication for surgical treatment is the presence of dysplasia or cancer. For patients with UC, regardless of the extent of disease, the entire colon must be removed. Historically, the initial operation for UC was a total proctocolectomy and Brooke ileostomy, but ileal pouch–anal anastomosis has become the procedure of choice in most patients. In this operation, the colon is removed and the small bowel is constructed into a reservoir (ileal pouch) that is anastomosed to the anus or a short segment of the rectum, allowing defecation through the anus. Complications include the development of inflammation of the rectum (cuffitis) or pouch (pouchitis), fecal incontinence, reduced fertility, and need for reoperation. Surgery is not curative in Crohn's disease. Many surgical procedures in patients with Crohn's disease are performed to manage complications of the disease, including segmental resection, stricturoplasty, fistulectomy, and abscess drainage.

PROGNOSIS

Approximately two thirds of patients with UC have at least one relapse in the 10 years after their diagnosis. About 20% to 30% of patients with extensive UC will require colectomy within their lifetime. Only 5% of individuals with proctitis undergo colectomy by 10 years after diagnosis. In contrast, more than 60% of Crohn's patients require surgery within the 10 years after their diagnosis although these data are based on patients treated in the pre-biologic era. The rate of recurrence in Crohn's disease is high, with 70% of patients having an endoscopic recurrence within 1 year after surgery and 50% having a symptomatic recurrence within 4 years. Predictors of a severe course in Crohn's disease include stricturing or penetrating disease and perianal disease.

The risk for colon cancer is increased in patients with UC, and its magnitude is related to the extent and duration of disease. The colon cancer risk is increased 10- to 20-fold after 8 to 10 years of disease in pancolitis, and after 15 to 20 years in left-sided colitis. The cumulative incidence of colorectal cancer is 2.5% after 20 years and 7.6% after 30 years of disease. Proctitis is not associated with an increased risk of colorectal cancer. In colonic Crohn's disease, the risk of colorectal cancer is equivalent to that in patients with UC of similar extent and duration. Patients with isolated small bowel Crohn's disease are not at increased risk for colorectal cancer. The rates of small bowel carcinoma and lymphoma are increased in patients with Crohn's disease but the absolute risk is very low.

Surveillance for dysplasia and colon cancer among patients with UC and Crohn's disease colitis should be performed by colonoscopy 8 to 10 years after the onset of symptoms. Surveillance examinations are performed every 1 to 3 years. Proctitis does not require endoscopic surveillance, but colonoscopy should be performed 8 years after diagnosis to look for evidence of proximal spread of the disease. Patients with IBD and PSC appear to have a particularly increased risk for colon cancer, and yearly surveillance is recommended after the initial diagnosis of PSC. UC associated with PSC may have minimal or no symptoms, so all patients with PSC should undergo colonoscopy with biopsy to look for evidence of UC. The classic approach for UC surveillance has been to take a minimum of 33 "random" mucosal biopsy samples during the colonoscopic examination, in addition to targeted samples of visible lesions. The use of chromoendoscopy (spraying of the colon surface with indigo carmine or methylene blue dye during colonoscopy) increases the detection of dysplastic lesions in patients with UC and has replaced the performance of random biopsies in some societal guidelines. Polypoid dysplasia entirely removed by polypectomy in the colon can be managed with continued surveillance colonoscopy. Colectomy is indicated in patients with unresectable dysplasia or evidence of colorectal cancer.

As understanding of the etiologic and pathophysiologic aspects of IBD increases, major advances in diagnosis and treatment are anticipated. These will be based on better use of molecular, genetic, and serologic tests to differentiate among the subtypes of disease; earlier and more targeted use of biologic agents to manage inflammation; and improvements in the detection and prevention of colorectal cancer in those at risk.

SUGGESTED READINGS

Abraham BP, Quigley EMM: Probiotics in inflammatory bowel disease, Gastroenterol Clin North Am 46(4):769–782, 2017.

Ananthakrishnan AN: Epidemiology and risk factors for IBD, Nat Rev Gastroenterol Hepatol 12(4):205–217, 2015.

Damas OM, Garces L, Abreu MT: Diet as adjunctive treatment for inflammatory bowel disease: review and update of the latest literature, Curr Treat Options Gastroenterol 17(2):313–325, 2019.

De Souza HSP, Fiocchi C, Iliopoulos D: The IBD interactome: an integrated view of aetiology, pathogenesis and therapy, Nat Rev Gastroenterol Hepatol 14(12):739–749, 2017.

Feuerstein JD, Cheifetz AS: Crohn disease: epidemiology, diagnosis, and management, Mayo Clin Proc 92(7):1088–1103, 2017.

Feuerstein JD, Moss AC, Farraye FA: Ulcerative colitis, Mayo Clin Proc 94(7):1357–1373, 2019.

Johnson CM, Dassopoulos T: Update on the use of thiopurines and methotrexate in inflammatory bowel disease, Curr Gastroenterol Rep 20(11):53, 2018.

Laine L, Kaltenbach T, Barkun A, McQuaid KR, Subramanian V, Soetikno R: SCENIC guideline development panel. SCENIC international consensus statement on surveillance and management of dysplasia in inflammatory bowel disease, Gastrointest Endosc 81(3):489–501, 2015.

Lichtenstein GR, Loftus EV, Isaacs KL, Regueiro MD, Gerson LB, Sands BE: ACG clinical guideline: management of crohn's disease in adults, Am J Gastroenterol 113(4):481–517, 2018.

会出现胆盐池耗竭，导致脂肪吸收不良。这些患者可能需要低脂饮食并补充中链甘油三酯，可适当使用止泻药，但不应使用胆盐树脂螯合剂。

营养支持是 IBD 治疗中非常重要的辅助治疗方法，但营养支持治疗作为一线治疗仅限于小肠型 CD，尤其是儿童 CD 患者。这些患者经过至少 4 周的营养支持治疗（包括全肠外营养和要素饮食）可以获得并维持缓解，并可避免使用皮质类固醇。许多 UC 或 CD 患者在病情加重期间会出现体重减轻，需要补充热量。维生素和矿物质可口服补充，如服用含多种维生素和叶酸的复合维生素制剂。对于广泛回肠病变或回肠切除的患者，需考虑肠外补充维生素 B_{12}。使用皮质类固醇的患者需补充钙和维生素 D。小肠广泛受累的患者可出现脂溶性维生素（维生素 A、D、E、K）、铁和微量元素（罕见）吸收不良。对疾病活动期或伴有狭窄的患者，低纤维饮食可能是必须的。观察性研究显示，特定碳水化合物饮食（SCD）在 IBD 患者中有一定疗效，但其在本质上限制性很强，因此在没有更多证据支持前，并未获得广泛推荐。

饮食作为 IBD 的治疗方法尚需更多研究证据的支持。IBD 患者经常使用补充和替代药物，因此医生需要仔细询问药物的使用情况。

外科手术

外科手术治疗适用于出现严重并发症的患者，如梗阻、穿孔、纤维性狭窄、消化道大出血和中毒性巨结肠，以及内科治疗无效的患者。出现异型增生或癌变也是外科手术指征，如 UC 患者出现异型增生或癌变，无论累及范围如何，均必须全结肠切除。从历史上看，UC 的初始手术方式是全结直肠切除术和布鲁克回肠造口术，但现在，回肠储袋肛管吻合术已成为大多数患者的首选。在这种术式中，全结肠被切除，末端回肠构建成储袋，与肛门或直肠残端吻合，患者可通过肛门排便。手术并发症包括封套炎、储袋炎、大便失禁、生育能力下降和需要再次手术。外科手术不能治愈 CD，手术主要用于治疗 CD 的各种并发症，主要术式包括部分肠切除、狭窄成形术、瘘管切除术和脓肿引流术等。

预后

约 2/3 的 UC 患者在确诊后的 10 年内至少有 1 次疾病复发，20%～30% 的广泛结肠型 UC 患者最终需接受结肠切除术，而直肠型 UC 患者 10 年手术切除率仅为 5%。相比之下，超过 60% 的 CD 患者在诊断后的 10 年内需接受手术治疗，尽管这些数据来自生物制剂时代之前。CD 的术后复发率很高，70% 的患者在术后 1 年出现内镜复发，50% 的患者在术后 4 年内出现临床复发。提示 CD 预后不良的因素包括出现狭窄性或穿透性病变和肛周病变。

UC 患者患结肠癌的风险增加，风险与病变范围和病程有关。起病 8～10 年后的全结肠型 UC 患者和起病 15～20 年后的左半结肠型 UC 患者，其结肠癌的发生风险增加 10～20 倍。UC 患者结直肠癌的累积发生率在起病 20 年后为 2.5%，30 年后为 7.6%。直肠型 UC 不增加结直肠癌的风险。结肠型 CD 患者结直肠癌的发生风险等同于病程和病变范围类似的 UC 患者。仅累及小肠的 CD 不增加结直肠癌的发生风险。CD 患者小肠癌和淋巴瘤的风险增加，但绝对风险非常低。

UC 和结肠型 CD 患者在起病 8～10 年后需行结肠镜监测异型增生和结直肠癌，其后每 1～3 年监测 1 次。直肠型 UC 患者无须进行结肠镜监测，但起病 8 年后需行结肠镜以明确病变范围是否有进展。IBD 合并 PSC 的患者结直肠癌的发生风险显著增加，建议 PSC 诊断明确后每年行结肠镜监测。UC 合并 PSC 的患者临床症状通常较轻，甚至无症状，因此所有 PSC 患者均应行结肠镜和活检，以寻找 UC 的证据。UC 癌变监测的经典方法为结肠镜检查时取至少 33 块样本随机活检，以及针对病变部位的靶向活检。色素内镜（即结肠镜检查时喷洒靛胭脂或亚甲蓝染料）可以提高 UC 患者异型增生的检出率，因此部分指南提倡用色素内镜取代随机活检。息肉型异型增生经完整息肉切除后，可继续行结肠镜随访。发现不可切除的异型增生或结直肠癌的患者，应行全结肠切除术。

随着对 IBD 病因和病理生理学的深入了解，未来在诊断和治疗方面将取得重大进展。例如，更好地利用分子检测、基因检测和血清学检查来鉴别疾病亚型，更早、更精准地使用生物制剂来控制炎症，改进对结直肠癌高危人群的监测和预防工作。

推荐阅读

Abraham BP, Quigley EMM: Probiotics in inflammatory bowel disease, Gastroenterol Clin North Am 46(4):769–782, 2017.

Ananthakrishnan AN: Epidemiology and risk factors for IBD, Nat Rev Gastroenterol Hepatol 12(4):205–217, 2015.

Damas OM, Garces L, Abreu MT: Diet as adjunctive treatment for inflammatory bowel disease: review and update of the latest literature, Curr Treat Options Gastroenterol 17(2):313–325, 2019.

De Souza HSP, Fiocchi C, Iliopoulos D: The IBD interactome: an integrated view of aetiology, pathogenesis and therapy, Nat Rev Gastroenterol Hepatol 14(12):739–749, 2017.

Feuerstein JD, Cheifetz AS: Crohn disease: epidemiology, diagnosis, and management, Mayo Clin Proc 92(7):1088–1103, 2017.

Feuerstein JD, Moss AC, Farraye FA: Ulcerative colitis, Mayo Clin Proc 94(7):1357–1373, 2019.

Johnson CM, Dassopoulos T: Update on the use of thiopurines and methotrexate in inflammatory bowel disease, Curr Gastroenterol Rep 20(11):53, 2018.

Laine L, Kaltenbach T, Barkun A, McQuaid KR, Subramanian V, Soetikno R: SCENIC guideline development panel. SCENIC international consensus statement on surveillance and management of dysplasia in inflammatory bowel disease, Gastrointest Endosc 81(3):489–501, 2015.

Lichtenstein GR, Loftus EV, Isaacs KL, Regueiro MD, Gerson LB, Sands BE: ACG clinical guideline: management of crohn's disease in adults, Am J Gastroenterol 113(4):481–517, 2018.

Ma C, Panaccione R, Khanna R, Feagan BG, Jairath V: IL12/23 or selective IL23 inhibition for the management of moderate-to-severe Crohn's disease? Best Pract Res Clin Gastroenterol 38–39, 2019.

Malik TA: Inflammatory bowel disease: historical perspective, epidemiology and risk factors, Surg Clin North Am 95(6):1105–1122, 2015.

McGovern DP, Kugathasan S, Cho JH: Genetics of inflammatory bowel diseases, Gastroenterology 149(5):1163–1176, 2015.

Rubin DT, Ananthakrishnan AN, Siegel CA, Sauer BG, Long MD: ACG clinical guideline: ulcerative colitis in adults, Am J Gastroenterol 114(3):384–413, 2019.

Weisshof R, El Jurdi K, Zmeter N, Rubin DT: Emerging therapies for inflammatory bowel disease, Adv Ther 35(11):1746–1762, 2018.

Windsor JW, Kaplan GG: Evolving epidemiology of IBD, Curr Gastroenterol Rep 21(8):40, 2019.

Ma C, Panaccione R, Khanna R, Feagan BG, Jairath V: IL12/23 or selective IL23 inhibition for the management of moderate-to-severe Crohn's disease? Best Pract Res Clin Gastroenterol 38–39, 2019.

Malik TA: Inflammatory bowel disease: historical perspective, epidemiology and risk factors, Surg Clin North Am 95(6):1105–1122, 2015.

McGovern DP, Kugathasan S, Cho JH: Genetics of inflammatory bowel diseases, Gastroenterology 149(5):1163–1176, 2015.

Rubin DT, Ananthakrishnan AN, Siegel CA, Sauer BG, Long MD: ACG clinical guideline: ulcerative colitis in adults, Am J Gastroenterol 114(3):384–413, 2019.

Weisshof R, El Jurdi K, Zmeter N, Rubin DT: Emerging therapies for inflammatory bowel disease, Adv Ther 35(11):1746–1762, 2018.

Windsor JW, Kaplan GG: Evolving epidemiology of IBD, Curr Gastroenterol Rep 21(8):40, 2019.

Diseases of the Pancreas

David R. Lichtenstein, Pushpak Taunk

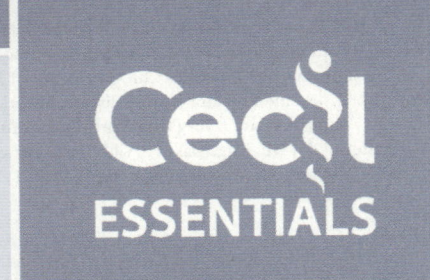

ACUTE PANCREATITIS

Definition and Epidemiology

Acute pancreatitis is an acute inflammatory process of the pancreas that may also involve peripancreatic tissues and remote organ systems. It is one of the leading causes of hospitalization for patients with gastrointestinal disorders in the United States, with more than 275,000 admissions annually. This translates into an overall incidence of 5 to 30 cases per 100,000 people in the general population. The aggregate cost of acute pancreatitis is more than $2.6 billion per year and the overall case fatality is roughly 5%. Approximately 80% of patients admitted with acute pancreatitis have mild, self-limited disease.

Pathology

The pancreas is located in the retroperitoneum and has exocrine and endocrine functions (Fig. 9.1) derived from the pancreatic acinus and the pancreatic islet, respectively. As an exocrine gland, the pancreas participates in normal digestion and nutrient absorption. The enzymes secreted by the pancreas digest starch (i.e., amylase), fats (i.e., lipase), and protein (i.e., trypsin and other proteolytic enzymes). Within acinar cells, proteolytic digestive enzymes are synthesized and packaged separately in the Golgi region into condensing vacuoles and transported in an inactive form referred to as zymogens to the apical portions of the cell. When stimulated, they are discharged into the central ductule of the acinus by exocytosis.

Normal physiology involves secretion of inactive enzymes into the duodenum, where they are converted to an active form by enterokinase, a brush border enzyme secreted by small bowel enterocytes. Trypsinogen conversion to active trypsin is the trigger enzyme that subsequently converts the other zymogens to active enzymes.

The pathogenesis of acute pancreatitis remains incompletely understood. Based on experimental models, the initiating event appears to involve intra-acinar activation of trypsin from trypsinogen, resulting in acute intracellular injury, pancreatic autodigestion, and the potential for profound systemic complications after activated enzymes are leaked into the bloodstream. The acinar cell injury results in a systemic inflammatory response that involves multiple cytokines, including platelet activating factor, tumor necrosis factor-α (TNF-α), and various interleukins. Initiating events may include obstruction of the pancreatic duct (e.g., gallstones, pancreatic tumor), overdistention of the pancreatic duct (e.g., from endoscopic retrograde cholangiopancreatography [ERCP]), reflux of biliary or duodenal juices into the pancreatic duct, changes in permeability of the pancreatic duct, ischemia of the organ, and toxin-induced cholinergic hyperstimulation (Fig. 9.2).

During the initial hospitalization for acute pancreatitis, reasonable attempts to determine the cause are appropriate, particularly those that may affect acute management. The cause of acute pancreatitis is readily identified in 70% to 90% of patients after an initial evaluation consisting of the history, physical examination, focused laboratory testing, and routine radiologic studies. Gallstones account for 45%, alcohol for 35%, miscellaneous causes for 10%, and idiopathic causes for 10% to 20% of acute pancreatitis cases (Table 9.1).

Gallstone Pancreatitis

Among patients with gallstones, the incidence of acute pancreatitis is about 0.17% per year. Gallstones increase the relative risk of pancreatitis 25- to 35-fold. Gallstone pancreatitis is more common in women than men. It is theorized that gallstone passage causes transient obstruction of the pancreatic duct, precipitating acute pancreatitis. Acute gallstone pancreatitis should be suspected when associated with a transient elevation in liver-associated enzymes, particularly alanine aminotransferase (ALT) levels greater than 150 IU/L. Most stones pass spontaneously from the ampulla and do not require intervention (discussed later).

Alcoholic Pancreatitis

Acute alcoholic pancreatitis is the second most common cause of pancreatitis in the United States. Approximately 10% of individuals with an alcohol use disorder develop attacks of pancreatitis that are indistinguishable from other forms of acute pancreatitis. Prolonged alcohol use (four to five drinks daily over a period of more than 5 years) is required for alcohol-associated pancreatitis. The type of alcohol does not affect risk, and binge drinking in the absence of long-term, heavy alcohol use infrequently precipitates acute pancreatitis. Alcoholics with acute pancreatitis most commonly have underlying chronic disease. However, some have true acute alcoholic pancreatitis because not all patients progress to chronic pancreatitis, even with continued alcohol use. The mechanism of pancreatic injury, the genetic and environmental factors that influence its development in alcoholics, and the reason only a small proportion of alcoholics develop pancreatitis are unclear (see "Chronic Pancreatitis").

Hypertriglyceridemia

Hypertriglyceridemia is the third most identifiable cause of pancreatitis, and serum triglyceride levels greater than 1000 mg/dL may precipitate attacks of acute pancreatitis. Patients may have lactescent (milky) serum owing to increased concentrations of chylomicrons. Both primary and secondary disorders of lipoprotein metabolism are associated with hypertriglyceridemic pancreatitis. Although the exact pathogenesis of hypertriglyceridemic pancreatitis is unclear, the release of free fatty acids by lipase may damage pancreatic acinar cells or capillary endothelium. The main treatment modalities for initial management of hypertriglyceridemia are apheresis with therapeutic plasma

胰腺疾病

李佳宁 译 吴颜延 谭蓓 校审 杨爱明 通审

急性胰腺炎

定义和流行病学

急性胰腺炎是一种胰腺的急性炎症病变，胰周组织及远处器官均可受累。急性胰腺炎是美国因胃肠疾病住院的主要原因之一，每年导致约 275 000 人住院。普通人群的总发病率为（5～30）/100 000。急性胰腺炎每年造成 26 亿美元的经济负担及约 5% 的病死率。因急性胰腺炎住院的患者中约 80% 为轻症患者，呈自限性。

病理学

胰腺位于腹膜后，胰腺腺泡和胰岛分别具有外分泌和内分泌功能（图 9.1）。作为外分泌腺，胰腺参与正常的消化与营养吸收过程。胰腺分泌的酶可消化淀粉（如淀粉酶）、脂肪（如脂肪酶）和蛋白质（如胰蛋白酶及其他蛋白水解酶）。在腺泡细胞内，蛋白水解酶在高尔基体区域被单独合成和包装成浓缩液泡，并以酶原的非活性形式被运输至细胞顶端。当受到刺激时，这些酶会通过胞吐作用被释放到腺泡的中央导管中。

正常生理情况下，非活性酶分泌至十二指肠，并被肠激酶（一种由小肠肠上皮细胞分泌的刷状缘酶）转化为活性形式。胰蛋白酶原被转化为具有活性的胰蛋白酶，胰蛋白酶作为触发酶，将其他酶原转化为活性酶形式。

急性胰腺炎的发病机制尚不完全清楚。根据实验动物模型，起始事件可能涉及胰蛋白酶原在腺泡细胞内被激活为胰蛋白酶，导致急性细胞内损伤、胰腺自消化，活性酶渗漏至血流后可能引发全身并发症。腺泡细胞损伤导致的全身炎症反应涉及多种细胞因子，包括血小板活化因子、肿瘤坏死因子α（TNF-α）及多种白介素。起始事件可能包括胰管梗阻（如胆石症、胰腺肿瘤），胰管过度扩张［如行内镜逆行胰胆管造影（ERCP）］，胆汁或十二指肠液反流至胰管，胰管通透性改变，器官缺血或毒素诱导的胆碱能过度刺激（图 9.2）。

患者因急性胰腺炎初次住院期间，应尽可能确定病因，特别是可能影响急性期管理的病因。在初步评估（包括病史、体格检查、特定实验室检查及常规影像学检查）后，70%～90% 的急性胰腺炎患者很容易明确病因。其中，胆石症占 45%，酒精占 35%，其他病因占 10%，而特发性胰腺炎占 10%～20%（表 9.1）。

胆源性胰腺炎

在胆石症患者中，急性胰腺炎的发病率约为每年 0.17%。胆石症可使胰腺炎的相对风险增加 25～35 倍。胆源性胰腺炎在女性中更为常见。理论上，胆结石通过导致胰腺导管暂时性梗阻，进而引发急性胰腺炎。当出现肝酶水平短暂升高，特别是丙氨酸转氨酶（ALT）> 150 IU/L 时，应怀疑急性胆源性胰腺炎。大多数结石会自发地从壶腹部通过，不需要特殊干预（见下文）。

酒精性胰腺炎

在美国，急性酒精性胰腺炎是胰腺炎的第二大病因。约 10% 的酒精使用障碍者会出现急性胰腺炎，且难以与其他类型的胰腺炎区分。诊断酒精相关胰腺炎需要患者满足长期饮酒的条件（每日饮酒 4～5 个标准杯，超过 5 年）。酒精种类不会影响急性胰腺炎的风险，在没有长期大量饮酒的情况下，短期内狂饮很少会引发急性胰腺炎。患有急性胰腺炎的酗酒者通常合并潜在的慢性疾病。然而，有些人患有真正的急性酒精性胰腺炎，因为即便持续饮酒，并非所有患者均会进展为慢性胰腺炎。目前尚不明确胰腺损伤的机制、影响酗酒者发生急性胰腺炎的基因和环境因素，以及仅有小部分酗酒者会发展为胰腺炎的原因（参见"慢性胰腺炎"）。

高甘油三酯血症

高甘油三酯血症是胰腺炎可识别的第三大病因。血清甘油三酯 > 1000 mg/dl 时，可能会引起胰腺炎急性发作。由于乳糜微粒浓度增加，患者血清可能呈乳白色（乳糜状）。原发性和继发性脂蛋白代谢异常均与高甘油三酯血症性胰腺炎相关。虽然高甘油三酯血症性胰腺炎的确切发病机制尚不清楚，但脂肪酶释放的游离脂肪酸可能会损伤胰腺腺泡细胞或毛细血管内皮。高甘油三酯血症初始治疗的主要方式是血浆置换和胰

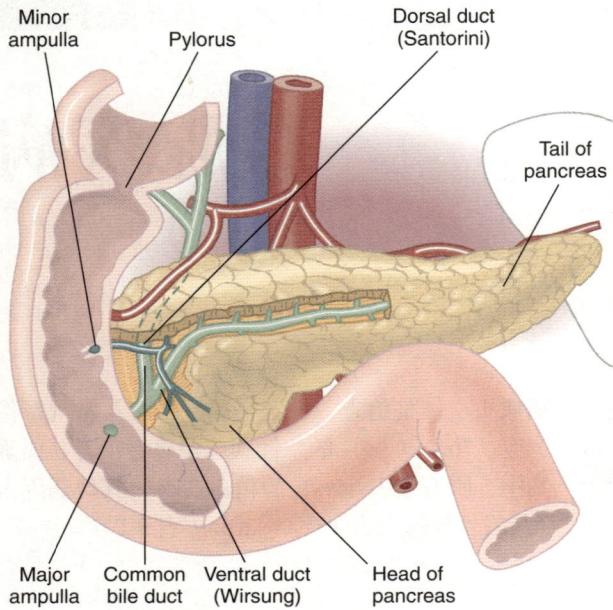

Fig. 9.1 Normal anatomy of the pancreas.

exchange and insulin. Lowering serum triglyceride levels to less than 200 mg/dL can prevent pancreatitis and is typically done with a combination of diet and medications.

Drug-Related Pancreatitis

Drugs appear to cause fewer than 5% of all cases of acute pancreatitis, although hundreds of medications have been implicated. The drugs most strongly associated with acute pancreatitis are azathioprine, 6-mercaptopurine, didanosine, valproic acid, angiotensin-converting-enzyme inhibitors, eluxadoline, and mesalamine. Though there are several potential pathogenic mechanisms of drug-induced pancreatitis, the most common is a hypersensitivity reaction. This tends to occur 4 to 8 weeks after starting the drug and is not dose related. On re-challenge with the drug, pancreatitis recurs within hours to days. The second mechanism is the presumed accumulation of a toxic metabolite that may cause pancreatitis, typically after several months of use. Pancreatitis caused by drugs is usually mild and self-limited.

Heredity

Hereditary causes of pancreatitis include mutations in the genes encoding cationic trypsinogen (*PRSS1*), pancreatic secretory trypsin inhibitor (serine protease inhibitor Kazal type 1 [*SPINK1*]), cystic fibrosis transmembrane conductance regulator (*CFTR*), chymotrypsin

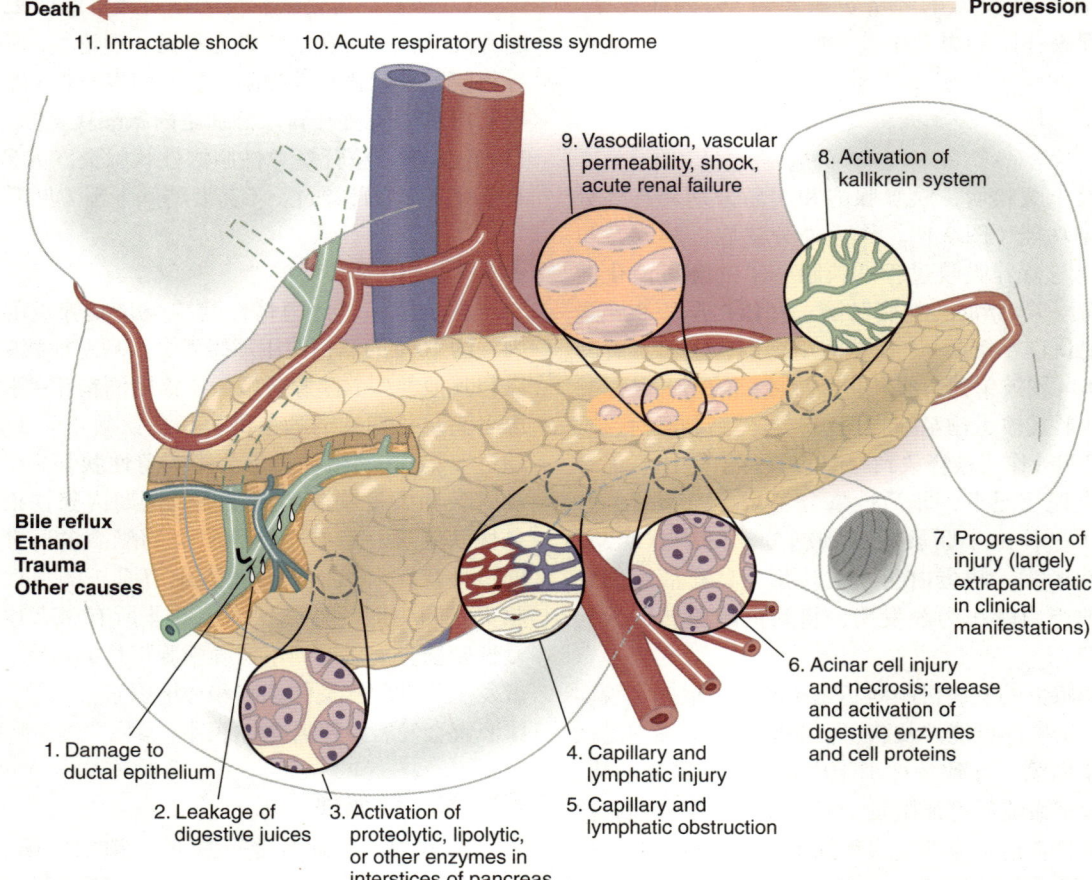

Fig. 9.2 The pathophysiology of acute pancreatitis is not fully understood, but as the schematic shows, a cascade of events seems likely, beginning with the release of toxic substances into the parenchyma and ending with shock and death. Damage to the ductal epithelium or acinar cell injury may result from bile reflux, increased intraductal pressure, alcohol, or trauma. (Modified from Grendell JH: The pancreas. In Smith LH Jr, Thier SO, editors: Pathophysiology: the biological principles of disease, ed 2, Philadelphia, 1985, WB Saunders, p 1228.)

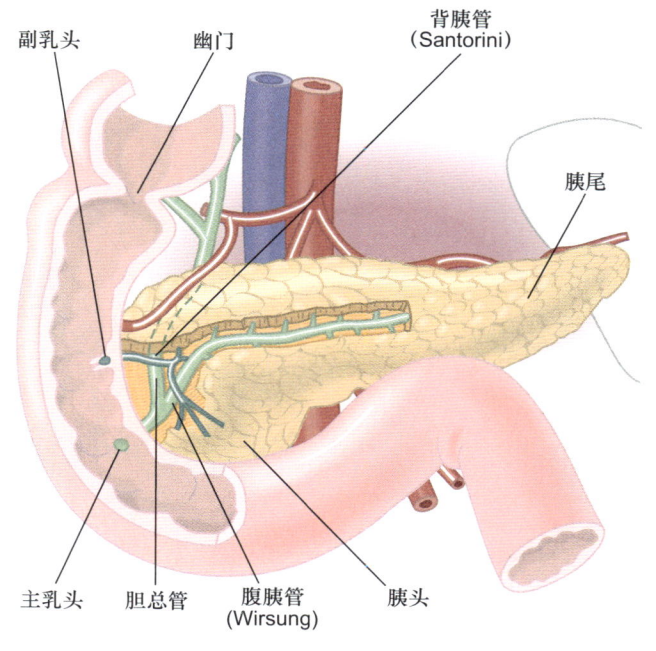

图 9.1 胰腺的正常解剖

岛素。将血清甘油三酯水平降至 200 mg/dl 以下可预防胰腺炎发作，这通常需要饮食结合药物来实现。

药物相关性胰腺炎

尽管有数百种药物与胰腺炎有关，但药物导致的胰腺炎占所有急性胰腺炎病例的 5% 以下。与急性胰腺炎相关性最强的药物包括硫唑嘌呤、6-巯基嘌呤、去羟肌苷、丙戊酸、血管紧张素转换酶抑制剂、艾沙度林和美沙拉嗪。药物相关性胰腺炎有多种潜在的发病机制，最常见的是超敏反应。药物相关性胰腺炎通常出现于用药后 4～8 周，且与剂量无关。再次使用同种药物后，胰腺炎可能在数小时至数天内再发。另一种机制是导致胰腺炎的有毒代谢产物的累积，通常在用药后数月出现。药物相关性胰腺炎通常症状轻微且呈自限性。

遗传

胰腺炎的遗传学病因包括编码阳离子胰蛋白酶原（*PRSS1*）、胰分泌型胰蛋白酶抑制剂［丝氨酸蛋白酶抑制剂 Kazal 1 型（*SPINK1*）］、囊性纤维化跨膜传导调

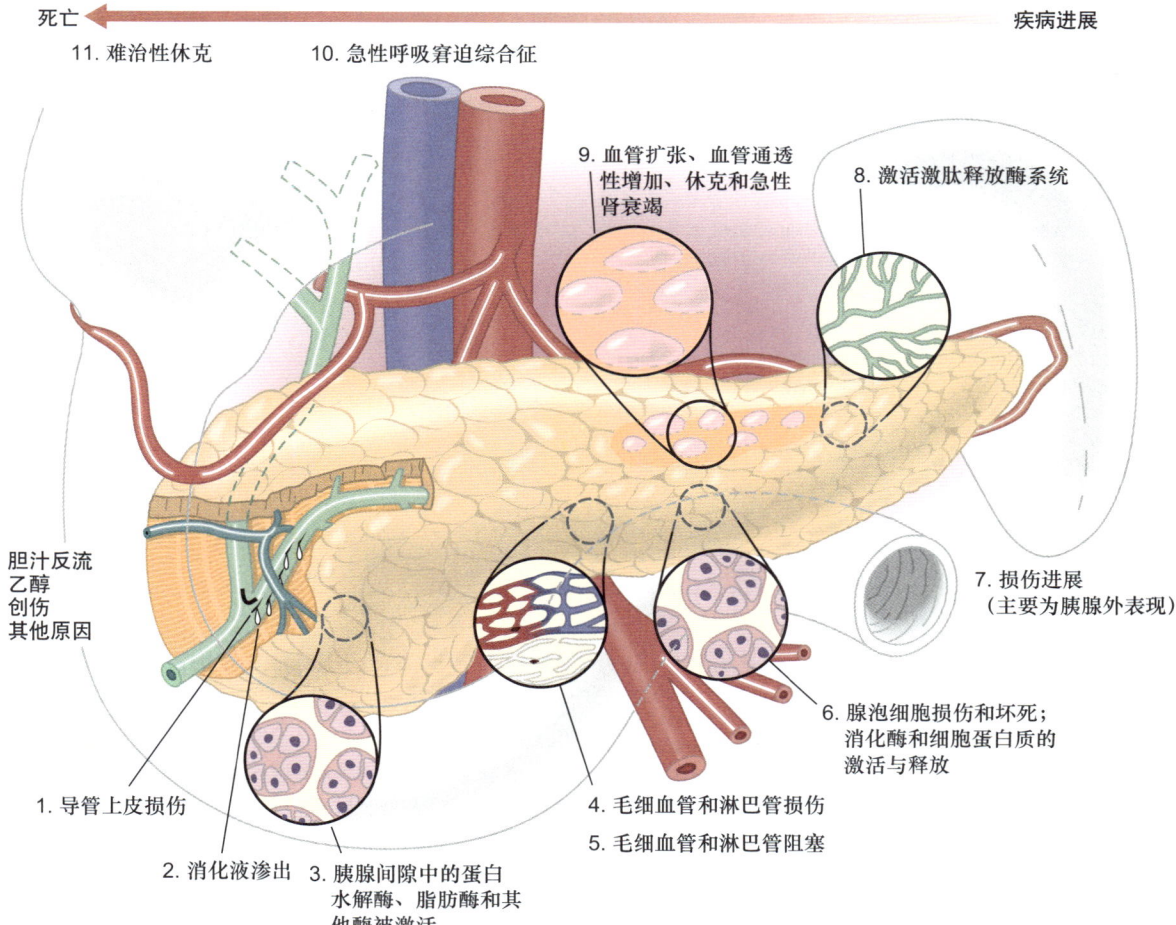

图 9.2 急性胰腺炎的病理生理学机制尚未完全明确，但如图所示，其可能包含一系列事件。从有毒物质释放到实质组织开始，以休克和死亡结束。胆汁反流、导管内压力升高、酒精或创伤可能导致导管上皮及腺泡细胞损伤（改编自 Grendell JH：The pancreas. In Smith LH Jr，Thier SO，editors：Pathophysiology：the biological principles of disease，ed 2，Philadelphia，1985，WB Saunders，p 1228.）

TABLE 9.1 Causes of Acute Pancreatitis

Obstruction
Gallstones
Tumors: ampullary or pancreatic tumors
Parasites: *Ascaris* or *Clonorchis* species
Developmental anomalies: pancreas divisum, choledochocele, annular pancreas
Periampullary duodenal diverticula
Hypertensive sphincter of Oddi
Afferent duodenal loop obstruction

Toxins
Ethyl alcohol
Methyl alcohol
Scorpion venom: excessive cholinergic stimulation causes salivation, sweating, dyspnea, and cardiac arrhythmias; seen mostly in the West Indies
Organophosphorus insecticides

Drugs
Definite associations (documented with rechallenges): azathioprine or 6-mercaptopurine, valproic acid, estrogens, tetracycline, metronidazole, nitrofurantoin, pentamidine, furosemide, sulfonamides, methyldopa, cytarabine, cimetidine, ranitidine, sulindac, dideoxycytidine
Probable associations: thiazides, ethacrynic acid, phenformin, procainamide, chlorthalidone, L-asparaginase

Metabolic Disorders
Hypertriglyceridemia, hypercalcemia, end-stage renal disease

Trauma
Accidental: blunt trauma to the abdomen (e.g., car accident, bicycle)
Iatrogenic: postoperative, endoscopic retrograde cholangiopancreatography

Infectious Diseases
Parasitic: ascariasis, clonorchiasis
Viral: mumps, rubella, hepatitis A, hepatitis B, hepatitis C, coxsackievirus B, echovirus, adenovirus, cytomegalovirus, varicella virus, Epstein-Barr virus, human immunodeficiency virus
Bacterial: mycoplasma, *Campylobacter jejuni*, tuberculosis, *Legionella* species, leptospirosis

Vascular Disorders
Ischemia: hypoperfusion (e.g., postcardiac surgery) or atherosclerotic emboli
Vasculitis: systemic lupus erythematosus, polyarteritis nodosa, malignant hypertension

Idiopathic Disorders
Accounts for 10–30% of patients with pancreatitis
Up to 60% have occult gallstone disease (e.g., biliary microlithiasis, gallbladder sludge)
Less common causes: sphincter of Oddi dysfunction, mutations in the cystic fibrosis transmembrane regulator

Miscellaneous Disorders
Penetrating peptic ulcer
Crohn's disease of the duodenum
Pregnancy-associated disorders
Pediatric associations: Reye's syndrome, cystic fibrosis
Autoimmune pancreatitis

C (i.e., caldecrin) *(CTRC)*, the calcium-sensing receptor *(CASR)*, and claudin-2. Aside from acute pancreatitis, mutations in these genes may increase the risk of development of diabetes and pancreatic cancer.

The role of genetic testing in idiopathic acute pancreatitis is controversial. Diagnosis of these genetic disorders contributes little to direct management because specific therapy is unavailable. Similarly, inadvertent disclosure of the results of genetic testing protects patients' health care insurance but may impact other financial decisions such as disability and life insurance. However, identification of an underlying genetic cause may obviate the need for further testing, allow more informed family planning, and enable better surveillance for complications, including pancreatic cancer. The decision to pursue genetic testing is one that should be made only with the advice and involvement of an experienced counselor.

Neoplasia

Primary pancreatic ductal adenocarcinoma, ampullary tumors, metastasis to the pancreas, and intraductal papillary mucinous neoplasms are uncommon causes of acute pancreatitis. The mechanism of pancreatitis is presumably secondary to obstruction of the pancreatic duct. These causes should be considered for patients older than 40 years. Pancreatitis has been reported in up to 10% of patients with pancreatic cancer.

表9.1 急性胰腺炎的病因
梗阻 胆石症 肿瘤：壶腹部或胰腺肿瘤 寄生虫：蛔虫或华支睾吸虫 发育异常：胰腺分裂、胆总管囊肿、环状胰腺 壶腹周围或十二指肠憩室 Oddi 括约肌高压 十二指肠输入袢梗阻
毒素 乙醇 甲醇 蝎毒：胆碱能过度刺激导致流涎、出汗、呼吸困难和心律失常；多见于西印度群岛 有机磷杀虫剂
药物 明确相关（再次使用后复发）：硫唑嘌呤或 6-巯基嘌呤、丙戊酸、雌激素、四环素、甲硝唑、呋喃妥因、喷他脒、呋塞米、磺胺类药物、甲基多巴、阿糖胞苷、西咪替丁、雷尼替丁、舒林酸、扎西他滨 可能相关：噻嗪类药物、依他尼酸、苯乙双胍、普鲁卡因胺、氯噻酮、L-天冬酰胺酶
代谢性疾病 高甘油三酯血症、高钙血症、终末期肾病
创伤 意外：腹部钝性创伤（如车祸、自行车事故） 医源性：术后损伤、内镜逆行胰胆管造影
感染性疾病 寄生虫：蛔虫病、华支睾吸虫病 病毒：腮腺炎病毒、风疹病毒、甲型肝炎病毒、乙型肝炎病毒、丙型肝炎病毒、柯萨奇病毒 B 组、埃可病毒、腺病毒、巨细胞病毒、水痘病毒、EB 病毒、人类免疫缺陷病毒 细菌：支原体、空肠弯曲菌、结核病、军团菌、钩端螺旋体病
血管疾病 缺血：低灌注（如心脏手术后）或动脉粥样硬化栓塞 血管炎：系统性红斑狼疮、结节性多动脉炎、恶性高血压
特发性疾病 占胰腺炎患者的 10%～30% 多达 60% 的患者有隐匿性胆石症（如胆道微结石、胆囊泥沙样结石） 较少见原因：Oddi 括约肌功能障碍、囊性纤维化跨膜传导调节蛋白基因突变
其他疾病 穿透性消化性溃疡 十二指肠克罗恩病 妊娠相关疾病 儿科相关疾病：瑞氏综合征、囊性纤维化 自身免疫性胰腺炎

节蛋白（$CFTR$）、糜蛋白酶 C（即降钙因子；$CTRC$）、钙离子感应受体（$CASR$）和密封蛋白 2 的基因突变。除了急性胰腺炎，这些基因突变还可能会增加患糖尿病和胰腺癌的风险。

基因检测在特发性胰腺炎中的作用存在争议。由于缺乏特定的治疗方法，这些遗传性疾病的诊断对疾病管理几乎没有帮助。同样，基因检测结果的无意披露虽然可以保障患者的医疗保险，但可能会影响其他财务决策，如残疾保险和人寿保险。然而，确定潜在的遗传学病因可避免进一步检测的需要，帮助更好地制订生育计划，并能够更好地监测并发症（如胰腺癌）。应在经验丰富的遗传学专家的建议和参与下决定是否进行基因检测。

肿瘤

原发性胰腺导管腺癌、壶腹部肿瘤、胰腺转移瘤和胰腺导管内乳头状黏液性肿瘤是急性胰腺炎的少见病因。胰腺炎可能由胰管梗阻所致。40 岁以上患者应考虑肿瘤病因。约 10% 的胰腺癌患者会出现胰腺炎。

Smoking

Smoking was once thought to be a risk factor due to its synergism with alcohol. However, studies have suggested that cigarette smoking is an independent risk factor for acute and chronic pancreatitis by mechanisms that are unclear.

Autoimmune Pancreatitis

Autoimmune pancreatitis (AIP) is a benign disease representing two distinct but overlapping immune-mediated inflammatory conditions of the pancreas referred to as type 1 and type 2 AIP. Type 1 is the classic and more common form of AIP. It is characterized histologically by a periductal lymphoplasmacytic infiltrate, storiform fibrosis, obliterative phlebitis, and abundant immunoglobulin G4 (IgG4) immunostaining (>10 IgG4-positive cells per high-power field).

The most common manifestation of AIP is obstructive jaundice, which closely mimics pancreatic cancer with focal enlargement of the pancreatic head. AIP can also manifest as acute pancreatitis in up to 15% to 30% of individuals, and about 5% of patients evaluated for acute or chronic pancreatitis have AIP. AIP has a peak incidence in the sixth or seventh decades of life and tends to affect men twice as often as women. Serum IgG4 levels are elevated to more than two times the upper limit of normal in most patients. Computed tomography (CT) typically demonstrates diffuse enlargement of the pancreas with delayed (rim) enhancement and a diffusely irregular, attenuated main pancreatic duct. More than 60% of individuals have clinical and histologic involvement of other organs, including the biliary tree, retroperitoneum, lacrimal and salivary glands, lymph nodes, periorbital tissues, kidneys, thyroid, lungs, meninges, aorta, breast, prostate, pericardium, and skin. Although a majority of patients initially respond to glucocorticoids, a significant portion of patients relapse once glucocorticoids are discontinued. Immunomodulator drugs have been used in those that fail steroids, relapse or cannot be weaned off steroids.

A less common form of AIP (type 2 AIP) has a similar clinical and radiographic presentation in the pancreas, but in contrast to type 1 disease, it requires histologic confirmation of an idiopathic duct centric pancreatitis lesion. Other hallmarks of type 1 disease are absent such that IgG4 levels are normal and other organs are not involved. Type 2 AIP is similarly steroid responsive but unlike type 1 disease, relapse is uncommon.

Pancreas Divisum

At approximately 4 weeks' gestation, the dorsal pancreas forms as an evagination from the duodenum, and shortly thereafter, the ventral pancreas forms from the hepatic diverticulum. At approximately the eighth intrauterine week of life, the ventral pancreas rotates posterior to the duodenum and comes to rest posterior and inferior to the head portion of the dorsal pancreas with associated fusion of the main ducts. If fusion is incomplete, the duct of Wirsung drains only the ventral pancreas through the major ampulla, and the duct of Santorini drains the bulk of the pancreas (i.e., dorsal pancreas) through the relatively small accessory (minor) ampulla. This anomaly, called *pancreas divisum*, occurs in 5% to 10% of the general population and is associated with acute and chronic pancreatitis.

Theories suggest that pancreatitis results from relative outflow obstruction of the main dorsal duct through the small accessory ampulla. Endoscopic papillotomy, stent placement across the minor papilla, and surgical sphincteroplasty are therapeutic maneuvers that may reduce the incidence of recurrent pancreatitis by increasing drainage through the accessory papilla. While there are studies that appear to show an association between pancreas divisum and pancreatitis, there is controversy as to whether pancreas divisum is truly a cause of acute recurrent pancreatitis.

Clinical Presentation

The hallmark of acute pancreatitis is persistent abdominal pain. In atypical cases, patients may have unexplained organ failure or postoperative ileus. The onset of pain is typically sudden, severe, and worse when supine. Pain is usually located in the upper abdomen and may radiate to the back, chest, and flanks. Nausea and vomiting are common. Physical examination usually reveals severe upper abdominal tenderness that is sometimes associated with guarding.

Pancreatic enzymes, vasoactive substances (e.g., kinins), and other toxic substances (e.g., elastase, phospholipase A_2) are liberated by the inflamed pancreas and extravasate along fascial planes in the retroperitoneal space, lesser sac, and peritoneal cavity. These materials cause chemical irritation and contribute to the development of ileus, chemical peritonitis, third-space losses of protein-rich fluid, hypovolemia, and hypotension. The toxic molecules may reach the systemic circulation by lymphatic and venous pathways and contribute to subcutaneous fat necrosis and end-organ damage, including shock, renal failure, and respiratory insufficiency (i.e., atelectasis, effusions, and acute respiratory distress syndrome [ARDS]). Grey Turner sign (i.e., ecchymosis of the flank) or Cullen sign (i.e., ecchymosis in the periumbilical region) may be associated with hemorrhagic pancreatitis.

Metabolic problems, which are common in severe disease, include hypocalcemia, hyperglycemia, and acidosis. Hypocalcemia is most commonly caused by concomitant hypoalbuminemia. Other mechanisms include complexing of calcium to released free fatty acids, protease-induced degradation of circulating parathyroid hormone (PTH), and failure of PTH to release calcium from bone.

Acute pancreatitis is associated with a variety of local and vascular complications, including local spread of inflammation to contiguous organs. The most common include peripancreatic fluid collections, pseudocyst formation, obstruction of the duodenum or bile duct, and exocrine or endocrine insufficiency. Less common complications include pancreatic fistula formation, vascular thrombosis (i.e., splenic, portal and superior mesenteric veins), colonic necrosis, and development of an arterial pseudoaneurysm. Trypsin can activate plasminogen to plasmin and induce clot lysis. However, trypsin also can activate prothrombin and thrombin and produce thrombosis leading to disseminated intravascular coagulation.

Acute peripancreatic fluid collections are pools of peripancreatic fluid confined by normal peripancreatic fascial planes without a definable wall encapsulating the collection. These fluid collections occur during the first 4 weeks after interstitial pancreatitis. When a localized acute peripancreatic fluid collection persists beyond 4 weeks, it is likely to develop into a pancreatic pseudocyst.

Pancreatic pseudocysts are encapsulated fluid collections with well-defined inflammatory walls and are usually located outside the pancreas with minimal or no necrosis. They occur a minimum of 4 weeks after the onset of acute pancreatitis. Although most pseudocysts remain asymptomatic, presenting symptoms may include abdominal pain, early satiety, nausea, and vomiting due to compression of the stomach or gastric outlet. Rapidly enlarging pseudocysts may rupture, hemorrhage, obstruct the extrahepatic biliary tree, erode into surrounding structures, and become infected.

The term *acute necrotic collection* describes a nonorganized accumulation of heterogeneous fluid and necrotic material in the setting of necrotizing pancreatitis. The necrosis may involve the pancreatic parenchyma or peripancreatic tissue, or both. Walled-off pancreatic necrosis is a mature, encapsulated collection of pancreatic or peripancreatic necrosis that usually occurs more than 4 weeks after the onset of necrotizing pancreatitis.

Abdominal compartment syndrome is diagnosed when the intra-abdominal pressure exceeds 20 mm Hg and there are signs of new

吸烟

吸烟既往因与酒精的协同作用而被认为是胰腺炎的危险因素。然而，研究表明，吸烟是急性和慢性胰腺炎的独立危险因素，其机制尚不清楚。

自身免疫性胰腺炎

自身免疫性胰腺炎（AIP）是一种良性疾病，表现为两种不同但相互重叠的免疫介导的胰腺炎症状态，即1型和2型AIP。1型是经典且更常见的AIP形式。其组织学特征为导管周围大量淋巴浆细胞浸润、席纹状纤维化、闭塞性静脉炎和大量免疫球蛋白G4（IgG4）免疫组织化学染色阳性（IgG4阳性细胞＞10个/高倍视野）。

AIP最常见的临床表现是梗阻性黄疸，这与伴有胰头局部增大的胰腺癌非常相似。15%～30%的AIP患者可表现为急性胰腺炎，约5%因急性胰腺炎或慢性胰腺炎而接受评估的患者被诊断为AIP。AIP的发病高峰年龄为50～70岁，男性患病率是女性的2倍。大多数患者的血清IgG4水平＞正常值上限的2倍。AIP的CT表现通常为胰腺弥漫性肿大伴延迟（边缘）强化及弥散不均、主胰管狭窄等。超过60%的AIP患者有其他器官的临床及组织学受累表现，包括胆道系统、腹膜后、泪腺及唾液腺、淋巴结、眶周组织、肾、甲状腺、肺、脑膜、主动脉、乳腺、前列腺、心包和皮肤。尽管绝大多数患者最初对糖皮质激素治疗的反应良好，但很大一部分患者停用糖皮质激素后会出现疾病复发。对于激素治疗无效、复发或无法停用激素的患者，可使用免疫调节剂。

2型AIP（较少见）具有相似的临床和胰腺影像学改变，但与1型AIP不同的是，2型AIP的诊断需要组织学检查确认具有特发性导管中心性胰腺炎改变。2型AIP不存在1型AIP的其他特征性改变，如2型AIP患者的血清IgG4水平通常在正常范围，且无其他脏器受累。2型AIP对激素治疗有反应，但与1型不同的是，疾病复发不常见。

胰腺分裂

在妊娠约第4周时，十二指肠突起形成背侧胰腺，随后腹侧胰腺自肝憩室形成。在妊娠第8周，腹侧胰腺旋转至十二指肠后方，并在背侧胰腺头部的后方和下方与主胰管融合。若融合不完全，腹胰管（Wirsung）将只通过主乳头引流腹侧胰腺区，而背胰管（Santorini）通过壶腹部相对较小的副乳头引流大部分胰腺区（如背侧胰腺）。这种解剖学异常被称为胰腺分裂，普通人群的发生率为5%～10%，与急性和慢性胰腺炎的发生相关。

研究表明，胰腺炎与较小的副乳头引流较大的背侧胰腺区域引发的相对梗阻有关。内镜下乳头切开术、经副乳头置入胰管支架和外科括约肌成形术可能通过增加副乳头引流而降低胰腺炎复发率。虽然有研究显示胰腺分裂与胰腺炎相关，但对于胰腺分裂是否真的是导致急性复发性胰腺炎的原因仍存在争议。

临床表现

急性胰腺炎的特征性表现是持续性腹痛。在非典型病例中，患者可能出现不明原因的器官功能衰竭或术后肠梗阻。疼痛通常突发而剧烈，仰卧位时加剧。疼痛部位通常位于上腹部，可能放射至背部、胸部或侧腹部。常见症状包括恶心和呕吐。体格检查常提示严重的上腹部压痛，甚至伴有肌卫。

胰腺在炎症状态下会释放胰酶、血管活性物质（如激肽）和其他有毒物质（如弹性蛋白酶、磷脂酶A_2），并沿着腹膜后间隙、小网膜囊和腹膜腔的筋膜平面渗出。这些物质会引起化学刺激，并导致肠梗阻、化学性腹膜炎、富含蛋白质的液体丢失至第三间隙、低血容量和低血压。这些毒性分子可能通过淋巴和静脉途径进入全身循环，导致皮下脂肪坏死和终末器官损伤，包括休克、肾衰竭、呼吸功能不全［如肺不张、胸腔积液、急性呼吸窘迫综合征（ARDS）］。格雷-特纳征（Grey Turner征；即侧腹瘀斑）和卡伦征（Cullen征；即脐周瘀斑）可能与出血性胰腺炎有关。

代谢异常（包括低钙血症、高血糖和酸中毒）常见于重症病例。低钙血症最常见的原因是伴随的低白蛋白血症，其他机制包括钙离子与游离脂肪酸形成复合物、蛋白酶诱导的循环甲状旁腺激素（PTH）降解及PTH未能从骨骼中释放钙。

急性胰腺炎与多种局部及血管并发症有关，包括炎症局部扩散至邻近器官。最常见的并发症包括胰周液体积聚、假性囊肿形成、十二指肠或胆道梗阻，以及外分泌和内分泌功能不全。较少见的并发症包括胰瘘形成，血管栓塞形成（如脾静脉、门静脉和肠系膜上静脉），结肠坏死和假性动脉瘤等。胰蛋白酶可将纤溶酶原激活为纤溶酶，并诱导血栓溶解。然而，胰蛋白酶同样可以激活凝血酶原和凝血酶，导致血栓产生，进而引发弥散性血管内凝血。

急性胰周液体积聚是指胰腺周围液体被正常的胰腺周围筋膜平面所限制，且没有明确的囊壁包裹。这些液体积聚发生在间质性胰腺炎后的前4周内。当局部急性胰周液体积聚持续超过4周时，可能会发展为胰腺假性囊肿。

胰腺假性囊肿是具有明确炎症囊壁的包裹性液体积聚，通常位于胰腺外，伴有轻微坏死或无坏死。胰腺假性囊肿见于急性胰腺炎发病4周之后。尽管大多数假性囊肿无症状，但患者仍可由于胃或胃出口受压而表现为腹痛、早饱、恶心和呕吐。快速增大的假性囊肿可能会破裂、出血、梗阻肝外胆道、侵蚀周围结构并发生感染。

急性坏死物积聚是指坏死性胰腺炎时异质性液体和坏死物的非组织化积聚。坏死物可能累及胰腺实质和（或）胰腺周围组织。胰腺包裹性坏死是指胰腺或胰腺周围坏死物的包裹性积聚，通常出现在坏死性胰腺炎发病4周之后。

当腹腔内压力超过20 mmHg且新发呼吸衰竭、肾衰竭或循环不稳定的征象时，即可诊断腹腔间室综合

respiratory, renal, or vascular organ failure. Intra-abdominal hypertension typically occurs early and is the result of pancreatic inflammation and fluid third spacing. Abdominal compartment syndrome is associated with mortality rates ranging up to 50% to 75% in various reports. Suggested treatment includes analgesics, sedation, nasogastric tube decompression, and fluid restriction. If these measures do not result in improvement, percutaneous catheter decompression followed if unsuccessful by a surgical laparotomy is recommended. The ability of this approach to improve outcomes is the focus of ongoing research.

Diagnosis and Differential Diagnosis

The diagnosis of acute pancreatitis is based on a combination of clinical, biochemical, and radiologic factors. A diagnosis of acute pancreatitis requires two of the following three features: abdominal pain characteristic of acute pancreatitis; serum amylase or lipase levels, or both, at least three times the upper limit of normal; and characteristic findings of acute pancreatitis on imaging.

Elevated serum amylase levels may occur in a wide variety of other conditions, including bowel perforation, intestinal obstruction or ischemia, acute appendicitis, cholecystitis, tubo-ovarian disease, and renal failure. Serum amylase levels may be normal in patients with hypertriglyceridemia or alcohol-induced acute pancreatitis. Serum lipase is preferred because it is more sensitive and specific than serum amylase for the diagnosis of acute pancreatitis. The serum lipase level remains normal in some nonpancreatic conditions associated with an elevated serum amylase level, including macroamylasemia (i.e., formation of large molecular complexes between amylase and abnormal immunoglobulins), salivary gland disorders, and tubo-ovarian disease, but it may similarly rise in appendicitis, renal disease, and cholecystitis. The serum lipase concentration is more sensitive than that of amylase because it remains elevated longer and may be diagnostic even for patients seeking medical attention several days after symptom onset. Repeated measurements of serum pancreatic enzymes have little value in assessing clinical progress, and the magnitude of serum amylase or lipase elevation does not correlate with the severity of pancreatitis.

Contrast-enhanced computed tomography (CECT) or magnetic resonance imaging (MRI) of the pancreas should be used for patients whose diagnosis is unclear or who fail to improve within the first 48 to 72 hours after hospital admission. Imaging findings supporting acute pancreatitis include pancreatic enlargement, peripancreatic inflammatory changes, and extrapancreatic fluid collections. Imaging does not exclude the diagnosis of acute pancreatitis because the pancreas appears normal in 15% to 30% of those with mild disease. CECT is also useful for assessing disease severity based on the presence and extent of complications such as pancreatic necrosis and acute peripancreatic fluid collections. Pancreatic imaging should be performed after adequate fluid resuscitation to minimize the risk of contrast-induced nephrotoxicity.

MRI is preferred for patients with a contrast allergy and renal insufficiency because T2-weighted images without gadolinium contrast can similarly diagnose pancreatic necrosis. Early imaging (within 72 hours of symptom onset) can underestimate the existence and extent of pancreatic necrosis. Gallstone pancreatitis should be suspected in patients with transient elevation in liver function test results, particularly a serum ALT level elevated more than 3-fold. Transabdominal ultrasonography should be performed in all patients with acute pancreatitis when considering a diagnosis of gallstone pancreatitis.

Prognosis

The distinction between interstitial and necrotizing acute pancreatitis has important prognostic implications (Fig. 9.3). *Interstitial pancreatitis* is characterized by an intact microcirculation and uniform enhancement of the gland on CECT. *Necrotizing pancreatitis* is characterized by disruption of the pancreatic microcirculation so that large areas (>3 cm or >30%) of pancreatic parenchyma do not enhance on CECT. Approximately 20% to 30% of patients with acute pancreatitis have necrotizing pancreatitis.

The finding of pancreatic necrosis predicts a more severe course, particularly infection in the necrotic pancreatic tissue, also called *infected necrosis*. Infection is a strong determinant of the severity of illness and accounts for a large percentage of the deaths from acute pancreatitis. Infected necrosis develops in 30% to 50% of patients with acute necrotizing pancreatitis but not in those with interstitial disease. Infected necrosis should be suspected in patients with persistent systemic inflammatory response syndrome (SIRS) or organ dysfunction. The diagnosis can be made if extraluminal gas is seen on CECT. More commonly, CT-guided needle aspiration is obtained for Gram stain and culture of necrotic material, or antibiotics are given empirically based on clinical suspicion after appropriate cultures are obtained. Antibiotics that penetrate pancreatic tissue, including cephalosporins, carbapenems, quinolones, and metronidazole, are used for treatment of infected necrosis.

Risk assessment should be performed for all patients to stratify the severity of illness. The current classification includes mild, moderate, and severe forms. Mild acute pancreatitis, the most common form, is characterized by the absence of organ failure and pancreatic necrosis. Mild pancreatitis usually does not require pancreatic imaging, and patients recover within several days with restoration of normal pancreatic function and gland architecture. Patients with mild acute pancreatitis account for 80% of all attacks and less than 5% of the overall mortality rate.

Moderately severe pancreatitis is characterized by local complications and/or transient organ failure over a time period of less than 48 hours. Local complications include pancreatic necrosis (with or without infection) and acute peripancreatic fluid collections or pancreatic pseudocysts. Death from moderately severe pancreatitis is much less common than in cases of severe pancreatitis.

Severe acute pancreatitis is defined by persistent organ failure extending for more than 48 hours. Severe acute pancreatitis occurs in 15% to 20% of patients. Most individuals with persistent organ failure have underlying necrotizing disease. The respiratory, cardiovascular, and renal systems are most commonly affected. Early deaths (within the first week) are most often the result of multiple organ failure caused by the release of inflammatory mediators and cytokines. Late deaths are more likely to result from local or systemic infection. The risks of infection and death correlate with disease severity and pancreatic necrosis. The overall mortality approaches 30% among patients with persistent organ failure.

Despite the importance of recognizing severe disease, most patients are initially admitted to the hospital without necrosis or organ failure, and methods to predict individuals more likely to progress to severe disease during the initial several days of hospitalization have been defined. A combination of clinical assessment, scoring systems, serum markers, and CECT scanning provides the most useful prognostic information (Table 9.2). Regardless of the prognostic factor chosen, there are significant limitations in predicting disease severity.

Clinical predictors of a poor outcome include severe comorbid illnesses, older age (≥60 years), obesity, and long-term, heavy alcohol use. Laboratory findings associated with increased mortality include blood urea nitrogen elevation (>20 mg/dL) on admission or a rise during the first 24 hours of admission, hemoconcentration from third spacing of fluids reflected by an elevated hematocrit of 44 or greater on admission, and serum markers reflecting a robust systemic inflammatory response, such as a C-reactive protein level greater than

征。腹腔内高压通常在早期发生，常由胰腺炎症和第三间隙积液导致。多项研究报道，腹腔间室综合征的死亡率为50%～75%。推荐的治疗包括镇痛药、镇静药、鼻胃管减压和限制性输液。如果这些措施未能改善病情，建议进行经皮穿刺置管减压术，如果仍无效，建议进行开腹手术。该方法能否改善预后是当前研究的重点。

诊断和鉴别诊断

急性胰腺炎的诊断需基于临床表现、生化特点和影像学检查结果进行综合判断。诊断急性胰腺炎需要具备以下3项特征中至少2项：①急性胰腺炎特征性腹痛；②血清淀粉酶和（或）脂肪酶≥正常值上限的3倍；③影像学检查显示急性胰腺炎的特征性表现。

血清淀粉酶水平升高可见于多种疾病，包括肠穿孔、肠梗阻或缺血、急性阑尾炎、胆囊炎、输卵管-卵巢疾病和肾衰竭。高甘油三酯血症或酒精诱发的急性胰腺炎患者的血清淀粉酶水平可能在正常范围内。血清脂肪酶在诊断急性胰腺炎方面比血清淀粉酶更加敏感和特异。在伴有血清淀粉酶水平升高的部分非胰腺疾病中，血清脂肪酶水平通常正常，包括巨淀粉酶血症（即淀粉酶与异常免疫球蛋白形成大分子复合物）、唾液腺疾病和输卵管-卵巢疾病，但在阑尾炎、肾病和胆囊炎中，脂肪酶水平也可能升高。血清脂肪酶浓度比淀粉酶更敏感，因为它升高的持续时间更长，即使患者在症状出现数天后就诊，也可能具有诊断价值。反复检测胰酶在评估临床进展方面价值不大，血清淀粉酶或脂肪酶升高的幅度与胰腺炎的严重程度无关。

对于诊断不明确或入院后48～72 h内未见好转的患者，应进行胰腺增强计算机断层成像（CECT）或MRI。支持诊断急性胰腺炎的影像学检查结果包括胰腺肿大、胰腺周围炎症性改变和胰腺外液体积聚。影像学检查不能排除急性胰腺炎的诊断，因为在15%～30%的轻症患者中，胰腺可能无异常影像学表现。CECT还可用于根据并发症（如胰腺坏死和急性胰周液体积聚）的存在和程度来评估疾病严重性。胰腺影像学检查应在充分的液体复苏后进行，以尽量减少造影剂引起的肾毒性风险。

对于造影剂过敏和肾功能不全患者，首选MRI，因为无需钆造影剂的T2加权像也能诊断胰腺坏死。早期影像学检查（症状出现72 h内）可能会低估胰腺坏死的存在和范围。对于短暂性肝功能指标升高（尤其是血清ALT水平升高超过3倍）的患者，应怀疑胆源性胰腺炎。所有考虑诊断急性胆源性胰腺炎的急性胰腺炎患者均应进行经腹部超声检查。

预后

区分间质性急性胰腺炎和坏死性急性胰腺炎对预后具有重要意义（图9.3），间质性胰腺炎的特征是微循环完整，CECT可见胰腺呈均匀强化。坏死性胰腺炎的特征是胰腺微循环中断，导致大面积（>3 cm或>30%）的胰腺实质在CECT中不增强。20%～30%的急性胰腺炎患者为坏死性胰腺炎。

发现胰腺坏死通常预示着病程更严重，特别是坏死的胰腺组织中合并感染，又称感染性坏死。感染是疾病严重程度的重要决定因素，在急性胰腺炎死亡病例中占很大比例。30%～50%的急性坏死性胰腺炎患者会发生感染性坏死，而间质性胰腺炎的患者则不会。对于持续存在全身炎症反应综合征（SIRS）或器官功能障碍的患者，应怀疑感染性坏死。若CECT可见肠外气体，即可诊断感染性坏死。更常用的方法是CT引导下针吸活检吸取坏死物质进行革兰氏染色和培养，或在获取合适的培养物后根据临床怀疑启动经验性抗生素治疗。应选择可穿透胰腺组织的抗生素治疗感染性坏死，包括头孢菌素、碳青霉烯类、喹诺酮类和甲硝唑。

所有患者均应进行风险评估，以对疾病严重程度进行分类。目前分类包括轻度、中度和重度。轻度急性胰腺炎最常见，其特征是无器官衰竭和胰腺坏死。轻度胰腺炎通常无须进行胰腺影像学检查，患者的胰腺功能和腺体结构常在数天内恢复正常。轻度急性胰腺炎占所有患者的80%，在总体死亡率中的占比<5%。

中度重症胰腺炎的特点是有局部并发症和（或）持续时间<48 h的短暂器官衰竭。局部并发症包括胰腺坏死（伴或不伴感染）和急性胰周液体积聚或胰腺假性囊肿。中度重症胰腺炎患者的死亡率显著低于重度胰腺炎。

重度急性胰腺炎的特征性表现是持续性器官功能衰竭（>48 h）。15%～20%的急性胰腺炎患者会进展至重症。大多数具有持续性器官功能衰竭的患者均有潜在的坏死性疾病。呼吸系统、心血管系统和肾最常受累。早期死亡（起病1周内）通常是由炎症介质和细胞因子释放导致的多器官衰竭引起。晚期死亡多由局部或全身感染导致。感染和死亡的风险与疾病严重程度及胰腺坏死相关。持续性器官衰竭患者的总体死亡率接近30%。

尽管识别重症病例非常重要，但大多数患者入院时并无胰腺坏死或器官功能衰竭，多种工具有助于预测在住院最初几天内可能进展为重症的患者。临床评估、评分系统、血清标志物和CECT的结合可提供最有用的预后信息（表9.2）。所有预后因素在预测疾病严重程度方面都有显著的局限性。

不良预后的临床预测因素包括严重共病、高龄（≥60岁）、肥胖症和长期大量饮酒。与死亡率升高相关的实验室检查结果包括入院时或入院后24 h内血尿素氮水平升高（>20 mg/dl）、入院时血细胞比容≥44%（反映体液向第三间隙渗漏引起的的血液浓缩），以及提示强烈全身炎症反应的血清标志物升高［如C反应蛋白

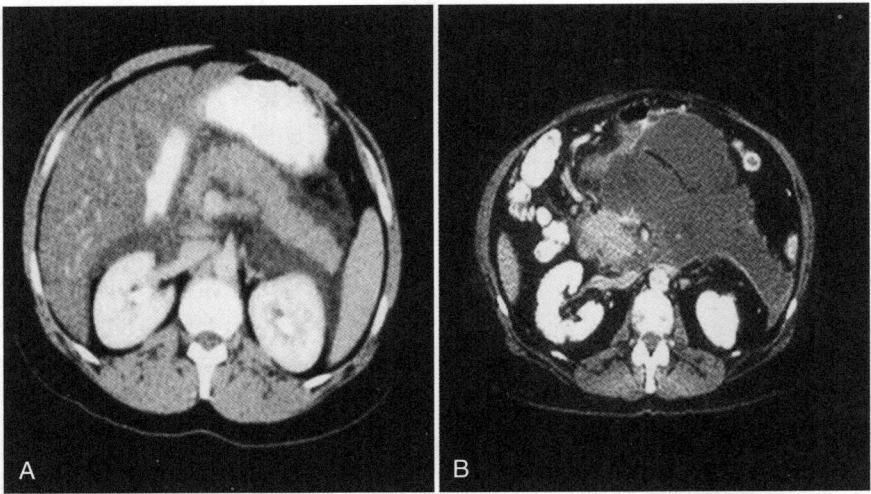

Fig. 9.3 Contrast-enhanced computed tomography demonstrates interstitial pancreatitis (A) and necrotizing pancreatitis (B).

TABLE 9.2 Predictors of Severe Pancreatitis

Criteria	Prognostic Indicators
Signs[a]	Heart rate: >90 beats/min Temperature: >38° C or <36° C White blood cell count: >12,000 or <4,000 cells/μL or >10% bands Respiratory rate >20 beats/min or Pa_{CO_2} <32 mm Hg
Patient characteristics	Comorbid illnesses Age >55 yr Obesity (BMI >30 kg/m²)
Laboratory values	BUN level of 20 mg/dL or higher and any rise in BUN during the first 24 hr of admission associated with increased mortality Serum creatinine >1.8 mg/dL within first 24 hr Hemoconcentration with Hct ≥44 on admission or failure of Hct to decrease in first 24 to 48 hr with volume resuscitation predicts severe pancreatitis Serum marker reflecting a systemic inflammatory response, CRP >150 mg/dL
Imaging findings	Pleural effusion Pancreatic necrosis Acute extrapancreatic fluid collections
Scoring systems	
Ranson's criteria	Eleven prognostic indicators, including five available on admission (age >55 yr, WBC >16,000/mm³, glucose >200 mg/dL, LDH >350 IU/L, AST >250 U/L) and six measured at the end of the first 48 hr (Hct decreased >10, BUN >5 mg/dL, P_{O_2} <60 mm Hg, base deficit >4 mEq/L, serum calcium <8 mg/dL, estimated fluid sequestration >6 L); mortality rate of 10–20% for three to five signs and >50% for six or more signs
Acute Physiologic and Chronic Health Evaluation (APACHE II) system	Calculated by assigning points based on age, heart rate, temperature, respiratory rate, mean arterial pressure, Pa_{O_2}, pH, potassium, sodium, creatinine, Hct, WBC, GCS, and previous health status
Bedside Index for Severity of Acute Pancreatitis (BISAP)	Five variables available in initial 24 hr: BUN >25 mg/dL, impaired mental status (GCS score <15), finding of SIRS, age >60 yr, and pleural effusion on imaging. Each variable adds 1 point to the total score, and scores of 3, 4, and 5 correspond to mortality rates of 5.3%, 12.7%, and 22.5%, respectively.

AST, Aspartate aminotransferase; *BMI*, body mass index; *BUN*, blood urea nitrogen; *CRP*, C-reactive protein; *GCS*, Glasgow Coma Scale; *Hct*, hematocrit; *LDH*, lactate dehydrogenase; *SIRS*, systemic inflammatory response syndrome; *WBC*, white blood cells.
[a]SIRS predisposes to multiple organ dysfunction and pancreatic necrosis. SIRS is defined by two or more of these criteria persisting for more than 48 hours.

150 mg/dL (sensitivity of 80%, specificity of 76%, positive predictive value of 67%, and negative predictive value of 86%). Imaging studies predicting a severe outcome include a pleural effusion seen on chest radiography within the first 24 hours or pancreatic imaging identifying necrosis. Unfortunately, CT evidence of severe acute pancreatitis lags behind clinical findings, and an early CT study can underestimate the severity of the disorder.

Severe pancreatitis is predicted by organ dysfunction, including shock (systolic blood pressure <90 mm Hg), respiratory failure (Pa_{O_2} ≤60 mm Hg), and acute renal injury (creatinine >2.0 mg/L after

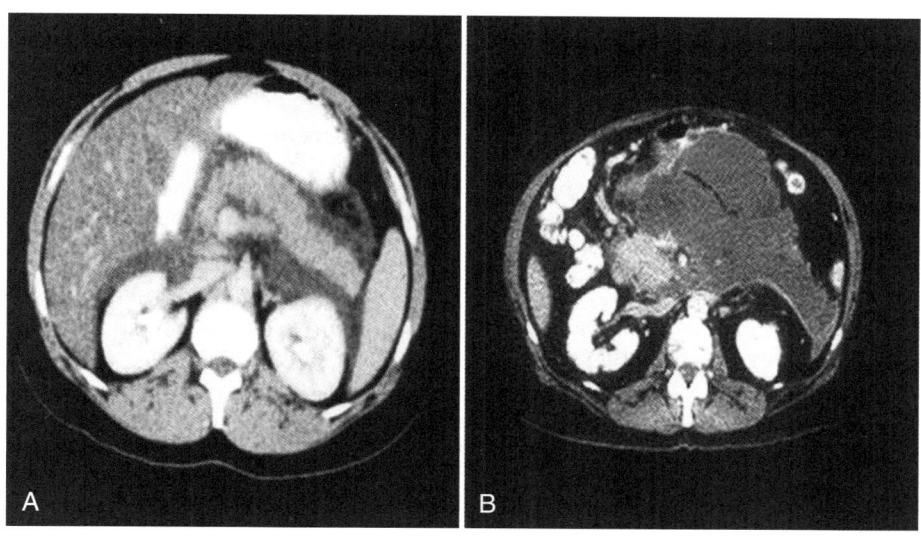

图 9.3　CECT 显示间质性胰腺炎（A）和坏死性胰腺炎（B）

表 9.2　重症胰腺炎的预后预测因素

指标	预后因素
体征 [a]	心率：> 90 次 / 分 体温：> 38℃ 或 < 36℃ WBC：> $12×10^9$/L 或 < $4×10^9$/L，或杆状核粒细胞 > 10% 呼吸频率：> 20 次 / 分或 PaO_2 < 32 mmHg
患者特征	共病 年龄 > 55 岁 肥胖（BMI > 30 kg/m^2）
实验室指标	入院后 24 h 内 BUN ≥ 20 mg/dl 或 BUN 水平升高，均与死亡率升高相关 入院后 24 h 内血清肌酐 > 1.8 mg/dl 入院时 HCT ≥ 44%，或在入院后 24～48 h 内经容量复苏后 HCT 未下降，可预测重症胰腺炎 反映全身炎症反应的血清标志物水平升高，如 CRP > 150 mg/dl
影像学检查	胸腔积液 胰腺坏死 急性胰腺外液体积聚
评分系统	
Ranson 评分	11 项预后指标，包括 5 项入院时可获得的指标（年龄 > 55 岁、WBC > $16×10^9$/L、葡萄糖 > 200 mg/dl、LDH > 350 IU/L、AST > 250 U/L）和 6 项在入院后 48 h 内测量的指标（HCT 降低 > 10%、BUN > 5 mg/dl、PaO_2 < 60 mmHg、碱剩余 > 4 mmol/L、血清钙 < 8 mg/dl、估计液体积聚量 > 6 L）。具有 3～5 项指标的患者死亡率为 10%～20%，具有 ≥ 6 项指标的患者死亡率 > 50%
急性生理和慢性健康评估 Ⅱ（APACHE Ⅱ）系统	根据年龄、心率、体温、呼吸频率、平均动脉压、PaO_2、pH 值、血钾、血钠、肌酐、HCT、WBC、GCS 和既往健康状况等指标分配分数进行计算
急性胰腺炎严重程度床旁指数（BISAP）	5 项在入院后 24 h 内可获得的变量：BUN > 25 mg/dl、精神状态受损（GCS 评分 < 15）、SIRS 表现、年龄 > 60 岁、影像学检查显示胸腔积液。每个变量计 1 分，得分为 3 分、4 分和 5 分的患者，其死亡率分别为 5.3%、12.7% 和 22.5%

AST，天冬氨酸转氨酶；BMI，体重指数；BUN，血尿素氮；CRP，C 反应蛋白；GCS，格拉斯哥昏迷评分；HCT，血细胞比容；LDH，乳酸脱氢酶；SIRS，全身炎症反应综合征；WBC，白细胞计数。
[a] SIRS 患者更易出现多器官功能障碍和胰腺坏死。SIRS 的定义是存在 ≥ 2 项指标且持续时间 > 48 h。

> 150 mg/dl（敏感性 80%，特异性 76%，阳性预测值 67%，阴性预测值 86%）]。提示重症的影像学检查结果包括在入院后 24 h 内胸部 X 线检查显示胸腔积液或胰腺影像学检查显示胰腺坏死。但是，重度急性胰腺炎的 CT 表现滞后于临床发现，早期 CT 检查可能低估疾病的严重程度。

重度胰腺炎的预测指标包括器官功能障碍，如休克（收缩压 < 90 mmHg）、呼吸衰竭（PaO_2 ≤ 60 mmHg）和急性肾损伤（补液后肌酐 > 2.0 mg/L）。SIRS 患者更

rehydration). SIRS predisposes to multiple organ dysfunction and pancreatic necrosis.

Well-established scoring systems include Ranson's criteria, Acute Physiologic and Chronic Health Evaluation II (APACHE II), APACHE combined with scoring for obesity (APACHE-O), the Glasgow Scoring System, and Bedside Index for Severity of Acute Pancreatitis (BISAP). With increasing scores, the likelihood of a complicated, prolonged, and fatal outcome increases. Unfortunately, because these scoring systems have a high false-positive rate (i.e., in many patients with high score, severe pancreatitis does not develop), they are not universally used. During the first 48 to 72 hours, a rising hematocrit or BUN, persistent SIRS after fluid resuscitation or the presence of pancreatic or peripancreatic necrosis on cross-sectional imaging constitute evidence of evolving severe pancreatitis.

Treatment

Early steps in the management of patients with acute pancreatitis can decrease severity, morbidity, and mortality (Fig. 9.4). Prevention of complications depends largely on monitoring, vigorous hydration, and early recognition of pancreatic necrosis and choledocholithiasis. Patients with multiorgan dysfunction and those with predicted development of severe disease are at greatest risk for adverse outcomes and should be treated when possible in a care unit with intensive monitoring capability and multidisciplinary input.

Supportive Care

Patients with acute pancreatitis are treated supportively with aggressive intravenous hydration, parenteral analgesics, and bowel rest. Supplemental oxygen is recommended initially for all patients. Nasogastric tube suction is indicated for symptomatic relief in patients with nausea, vomiting, and ileus. No specific treatments are effective in limiting systemic complications. Agents that put the pancreas to rest (e.g., somatostatin, calcitonin, glucagon, H_2-receptor antagonists) and enzyme inhibitors (e.g., aprotinin, gabexate mesylate) have not been shown to lower disease-related morbidity and mortality.

Antibiotics

Antibiotic therapy is no longer recommended for patients with sterile necrosis due to the lack of proven benefit. For patients with suspected infected necrosis, appropriate antibiotics are initiated before the confirmatory diagnosis, with the initial choice taking into consideration the likely pathogenic organisms and the ability of the antimicrobials to penetrate into necrotic pancreatic tissues. After culture results are available, the antibiotics can be tailored appropriately.

Fluid Management

Vigorous fluid resuscitation is important for maintaining the microcirculation and perfusion of the pancreas during the early phase of acute pancreatitis. Early aggressive intravenous hydration during the first 12 to 24 hours after the onset of symptoms translates into a potential benefit of reduced pancreatic necrosis and organ failure. Vigorous fluid therapy is of little value after 24 hours. Crystalloid, the preferred intravenous fluid, is administered at an initial rate of 250 to 500 mL/hour or 5 to 10 mL/kg/hr with a preceding bolus infusion for individuals with severe volume depletion. Lactated Ringer's solution may be the preferred crystalloid replacement because in one comparative study, it reduced the incidence of inflammatory markers by more than 80% compared with normal saline infusion. Goal-directed fluid therapy is recommended for patients with acute pancreatitis. Goal-directed therapy is defined as titration of intravenous fluids every few hours to specific clinical and biochemical targets of perfusion (e.g., heart rate, blood pressure, urine output, BUN, and hematocrit). Caution must be used for the elderly and those with underlying cardiovascular or renal impairment.

Analgesia

Despite the theoretical concern that narcotic analgesia may result in sphincter of Oddi spasm and worsening pancreatitis, there is no evidence to support withholding narcotics from patients with acute pancreatitis. The physician should consider liberal use of patient-controlled analgesia, although this approach has not been compared prospectively with on-demand analgesia. There is no evidence to indicate superiority of a specific opiate. Patients administered repeated doses of narcotic analgesics should have oxygen saturation monitored due to risks of unrecognized hypoxia.

Nutritional Care

Patients with mild acute pancreatitis can begin oral feeding within 24 hours of admission without waiting for resolution of pain or normalization of serum pancreatic enzyme levels. Early introduction of a low-fat solid diet is as safe as the traditional approach of progressive advancement from a clear liquid diet and is associated with a shorter length of hospital stay.

For patients with predicted severe pancreatitis or small bowel ileus, early introduction of oral intake may not be tolerated due to postprandial abdominal pain, nausea, and vomiting. These individuals can have nutrition introduced as nasoenteric or nasogastric feeding. Enteral feeding is preferable to total parenteral nutrition (TPN) because it is less expensive than TPN and is associated with a reduction in systemic infection, need for surgical intervention, organ failure, and mortality. Enteral feeding is usually well tolerated, even by patients with an ileus. Nasogastric feeding offers a safe alternative to nasojejunal feeding because it appears to be equally safe and effective. Parenteral nutrition should be reserved for patients who cannot achieve sufficient caloric intake through the enteral route or those in whom enteral access cannot be maintained.

Management of Recurrence and Necrosis

Gallstone pancreatitis. The risk of gallstone pancreatitis (see also Chapter 15) recurrence is as high as 50% to 75% within 6 months of the initial episode, and cholecystectomy before discharge is recommended for patients with mild attacks of pancreatitis. Cholecystectomy performed during the initial admission for patients with suspected biliary pancreatitis is associated with substantial reductions in mortality and gallstone-related complications, readmission for recurrent pancreatitis, and pancreaticobiliary complications. Cholecystectomy is often delayed in patients with severe pancreatitis to allow for better exposure of the ductal anatomy at the time of surgery. Urgent ERCP with identification and clearance of bile duct stones is recommended for patients with documented choledocholithiasis on imaging, cholangitis or strong evidence of ongoing biliary obstruction, as suggested by imaging and laboratory data. Biliary sphincterotomy leaving the gallbladder in situ is considered an effective alternative for those who are not candidates for cholecystectomy.

Acute fluid collections and pseudocysts. Acute peripancreatic fluid collections do not require any specific therapy, other than supportive therapy that is standard for acute pancreatitis. Most remain sterile and are reabsorbed spontaneously during the first several weeks after the onset of acute pancreatitis. When a localized acute peripancreatic fluid collection persists beyond 4 weeks, it is likely to develop into a pancreatic pseudocyst. While patients with asymptomatic pseudocysts should be followed, for those who are symptomatic, pseudocyst drainage should be considered. Indications for pseudocyst drainage include suspicion of infection or progressive

易出现多器官功能障碍和胰腺坏死。

公认的评分系统包括 Ranson 评分、急性生理和慢性健康评估 Ⅱ（APACHE Ⅱ）、APACHE 结合肥胖评分（APACHE-O）、格拉斯哥评分系统和急性胰腺炎严重程度床旁指数（BISAP）。随着评分的增大，发生复杂、持久和致命结局的可能性也随之增加。但是，由于这些评分系统的假阳性率较高（即许多高评分患者未发展为重度胰腺炎），它们并未被普遍使用。在入院后 48～72 h 内，提示会进展至重度胰腺炎的证据包括血细胞比容或 BUN 水平升高、液体复苏后 SIRS 持续存在，以及断层成像检查显示胰腺或胰周坏死。

治疗

急性胰腺炎患者的早期管理可降低疾病的严重程度、发病率和死亡率（图 9.4）。并发症的预防主要依赖于监测、积极补液，以及早期识别胰腺坏死和胆总管结石。多器官功能障碍患者和预计会发展为重症的患者预后不良的风险最大，应尽可能在具有强化监测能力和多学科协作的监护病房进行治疗。

支持治疗

急性胰腺炎患者的支持治疗包括积极静脉补液、肠外应用镇痛药和肠道休息。初期建议所有患者吸氧。对于有恶心、呕吐和肠梗阻症状的患者，鼻胃管胃肠减压可以缓解症状。目前没有特定的治疗方法可有效改善全身并发症。抑制胰腺分泌的药物（如生长抑素、降钙素、胰高血糖素、H_2 受体拮抗剂）和酶抑制剂（如抑肽酶、甲磺酸加贝酯）未被证明能降低疾病相关的并发症发生率和死亡率。

抗生素

由于缺乏明确获益，对于无菌性坏死的患者，不再推荐抗生素治疗。对于疑似感染性坏死的患者，在确诊前应开始使用适当的抗生素，初步选择应考虑可能的致病微生物及抗菌药物穿透坏死胰腺组织的能力。在获得病原体培养结果后，应适当调整抗生素方案。

液体管理

在急性胰腺炎的早期阶段，积极的液体复苏对于维持胰腺的微循环和灌注非常重要。在症状出现后 12～24 h 内进行积极静脉补液可减少胰腺坏死和器官功能衰竭。起病 24 h 后积极静脉补液几乎没有价值。静脉补液首选晶体液，初始输液速率为 250～500 ml/h 或 5～10 ml/(kg·h)。对于严重容量不足的个体，需先进行快速输液。乳酸林格液是首选的晶体液，因为一项比较研究表明，与输注生理盐水相比，它可将炎症标志物水平降低 80% 以上。建议对急性胰腺炎患者进行目标导向的液体治疗。目标导向的治疗是指每隔几小时根据特定的临床和生化灌注指标（如心率、血压、尿量、BUN 和血细胞比容）来调整静脉输液量。对于老年患者和有心血管疾病或肾功能不全的患者，必须谨慎补液。

镇痛

尽管理论上麻醉性镇痛药可能导致 Oddi 括约肌痉挛并加重胰腺炎，但没有证据支持急性胰腺炎患者禁用麻醉性镇痛药。医生应考虑广泛使用患者自控镇痛，尽管这种方法尚未与按需镇痛进行前瞻性比较。尚无证据表明某种特定的阿片类药物优于其他药物。对于反复使用麻醉性镇痛药的患者，应监测其氧饱和度，因其存在未识别的缺氧风险。

营养治疗

轻度急性胰腺炎患者在入院后 24 h 内即可开始口服进食，无须等待疼痛消退或血清胰酶水平恢复正常。早期引入低脂固体饮食与传统的从清淡流质饮食逐步过渡的方法同样安全，并可缩短住院时间。

对于预计进展为重度胰腺炎或小肠梗阻的患者，早期经口进食可能会因餐后腹痛、恶心和呕吐而无法耐受。这些患者可通过鼻肠管或鼻胃管进行营养支持。肠内营养优于全肠外营养（TPN），因其成本较低，且可减少全身感染、对手术干预的需求和器官衰竭，以及降低死亡率。即便是肠梗阻患者，通常也能很好地耐受肠内营养。鼻胃管喂养是鼻空肠管喂养的替代方案，因为它同样安全有效。肠外营养应作为无法通过肠内途径摄取足够热量或无法维持肠内通道的患者的治疗方案。

复发和坏死的管理

胆源性胰腺炎　胆源性胰腺炎（见第 15 章）的复发风险在初次发作后的 6 个月内高达 50%～75%，对于轻度胰腺炎患者，建议在出院前进行胆囊切除术。对于疑似胆源性胰腺炎的患者，在首次住院期间进行胆囊切除术亦可使死亡率、与胆石症相关的并发症发生率、因复发性胰腺炎再入院率和胰胆并发症发生率显著降低。对于重度胰腺炎患者，胆囊切除术通常会择期进行，以便在手术时更好地暴露导管解剖结构。对于影像学检查证实胆总管结石、胆管炎，或影像学和实验室检查强烈提示有持续胆道梗阻的患者，建议行急诊 ERCP，以识别和清除胆管结石。对于不适合进行胆囊切除术的患者，行胆道括约肌切开术并原位保留胆囊被认为是有效的替代方案。

急性液体积聚和假性囊肿　除了急性胰腺炎的标准支持治疗外，急性胰周液体积聚不需要任何特定治疗。大多数液体为无菌性，并在急性胰腺炎发作后数周内自发重吸收。当局限性急性胰周液体积聚持续超过 4 周时，可能会发展为胰腺假性囊肿。对于无症状的假性囊肿患者，应进行随访。对于有症状的患者，应考虑假性囊肿引流。假性囊肿引流的指征包括怀疑

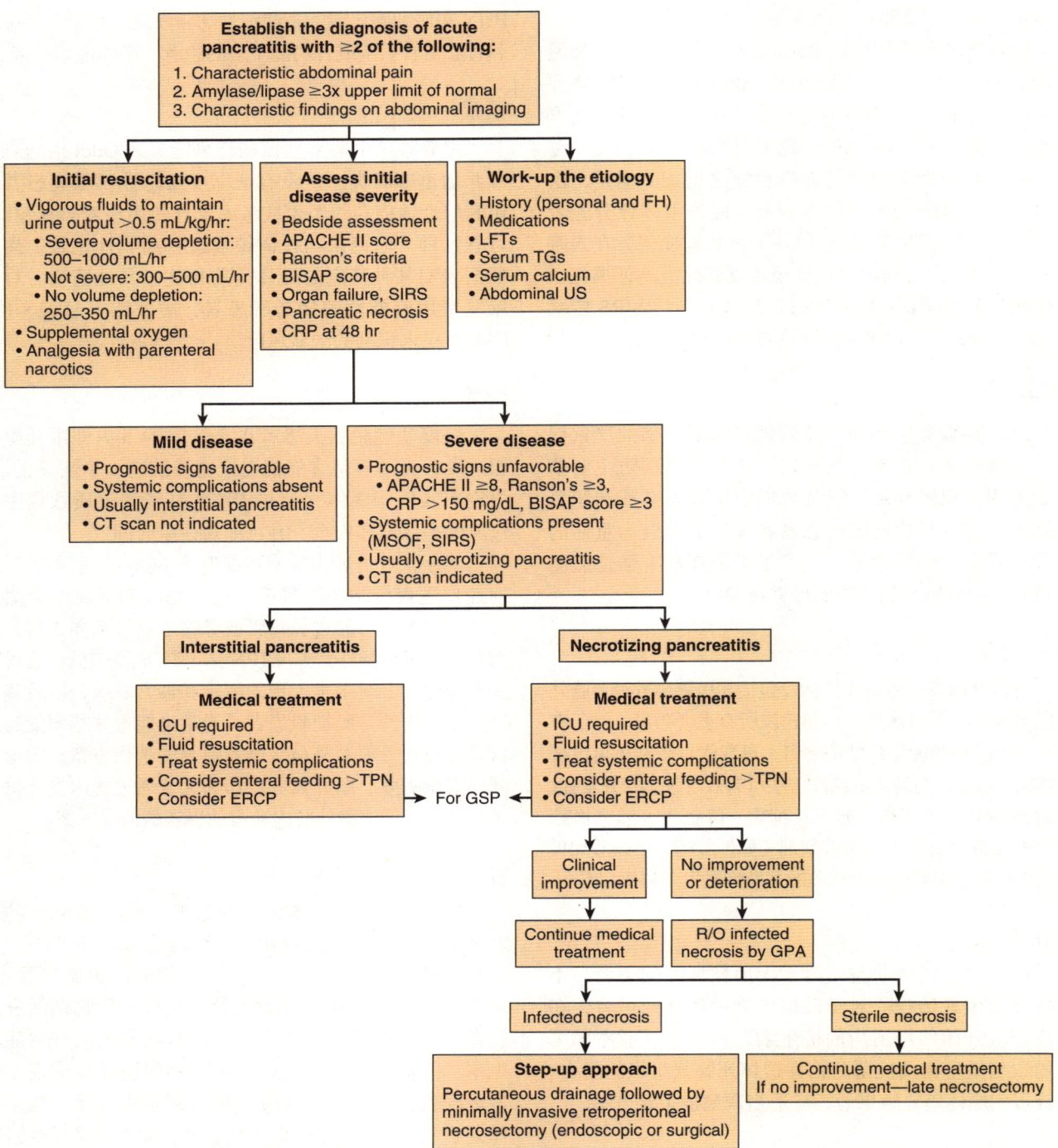

Fig. 9.4 Management algorithm for acute pancreatitis. Some of the guidelines, such as the diagnostic utility of the C-reactive protein (CRP) level, require further validation. Antibiotic use, including the type and duration of treatment, continues to be examined, and these suggested approaches will likely be modified by the findings of future studies. *APACHE II*, Acute Physiologic and Chronic Health Evaluation II; *BISAP*, Bedside Index for Severity of Acute Pancreatitis; *CT*, computed tomography; *ERCP*, endoscopic retrograde cholangiopancreatography; *FH*, family history; *GPA*, CT-guided percutaneous aspiration; *GSP*, gallstone pancreatitis; *ICU*, intensive care unit; *LFTs*, liver function tests; *MSOF*, multiple system organ failure; *R/O*, rule out; *SIRS*, systemic inflammatory response syndrome; *TGs*, triglycerides; *TPN*, total parenteral nutrition; *US*, ultrasound.

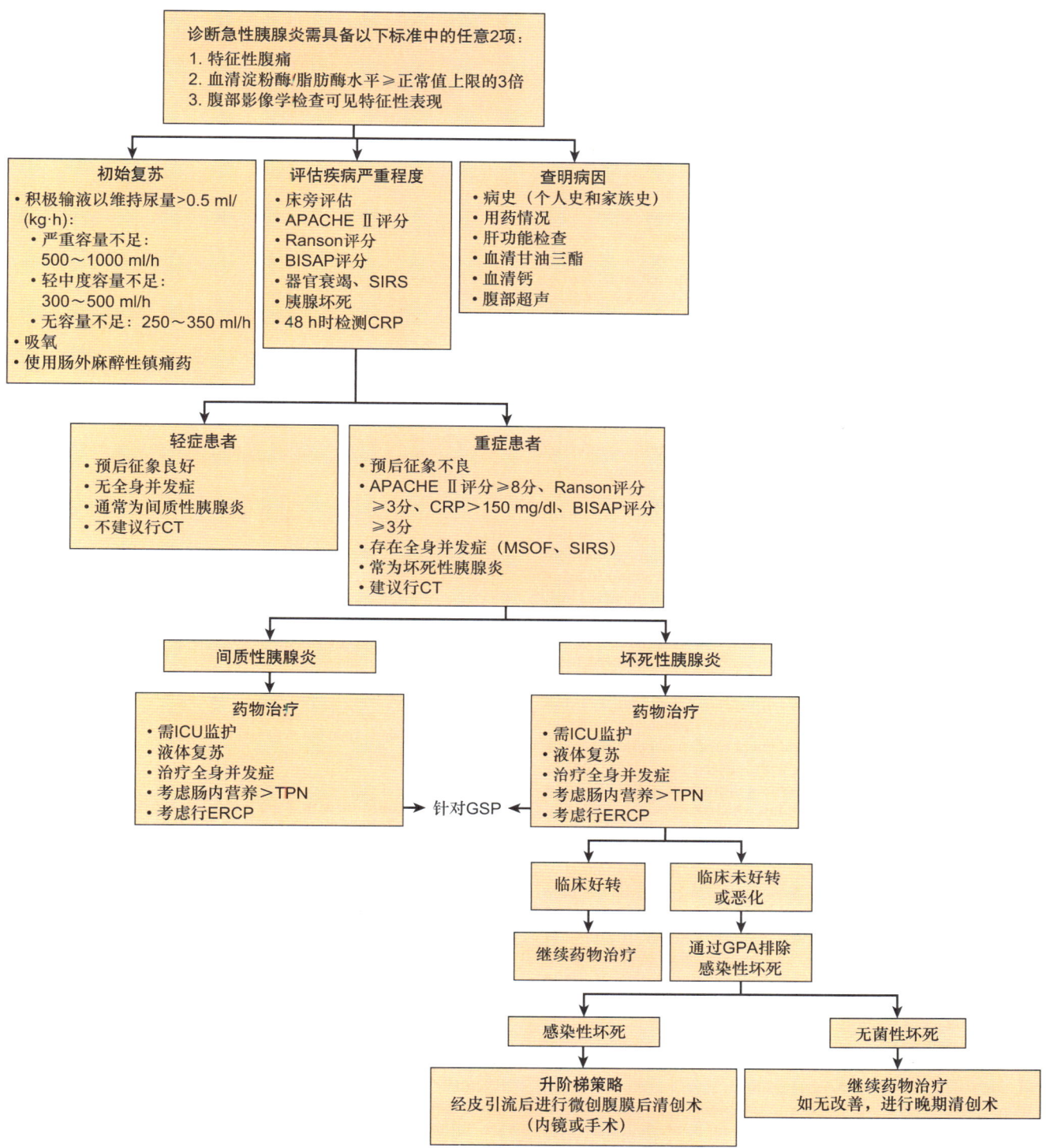

图 9.4 急性胰腺炎的管理流程。部分建议［如 C 反应蛋白（CRP）的诊断效能］需进一步验证。抗生素的使用类型和治疗持续时间仍在研究中，这些建议可能会随着未来研究结果而进行修改。APACHE Ⅱ，急性生理和慢性健康评估 Ⅱ；BISAP，急性胰腺炎严重程度床旁指数；CT，计算机断层成像；ERCP，内镜逆行胰胆管造影；GPA，CT 引导下经皮抽吸；GSP，胆源性胰腺炎；ICU，重症监护病房；MSOF，多器官功能衰竭；SIRS，全身炎症反应综合征；TPN，全肠外营养

enlargement with associated symptoms including biliary obstruction, abdominal pain, early satiety, and nausea and vomiting due to stomach compression or gastric outlet obstruction. In symptomatic patients, if the pseudocyst is mature and encapsulated, treatment can involve endoscopic, surgical, or percutaneous drainage. Based on available expertise, endoscopic ultrasound (EUS) guided drainage is preferred with cystogastrostomy or cystoduodenostomy.

Sterile pancreatic and extrapancreatic necrosis. Sterile pancreatic necrosis usually is treated with supportive medical care during the first several weeks, even in patients with multiple organ failure. After the acute pancreatic inflammatory process has subsided and coalesced into an encapsulated structure (e.g., walled-off pancreatic necrosis), débridement may be required for intractable abdominal pain, vomiting caused by extrinsic compression of stomach or duodenum, biliary obstruction, failure to thrive or persistent systemic toxicity. Débridement is delayed for at least 4 to 6 weeks after the onset of pancreatitis and can be performed by a combination of endoscopic, radiologic, and surgical techniques. Asymptomatic pancreatic necrosis does not warrant intervention, regardless of the extent and location.

Infected pancreatic and extrapancreatic necrosis. The development of infection in the necrotic collection is the main indication for therapy. The development of fever leukocytosis and increasing abdominal pain suggests infection of the necrotic tissue. A CT scan may reveal evidence of air bubbles in the necrotic cavity.

Infected pancreatic necrosis is best treated with drainage or débridement, or both. Routine CT-guided fine-needle aspiration to diagnose infected necrosis is not recommended given that clinical and imaging signs are accurate in the majority of patients. In addition, there is a high false-negative rate of the samples. Thus, débridement warrants consideration when infected necrosis is suspected, even if infection is not documented. The consensus is that the best outcomes are achieved when invasive interventions are delayed for a minimum of 4 weeks after the onset of disease to allow liquefaction of necrotic tissues and a fibrous rim to form around the necrosis (i.e., walled-off pancreatic necrosis). This delay makes drainage end débridement easier and reduces the risk of complications or death. Patients with infected necrosis are initially treated with broad-spectrum antibiotics and medical support to allow encapsulation of the necrotic collections, which may facilitate intervention and reduce complications of bleeding and perforation. When there is dramatic clinical deterioration, patients are not stable and delay is not feasible, and early intervention with a percutaneous drain is required.

Traditional management of infected pancreatic necrosis has been open surgical necrosectomy with closed irrigation by indwelling catheters, necrosectomy with closed drainage without irrigation, or necrosectomy and open packing. The open surgical approaches are associated with a high morbidity (34% to 95%) and mortality (11% to 39%) rates. A more conservative step-up approach using percutaneous catheter drainage as the initial treatment has gained favor, and a delay in invasive treatment is now standard. The step-up approach consists of antibiotic administration, percutaneous drainage as needed, and after a delay of several weeks, minimally invasive débridement, if required. This approach is superior to traditional open necrosectomy with respect to the risk of major complications or death. If the percutaneous approach fails, it is followed by a less invasive, video-assisted retroperitoneal débridement (VARD) or endoscopic transluminal drainage with or without necrosectomy, provided expertise is available.

CHRONIC PANCREATITIS

Definition and Epidemiology

Chronic pancreatitis is characterized by inflammation, fibrosis, and irreversible loss of acinar (exocrine) and islet (endocrine) cell function.

TABLE 9.3 Causes of Chronic Pancreatitis (TIGAR-O)

Toxic-Metabolic
Alcohol
Tobacco
Hypercalcemia
Hypertriglyceridemia
Chronic renal failure

Idiopathic
Early onset
Late onset
Tropical

Genetic
Autosomal dominant-cationic trypsinogen (PRSS1)
Autosomal recessive-CFTR, SPINK1, chymotrypsin C

Autoimmune
Isolated (types 1 and 2)
Syndromic (Sjögren's, inflammatory bowel disease, primary biliary cholangitis)

Recurrent Acute Pancreatitis
Postnecrotic severe acute pancreatitis
Post-irradiation
Ischemic vascular

Obstructive
Benign-pancreas divisum, sphincter of Oddi dysfunction, post-traumatic pancreatic duct stricture
Neoplastic-pancreatic ductal adenocarcinoma, IPMN, ampullary tumor

CFTR, Cystic fibrosis transmembrane conductance regulator; *IPMN,* intraductal papillary mucinous neoplasia; *PRSS1,* serine protease 1; *SPINK1,* serine peptidase inhibitor Kazal type 1.

This disorder contrasts with acute pancreatitis, which is usually nonprogressive. The two conditions may overlap because recurrent attacks of acute pancreatitis may lead to chronic pancreatitis, and individuals with chronic pancreatitis may experience exacerbations of acute pancreatitis. The annual incidence of chronic pancreatitis ranges from 5 to 12 cases per 100,000 people, and the prevalence is about 50 cases per 100,000 people.

Pathology

Chronic pancreatitis can be classified using a system termed "TIGAR-O," which refers to *t*oxic-metabolic, *i*diopathic, *g*enetic, *a*utoimmune, *r*ecurrent and severe acute pancreatitis, and *o*bstructive (Table 9.3). The most common cause of chronic pancreatitis is chronic alcoholism, accounting for 45% to 65% of cases. Alcohol can cause episodes of acute pancreatitis, but at the time of the initial attack, structural and functional abnormalities often indicate underlying chronic pancreatitis. Because most alcohol users do not develop pancreatitis, the presumption is that unidentified genetic, dietary, or environmental influences must coexist with alcohol use. Smoking is a causal, dose-dependent risk factor for chronic pancreatitis. The effect of smoking is synergistic with alcohol consumption and contributes profoundly to the development and progression of the disease.

Twenty percent of US patients with chronic pancreatitis have no immediately demonstrable cause. Gallstone pancreatitis, the major cause of acute pancreatitis, rarely leads to chronic pancreatitis. Calcific

感染或囊肿逐渐增大并伴有以下症状：胆道梗阻、腹痛、早饱，以及由于胃被压迫或胃出口梗阻引起的恶心和呕吐。在有症状的患者中，如果假性囊肿已经成熟且被包裹，可进行内镜、手术或经皮引流。根据现有经验，首选超声内镜（EUS）引导下引流，并进行囊肿-胃吻合术或囊肿-十二指肠吻合术。

无菌性胰腺和胰腺外坏死 无菌性胰腺坏死在最初几周内通常以支持治疗为主，即使是多器官衰竭的患者。在急性胰腺炎的炎症过程消退并融合成包裹性结构（胰腺包裹性坏死）后，可能需要进行清创术，以解决顽固性腹痛、呕吐（由胃或十二指肠受外部压迫引起）、胆道梗阻、发育不良或持续性全身毒性等问题。清创治疗应在胰腺炎发作至少4～6周后开展，可通过内镜、介入和外科技术组合的方式进行。无症状的胰腺坏死，无论程度和位置如何，都不需要进行干预。

感染性胰腺及胰腺外坏死 聚集的坏死物中出现感染是治疗的主要指征。发热伴白细胞增多、腹痛加剧均表明坏死物感染。CT 可能发现坏死物腔内有气泡。

感染性胰腺坏死的最佳治疗是引流和（或）清创。不推荐常规进行 CT 引导下细针穿刺来诊断感染性坏死，因为绝大多数患者的临床和影像学表现足以确诊。此外，样本的假阴性率较高。因此，当怀疑有感染性坏死时，即使未能明确感染，也应考虑进行清创。目前公认在发病至少 4 周后进行延迟侵入性干预的治疗效果最佳，因为此时坏死组织将液化并在坏死周围形成纤维边缘（即包裹性胰腺坏死），使得引流和清创更容易，并降低并发症或死亡的风险。感染性坏死的患者最初使用广谱抗生素和支持治疗，促进坏死组织形成包裹，有助于干预的实施并减少出血和穿孔等并发症。如果患者病情急剧恶化、不稳定且无法延迟干预，应尽早进行经皮引流。

感染性胰腺坏死的传统治疗方法包括开腹清创术配合留置引流管进行冲洗、开腹清创术后保留闭式引流而不进行冲洗或开腹清创并开放填塞。开腹手术与高并发症发病率（34%～95%）和高死亡率（11%～39%）相关。采用经皮穿刺置管引流作为初始治疗手段的升阶梯方案已获得认可，延迟侵入性治疗已成为标准治疗。升阶梯方案包括应用抗生素、按需经皮引流，以及在数周延迟后再进行微创清创（必要时）。这种方法在降低严重并发症或死亡风险方面优于传统开腹清创术。若经皮引流失败且具备相应的技术团队，接下来可进行创伤较小的视频辅助腹膜后清创（VARD）或内镜透壁引流（清创或不清创）。

慢性胰腺炎

定义和流行病学

慢性胰腺炎的特征是炎症、纤维化，以及不可逆的腺泡细胞（外分泌）和胰岛细胞（内分泌）功能丧

表 9.3 慢性胰腺炎的病因（TIGAR-O）

毒性-代谢性（Toxic-metabolic）
酒精
烟草
高钙血症
高甘油三酯血症
慢性肾衰竭

特发性（Idiopathic）
早发型
晚发型
热带型

遗传性（Genetic）
常染色体显性遗传：阳离子胰蛋白酶原（PRSS1）
常染色体隐性遗传：CFTR、SPINK1、糜蛋白酶 C

自身免疫性（Autoimmune）
孤立性（1 型和 2 型）
综合征性（干燥综合征、炎症性肠病、原发性胆汁性胆管炎）

复发性急性胰腺炎（Recurrent Acute Pancreatitis）
坏死后重症急性胰腺炎
放疗后
缺血性血管性

梗阻性（Obstructive）
良性：胰腺分裂、Oddi 括约肌功能障碍、创伤后胰腺导管狭窄
肿瘤性：胰腺导管腺癌、IPMN、壶腹部肿瘤

CFTR，囊性纤维化跨膜传导调节蛋白；IPMN，胰腺导管内乳头状黏液瘤；PRSS1，丝氨酸蛋白酶 1；SPINK1，丝氨酸肽酶抑制剂 Kazal 型 1。

失。慢性胰腺炎与急性胰腺炎不同，后者通常为非进展性。两种情况可能会重叠，因为反复发作的急性胰腺炎可能导致慢性胰腺炎，而慢性胰腺炎患者可能会出现急性加重。慢性胰腺炎的年发病率为（5～12）/100 000，患病率约为 50/100 000。

病理学

慢性胰腺炎可使用"TIGAR-O"系统进行分类，该系统是指毒性-代谢性（Toxic-metabolic）、特发性（Idiopathic）、遗传性（Genetic）、自身免疫性（Autoimmune）、复发性重症急性胰腺炎（Recurrent and severe acute pancreatitis）和梗阻性（Obstructive）（表 9.3）。慢性胰腺炎最常见的原因是慢性酒精中毒，占所有病例的 45%～65%。酒精可引发急性胰腺炎发作，但在首次发作时，结构和功能异常通常表明存在潜在的慢性胰腺炎。由于大多数饮酒者并不会发展为胰腺炎，因此推测尚未被明确的遗传、饮食或环境因素与饮酒同时发挥作用。吸烟是导致慢性胰腺炎的剂量依赖性危险因素。吸烟与饮酒具有协同作用，并对慢性胰腺炎的发生和发展具有深远影响。

美国约 20% 的慢性胰腺炎患者没有明确的病因。胆石症性胰腺炎是急性胰腺炎的主要原因，但很少导致慢性胰腺炎。钙化性胰腺炎是南印度及其他热带地区慢性胰腺炎的主要原因。自身免疫性胰腺炎，基因突变

pancreatitis is a major cause of chronic pancreatitis in South India and other parts of the tropics. Autoimmune pancreatitis, genetic mutations (*CFTR, SPINK1, PRSS1, CTRC, CASR*), obstruction (e.g., tumors, sphincter of Oddi dysfunction, pancreas divisum), hypertriglyceridemia, and hypercalcemia are potential causes of cases initially labeled idiopathic.

Clinical Presentation

Most patients with chronic pancreatitis experience episodic or continuous pain. Occasionally, patients exhibit exocrine or endocrine insufficiency in the absence of pain. Other patients are asymptomatic and are found to have chronic pancreatitis incidentally on imaging.

The pain of chronic pancreatitis is typically epigastric, often radiates to the back, is occasionally associated with nausea and vomiting, and may be partially relieved by sitting upright or leaning forward. The pain is often worse 15 to 30 minutes after eating. Early in the course of chronic pancreatitis, the pain may occur in discrete attacks; as the condition progresses, the pain tends to become continuous.

The pain of chronic pancreatitis is poorly understood. Possible causes include inflammation of the pancreas, increased intrapancreatic pressure, neural inflammation, and extrapancreatic causes, such as stenosis of the common bile duct and duodenum.

Glucose intolerance occurs with some frequency in chronic pancreatitis, but overt diabetes mellitus usually manifests late in the course of disease. Diabetes in patients with chronic pancreatitis is different from typical type 1 diabetes in that the pancreatic alpha cells, which produce glucagon, are also affected, increasing the risk of hypoglycemia.

Clinically significant endocrine or exocrine insufficiency (i.e., protein and fat deficiencies) does not occur until more than 90% of pancreatic function is lost. Steatorrhea usually occurs before protein deficiencies because lipolytic activity decreases faster than proteolysis. Mild pancreatic exocrine insufficiency (PEI) may take the form of abdominal bloating or malabsorption of fat-soluble vitamins (A, D, E, K) and vitamin B_{12}, although clinically symptomatic vitamin deficiency is uncommon. Because reduced vitamin D absorption can result in osteoporosis, osteopenia, and fractures, periodic assessment of vitamin D levels and bone densitometry are recommended. More severe PEI may lead to overt malabsorption and weight loss.

Diagnosis and Differential Diagnosis

Because direct biopsy of the pancreas has considerable risk, the diagnosis of chronic pancreatitis is typically based on indirect tests of pancreatic structure and function. Marked structural changes usually correlate with severe functional impairment. In early chronic pancreatitis, however, mild abnormalities of pancreatic function can precede the morphologic changes seen on imaging. Studies of pancreatic structure may remain normal even with advanced deterioration of pancreatic function.

Laboratory evaluations of serum pancreatic enzymes, such as amylase and lipase, are frequently normal in the setting of well-established chronic pancreatitis, even during painful exacerbations. Serum pancreatic enzymes neither confirm nor exclude the diagnosis.

Tests of Function

Function tests assess pancreatic secretory reserve of ductal function or acinar function by measuring secretion of bicarbonate ions (HCO_3^-) or digestive enzymes, respectively. Direct tests (e.g., secretin stimulation) involve stimulation of the pancreas through the administration of hormonal secretagogues. Indirect tests measure the consequences of pancreatic insufficiency, and although more widely available, the results usually are not abnormal until enzyme output has declined by more than 90%. Thus they are insensitive to early pancreatic insufficiency.

Clinicians have preferentially relied on noninvasive methods to circumvent the challenges associated with direct pancreatic function tests. Clinically available indirect tests of pancreatic function include analyses of fecal fat, fecal elastase, and serum trypsin.

The secretin stimulation test takes advantage of the normal response of pancreatic ductular cells to secrete HCO_3^- in response to physiologic and exogenously administered secretin. The observation that HCO_3^- production is impaired early in the course of chronic pancreatitis led to the use of this test to diagnose early-stage disease (sensitivity of 95%). The test involves oral placement of a double-lumen gastroduodenal catheter for aspiration and quantitative measurement of pancreatic enzyme and HCO_3^- production before and after stimulation with intravenous secretin. This test is primarily performed for patients with suspected chronic pancreatitis who have chronic abdominal pain but negative or equivocal results of imaging studies. Peak pancreatic fluid HCO_3^- concentrations of less than 80 mEq/L represent pancreatic insufficiency. The secretin stimulation test has been infrequently used in clinical practice because the study is labor intensive and is associated with discomfort. Endoscopic collection methods have simplified pancreatic fluid collection and made the test more suitable for clinical use.

The 72-hour fecal fat determination is sometimes used for detection of steatorrhea (fecal fat >7 g/24 hours), but the test is not specific for pancreatic exocrine insufficiency. The test also lacks sensitivity because steatorrhea occurs only in advanced chronic pancreatitis. Because the quantitative fecal fat test is inconvenient, unpleasant for patients, and prone to laboratory error, a qualitative assay is used preferentially in clinical practice to assess for malabsorption.

Determination of fecal elastase is the most commonly used noninvasive indirect test for the diagnosis of pancreatic exocrine insufficiency. Elastase, a protease synthesized by pancreatic acinar cells, is useful for evaluating insufficiency because it is stable in stool, unaffected by pancreatic enzyme replacement, and correlates well with stimulated pancreatic function test results. Moderate to severe exocrine insufficiency is based on fecal elastase values of less than 200 µg/g of stool. False-positive results can be seen with diarrheal illnesses, due to a dilutional effect.

Tests of Structure

Imaging findings with CT scan, ultrasound, and MRI may show changes of chronic pancreatitis include ductal abnormalities (e.g., dilation, stones, irregular beaded walls, and side branch ectasia), parenchymal abnormalities (e.g., calcification, inhomogeneity, atrophy), gland contour changes, and pseudocysts. Imaging studies are often normal or inconclusive in the early stages of disease. CT imaging and MRI are also helpful in identifying complications of chronic pancreatitis including pseudocysts, portosplenic venous thrombosis, arterial pseudoaneurysms, and pancreatic duct fistulas.

CT scanning is often considered the preferred initial test for diagnosis of chronic pancreatitis. Magnetic resonance cholangiopancreatography is a noninvasive diagnostic imaging modality that provides visualization of the pancreatic parenchyma similar to CT scanning but with improved duct imaging resulting in a greater sensitivity for diagnosis of chronic pancreatitis. MRI pancreatic duct images are similar to those obtained by ERCP but without the risk of precipitating acute pancreatitis. Stimulation of the pancreas using IV secretin enhances main and side branch pancreatic duct visualization, which may improve the diagnostic accuracy for chronic pancreatitis. ERCP provides reliable structural information about the pancreatic ductular system including ductal dilation, strictures, abnormal side branches, communicating pseudocysts, and ductal stones and fistulas. ERCP is highly effective for visualizing these ductal and duct-related findings,

（*CFTR*、*SPINK1*、*PRSS1*、*CTRC*、*CASR*），梗阻（如肿瘤、Oddi 括约肌功能障碍、胰腺分裂），高甘油三酯血症和高钙血症是最初被标记为特发性病例的潜在原因。

临床表现

大多数慢性胰腺炎患者会经历间歇性或持续性疼痛。患者偶尔在没有疼痛的情况下出现胰腺外分泌或内分泌功能不全的表现。部分患者无症状，仅在影像学检查中偶然发现慢性胰腺炎。

慢性胰腺炎的疼痛通常位于上腹部，常放射至背部，有时伴有恶心和呕吐，直立位或前倾位可部分缓解疼痛。疼痛通常在进食后 15～30 min 加重。在慢性胰腺炎早期，疼痛可能呈间歇性发作；随着病情进展，疼痛往往变为持续性。

目前人们对慢性胰腺炎的疼痛机制知之甚少。可能的病因包括胰腺炎症、胰腺内压力增加、神经炎症，以及胰腺外因素（如胆总管和十二指肠狭窄）等。

糖耐量异常在慢性胰腺炎患者中较为常见，但明显的糖尿病通常出现于疾病晚期。与典型的 1 型糖尿病不同，慢性胰腺炎相关性糖尿病患者的胰腺 α 细胞（分泌胰高血糖素）也会受到影响，从而增加了发生低血糖的风险。

临床明显的内分泌或外分泌功能不全（即蛋白质和脂肪缺乏）在胰腺功能丧失超过 90% 之前不会发生。由于脂肪分解活性下降比蛋白质水解更快，脂肪泻通常先于蛋白质缺乏出现。轻度胰腺外分泌功能不全（PEI）可能表现为腹胀或脂溶性维生素（维生素 A、D、E、K）和维生素 B_{12} 吸收不良，但症状明显的维生素缺乏并不常见。维生素 D 吸收减少可能导致骨量减少、骨质疏松症和骨折，建议定期评估维生素 D 水平和检测骨密度。重度 PEI 可能导致明显的吸收不良和体重减轻。

诊断和鉴别诊断

由于直接进行胰腺活检的风险较大，慢性胰腺炎的诊断通常基于对胰腺结构和功能的间接检查。显著的结构变化通常与严重的功能损害相关。然而，在慢性胰腺炎早期，胰腺功能的轻度异常可能先于影像学检查观察到的形态学改变出现。即使胰腺功能已经严重恶化，胰腺结构的检查结果也可能是正常的。

在明确诊断的慢性胰腺炎患者中，实验室检测血清胰酶（如淀粉酶和脂肪酶）水平通常是正常的，即使是在疼痛加剧期间。血清胰酶水平既不能确诊也不能排除慢性胰腺炎的诊断。

胰腺功能检查

功能检查是指分别通过检测碳酸氢盐（HCO_3^-）和消化酶的分泌来评估胰管功能和胰腺腺泡的分泌储备功能。直接检查（如胰泌素刺激）通过给予激素促泌剂来刺激胰腺。间接检查主要是检测胰腺功能不全的后果，尽管已得到广泛应用，但检测结果在酶输出功能下降超过 90% 之前不会出现明显异常。因此，这些检查对于早期胰腺功能不全并不敏感。临床医生倾向于使用无创性检查来规避进行直接胰腺功能检查的风险。目前临床可选择的间接胰腺功能检查方法包括粪便脂肪分析、粪便弹性蛋白酶分析及血清胰蛋白酶分析。

胰泌素刺激试验利用了胰腺导管细胞在生理性或外源性胰泌素刺激下分泌 HCO_3^- 的正常反应。在慢性胰腺炎的早期阶段可观察到 HCO_3^- 分泌受损，因此该检查可用于诊断早期慢性胰腺炎（敏感性为 95%）。检测过程为经口置入双腔胃十二指肠导管，在静脉注射胰泌素前后吸取及定量检测胰酶和 HCO_3^-。该检查适用于出现慢性腹痛、疑诊慢性胰腺炎但影像学检查结果为阴性或结论不明确的患者。胰液中 HCO_3^- 浓度峰值 < 80 mmol/L 提示胰腺功能不全。由于胰泌素刺激试验的工作量大且伴有不适感，该检查在临床实践中较少使用。内镜收集法简化了胰液的收集过程，使其更适合临床使用。

72 h 粪便脂肪分析有时用于检测脂肪泻（粪便脂肪 > 7 g/24 h），但该检测对胰腺外分泌功能不全的特异性较低。此外，由于脂肪泻仅在慢性胰腺炎进展期出现，该检测的敏感性也较低。由于定量粪便脂肪分析不方便、检查过程导致患者不适、实验室误差较大，因此在临床实践中优先使用定性分析来评估吸收不良。

粪便弹性蛋白酶分析是诊断胰腺外分泌功能不全最常用的无创性间接检查方法。弹性蛋白酶是一种由胰腺腺泡细胞合成的蛋白酶，由于其在粪便中十分稳定、不受胰酶替代治疗的影响，且与胰腺功能刺激试验结果的相关性良好，因此对评估胰腺功能不全非常有用。若粪便弹性蛋白酶 < 200 μg/g 粪便，可考虑诊断中重度外分泌功能不全。由于稀释效应，腹泻性疾病可能会导致假阳性结果。

胰腺结构检查

CT、超声和 MRI 可显示慢性胰腺炎的结构变化，包括导管异常（如扩张、结石、导管壁呈不规则串珠状和分支胰管扩张），实质异常（如钙化、不均质性、萎缩），腺体轮廓变化和假性囊肿。在早期阶段，影像学检查结果通常正常或结论不明确。CT 和 MRI 有助于识别慢性胰腺炎的并发症，包括假性囊肿、门静脉和脾静脉血栓、动脉假性动脉瘤及胰管瘘等。

CT 通常被认为是诊断慢性胰腺炎的首选初步检查。磁共振胰胆管成像（MRCP）是一种非侵入性诊断性影像学检查，可显示胰腺实质，但在显示胰管方面比 CT 更有优势，因此对诊断慢性胰腺炎的敏感性更高。MRI 与 ERCP 获得的图像相似，但没有诱发急性胰腺炎的风险。静脉注射胰泌素可提高主胰管及分支胰管的显影程度，进而提高慢性胰腺炎的诊断准确性。ERCP 可提供有关胰腺导管的可靠结构信息，可显示胰管扩张、胰管狭窄、异常分支、与假性囊肿交通、胰管内结石和胰瘘。ERCP 在显示这些导管系统及其相关异常方面非常有效，诊断慢性胰腺炎的敏感性为 71%～93%，特异性

with a sensitivity for the diagnosis of chronic pancreatitis of 71% to 93% and a specificity of 89% to 100%. The major limitation of ERCP is the development of procedure-related acute pancreatitis in up to 5% of patients. Thus, ERCP should not be used for diagnostic purposes but instead be reserved for patients with established chronic pancreatitis when endoscopic therapy is recommended (discussed later).

Endoscopic ultrasound (EUS) as a diagnostic imaging study for chronic pancreatitis relies on quantitative and qualitative parenchymal tissue and ductal findings. EUS appears to be equally or more sensitive than other tests of structure and function. An international consensus panel proposed the Rosemont criteria for diagnosing chronic pancreatitis. Major criteria include hyperechoic foci with shadowing that indicates pancreatic duct calculi and parenchymal lobularity with honeycombing. Minor criteria include cysts, a dilated main duct (≥3.5 mm in diameter), irregular pancreatic duct contour, dilated side branches (≥1 mm in diameter), hyperechoic duct wall, parenchymal strands, nonshadowing hyperechoic foci, and lobularity with noncontiguous lobules. In the absence of any of these criteria, chronic pancreatitis is unlikely, whereas with detection of four or more criteria, the disease is likely, even when other imaging and pancreatic function tests may still be normal.

Treatment
Malabsorption

Treatment of PEI is best achieved with pancreatic enzyme replacement therapy (PERT). Most commercial preparations consist of pancreatin, which is the shock-frozen powdered extract of porcine pancreas containing lipase, amylase, trypsin, and chymotrypsin.

In order to treat malabsorption due to PEI, it is necessary to provide approximately 10 percent of the normal pancreatic enzyme output. This translates into approximately 30,000 international units (IU) or the equivalent 90,000 United States Pharmacopeia units (USP) of lipase per meal. For most patients, the recommended dose depends on the size and nature of the meal (i.e., fat content), residual pancreatic function, and therapeutic goals (i.e., elimination of steatorrhea, reduction in the abdominal symptoms of maldigestion, or improvement in nutrition). Due to residual pancreatic lipase secretion and physiologic gastric lipase secretion, it is appropriate to begin therapy with 40,000 to 50,000 USP of lipase with each meal and one half of that amount with snacks. Administration of acid-stable, encapsulated microspheres or microtablets filled with pancreatic enzymes has greatly increased the efficacy of enzyme supplementation. Enzyme preparations should be taken with meals. If more than one capsule/tablet per meal must be taken, it may be beneficial to take one part of the dose at the beginning and the rest during the meal.

Other factors may accentuate steatorrhea, including concomitant small bowel bacterial overgrowth, which can occur in up to 25% of patients with chronic pancreatitis. Bacterial overgrowth may be caused by hypomotility due to pancreatic inflammation or chronic use of narcotic analgesics.

Pain

The greatest challenge in treating chronic pancreatitis is controlling abdominal pain. Pain may improve over time, but the course is not predictable and improvement may take years. Therapy targets the mechanisms responsible for pancreatic pain, including pancreatic hyperstimulation, ischemia, obstruction of ducts, inflammation, and neuropathic hyperalgesia. Pain can develop in the early stages of chronic pancreatitis before morphologic changes can be demonstrated on imaging studies. Patients with chronic pancreatitis are at increased risk for pancreatic cancer, which may cause a change in the pain pattern, and extrapancreatic causes of pain must always be considered.

Pain management should proceed in a stepwise fashion and begin with lifestyle modifications such as alcohol and tobacco abstinence, a low-fat diet, and pancreatic enzyme supplementation, followed by a sequentially more aggressive and invasive approach for symptomatic failures, although it should be recognized that placebo alone is effective for up to 30% of patients. Several approaches can be considered for chronic pain relief.

1. Tobacco and alcohol abstinence. Abstention may decrease the frequency of painful attacks and reduce the likelihood of pancreatic function deterioration and development of pancreatic cancer.
2. Analgesics. Most patients with chronic pain require analgesics. Nonopioid analgesics such as acetaminophen and nonsteroidal anti-inflammatory drugs are used as initial treatment. If possible, the use of opioids should be avoided due to the risk of abuse, tolerance, and addiction. When deemed necessary, weak opioids (e.g., tramadol or codeine) are initially prescribed before escalation to stronger opioids (e.g., morphine, oxycodone, fentanyl) for poorly controlled pain. The risk of dependence to opioids is not known in this setting; however, patients with previous addictive behaviors such as substance use with alcohol or tobacco are at greater risk for analgesic dependence and addiction. Safe opioid prescribing practices are necessary with close monitoring of patients' symptoms and adherence to a well-defined plan that includes a patient agreement, regular follow-up, urine drug testing, and query of the state's online prescription monitoring program.
3. Secretion suppression. Oral pancreatic enzyme replacement, somatostatin analogue, and enteral nutrition are proposed treatments to blunt pain by reducing pancreatic secretion. These therapies are of unproven benefit and not routinely recommended as adjuncts to pain therapy. When PERT is initiated for pain management, the non–enteric-coated pancrelipases (i.e., pancreatic enzyme preparations) are preferred because the enteric-coated preparations theoretically release their enzymes further down the intestine, away from the stimulatory cholecystokinin (CCK) enterocytes.
4. Neural transmission modification. Gabapentinoids, including pregabalin, have been used effectively to treat neuropathic pain disorders, including diabetic neuropathy and neuropathic pain of central origin. Based on the finding that pancreatic pain is accompanied by similar alterations of central pain processing, studies suggest a benefit with pregabalin as an adjuvant treatment to decrease pain associated with chronic pancreatitis. Similarly, tricyclic antidepressants, selective serotonin reuptake inhibitors, and serotonin-norepinephrine reuptake inhibitors can be administered on a trial basis.
5. Neuroablative techniques such as celiac plexus blockade can be performed by injection of a local anesthetic and a steroid into the region of the celiac ganglia. This can be accomplished through endoscopic (i.e., EUS) or percutaneous radiologic guidance. The results are disappointing with a pain reduction in a minority of individuals (15% to 50%) that is not durable with pain reduction or relief of up to 1 to 6 months.
6. Antioxidants. Oxidative stress can cause direct pancreatic acinar cell damage through several pathways. Supplementation with antioxidants, such as selenium, vitamins C and E, and methionine, may relieve pain and reduce oxidative stress. In a randomized trial, the reduction in the number of painful days per month was higher for the patients who received antioxidants compared with those who received placebo (7.4 vs. 3.2 days). Patients who received antioxidants also were more likely to become pain free (32% vs. 13%).
7. Endoscopic decompression. Endoscopic decompression of the pancreatic duct is an option for obstruction caused by strictures, stones, or sphincter of Oddi dysfunction. Endoscopic therapies include pancreatic sphincterotomy, stricture dilation, stone

高达89%～100%。ERCP的主要应用限制是约5%的患者可能出现与操作相关的急性胰腺炎。因此，ERCP不应用于诊断，而是用于已确诊为慢性胰腺炎且需要内镜治疗的患者（见下文）。

超声内镜（EUS）依赖于对胰腺实质和胰管的定量及定性结果，可作为诊断慢性胰腺炎的影像学检查。EUS在结构和功能检查方面的敏感性似乎与其他检查相当或更高。国际共识小组提出采用Rosemont标准诊断慢性胰腺炎。主要标准包括提示胰管结石的高回声影伴后方声影衰减，以及蜂窝状实质小叶结构。次要标准包括囊肿、主胰管扩张（直径 ≥ 3.5 mm）、胰管轮廓不规则、分支胰管扩张（直径 ≥ 1 mm）、胰管高回声、实质纤维束、不伴有后方衰减的高回声影、不连续的实质小叶结构。如果不存在这些标准中的任何一项，则诊断慢性胰腺炎的可能性很小，而当满足 ≥ 4项标准时，即使其他影像学检查和胰腺功能检查结果正常，慢性胰腺炎的可能性仍然很大。

治疗

吸收不良

胰腺外分泌功能不全（PEI）的最佳治疗方法是胰酶替代治疗（PERT）。大多数市售制剂由猪胰腺冷冻粉末提取物中提取的胰酶组成，包含脂肪酶、淀粉酶、胰蛋白酶和糜蛋白酶。

治疗由PEI引起的吸收不良时，需提供约10%的正常胰酶输出量。这对应于每餐约30 000国际单位（IU）或90 000美国药典单位（USP）的脂肪酶。对于大多数患者，推荐的剂量取决于每餐的量和性质（即脂肪含量）、残余胰腺功能和治疗目标（即消除脂肪泻、减少消化不良引起的腹部症状或改善营养状况）。由于存在残留的胰腺脂肪酶分泌和生理性胃脂肪酶分泌，初始治疗可给予每餐40 000～50 000 USP脂肪酶，并在摄入零食时给予该量的1/2。胰酶的耐酸包封微球或微片剂极大地提高了酶补充治疗的疗效。胰酶应随餐口服。如果每餐需要服用1粒以上的胶囊或片剂，建议餐前服用一部分，剩余部分于餐时服用，以使疗效更佳。

其他因素可能会加重脂肪泻，如合并小肠细菌过度生长，这可见于多达25%的慢性胰腺炎患者。细菌过度生长可能是胰腺炎或长期使用麻醉性镇痛药引起的肠道蠕动减慢的结果。

疼痛

镇痛是慢性胰腺炎治疗中最大的挑战。虽然腹痛可能会随时间推移而有所改善，但其过程难以预测，可能需要数年时间才能缓解。治疗目标主要针对导致胰腺疼痛的病因，包括胰腺过度刺激、缺血、胰管阻塞、炎症和神经性痛觉过敏。疼痛可出现在影像学检查未显示形态改变的慢性胰腺炎早期阶段。慢性胰腺炎患者患胰腺癌的风险增加，这可能导致疼痛模式的改变，且应始终注意疼痛的胰腺外原因。

疼痛管理应分阶梯进行，首先应从调整生活方式开始，如戒酒、戒烟、低脂饮食和胰酶补充。对于经以上治疗后症状未能缓解的患者，应逐步采取更积极和侵入性的方法。然而，仅使用安慰剂对多达30%的患者有效。为缓解慢性疼痛，可考虑以下几种方法。

1. 戒烟、戒酒。可能减少疼痛发作的频率，并降低胰腺功能恶化和进展为胰腺癌的可能性。

2. 镇痛药。大多数慢性疼痛患者需要使用镇痛药。初始治疗通常使用非阿片类镇痛药［如对乙酰氨基酚和非甾体抗炎药（NSAID）］。考虑到滥用、耐药性和成瘾的风险，应尽量避免使用阿片类药物。必要时，首先应给予弱效阿片类药物（如曲马多或可待因），疼痛控制不佳时再逐渐升级为强效阿片类药物（如吗啡、羟考酮、芬太尼）。在这种情况下，阿片类药物依赖的风险尚不明确，然而，既往有成瘾行为（如酒精或烟草滥用）的患者，镇痛药依赖和成瘾的风险较高。采取安全的阿片类药物处方实践是必要的，需密切监测患者的症状，并遵循明确的计划，包括患者协议、定期随访、尿液药物检测、查询在线处方监控程序。

3. 分泌抑制。口服胰酶替代、生长抑素类似物和肠内营养可通过减少胰腺分泌来缓解疼痛。然而，这些治疗的益处尚未得到证实，不作为疼痛治疗的常规辅助措施。当启动PERT用于疼痛管理时，首选非肠溶性胰酶制剂，因为肠溶性制剂理论上会在更远的肠道部位释放消化酶，这些部位距离分泌刺激性胆囊收缩素（CCK）的肠上皮细胞较远。

4. 神经传导调节。加巴喷丁类药物（如普瑞巴林）已被用于治疗神经性疼痛疾病，如糖尿病神经病变和中枢性神经性疼痛。由于胰腺疼痛伴随着与中枢性疼痛过程类似的改变，研究表明普瑞巴林作为辅助治疗有助于减少与慢性胰腺炎相关的疼痛。同样，三环类抗抑郁药、选择性5-羟色胺再摄取抑制剂（SSRI）和5-羟色胺-去甲肾上腺素再摄取抑制剂（SNRI）也可作为试验性用药。

5. 神经消融技术（如腹腔丛阻滞）可通过向腹腔神经节区域注射局部麻醉剂和类固醇来实现。该治疗可在内镜（如EUS）或放射引导下经皮操作来完成。但治疗效果令人失望，仅有少数患者（15%～50%）实现了疼痛缓解，但效果不持久，缓解时间通常为1～6个月。

6. 抗氧化剂。氧化应激可通过多种途径直接损伤胰腺腺泡细胞。补充抗氧化剂（如硒、维生素C和E、甲硫氨酸）可能有助于缓解疼痛并减少氧化应激。在一项随机试验中，与接受安慰剂的患者相比，接受抗氧化剂的患者每月减少的疼痛天数更多（7.4天 *vs.* 3.2天）。接受抗氧化剂的患者更可能完全摆脱疼痛（32% *vs.* 13%）。

7. 内镜减压。对于由狭窄、结石或Oddi括约肌功能障碍引起的胰管梗阻，内镜减压是一种治疗

removal with intracorporeal or extracorporeal shock wave lithotripsy, and temporary plastic stent placement. Complete or partial pain relief is reported for approximately 50% to 80% of carefully selected patients during follow-up extending as long as 3 to 4 years.

8. **Surgery.** Surgical pancreatic ductal drainage, usually with lateral pancreaticojejunostomy (i.e., Puestow procedure), can be offered to those with a dilated (>6 mm in diameter) main pancreatic duct. Pain reduction is reported by approximately 80% of patients. This procedure is safe and has an operative mortality rate of less than 5%; however, only 35% to 60% of patients are free of pain at the 5-year follow-up. Individuals with nonobstructed, nondilated pancreatic ductal systems with disease predominating in the pancreatic head may be offered resection of the focally diseased portion of the gland with a pancreaticoduodenectomy or a duodenum-preserving pancreatic head resection also referred to as a Frey or Beger procedure. Highly selected patients with diffuse pancreatic parenchymal disease refractory to other forms of therapy may benefit from a total pancreatectomy with islet cell autotransplantation.

Management of Complications

The complications of chronic pancreatitis include pseudocysts, pancreatic fistulas, biliary obstruction, pancreatic cancer, small bowel bacterial overgrowth, and isolated gastric varices due to splenic vein thrombosis.

Pancreatic fistulas. Pancreatic fistulas occur as a result of duct disruption resulting in localized fluid collections, ascites, or pleural effusions. Treatment consists of bowel rest, endoscopic pancreatic duct stenting, and administration of a somatostatin analogue. Surgical intervention may be needed if this conservative approach is unsuccessful.

Vascular complications. The splenic vein courses along the posterior surface of the pancreas, where it can be affected by inflammation from pancreatitis or malignancy that leads to thrombosis. Splenic vein thrombosis can result in isolated fundal gastric varices. Splenectomy is usually curative for patients who develop bleeding from gastric varices.

Pseudoaneurysm formation is a complication of acute and chronic pancreatitis. Affected vessels, including the hepatic, splenic, pancreaticoduodenal, and gastroduodenal arteries, lie close to the pancreas. CT or MR imaging shows the pseudoaneurysm as a cystically dilated vascular structure in or adjacent to the pancreas. EUS with Doppler imaging can show blood flow within the pseudoaneurysm. Mesenteric angiography permits confirmation of the diagnosis and provides a means of therapy because selective embolization of the pseudoaneurysm can be accomplished during the procedure. Surgery for bleeding pseudoaneurysms is difficult and associated with high morbidity and mortality rates.

Biliary and duodenal obstruction. Symptomatic obstruction of the bile duct or duodenum, or both, develops in a few patients with chronic pancreatitis. Postprandial pain and early satiety are characteristic of duodenal obstruction, whereas pain and cholestasis (sometimes with resultant cholangitis) suggest a bile duct stricture. These complications most commonly result from inflammation or fibrosis in the head of the pancreas or an adjacent pseudocyst.

Endoscopic stenting may be attempted for bile duct strictures, but they are often refractory and typically require prolonged treatment. Endoscopic failures can be treated with surgical biliary decompression. The importance of decompression is underscored by the observation that it can reverse secondary biliary fibrosis associated with bile duct obstruction.

CARCINOMA OF THE PANCREAS

Definition and Epidemiology

Pancreatic ductal adenocarcinoma (PDAC) is the fourth leading cause of cancer-related death in the United States, with approximately 45,000 new cases diagnosed annually. The peak incidence of PDAC occurs in the seventh decade of life. There is a modest male-to-female predominance (relative risk of 1.4:1), and blacks have a 30% to 40% higher incidence of PDAC than white individuals in the United States.

Many environmental factors have been implicated as increasing the risk for pancreatic cancer. Cigarette smoking is the most consistent factor, with the increased risk attributed to the aromatic amines found in cigarette smoke. Other risk factors include obesity, lack of physical activity, and diabetes mellitus. Studies evaluating the relationship between diet and pancreatic cancer are inconclusive. A Western diet (i.e., high intake of fat and meat, particularly smoked or processed meats) has been linked to the development of pancreatic cancer in many studies. Chronic pancreatitis also increases the risk of PDAC (relative risk as high as 13-fold), particularly in those individuals with hereditary pancreatitis and tropical pancreatitis. Epidemiologic studies have failed to find a consistent association between alcohol or coffee consumption and the development of pancreatic cancer.

Up to 10% of patients with pancreatic cancer have a family history of the disease, but most cannot be identified with a known genetic disorder. Recognized genetic disorders that predispose to pancreatic cancer include hereditary pancreatitis (*PRSS1* gene), hereditary nonpolyposis colorectal cancer, familial adenomatous polyposis, hereditary breast and ovarian cancers (*PALB2* and *BRCA2* genes), Peutz-Jeghers syndrome (*STK11* gene), familial atypical mole melanoma syndrome (*CDKN2A* gene), ataxia telangiectasia (*ATM* gene), and the Von Hippel–Lindau syndrome (*VHL* gene). Screening to detect precancerous lesions or early cancers should be considered for individuals with a cumulative predicted risk of PDAC greater than 5% or relative risk (RR) of 5 or greater (having ≥2 relatives with PDAC including ≥1 a first degree, or having a germline mutation of a predisposing gene and ≥2 relatives with PDAC or ≥1 a first degree, or Peutz–Jeghers syndrome even in the absence of a family history) and eligible for a possible pancreatic resection after discussion of the risks and benefits of such screening. Although imaging surveillance of high-risk family cohorts is practiced at some centers of expertise, there is no consensus about the optimal methods or frequency of pancreatic cancer screening. Screening with EUS and/or MRI can be considered but has not been shown to improve survival rates.

Pathology

More than 95% of malignant neoplasms of the pancreas arise from the exocrine pancreas. The term *pancreatic cancer* usually refers to ductal adenocarcinoma of the pancreas, representing 85% to 90% of all pancreatic neoplasms. *Exocrine pancreatic neoplasm* is a more inclusive term that includes neoplastic pancreatic ductal and acinar cells and their stem cells (e.g., pancreatoblastoma). Other, less common exocrine cancers include adenosquamous carcinomas, squamous cell carcinomas, signet ring cell carcinomas, and undifferentiated carcinomas. Neoplasms arising from the endocrine pancreas (i.e., islet cell or neuroendocrine tumors) comprise no more than 5% of pancreatic neoplasms.

Pancreatic cancers are composed of several distinct elements, including pancreatic cancer cells, tumor stroma, and stem cells. The precursor lesion of pancreatic cancer is pancreatic intraepithelial neoplasia, which progresses from mild dysplasia (PanIN grade 1) to more severe dysplasia (PanIN grades 2 and 3) and eventually to invasive carcinoma.

选择。内镜治疗包括胰腺括约肌切开术、狭窄扩张术、使用体内或体外冲击波碎石术进行结石清除或放置临时塑料支架。在长达 3～4 年的随访期间，50%～80% 的经过仔细筛选入组的患者实现了部分或完全疼痛缓解。

8. 手术。对于主胰管扩张（直径 > 6 mm）的患者，可进行手术胰管引流，常用术式为胰管空肠侧侧吻合术（即 Puestow 手术）。约 80% 的患者可获得疼痛缓解。这种手术是安全的，手术死亡率 < 5%。然而，在 5 年的随访中，只有 35%～60% 的患者未出现疼痛。对于以胰头疾病为主且胰管系统无阻塞或未扩张的患者，可考虑进行胰十二指肠切除术或保留十二指肠的胰头切除术（又称 Frey 或 Beger 手术）切除胰腺病变部位。经严格筛选的其他治疗无效的弥漫性胰腺实质疾病患者，可能获益于全胰腺切除术结合胰岛细胞自体移植。

并发症管理

慢性胰腺炎的并发症包括假性囊肿、胰瘘、胆道梗阻、胰腺癌、小肠细菌过度生长，以及由脾静脉血栓引起的孤立性胃静脉曲张。

胰瘘 胰瘘由胰管破裂引起，导致局部液体积聚、腹腔积液或胸腔积液。治疗包括肠道休息、内镜下胰管支架置入及使用生长抑素类似物。若保守治疗不成功，可能需要进行手术干预。

血管并发症 脾静脉沿胰腺背部走行，可能受胰腺炎或恶性肿瘤引起的炎症的影响，形成脾静脉血栓，进而导致孤立性胃底静脉曲张。脾切除术对胃静脉曲张出血患者通常有治愈效果。

急性和慢性胰腺炎均可导致假性动脉瘤形成。胰腺周围血管（如肝动脉、脾动脉、胰十二指肠动脉和胃十二指肠动脉）均可受累。假性动脉瘤的 CT 或 MRI 表现为胰腺内或胰腺周围囊性扩张的血管结构。EUS 多普勒成像可显示假性动脉瘤内的血流。肠系膜血管造影可确认诊断并提供治疗，因为检查期间可同时进行假性动脉瘤选择性栓塞。对于伴有出血的假性动脉瘤，手术治疗困难且并发症发生率和死亡率均较高。

胆道及十二指肠梗阻 少数慢性胰腺炎患者会出现症状性胆管梗阻和（或）十二指肠梗阻。餐后腹痛和早饱是十二指肠梗阻的典型特征，而疼痛和胆汁淤积（有时伴有胆管炎）则提示胆管狭窄。这些并发症通常由胰头炎症和纤维化或邻近的假性囊肿引起。

对于胆管狭窄，可尝试内镜下置入支架，但这些狭窄通常较顽固，且需要长期治疗。内镜治疗失败的患者可选择外科胆道减压手术。观察结果强调了胆道减压的重要性，其可逆转胆道梗阻引起的继发性胆道纤维化。

胰腺肿瘤

定义和流行病学

在美国，胰腺导管腺癌（PDAC）是癌症相关死亡的第四大原因，每年新诊断约 45 000 例患者。PDAC 的发病高峰年龄为 60～70 岁。男性发病率略高于女性（相对风险 1.4 : 1），美国黑人 PDAC 的发病率比白人高 30%～40%。

许多环境因素被认为可增加胰腺癌的风险。最公认的因素是吸烟，其增加 PDAC 风险的作用被归因于香烟烟雾中的芳香胺。其他危险因素包括肥胖、缺乏运动和糖尿病。针对饮食与胰腺癌相关性的研究结果尚不明确。许多研究发现，西方饮食（即摄入大量脂肪和肉类，特别是熏肉或加工肉类）与胰腺癌的发展有关。慢性胰腺炎也会增加 PDAC 的风险（相对风险增加 13 倍），特别是遗传性胰腺炎和热带性胰腺炎患者。流行病学研究未发现酒精或咖啡摄入与胰腺癌之间的一致性关联。

高达 10% 的胰腺癌患者有家族史，但大多数无法与已知的遗传病关联。已知易导致胰腺癌的遗传病包括遗传性胰腺炎（*PRSS1* 基因）、遗传性非息肉性结直肠癌、家族性腺瘤性息肉病、遗传性乳腺癌-卵巢癌（*PALB2* 基因和 *BRCA2* 基因）、黑斑息肉综合征（Peutz-Jeghers 综合征；*STK11* 基因）、家族性非典型痣黑色素瘤综合征（*CDKN2A* 基因）、共济失调毛细血管扩张症（*ATM* 基因）和希佩尔-林道综合征（Von Hippel-Lindau 综合征；*VHL* 基因）。对于 PDAC 累积预测风险 > 5% 或相对危险度（RR）≥ 5（如 ≥ 2 名亲属罹患 PDAC 且其中包括 ≥ 1 名一级亲属；携带易感基因突变，且 ≥ 2 名亲属罹患 PDAC 或 ≥ 1 名一级亲属罹患 PDAC；患有 Peutz-Jeghers 综合征，即使没有家族史）的个体，应考虑筛查癌前病变或早期胰腺癌，并在讨论此类筛查的风险和获益后决定是否进行胰腺切除术。虽然一些专科中心对高风险家族群体进行了影像学监测，但关于胰腺癌筛查的最佳方法或频率尚无共识。可考虑使用 EUS 和（或）MRI 进行筛查，但尚未证明其能提高生存率。

病理学

95% 以上的胰腺恶性肿瘤起源于胰腺的外分泌部分。胰腺癌这一术语通常是指 PDAC，其占所有胰腺肿瘤的 85%～90%。胰腺外分泌肿瘤是一个更广泛的概念，包括胰腺导管细胞、腺泡细胞及其干细胞的肿瘤（如胰母细胞瘤）。其他较少见的外分泌癌包括腺鳞癌、鳞状细胞癌、印戒细胞癌和未分化癌。起源于胰腺内分泌部分的肿瘤（即胰岛细胞肿瘤或神经内分泌肿瘤）在胰腺肿瘤中的占比不足 5%。

胰腺癌由数个不同成分组成，包括胰腺癌细胞、肿瘤间质和干细胞。胰腺癌的前驱病变是胰腺上皮内瘤变（PanIN），其从轻度异型增生（PanIN 1 级）进展到更严重的异型增生（PanIN 2 级和 3 级），最终发展为浸润性癌。

TABLE 9.4 Definitions of Pancreatic Ductal Adenocarcinoma Treatment Categories

Resectable	No evidence of tumor spread outside the pancreas
	No involvement of the superior mesenteric artery (SMA), celiac, or common hepatic artery (CHA)
	No invasion of the superior mesenteric vein (SMV) or portal vein (PV)
Metastatic	Evidence of spread to other organs (typically liver, lung, or peritoneum)
Borderline resectable	Tumor abutment (<50% of vessel circumference) of celiac, SMA or CHA
	Involvement but patent SMV or PV or short-segment occlusion with option for reconstruction
Locally advanced	Arterial encasement (>180 degrees or 50% of vessel circumference) of SMA, celiac or CHA
	SMV/PV occlusion without ability to surgically reconstruct

Clinical Presentation

The clinical manifestations of pancreatic carcinoma may be nonspecific and are often insidious. The clinical presentation is dependent to a great extent on tumor location and stage. PDAC localized to the head of the pancreas (70% to 80%) are more frequently symptomatic than those located in the body or tail (20% to 30%). Most PDAC has reached an advanced stage by the time of diagnosis. Common presenting signs and symptoms of pancreatic cancer include jaundice, weight loss, and abdominal pain. The pain is usually constant, with radiation to the back. Because most cancers begin in the pancreatic head, patients may exhibit obstructive jaundice or a large, palpable gallbladder (i.e., Courvoisier's sign).

Painless jaundice is the most common manifestation in patients with a potentially resectable and curable lesion. Anorexia, nausea, and vomiting may also occur, along with emotional disturbances such as depression. Less common manifestations include superficial thrombophlebitis (i.e., Trousseau sign), acute pancreatitis, diabetes mellitus, ascites, paraneoplastic syndromes (e.g., Cushing's syndrome), hypercalcemia, gastrointestinal bleeding, splenic vein thrombosis, and a palpable abdominal mass.

Diagnosis and Staging

The goal of imaging in the evaluation of suspected pancreatic carcinoma is to establish the diagnosis with a high degree of certainty and to determine resectability in patients who are otherwise candidates for operative resection. The diagnosis of pancreatic cancer is frequently suggested by a pancreatic mass seen on imaging studies. Evidence of a dilated pancreatic duct, hepatic metastases, invasion of vessels, or a dilated common bile duct in the setting of biliary obstruction may also be found. The imaging appearance may be impossible to distinguish from benign causes of pancreatic masses such as focal pancreatitis or autoimmune pancreatitis. Pancreas protocol triple phase (i.e., arterial, late arterial, and venous phases) cross-sectional multidetector CT scanning is the best initial study to diagnose and stage pancreatic cancer by identifying a mass lesion and assessing for liver metastasis or vascular invasion. CT is reported to have a sensitivity of 90% to 97% for identifying PDAC, although it is less sensitive for diagnosing small (<2 cm) lesions, with a sensitivity of 65% to 75%. CT is not sensitive for detecting nodal metastases. MRI is an alternative imaging modality that has similar accuracy to CT scanning for the diagnosis and staging of PDAC. EUS is superior to CT and MRI for detecting small lesions of the pancreas and should be performed when there is strong suspicion of PDAC despite the absence of a mass lesion by other imaging modalities. EUS-guided fine-needle aspiration (sensitivity of 85% to 90% and specificity approaching 100%) is recommended when histologic confirmation will alter management such as confirming malignancy in unresectable disease prior to initiating palliative care, confirming a potentially resectable tumor prior to neoadjuvant therapy, and for a suspected mass not visible on cross-sectional imaging.

The imaging techniques are highly accurate for recognizing unresectable disease, but they are somewhat limited for identifying resectable disease because occult metastases (<1 cm in diameter) may be on the surface of the liver or peritoneum. Staging laparoscopy may reduce morbidity and cost from open surgical tumor resection; it should be considered for patients with the highest likelihood of occult metastatic disease (i.e., those with tumors of the body or tail of the pancreas) who appear to have potentially resectable disease by CT (one half of whom have occult peritoneal metastases), those with large (>3 cm) primary tumors, those for whom imaging suggests occult metastatic disease, and those with a very high initial CA 19-9 level (>1000 units/mL).

The use of tumor markers to diagnose carcinoma of the pancreas has yielded disappointing results. The tumor marker CA 19-9 has a sensitivity of 70% to 80% and a specificity of 85% to 95% for diagnosing selected patients already exhibiting signs and symptoms that suggest pancreatic cancer. However, for early-stage cancers, CA 19-9 has limited sensitivity. Use of CA 19-9 requires the Lewis blood group antigen, which is absent in 5% to 10% of the population. The greatest utility for CA 19-9 is to identify occult metastasis in patients with seemingly resectable tumors, for monitoring patients after apparently curative surgery, and for following those receiving chemotherapy for advanced disease. Rising CA 19-9 levels suggest recurrent disease even in the absence of radiographically detectable lesions.

Treatment

Dividing patients with PDAC into resectable, borderline resectable, locally advanced, and metastatic categories is clinically useful (Table 9.4).

Resectable Disease

Unfortunately, only 10% to 20% of carcinomas in the head of the pancreas and rare cancers of the body and tail are resectable for cure. Current criteria for resectability include the absence of distant metastases and the absence of tumor involvement of major arteries (superior mesenteric, celiac, and common hepatic). Venous involvement requires vascular patency and criteria for resectability will depend on the surgeon's experience and ability to perform vascular reconstruction.

Universal preoperative ERCP for patients with biliary obstruction is not recommended due to lack of proven benefit and the potential to increase adverse events. Selective use of ERCP with biliary stent placement is recommended for those patients with biliary obstruction and a clinical presentation of either cholangitis, intractable pruritus, marked hyperbilirubinemia, or when surgery is delayed for neoadjuvant therapy. Technical success of ERCP is achieved in over 90% of such patients with an acceptable complication rate of under 5%. At the

表 9.4	胰腺导管腺癌治疗类别的定义
可切除病变	无肿瘤扩散至胰腺外的证据 未累及肠系膜上动脉（SMA）、腹腔动脉或肝总动脉（CHA） 未侵犯肠系膜上静脉（SMV）或门静脉（PV）
转移性病变	扩散至其他器官（通常是肝、肺或腹膜）
交界可切除病变	肿瘤贴近（＜血管周长的50%）腹腔动脉、SMA 或 CHA 累及 SMV 或 PV 但保持通常，或短段闭塞且可进行重建
局部晚期病变	SMA、腹腔动脉或 CHA 包绕（＞180° 或＞血管周长的50%） SMV/PV 闭塞且无法进行手术重建

临床表现

胰腺癌的临床表现可能无特异性，通常比较隐匿。临床表现在很大程度上取决于肿瘤的位置和分期。局限于胰头的 PDAC（占 70%～80%）比位于胰体或胰尾的 PDAC（占 20%～30%）更易出现症状。大多数 PDAC 患者在诊断时已处于晚期。胰腺癌常见的症状和体征包括黄疸、体重减轻和腹痛。腹痛通常为持续性且向背部放射。由于大多数癌症始于胰头，患者可能出现梗阻性黄疸或大的、可触及的胆囊（即 Courvoisier 征）。

无痛性黄疸是具有潜在可切除或可治愈病变患者最常见的表现。患者还可能出现厌食、恶心和呕吐，伴有抑郁等情绪障碍。较少见的表现包括浅表性血栓性静脉炎（即 Trousseau 征）、急性胰腺炎、糖尿病、腹腔积液、副肿瘤综合征（如库欣综合征）、高钙血症、消化道出血、脾静脉血栓形成和可触及的腹部肿块。

诊断和分期

在评估疑似胰腺癌患者时，影像学检查的目标是建立高度确定性的诊断，并确定哪些患者适合进行切除术。影像学检查中发现胰腺肿块通常提示胰腺癌的诊断。此外，还可能发现胰管扩张、肝转移、血管侵犯或在胆道梗阻的情况下出现胆总管扩张。然而，影像学表现有时难以将胰腺癌与表现为胰腺肿块的良性疾病（如局灶性胰腺炎或自身免疫性胰腺炎）区分开来。3 期时相（即动脉期、延迟期和静脉期）胰腺多排 CT 可识别病灶并评估肝转移或血管侵犯，是胰腺癌诊断和分期的最佳初始检查方法。据报道，CT 对识别 PDAC 的敏感性为 90%～97%，但对小病灶（＜2 cm）的敏感性较低，仅为 65%～75%。CT 对识别淋巴结转移的敏感性较低。MRI 是一种替代影像学方法，其在 PDAC 诊断和分期方面的准确性与 CT 相似。EUS 在识别胰腺小病灶方面优于 CT 和 MRI，当其他影像学检查未能显示病灶但高度怀疑 PDAC 时，应进行 EUS。当组织学确诊将会改变管理策略时，推荐进行 EUS 引导下细针穿刺（敏感性为 85%～90%，特异性接近 100%），如在开始姑息治疗前确认恶性肿瘤不可切除、在开始新辅助治疗前确认肿瘤为潜在可切除，以及确认在断层影像学检查中未能显示的疑似病灶情况。

影像学技术在识别不可切除的肿瘤方面非常准确，但在识别可切除的肿瘤时存在一定局限性，因为隐匿性转移灶（直径＜1 cm）可能位于肝或腹膜表面。分期腹腔镜检查可减少开放性外科肿瘤切除术的并发症发生率和成本；对于隐匿性转移发生风险最高（如 CT 显示潜在可切除的胰体或胰尾肿瘤，其中 1/2 存在隐匿性腹膜转移）、原发肿瘤较大（＞3 cm）、影像学提示存在隐匿性转移，以及初始 CA19-9 水平非常高（＞1000 U/ml）的患者，应考虑进行分期腹腔镜检查。

利用肿瘤标志物来诊断胰腺癌的效果令人失望。在诊断已表现出胰腺癌相关症状和体征的特定患者时，肿瘤标志物 CA19-9 的敏感性为 70%～80%，特异性为 85%～95%。然而，对于早期胰腺癌，CA19-9 的敏感性较低。使用 CA19-9 需要 Lewis 血型抗原，而人群中 5%～10% 的个体缺乏这种抗原。CA19-9 的最大作用在于识别看似为可切除肿瘤的患者的隐匿性转移、监测治愈性手术后的患者，以及随访接受化疗的癌症晚期患者。即使影像学检查未检测到病灶，CA19-9 水平升高也能提示疾病复发。

治疗

将 PDAC 患者分为可切除、交界可切除、局部晚期和转移性四类具有临床意义（表 9.4）。

可切除病变

遗憾的是，仅有 10%～20% 的胰头癌和少数胰体癌及胰尾癌可通过手术切除达到治愈的目的。可切除的现行标准包括无远处转移和未累及主要动脉（如肠系膜上动脉、腹腔动脉和肝总动脉）。对于静脉受累患者，则要求血管通畅，且可切除的标准主要取决于外科医生的经验及进行血管重建的能力。

由于缺乏确凿的获益证据，且可能增加不良事件的风险，不推荐对有胆道梗阻的患者常规进行术前 ERCP。对于存在胆道梗阻并伴有胆管炎、顽固性瘙痒、严重高胆红素血症、因新辅助治疗而延迟手术的患者，建议选择性进行 ERCP 并放置胆道支架。在这些患者中，ERCP 的技术成功率超过 90%，可接受的并发症发生率＜5%。

time of stent placement, ERCP tissue sampling techniques can confirm a diagnosis of pancreatic malignancy (sensitivity of 30% to 60% and specificity 100%).

The standard operation for pancreatic cancer of the head or uncinate process is the Whipple procedure (i.e., pancreaticoduodenectomy). Whipple resection consists of removal of the pancreatic head, distal common bile duct, gallbladder, duodenum, proximal jejunum, gastric antrum, and regional lymph nodes. Reconstruction requires pancreaticojejunostomy, hepaticojejunostomy, and gastrojejunostomy. The pylorus-preserving version of the Whipple procedure leaves the stomach intact. The surgical mortality rate for this procedure is approximately 3% when performed by experienced pancreatic surgeons. Adjuvant therapy is indicated in all patients following resection of PDAC, irrespective of the pTNM stage, as it improves progression-free and overall survival rates.

Locally Advanced and Borderline Resectable

The term *borderline resectable* is reserved for patients with focal tumor abutment of the visceral arteries (celiac, superior mesenteric artery [SMA], or common hepatic), defined as contact of the tumor with less than one half circumference of the vessel wall, or short-segment occlusion of the superior mesenteric vein (SMV) or SMV–portal vein confluence. The latter is considered a relative rather than absolute contraindication to curative resection as some surgeons are performing resection with vascular reconstruction for selected individuals under these circumstances. Also, for tumors of the tail of the pancreas, encasement of the splenic vein does not necessarily obviate resectability. Locally advanced disease refers to individuals with unresectable cancer due to arterial encasement (>180° or >50% vessel circumference) of SMA, celiac or common hepatic arteries or SMV/PV occlusion without an option for reconstruction.

The use of preoperative neoadjuvant chemoradiation therapy in an effort to convert patients with unresectable borderline or locally advanced disease to a resectable status has increased the overall resection rate, but no difference in survival has been demonstrated.

Metastatic or Unresectable Disease

Although practice varies across institutions, most surgeons consider a pancreatic cancer to be categorically unresectable if there is extrapancreatic involvement, including extensive peripancreatic lymphatic extension, nodal involvement beyond the peripancreatic tissues, or distant metastases (e.g., liver, peritoneum, omentum, extra-abdominal sites). Other indications of unresectability include vascular encasement (i.e., tumor contact with more than one-half of the vessel's circumference), or direct involvement of the superior mesenteric artery, aorta, celiac artery, or hepatic artery, as defined by the absence of a fat plane between the tumor and these structures on CT imaging.

Patients with metastatic or inoperable pancreatic cancer should be offered treatment with multidisciplinary input based on goals of care, patient preferences, performance status (PS) and social support systems. If protocol enrollment is not available or is declined, conventional systemic chemotherapy should be offered because it provides benefit improving disease-related symptoms and overall survival.

- Patients under age 75 years with an ECOG PS 0 to 1 and bilirubin less than 1.5 mg/dL should be offered FOLFIRINOX or gemcitabine plus nab-paclitaxel;
- Patients with an ECOG PS 2 and bilirubin less than 1.5 ULN should be offered gemcitabine plus nab-paclitaxel or gemcitabine;
- Patients with an ECOG PS 0 to 2 and bilirubin 1.5 ULN or greater or comorbidities should be offered gemcitabine; and
- Patients with an ECOG PS 3 to 4 should be offered best supportive care.

For patients with inoperable cancers and poor performance status, palliative interventions to alleviate jaundice, pain, and intestinal obstruction often become the focus of therapy. When advanced disease is observed operatively, the surgeon must determine whether to perform additional palliative surgery. Biliary bypass is indicated in patients with obstructive jaundice. Duodenal bypass is indicated when features suggest impending gastric outlet obstruction. Alternative palliative endoscopic approaches are available for patients not undergoing exploratory surgery.

Prognosis

Carcinoma of the pancreas accounts for approximately 5% of cancer deaths in the United States. The overall prognosis is poor because less than 20% of patients are alive beyond the first year after diagnosis, and only 7% survive to the fifth year. Although 15% to 20% of patients have resectable disease at initial diagnosis, most have locally advanced or metastatic cancer. Median survival is 8 to 12 months for patients with locally advanced unresectable disease and 3 to 6 months for those with metastases at diagnosis.

A Whipple resection for pancreatic head cancers is the only chance for cure; however, the median survival after surgery is 15 to 20 months. Five-year survival after margin negative (R0) pancreaticoduodenectomy is approximately 25% to 30% following node-negative resection and 10% for node-positive disease. The overall 5-year survival rate is 10% to 25%, and up to 50% of those who survive 5 years ultimately die of recurrent cancer. Poor prognostic factors include a high tumor grade, a large tumor, high levels of CA 19-9 before and after surgery, tumor-positive surgical margins, and lymph node metastases.

For a deeper discussion of these topics, please see Chapter 135, "Pancreatitis," and Chapter 185, "Pancreatic Cancer," in *Goldman-Cecil Medicine*, 26th Edition.

SUGGESTED READINGS

Baron TE, DiMaio CJ, Wang AY, et al: American Gastroenterological Association Clinical Practice update: management of pancreatic necrosis, Gastroenterology 158:67–75, 2020.

Fogel EL, Shahda S, Sandrasegaran K, et al: A multidisciplinary approach to pancreas cancer in 2016: a review, Am J Gastroenterol 112:537–554, 2017.

Forsmark CE: Management of chronic pancreatitis, Gastroenterology 144:1282–1291, 2013.

Gardner TB, Adler DG, Forsmark CE: ACG clinical guideline: chronic pancreatitis, Am J Gastroenterol, 2020.

Hidalgo M: Pancreatic cancer, N Engl J Med 362:1605–1617, 2010.

Paulson AS, Cao HS, Tempero MA, et al: Therapeutic advances in pancreatic cancer, Gastroenterology 144:1316–1326, 2013.

Singh VK, Yadav D, Garg PK: Diagnosis and management of chronic pancreatitis: a review, JAMA 322:2422–2434, 2019.

Tenner S, Baillie J, DeWitt J, et al: American College of Gastroenterology guideline: management of acute pancreatitis, Am J Gastroenterol 108:1400–1415, 2013.

Vege SS, DiMagno MJ, Forsmark CE, et al: Initial medical treatment of acute pancreatitis: American Gastroenterological Association Institute Technical review, Gastroenterology 154:1103–1139, 2018.

Whitcomb DC: Genetic risk factors for pancreatic disorders, Gastroenterology 144:1292–1302, 2013.

Yadav D, Lowenfels AB: The epidemiology of pancreatitis and pancreatic cancer, Gastroenterology 144:1252–1261, 2013.

在放置支架时，ERCP 的组织采样技术可确认胰腺恶性肿瘤的诊断，其敏感性为 30%～60%，特异性为 100%。

对于位于胰头或钩突的胰腺癌，标准术式是 Whipple 手术（即胰十二指肠切除术）。Whipple 手术将切除胰头、远端胆总管、胆囊、十二指肠、近端空肠、胃窦和区域淋巴结。重建手术则需要进行胰空肠吻合、肝空肠吻合和胃空肠吻合。保留幽门的 Whipple 手术会保留完整的胃。由经验丰富的胰腺外科医生进行该手术的围术期死亡率约为 3%。无论 pTNM 分期如何，所有 PDAC 切除术后的患者均应接受辅助治疗，因其可提高无进展生存率和总生存率。

局部晚期和交界可切除病变

"交界可切除"这一术语适用于肿瘤局部紧邻内脏动脉〔如腹腔动脉、肠系膜上动脉（SMA）或肝总动脉〕的患者，定义为肿瘤与血管壁的距离＜血管周长的 50%，或肠系膜上静脉（SMV）或 SMV-门静脉汇合处有短段闭塞。后者被认为是手术的相对禁忌证而非绝对禁忌证，因为一些外科医生在这种情况下可为特定患者进行血管重建手术。此外，对于胰尾肿瘤，脾静脉包绕并不一定意味着不可切除。局部晚期是指由于 SMA、腹腔动脉或肝总动脉包绕（＞180° 或＞血管周长的 50%）或 SMV/PV 闭塞且无法重建，导致病变不可切除。

术前新辅助放化疗旨在将不可切除的交界可切除或局部晚期病变转化为可切除病变，新辅助放化疗可提高总体切除率，但尚未显示出对生存率的明显改善。

转移性或不可切除病变

尽管各机构的临床实践有所不同，但大多数外科医生认为，如果累及胰腺外，包括广泛的胰腺周围淋巴结肿大、胰腺周围组织以外的淋巴结受累或远处转移（如肝、腹膜、大网膜或腹腔外部位），则认为胰腺癌不可切除。其他不可切除的指征包括血管包绕（即肿瘤接触血管周长的 50% 以上），或直接累及 SMA、主动脉、腹腔动脉或肝动脉，CT 表现为肿瘤与这些结构之间缺乏脂肪间隙。

对于转移性或不可切除的胰腺癌患者，应基于治疗目标、患者偏好、体能状态（PS）和社会支持系统，提供多学科协作治疗。如果患者无法参与或拒绝参加临床试验，应提供常规的全身化疗，因其有助于改善与疾病相关的症状和总生存率。

- 年龄＜75 岁、ECOG PS 评分为 0～1 分且胆红素＜1.5 mg/dl 的患者，应给予 FOLFIRINOX 或吉西他滨联合纳米白蛋白结合型紫杉醇（nab-paclitaxel）
- ECOG PS 评分为 2 分且胆红素＜1.5 倍正常值上限（ULN）的患者，应给予吉西他滨联合纳米白蛋白结合型紫杉醇或单用吉西他滨
- ECOG PS 评分为 0～2 分且胆红素水平≥1.5 倍 ULN，或有合并症的患者，应给予吉西他滨
- ECOG PS 评分为 3～4 分的患者，应给予最佳支持治疗

对于无法手术且体能状态较差的患者，缓解黄疸、疼痛和肠梗阻的姑息性干预通常是治疗的重点。当在术中发现晚期病变时，外科医生必须决定是否进行额外的姑息性手术。对于有阻塞性黄疸的患者，建议进行胆道旁路手术。对于有提示即将发生胃出口梗阻征象的患者，建议进行十二指肠旁路手术。对于不接受探查性手术的患者，可选择其他姑息性内镜治疗方法。

预后

在美国，胰腺癌约占癌症死亡人数的 5%。总体预后较差，因为诊断后生存时间超过 1 年的患者不足 20%，而只有 7% 的患者能够存活至诊断后第 5 年。虽然在初次诊断时有 15%～20% 的患者病情评估为可切除病变，但大多数患者在确诊时已处于局部晚期或转移状态。局部晚期无法切除的患者的中位生存期为 8～12 个月，而诊断时已有转移的患者的中位生存期为 3～6 个月。

对于胰头癌，Whipple 手术是唯一可能治愈的机会；然而，术后的中位生存期为 15～20 个月。在 Whipple 手术后切缘阴性（R0）的患者中，淋巴结阴性患者的 5 年生存率为 25%～30%，而淋巴结阳性患者的 5 年生存率为 10%。5 年总生存率为 10%～25%，其中多达 50% 的存活 5 年的患者最终因癌症复发而死亡。预后不良的因素包括肿瘤级别高、肿瘤较大、术前和术后 CA19-9 水平高、手术切缘阳性和淋巴结转移。

有关此专题的深入讨论，请参阅 *Goldman-Cecil Medicine* 第 26 版第 135 章 "胰腺炎" 和第 185 章 "胰腺癌"。

推荐阅读

Baron TE, DiMaio CJ, Wang AY, et al: American Gastroenterological Association Clinical Practice update: management of pancreatic necrosis, Gastroenterology 158:67–75, 2020.

Fogel EL, Shahda S, Sandrasegaran K, et al: A multidisciplinary approach to pancreas cancer in 2016: a review, Am J Gastroenterol 112:537–554, 2017.

Forsmark CE: Management of chronic pancreatitis, Gastroenterology 144:1282–1291, 2013.

Gardner TB, Adler DG, Forsmark CE: ACG clinical guideline: chronic pancreatitis, Am J Gastroenterol, 2020.

Hidalgo M: Pancreatic cancer, N Engl J Med 362:1605–1617, 2010.

Paulson AS, Cao HS, Tempero MA, et al: Therapeutic advances in pancreatic cancer, Gastroenterology 144:1316–1326, 2013.

Singh VK, Yadav D, Garg PK: Diagnosis and management of chronic pancreatitis: a review, JAMA 322:2422–2434, 2019.

Tenner S, Baillie J, DeWitt J, et al: American College of Gastroenterology guideline: management of acute pancreatitis, Am J Gastroenterol 108:1400–1415, 2013.

Vege SS, DiMagno MJ, Forsmark CE, et al: Initial medical treatment of acute pancreatitis: American Gastroenterological Association Institute Technical review, Gastroenterology 154:1103–1139, 2018.

Whitcomb DC: Genetic risk factors for pancreatic disorders, Gastroenterology 144:1292–1302, 2013.

Yadav D, Lowenfels AB: The epidemiology of pancreatitis and pancreatic cancer, Gastroenterology 144:1252–1261, 2013.

SECTION II

Diseases of the Liver and Biliary System

10 Laboratory Tests in Liver Diseases, 152

11 Jaundice, 158

12 Acute and Chronic Hepatitis, 170

13 Acute Liver Failure, 186

14 Cirrhosis of the Liver and Its Complications, 192

15 Disorders of the Gallbladder and Biliary Tract, 214

第 2 篇

肝脏与胆道系统疾病

10　肝脏疾病的实验室检查，153

11　黄疸，159

12　急性和慢性肝炎，171

13　急性肝衰竭，187

14　肝硬化及其并发症，193

15　胆囊和胆道疾病，215

10

Laboratory Tests in Liver Diseases

Michael B. Fallon, Ester Little

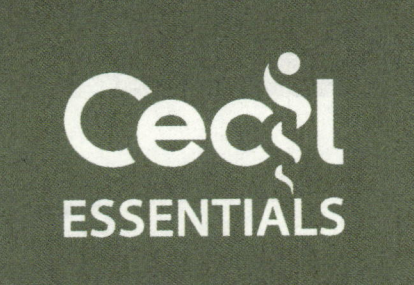

INTRODUCTION

The liver is a large and complex organ, involved in major metabolic, secretory, and nutritional functions. It plays a central role in glucose homeostasis, synthesis and secretion of bile, and synthesis of lipoproteins and plasma proteins, including clotting factors and vitamin storage (vitamins B_{12}, A, D, E, and K). It is also the site of biotransformation, detoxification, and excretion of a multitude of endogenous and exogenous compounds.

Given the diversity of the liver roles, the clinical manifestation of liver diseases is varied and can be quite subtle. The first step in evaluating a patient with liver disease is the clinical history, and signs of liver disease can also be seen on physical exam (e.g., jaundice, dark urine, light colored stools, gastrointestinal bleeding, spider angiomas, palmar erythema, hepatomegaly, splenomegaly, ascites, and asterixis). The history and physical findings guide the initial set of laboratory tests ordered.

LIVER CHEMISTRY TESTS

The most widely used tests to evaluate the liver are aspartate and alanine aminotransferases (AST and ALT), alkaline phosphatase (ALP), gamma glutamyl transpeptidase (GGT), bilirubin, albumin, and prothrombin time. They are commonly referred to as "liver function tests." However, this is misleading because (1) they do not accurately reflect the function of the liver, (2) abnormal levels can indicate diseases affecting other organs, and (3) they may be normal in patients with advanced liver disease. A better terminology is liver chemistry tests. These tests reflect patterns of abnormalities seen in liver and biliary cell injury.

Patterns of Abnormalities in Liver Chemistry Tests

There are primarily three patterns of abnormalities in liver chemistry tests: one that reflects damage of the hepatocytes or hepatocellular damage (AST and ALT), one that reflects cholestasis and damage of the biliary cells (ALP and GGT), and one when patients have isolated elevation in bilirubin.

The tests are interpreted based on limits of normality and may vary between different laboratories. However, for ALT, it is now recognized that the limit of normality should be the same for all, and many professional societies have included the following levels in their guidelines: normal ALT ranges from 29 to 33 units/L in adult men and 19 to 25 units/L in adult women. Table 10.1 depicts the most common liver chemistry tests and the disease processes associated with each set of tests.

Hepatocellular Damage

ALT and AST are intracellular enzymes that catalyze the transfer of the α-amino group of aspartate or alanine to the α-keto group of ketoglutaric acid, resulting in formation of pyruvate or oxaloacetic acid, respectively. Vitamin B_6 is required to carry out this reaction. In the presence of cell injury or death, AST and ALT are released into circulation. ALT is found predominantly in hepatocytes and is more specific, whereas AST is also found in the heart, lungs, kidney, pancreas, brain, and skeletal muscle.

In most hepatocellular disorders (i.e., viral hepatitis, autoimmune hepatitis, hemochromatosis, Wilson's disease and some drug-induced liver injury) ALT is higher than or equal to AST. However, in alcoholic liver disease this ratio is reversed. A ratio greater than 2 is seen in 70% and greater than 3 in 96% of the patients with known alcoholic liver disease. Chronic and heavy alcohol consumption leads to vitamin B deficiency. The effect of vitamin B_6 deficiency is more prominent on ALT than AST activity, causing the increase in AST/ALT ratio. Not uncommonly, the AST is also higher than ALT in patients with nonalcoholic fatty liver disease (NAFLD), mimicking alcoholic liver disease.

The magnitude of elevation in aminotransferases also helps identify the possible cause of liver damage. Marked elevation, above 15 times the upper limit of normality (ULN), is seen in acute viral hepatitis, acetaminophen toxicity, hypoxic hepatopathy (shock, ischemia, hypoxemia) or acute bile duct obstruction. More modest elevations, usually 10 to 15 times the ULN, are seen in alcoholic hepatitis, autoimmune hepatitis, Wilson's disease, Budd-Chiari, and malignant infiltration of the liver (usually from breast cancer, small cell lung cancer, lymphoma, melanoma). In patients with chronic viral hepatitis, ALT and AST levels are rarely above 10 times the ULN, except during exacerbations of chronic hepatitis B. Elevations less than four times the ULN are more commonly seen in nonalcoholic fatty liver disease, hemochromatosis, α1-antitrypsin deficiency, celiac disease, and thyroid disease. Once the liver damage has progressed to cirrhosis, the elevation in aminotransferases is mild and can be normal. Conversely, ALT and AST can be massively elevated in diseases not related to the liver, such as rhabdomyolysis and heat stroke. In addition to acetaminophen, multiple medications can cause elevation in the aminotransferases at different levels of magnitude, including diclofenac, fluoxetine, isoniazid, ketoconazole, lisinopril, phenytoin, rifampin, ritonavir, and statins.

The rate at which the AST and ALT levels decrease as the patient improves can also help in identifying the cause. More rapid decline suggests ischemia or resolution of an acute biliary obstruction.

Cholestasis

The tests that indicate cholestasis and biliary cell damage are ALP and GGT. Serum ALP comprises a group of isoenzymes derived from the liver, intestine, bone, and placenta. The liver isoenzyme (ALP-1) is present in the mucosal cells lining the bile ducts and increases in response to bile duct damage from inflammation or obstruction. In these circumstances,

肝脏疾病的实验室检查

谢思 译　魏来 审校　贾继东 通审

引言

肝脏是一个大而复杂的器官，主要参与机体的代谢、分泌和营养功能。肝脏还在维持血糖稳定、合成和分泌胆汁、合成脂蛋白和血浆蛋白（包括凝血因子），以及储存维生素（维生素 B_{12}、A、D、E 和 K）等方面发挥重要作用。同时，肝脏也是众多内源性和外源性化合物进行生物转化、解毒和排泄的场所。

鉴于肝脏功能的多样性，肝脏疾病的临床表现也多种多样，且可能相当隐匿。临床病史是评估肝脏疾病患者的第一步，体格检查也可发现肝脏疾病相关体征（如黄疸、尿色加深、粪便颜色变浅、消化道出血、蜘蛛痣、肝掌、肝大、脾大、腹腔积液和扑翼样震颤）。病史和体格检查的发现可以指导进行初步的实验室检查。

肝脏化学试验

评估肝脏最常用的指标包括天冬氨酸转氨酶（AST）、丙氨酸转氨酶（ALT）、碱性磷酸酶（ALP）、γ-谷氨酰转移酶（GGT）、胆红素、白蛋白和凝血酶原时间（PT）。这些指标常被称为"肝功能检查"，但该术语可能造成误解，因为：①这些指标不能准确反映肝脏功能；②这些指标异常可能由其他器官或组织损伤所致；③进展期肝病患者的这些指标可能在正常范围内。因此，肝脏化学试验是更合适的术语。这些指标反映了肝脏和胆管细胞损伤。

肝脏化学试验异常的类型

肝脏化学试验异常主要分为 3 类：①反映肝细胞损伤（AST 和 ALT）；②反映胆汁淤积和胆管细胞损伤（ALP 和 GGT）；③孤立性胆红素水平升高。

肝脏化学试验指标需根据其正常值范围进行解读，不同实验室的参考值范围可能存在差异。但是，目前 ALT 的正常值范围是统一的，许多专业学会指南均提出以下正常值范围：成年男性 29～33 U/L，成年女性 19～25 U/L。表 10.1 列出了常用的肝脏化学试验指标及其相关疾病。

肝细胞损伤

ALT 和 AST 是胞内酶，可催化丙氨酸或天冬氨酸的 α-氨基转移到酮戊二酸的 α-酮基上，分别生成丙酮酸或草酰乙酸。这一反应需要维生素 B_6 的参与。当细胞损伤或死亡时，AST 和 ALT 被释放到血液循环中。ALT 主要存在于肝细胞中，因此更具肝特异性，而 AST 也可存在于心脏、肺、肾、胰腺、大脑和骨骼肌中。

在大多数肝细胞性疾病（如病毒性肝炎、自身免疫性肝炎、血色病、肝豆状核变性和部分药物性肝损伤）中，ALT ≥ AST。然而，在酒精性肝病中，ALT < AST。70% 确诊酒精性肝病的患者 AST/ALT 比值 > 3，96% 的患者 AST/ALT 比值 > 2［译者注：原文有误，已更正］。长期大量饮酒会导致维生素 B 缺乏。维生素 B_6 缺乏对 ALT 活性的影响较其对 AST 的影响更显著，因此会导致 AST/ALT 比值升高。与酒精性肝病类似，非酒精性脂肪性肝病（NAFLD）患者通常 AST 高于 ALT。

转氨酶水平升高的程度有助于鉴别肝损伤的原因。转氨酶水平显著升高［>正常值上限（ULN）的 15 倍］主要见于急性病毒性肝炎，对乙酰氨基酚中毒，低氧性肝病（休克、缺血、低氧血症）或急性胆道梗阻。转氨酶水平中度升高（通常为 ULN 的 10～15 倍）主要见于酒精性肝炎，自身免疫性肝炎，肝豆状核变性，布-加综合征和恶性肿瘤肝浸润（通常来源于乳腺癌、小细胞肺癌、淋巴瘤、黑色素瘤）。在慢性病毒性肝炎患者中，ALT 和 AST 水平很少超过 10 倍 ULN，除非在慢性乙型肝炎急性加重时。转氨酶水平升高 < 4 倍 ULN 更常见于 NAFLD、血色病、$α_1$-抗胰蛋白酶缺乏症、乳糜泻和甲状腺疾病。一旦肝损伤进展为肝硬化，转氨酶通常仅轻微升高，甚至可能正常。相反，ALT 和 AST 在非肝脏疾病中也可能显著升高，如横纹肌溶解和热射病。除对乙酰氨基酚外，多种药物（如双氯芬酸、氟西汀、异烟肼、酮康唑、赖诺普利、苯妥英、利福平、利托那韦和他汀类药物）可引起不同程度的转氨酶水平升高。

患者病情好转时 AST 和 ALT 水平下降的速度也有助于鉴别病因。转氨酶水平迅速下降常提示缺血或急性胆道梗阻的解除。

胆汁淤积

ALP 和 GGT 是提示胆汁淤积和胆管细胞损伤的指标。血清 ALP 由来源于肝、肠道、骨骼和胎盘的一组同工酶组成。肝脏同工酶（ALP-1）存在于胆管黏膜细胞中，当炎症或梗阻导致胆管损伤时，ALP-1 水平升高。在这种情况下，GGT 和 5′-核苷酸酶（5′-NT）同

153

TABLE 10.1 Liver Chemistry Tests

Liver Chemistry Test	What It Reflects	Associated Diseases
Aspartate aminotransferase and alanine aminotransferase	Hepatocellular damage	Viral hepatitis, autoimmune hepatitis (AIH), alcoholic hepatitis, hemochromatosis, ischemic hepatitis, Budd-Chiari syndrome, α1-antitrypsin deficiency, Wilson's disease, and drugs
Alkaline phosphatase and γ-glutamyl transpeptidase	Cholestasis, biliary cell damage, and infiltrative processes	Primary biliary cholangitis (PBC), primary sclerosing cholangitis (PSC), familial cholestatic syndromes, AIDS cholangiopathy, cholestasis of pregnancy, biliary obstruction by stones or cancer, drugs, sarcoidosis, amyloidosis, and malignancy infiltration
Isolated bilirubin elevation	Increased production and impaired uptake, conjugation or excretion of bilirubin	Hemolysis, Gilbert, Crigler-Najjar, Dubin-Johnson, and Rotor syndromes
Decreased albumin and prolonged prothrombin time	Impaired synthetic liver function	Liver failure, severe acute hepatitis, and advanced liver disease with cirrhosis

GGT and 5′-nucleotidase (5′-NT) are simultaneously released. Thus, an elevation of ALP without elevation of GGT and 5′-NT indicates a nonhepatic cause. Fractionation of the different ALP isoenzymes by electrophoresis can be useful in determining alternative sources.

ALP does not differentiate intrahepatic from extrahepatic cholestasis. Examples of disorders that cause *intrahepatic cholestasis* are primary biliary cholangitis (PBC), primary sclerosing cholangitis (PSC), infections (AIDS cholangiopathy), familial cholestatic syndromes, cholestasis of pregnancy, total parenteral nutrition, ischemic cholangiopathy, liver allograft rejection, congestive hepatopathy (liver congestion secondary to right-sided heart failure), some medications (amiodarone, anabolic steroids, amoxicillin clavulanate, carbamazepine, estrogens, naproxen, phenytoin, rifampin), and infiltrative diseases (sarcoidosis, amyloidosis, malignant infiltration of the liver). Causes of *extrahepatic cholestasis* include bile duct stones or tumors, diverticulum of the ampulla of Vater, chronic pancreatitis, and pancreatic cancer.

ALP is frequently below normal range in patients with Wilson's disease, particularly those presenting with acute liver failure, in whom bilirubin is disproportionally elevated compared to alkaline phosphatase.

GGT is very nonspecific, and in addition to liver diseases it can be elevated in pancreatic diseases, myocardial infarction, renal failure, alcoholism, chronic obstructive pulmonary disease, and from several medications. As noted above, 5′-NT would not be elevated in these conditions.

Isolated Bilirubin Elevation

Patients with both hepatocellular diseases and cholestasis frequently also have bilirubin elevation secondary to leakage of bilirubin into the serum. However, some patients have elevated bilirubin with normal ALT, AST, ALP and GGT, which is termed *isolated bilirubin elevation*. In such cases, the first step is to fractionate the bilirubin to determine if it is caused by an elevation in the unconjugated (indirect) or conjugated (direct) bilirubin. An increase in *unconjugated bilirubin* results from overproduction (hemolysis), impaired uptake (Gilbert's disease) or impaired conjugation (Crigler-Najjar syndrome). An increase in *conjugated bilirubin* is due to decreased excretion in the bile ducts (Dubin-Johnson and Rotor syndromes) or leakage of the pigment from hepatocytes into serum.

More detailed discussion on cholestasis and isolated elevation of bilirubin can be found in Chapter 11.

LIVER SYNTHETIC FUNCTION

Albumin

From 300 g to 500 g of albumin is distributed in body fluids, and the adult liver synthesizes 15 g of albumin per day. Serum albumin concentration reflects the rate of synthesis, degradation, and volume of distribution. The synthesis of albumin is influenced by several factors including nutritional status, serum oncotic pressure, hormones, and cytokines.

The half-life of albumin in serum is 14 to 20 days. Low albumin is seen in prolonged liver dysfunction or acute liver impairment, and a decrease in albumin concentration reflects a reduction in albumin synthesis.

Hypoalbuminemia does not always reflect liver synthetic dysfunction. Several other conditions may decrease albumin, including malnutrition, nephrotic syndrome, protein losing enteropathy, and systemic inflammation.

Coagulation Factors and Prothrombin Time

The liver is the major site for the synthesis of 11 coagulation factors, including factors I, II, V, VII, IX, X, XII, and XIII. Deficiency in clotting factors occurs in more severe or more advanced stages of liver diseases. These factors can be measured individually or indirectly by determining the prothrombin time (PT).

The PT is dependent on factors II, V, VII and X, all of which are synthesized in the liver. Prolonged PT is not specific to liver diseases and can be seen in several congenital or acquired disorders. When these conditions are excluded, a prolonged PT is usually secondary to deficiency of vitamin K (inadequate dietary intake, prolonged obstructive jaundice, intestinal malabsorption or prolonged broad spectrum antibiotic use) or by poor utilization of vitamin K because of advanced liver disease. The administration of a single parenteral dose of vitamin K normalizes the PT in cases of vitamin K deficiency.

The magnitude of the prolongation of PT reflects the severity of the liver disease; however, PT does not correlate with the coagulation status or the risk of bleeding in patients with cirrhosis. In fact, in patients with cirrhosis there is also a decrease in synthesis of anti-hemostatic factors, and some patients become relatively hypercoagulable and have an increased risk of clot formation, despite having prolonged PT. This is an important and frequently misunderstood concept.

Gamma Globulins

Elevation of individual gamma globulins can be suggestive of specific liver diseases. Some examples include elevation of immunoglobulin G (IgG) in patients with autoimmune hepatitis, elevation of immunoglobulin M (IgM) in PBC, and elevation of immunoglobulin A (IgA) in patients with alcoholic cirrhosis. IgG4-related disease is an autoimmune phenomenon in which increased IgG4 levels cause dysfunction in multiple organs, including bile ducts (IgG4-related cholangiopathy).

Specific Markers of Liver Diseases

Specific laboratory tests are required for the diagnosis of some liver diseases.

- **α1-Antitrypsin (α1AT):** it can be quantified and, if decreased, the A1AT phenotype can be determined
- **Autoimmune hepatitis:** antinuclear antibody (ANA), anti–smooth muscle antibody (ASMA), anti–liver/kidney microsomal antibody type 1 (anti-LKM1)

表 10.1 肝脏化学试验		
肝脏化学试验	反映的异常类型	相关疾病
天冬氨酸转氨酶和丙氨酸转氨酶	肝细胞损伤	病毒性肝炎、自身免疫性肝炎（AIH）、酒精性肝炎、血色病、缺血性肝炎、布-加综合征、α_1-抗胰蛋白酶缺乏症、肝豆状核变性、药物
碱性磷酸酶和 γ-谷氨酰转移酶	胆汁淤积、胆管细胞损伤、浸润性疾病	原发性胆汁性胆管炎（PBC）、原发性硬化性胆管炎（PSC）、家族性胆汁淤积综合征、艾滋病相关胆管病变、妊娠期胆汁淤积、结石或肿瘤所致的胆道梗阻、药物、结节病、淀粉样变性、恶性肿瘤肝浸润
孤立性胆红素水平升高	胆红素生成过多，以及摄取、结合、排泄障碍	溶血、吉尔伯特综合征（Gilbert综合征）、克-纳综合征（Crigler-Najjar综合征）、杜-约综合征（Dubin-Johnson综合征）、罗托综合征（Rotor综合征）
白蛋白水平下降和凝血酶原时间延长	肝合成功能障碍	肝衰竭、严重急性肝炎、进展期肝病伴肝硬化

时被释放。因此，如果 ALP 水平升高而 GGT 和 5′-NT 正常，则提示由非肝脏原因所致。通过电泳法分离不同的 ALP 同工酶有助于确定其不同的来源。

ALP 水平无法区分肝内和肝外胆汁淤积。可引起肝内胆汁淤积的原因包括原发性胆汁性胆管炎（PBC），原发性硬化性胆管炎（PSC），感染（艾滋病相关胆管病变），家族性胆汁淤积综合征，妊娠期胆汁淤积，全肠外营养，缺血性胆管病，肝移植排斥反应，充血性肝病（继发于右心衰竭的肝充血），某些药物（胺碘酮、合成类固醇、阿莫西林-克拉维酸、卡马西平、雌激素、萘普生、苯妥英、利福平）和浸润性疾病（结节病、淀粉样变性、恶性肿瘤肝浸润）。可引起肝外胆汁淤积的原因包括胆管结石或肿瘤、肝胰壶腹憩室、慢性胰腺炎和胰腺癌。

肝豆状核变性患者的 ALP 常低于正常范围，尤其是在表现为急性肝衰竭的患者中，胆红素水平的升高与 ALP 不成比例。

GGT 的特异性非常低，除肝脏疾病外，胰腺疾病、心肌梗死、肾衰竭、酒精中毒、慢性阻塞性肺疾病和多种药物均可导致 GGT 水平升高。如上所述，5′-NT 水平在这些情况下不会升高。

孤立性胆红素水平升高

肝细胞损伤和胆汁淤积的患者常因胆红素反流入血而同时出现胆红素水平升高。然而，一些患者胆红素水平升高但 ALT、AST、ALP 和 GGT 正常，被称为孤立性胆红素水平升高。这种情况下，首先应区分胆红素水平升高是由非结合（间接）胆红素还是结合（直接）胆红素升高所致。非结合胆红素升高由胆红素生成过多（溶血）、摄取障碍（Gilbert 综合征）或结合障碍（Crigler-Najjar 综合征）所致。结合胆红素升高由胆红素排泄障碍（Dubin-Johnson 综合征和 Rotor 综合征）或肝细胞色素反流入血所致。

关于胆汁淤积和孤立性胆红素水平升高的详细讨论见第 11 章。

肝脏合成功能

白蛋白

正常人体液中含有 300 ~ 500 g 白蛋白，成人肝脏每天合成 15 g 白蛋白。血清白蛋白浓度反映了其合成速率、降解速率及分布容积。白蛋白的合成受营养状态、血清渗透压、激素和细胞因子等多种因素的影响。血清中白蛋白的半衰期为 14 ~ 20 天。白蛋白水平降低见于长期肝功能障碍或急性肝损伤，白蛋白浓度下降反映了白蛋白合成减少。

低白蛋白血症并不一定反映肝脏合成功能障碍。营养不良、肾病综合征、蛋白质丢失性肠病和全身炎症等其他情况也可能导致白蛋白水平下降。

凝血因子和凝血酶原时间

肝脏是 11 种凝血因子合成的主要场所，包括凝血因子 I、II、V、VII、IX、X、XII 和 XIII。凝血因子缺乏主要见于较严重或较晚期的肝脏疾病。这些凝血因子可以单独检测或通过凝血酶原时间（PT）来间接检测。

PT 取决于凝血因子 II、V、VII 和 X，这些凝血因子均在肝脏中合成。PT 延长并不是肝脏疾病特有的表现，可见于多种先天性或获得性疾病。排除上述情况后，PT 延长通常继发于维生素 K 缺乏（饮食摄入不足、长期阻塞性黄疸、肠道吸收不良或长期使用广谱抗生素）或进展期肝病所致的维生素 K 利用障碍。在维生素 K 缺乏的情况下，单次注射维生素 K 即可使 PT 恢复正常。

PT 延长的程度可反映肝脏疾病的严重程度；然而，PT 和肝硬化患者的凝血状态或出血风险并不完全相关。事实上，肝硬化患者抗凝血因子的合成也会减少，部分患者虽然 PT 延长，但处于相对高凝状态，其血栓形成风险反而增加。这是一个重要且经常被误解的概念。

丙种球蛋白

单项丙种球蛋白水平升高可能提示特定的肝脏疾病。例如，自身免疫性肝炎（AIH）患者免疫球蛋白 G（IgG）水平升高，PBC 患者免疫球蛋白 M（IgM）水平升高，酒精性肝硬化患者免疫球蛋白 A（IgA）水平升高。IgG4 相关性疾病是一类自身免疫病，IgG4 水平升高可导致多器官功能障碍，包括胆道（IgG4 相关性胆管病变）。

肝脏疾病的特异性标志物

部分肝脏疾病的诊断需要进行特定的实验室检查。

- **α_1-抗胰蛋白酶（α_1-AT）**：可定量检测，若 α_1-AT 水平降低，可测定其表型
- **AIH**：抗核抗体（ANA）、抗平滑肌抗体（ASMA）、抗肝肾微粒体抗体 1 型（抗 LKM-1）

- **Primary biliary cholangitis:** antimitochondrial antibody (AMA)
- **Hemochromatosis:** iron panel (serum iron, total iron binding capacity, transferrin saturation and ferritin) and HFE gene mutations
- **Wilson's disease:** serum ceruloplasmin and urinary copper levels
- **Viruses:** different viruses (e.g., hepatitis A, B, C, D, E, Epstein-Barr virus, cytomegalovirus, and herpes virus) that cause hepatitis are detected using polymerase chain reaction.

Biomarkers of Liver Fibrosis

Liver biopsy is the "gold standard" for evaluation of liver histopathology. Although the complications are few, it is an invasive test and the need for less invasive means to evaluate fibrosis led to several studies in search of surrogate markers for hepatic fibrosis. Many such tests combine clinical and serum markers and have been validated in specific populations, particularly chronic hepatitis C and nonalcoholic fatty liver disease. Caution is needed when using the results in other patient populations. In addition, serum markers are not liver specific and concurrent sites of inflammation may contribute to deranged serum levels.

These tests are used to differentiate patients with more significant stages of fibrosis and cirrhosis (stages 3 and 4), from those with minimal or no fibrosis (stages 0 and 1). The stages are based on the METAVIR score and range from 0 to 4, where stage 4 corresponds to cirrhosis.

Examples of such tests include the following:

- **APRI Score** is based on the AST and platelet count (AST elevation/platelet count) × 100. It has been mostly studied in patients with HCV, HCV and HIV co-infection, alcoholic liver disease, and NAFLD.
- **FibroSure or FibroTest** uses the measurement of α2-macroglobulin, α2-globulin, γ-globulin, apolipoprotein A1, GGT, and total bilirubin. It also utilizes the patient's age and sex. The results classify the patients as having mild fibrosis, indeterminate fibrosis or significant fibrosis. It has been better studied in patients with HCV and has a better specificity than sensitivity.
- **HepaScore** utilizes the combination of bilirubin, GGT, hyaluronic acid, α2-macroglobulin, age, and sex. Its performance is similar to the FibroTest.
- **FIB 4 index** combines platelet count, ALT, AST, and age. Better studied in HCV and NAFLD.
- **NAFLD fibrosis score** considers the patient's age, body mass index, blood glucose, aminotransferases, platelet count, and albumin.

Other panel tests have included products of collagen synthesis or degradation, enzymes involved in matrix biosynthesis or degradation, extracellular matrix glycoproteins, and proteoglycans/glycosaminoglycans.

The routine use of these panels in clinical practice is not clearly established and some suggest their use in combination with image modalities.

Image tests applying mechanical waves and measuring their propagation speed through liver tissue using ultrasound and MRI have become more readily available. They have been studied in a broader spectrum of liver diseases and have better sensitivity and specificity than the serologic tests. Nevertheless, at this point none of these tests fully substitute for liver biopsy.

SUGGESTED READINGS

Gao Y, Zheng J, Liang P, et al: Liver fibrosis with two-dimensional US shear-wave elastography in participants with chronic hepatitis B: a prospective multicenter study, Radiology 289:407–415, 2018.

Newsome PN, Cramb R, Davison SM, et al: Guidelines on the management of abnormal liver blood tests, Gut 67:6–19, 2018.

Northup PG, Caldwell SH: Coagulation in liver disease: a guide for the clinician, Clin Gastroenterol Hepatol 11:1064–1074, 2013.

Poynard T, De Ledinghen V, Zarski JP, et al: Relative performances of FibroTest, Fibroscan, and biopsy for the assessment of the stage of liver fibrosis in patients with chronic hepatitis C: a step toward the truth in the absence of a gold standard, J Hepatol 56:541–548, 2012.

Rockey D, Caldwell SH, Goodman ZD, et al: AASLD position paper: liver biopsy, Hepatology 49:1017–1044, 2009.

Sebastiani G, Halfon P, Castera L, et al: Comparison of three algorithms of non-invasive markers of fibrosis in chronic hepatitis C, Aliment Pharmacol Ther 35:92–104, 2012.

Tapper EB, Saini SC, Sengupta N: Extensive testing or focused testing of patients with elevated liver enzymes, J Hepatol 66:313–319, 2017.

- **PBC**：抗线粒体抗体（AMA）
- **血色病**：铁代谢检查（血清铁、总铁结合力、转铁蛋白饱和度和铁蛋白）和 *HFE* 基因突变
- **肝豆状核变性**：血清铜蓝蛋白和尿铜水平
- **病毒**：通过聚合酶链反应（PCR）检测可引起肝炎的不同病毒（如甲型、乙型、丙型、丁型、戊型肝炎病毒，以及 EB 病毒、巨细胞病毒和疱疹病毒）

肝纤维化的生物标志物

肝活检是评价肝组织病理学的"金标准"。尽管并发症很少，但肝活检是一种侵入性检查。对无创性评估肝纤维化的需求促使人们开展了多项探索肝纤维化替代标志物的研究。许多检测将临床和血清学标志物结合在一起，并在特定人群中得到了验证，特别是在慢性丙型肝炎和 NAFLD 患者中。在将这些研究结果用于其他患者人群时需谨慎。此外，血清学标志物并不是肝脏特异性的，合并其他部位炎症也可能影响其血清水平。

这些检测可用于鉴别显著纤维化和肝硬化（3 期和 4 期）的患者与轻微肝纤维化或无肝纤维化（0 期和 1 期）的患者。METAVIR 评分将肝纤维化分为 0～4 期，其中 4 期为肝硬化。

这类检测包括：

- **APRI 评分**基于 AST 和血小板计数 [计算公式为：AST 升高的倍数 / 血小板计数（10^9/L）] × 100。有关 APRI 评分的研究主要在丙型肝炎病毒（HCV）、HCV 与人类免疫缺陷病毒（HIV）重叠感染、酒精性肝病和 NAFLD 患者中进行。
- **FibroSure 或 FibroTest** 通过检测 α_2- 巨球蛋白、α_2- 球蛋白、γ- 球蛋白、载脂蛋白 A1、GGT 和总胆红素来进行评估。同时，它还需要用到患者的年龄和性别。其结果将患者分为轻度纤维化、不确定纤维化和显著纤维化。它在 HCV 感染患者中的研究更为深入，其特异性高于敏感性。
- **HepaScore** 通过结合胆红素、GGT、透明质酸、α_2- 巨球蛋白、年龄和性别来进行评估。其诊断效能和 FibroTest 相似。
- **FIB 4 指数**综合了血小板计数、ALT、AST 和年龄。在 HCV 感染和 NAFLD 患者中的研究更深入。
- **NAFLD 纤维化评分**综合了患者的年龄、体重指数、血糖、转氨酶、血小板计数和白蛋白。

其他检测模型中还包含了胶原蛋白合成或降解产物、参与基质生物合成或降解的酶、细胞外基质糖蛋白、蛋白聚糖 / 糖胺聚糖等指标。

这些检测模型在临床实践中的常规应用尚未得到公认，有人建议将其与影像学检查联合使用。

采用超声和 MRI 测量机械波在肝组织中的传播速度的影像学检查越来越普及。这些检查已在更广泛的肝脏疾病中进行了研究，且比血清学检测具有更高的敏感性和特异性。尽管如此，目前为止仍没有任何检查能够完全替代肝活检。

推荐阅读

Gao Y, Zheng J, Liang P, et al: Liver fibrosis with two-dimensional US shear-wave elastography in participants with chronic hepatitis B: a prospective multicenter study, Radiology 289:407–415, 2018.

Newsome PN, Cramb R, Davison SM, et al: Guidelines on the management of abnormal liver blood tests, Gut 67:6–19, 2018.

Northup PG, Caldwell SH: Coagulation in liver disease: a guide for the clinician, Clin Gastroenterol Hepatol 11:1064–1074, 2013.

Poynard T, De Ledinghen V, Zarski JP, et al: Relative performances of FibroTest, Fibroscan, and biopsy for the assessment of the stage of liver fibrosis in patients with chronic hepatitis C: a step toward the truth in the absence of a gold standard, J Hepatol 56:541–548, 2012.

Rockey D, Caldwell SH, Goodman ZD, et al: AASLD position paper: liver biopsy, Hepatology 49:1017–1044, 2009.

Sebastiani G, Halfon P, Castera L, et al: Comparison of three algorithms of non-invasive markers of fibrosis in chronic hepatitis C, Aliment Pharmacol Ther 35:92–104, 2012.

Tapper EB, Saini SC, Sengupta N: Extensive testing or focused testing of patients with elevated liver enzymes, J Hepatol 66:313–319, 2017.

11

Jaundice

Mohanad T. Al-Qaisi, Mashal Batheja, Michael B. Fallon

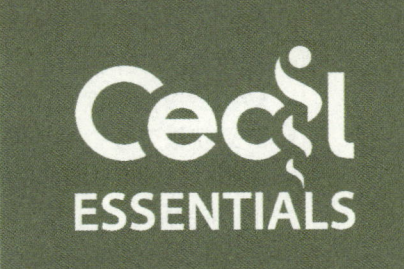

INTRODUCTION

Jaundice is the condition of yellowish pigmentation of the skin, the conjunctival membranes over the sclera, and other mucous membranes that is caused by elevated serum bilirubin levels (hyperbilirubinemia). The term jaundice is derived from *jaune*, the French word for "yellow," and the condition is also known as *icterus* (Greek for "yellow"). Normal serum bilirubin levels range from 0.5 to 1.0 mg/dL, and plasma bilirubin concentrations typically must exceed 2.5 mg/dL before jaundice becomes evident clinically.

Although jaundice is commonly due to liver and biliary tract disease, it has many causes, so it is not surprising that the diagnosis and management of jaundice have challenged clinicians for centuries. In most cases, jaundice or hyperbilirubinemia per se is not a pathologic condition but rather a sign of one or more illnesses originating from or affecting the liver and blood. However, there is one notable exception: In newborns, high bilirubin levels can lead to pathologic cerebral changes. In this condition, which is known as *kernicterus* (*kern* is the German word for "nucleus"), persistent elevation of unconjugated bilirubin leads to its deposition in the cerebral basal ganglia (or nuclei). This process can be prevented and treated and therefore merits special recognition to prevent damage to the developing brain.

BILIRUBIN METABOLISM

Hyperbilirubinemia can be classified based on the three phases of hepatic bilirubin metabolism: uptake, conjugation, and excretion into the bile (the rate-limiting step). In addition, jaundice can be classified into prehepatic, hepatic, and posthepatic causes (Table 11.1). Although the approaches are complementary, the latter classification may be more useful for the practicing clinician.

The main source of bilirubin is the hemoglobin released from senescent red blood cells, and the liver serves as its primary site of metabolism and excretion. Abnormalities at any step in bilirubin production, metabolism, or excretion can lead to an increase in the serum bilirubin and clinical jaundice. Under normal conditions, human red blood cells have a lifespan of about 120 days. As they age, erythrocytes are broken down and removed from the circulation by phagocytes. Most bilirubin (80%) is derived from the breakdown of hemoglobin released from these cells; the remainder is derived from ineffective erythropoiesis in the bone marrow and from catabolism of myoglobin and hepatic hemoproteins such as the cytochrome P-450 isoenzymes. The normal rate of bilirubin production is approximately 4 mg/kg body weight per day.

As erythrocytes are destroyed within the reticuloendothelial system, free hemoglobin is ingested by macrophages and then split into heme and globin moieties. The heme ring is cleaved by the enzyme microsomal heme oxygenase to form biliverdin (*verde* = "green"), which is then converted to the tetrapyrrole pigment bilirubin by the cytosolic enzyme biliverdin reductase. This unconjugated (or "indirect") bilirubin is released into the plasma, where it is tightly bound to albumin. Because unconjugated bilirubin is insoluble in water, it cannot be excreted in urine or bile. However, it is permeable across lipid-rich environments and therefore can traverse the blood-brain barrier and the placenta.

The unconjugated bilirubin-albumin complex is transported to the liver. Once in the space of Disse, this complex dissociates; unconjugated bilirubin is transported across the basolateral plasma membrane of liver cells and attaches to intracellular binding proteins (ligandins). It is then conjugated with glucuronic acid by the enzyme uridine diphosphate glucuronyl transferase (UDP-GT) to form bilirubin monoglucuronide and diglucuronide, making the molecule water soluble. This conjugated (or "direct") bilirubin is excreted into bile via active transport across the canalicular membrane by means of a multispecific canalicular transport protein. In healthy persons, most bilirubin circulates in its unconjugated form with less than 5% of circulating bilirubin appearing in its conjugated form. If biliary excretion of conjugated bilirubin is impaired, it can exit the basolateral membrane and reenter the circulation, causing an increase in plasma levels. Because conjugated bilirubin is water soluble and less tightly bound to albumin than its unconjugated form, it is readily filtered by the glomerulus and appears in the urine, giving it a dark color (choluria). Once in bile, bilirubin enters the intestine, where bacteria convert it to colorless tetrapyrroles (urobilinogens) that are excreted in feces. Up to 20% of urobilinogen is reabsorbed and undergoes enterohepatic circulation or excretion in urine.

LABORATORY MEASUREMENT OF BILIRUBIN

The *van den Bergh reaction,* which is the most commonly used test for detecting bilirubin in biologic fluids, combines bilirubin with diazotized sulfanilic acid to form a colored compound. The direct-reacting fraction is roughly equivalent to conjugated bilirubin and the indirect-reacting fraction (total minus direct fraction) to unconjugated bilirubin. This characteristic provides a means for classifying jaundice into two categories: unconjugated hyperbilirubinemia and conjugated hyperbilirubinemia.

UNCONJUGATED HYPERBILIRUBINEMIA

Mechanisms that cause unconjugated hyperbilirubinemia include overproduction, impaired hepatic uptake, and decreased conjugation

黄疸

武丽娜 译　王晓明　马红 审校　贾继东 通审

引言

黄疸是指由血清胆红素水平升高（高胆红素血症）引起皮肤、巩膜及黏膜等出现黄染的现象。"jaundice"一词来源于法语的"jaune"，同希腊语的"icterus"，意为"黄色"。正常血清胆红素浓度为 0.5～1.0 mg/dl，通常仅在血清胆红素浓度 > 2.5 mg/dl 时，才会出现临床显性黄疸。

虽然黄疸通常由肝脏疾病和胆道疾病引起，但其原因繁多，因此数百年来黄疸的诊断和治疗一直是临床医生面临的挑战。大多数情况下，黄疸或高胆红素血症并不是一个独立疾病，而是由原发性或继发性肝脏疾病或血液疾病引起的症状。但有一个需特别注意的例外：新生儿高胆红素血症可引起核黄疸（kernicterus，"kern"在德语中意为"核"）。它是由于持续升高的血清非结合胆红素沉积在大脑基底神经节（或神经核），导致大脑病理性改变。核黄疸是可防和可治的，因此，需要临床注意识别，防止新生儿大脑受损。

胆红素代谢

肝脏胆红素代谢涉及 3 个阶段：胆红素摄取、结合和排泄入胆汁，其中排泄是限速步骤，据此可对高胆红素血症进行分类。此外，根据病因可将黄疸分为肝前性、肝细胞性和肝后性（表 11.1）。后一种分类对临床医生来说可能更为实用。

胆红素主要来源于衰老红细胞释放的血红蛋白，肝脏是胆红素代谢和排泄的主要场所。胆红素生成、代谢或排泄过程中出现任何异常都可能导致血清胆红素水平升高，引起黄疸。正常情况下，人类红细胞的寿命约为 120 天。红细胞衰老后，被吞噬细胞分解并清除出循环系统。大部分胆红素（约 80%）来源于吞噬细胞分解释放的血红蛋白；少部分则来源于骨髓中的无效造血，以及肌红蛋白和肝脏血红素蛋白（如细胞色素 P450 同工酶）的分解代谢。正常情况下，机体每天生成胆红素约 4 mg/kg。

当红细胞在网状内皮系统中被破坏，游离血红蛋白被巨噬细胞摄取并分解为血红素和珠蛋白。血红素环被微粒体中的血红素加氧酶切割而形成胆绿素，随后通过胞质胆绿素还原酶转化为胆红素。这种非结合胆红素（即间接胆红素）释放入血浆中，并与白蛋白紧密结合。由于非结合胆红素不溶于水，不能通过尿液或胆汁排出，但可透过脂质，因此能够穿过血脑屏障和胎盘。

非结合胆红素-白蛋白复合物被运输至肝脏。进入窦周隙（Disse 间隙）后，非结合胆红素与白蛋白分离，并通过肝细胞基底外侧膜转运，与细胞内的结合蛋白（Y 蛋白）结合。随后，在尿苷二磷酸-葡萄糖醛酸基转移酶（UDP-GT）的作用下，非结合胆红素与葡萄糖醛酸结合，形成具有水溶性的胆红素单葡糖醛酸和双葡糖醛酸。这种结合胆红素（即直接胆红素）通过特异性转运蛋白的主动转运，跨过毛细胆管膜并排泄至胆汁中。正常情况下，大多数胆红素以非结合形式存在，只有不足 5% 的胆红素以结合形式存在。如果胆汁排泄受损，结合胆红素可能脱离基底外侧膜，重新进入血液循环，导致血清胆红素水平升高。由于结合胆红素为水溶性，与白蛋白的结合不如非结合胆红素紧密，因此易被肾小球滤过，排入尿液中，使尿液颜色加深（胆汁尿）。胆红素进入胆管并排入肠道，在肠道细菌的作用下转化为无色的四吡咯（尿胆原），通过粪便排出。20% 的尿胆原可被重吸收，参与肠肝循环或通过尿液排出。

胆红素的实验室测定

范登贝赫反应（van den Bergh reaction）是被广泛用于检测体液中胆红素水平的检测方法。该方法通过将胆红素与对氨基苯磺酸的重氮化合物结合，形成有色产物。该检测的直接反应部分主要反映了结合胆红素的含量，而间接反应部分（即总反应减去直接反应部分）主要代表非结合胆红素水平。这种方法可将黄疸分为两大类：高非结合胆红素血症和高结合胆红素血症。

高非结合胆红素血症

多种机制可导致高非结合胆红素血症，包括胆红素生成过量、肝脏对胆红素的摄取障碍和胆红素结合

TABLE 11.1 Classification of Jaundice and Representative Causes

Prehepatic Causes
Predominantly unconjugated hyperbilirubinemia
Hemolysis (e.g., sickle cell disease, autoimmune hemolytic anemia, mechanical cardiac valve with accelerated red cell destruction)
Microbe-induced hemolysis (malaria, leptospirosis)
Ineffective erythropoiesis (e.g., megaloblastic anemias)
Hematoma resolution

Hepatic Causes
Unconjugated hyperbilirubinemia
Decreased hepatic uptake
   Therapeutic drugs that interfere with bilirubin uptake (e.g., rifampin, metformin, methimazole, propylthiouracil, clopidogrel, sulfamethoxazole/trimethoprim)
   Herbal medicines (e.g., *Teucrium viscidum*, kava-kava, chaparral, greater celandine)
   Hyperthyroidism
   Diminished uptake and decreased cytosolic binding proteins (e.g., newborn or premature infants)
   Shunting of blood away from the liver (portal hypertension or surgical shunt)
Decreased conjugation due to limited glucuronyl transferase activity
   Gilbert syndrome
   Crigler-Najjar syndrome types I and II
   Neonatal jaundice
   Breast-milk jaundice
   Drug-induced inhibition (e.g., chloramphenicol)
Predominantly conjugated hyperbilirubinemia
Impaired hepatic excretion
   Familial cholestasis (Dubin-Johnson syndrome, Rotor syndrome, benign recurrent cholestasis, cholestasis of pregnancy)
   Hepatocellular injury from infiltrative disorders, hemochromatosis, α_1-antitrypsin deficiency, lymphoma, sarcoidosis, extensive metastases
   Liver cirrhosis
   Hepatitis
   Drug-induced cholestasis (chlorpromazine, erythromycin estolate, isoniazid, halothane, and many others)
   Primary biliary cirrhosis
   Congestive heart failure
   Sepsis

Posthepatic Causes
Extrahepatic biliary obstruction
   Common bile duct obstruction from gallstones
   Benign and malignant tumors of the pancreas
   Tumors of bile ducts (cholangiocarcinoma) and ampulla of Vater
   Biliary strictures (postsurgical, gallstone-related, primary sclerosing cholangitis)
   Congenital disorders (biliary atresia, cystic fibrosis)
   Infectious cholangiopathy
   Chronic pancreatitis (fibrosis of the head of the pancreas)

of bilirubin. These disorders are not usually associated with significant hepatic disease.

Etiology of Hyperbilirubinemia

There are many potential causes of hyperbilirubinemia, and the major categories are summarized in Table 11.1. It is helpful to consider them mechanistically as conditions affecting the balance of bilirubin production, liver metabolism, and excretion. The classic cause of bilirubin overproduction is hemolysis, whereas the most common cause of impaired bilirubin uptake and metabolism is cirrhosis or other liver disease (viral hepatitis, drugs, hepatotoxins or ischemia). Bile duct obstruction due to cancer (classically cholangiocarcinoma or pancreatic head cancer), stones, or strictures is the most common cause of obstructive jaundice. Because multiple mechanisms are often involved in an individual patient, the evaluation of jaundice can be complex.

Prehepatic Jaundice

Prehepatic jaundice is associated with excessive bilirubin production (Fig. 11.1), which most often results from hemolysis (intravascular or extravascular), resolution of large hematomas, or mechanical injury to red cells, as in disseminated intravascular coagulation. Certain genetic diseases can lead to increased red cell lysis and therefore hemolytic jaundice. Sickle cell anemia is the classic cause, but others include glucose 6-phosphate dehydrogenase deficiency and hereditary spherocytosis. Infectious diseases also can cause hemolysis, either directly (e.g., malaria) or indirectly (e.g., autoimmune injury). Jaundice resulting from hemolysis is characteristically mild in degree, and serum bilirubin levels rarely exceed 5 mg/dL in the absence of coexisting hepatic disease. Ineffective erythropoiesis, which may be significantly increased in megaloblastic anemia, also leads to mild jaundice.

表 11.1 黄疸的分类和典型病因

肝前性病因
主要为高非结合胆红素血症
溶血（如镰状细胞贫血、自身免疫性溶血性贫血、心脏机械瓣膜加速红细胞破坏）
微生物引起的溶血（疟疾、钩端螺旋体病）
无效造血（如巨幼红细胞贫血）
血肿消散

肝脏原因
高非结合胆红素血症
肝脏摄取减少
  影响胆红素摄取的药物（如利福平、二甲双胍、甲巯咪唑、丙硫氧嘧啶、氯吡格雷、磺胺甲噁唑/甲氧苄啶）
  草药（如山藿香、卡瓦、槲树、白屈菜）
  甲状腺功能亢进症
  摄取减少和胞质结合蛋白减少（如新生儿或早产儿）
  血液分流（门静脉高压或外科分流）
葡萄糖醛酸基转移酶活性降低，胆红素结合减少
  Gilbert 综合征
  Crigler-Najjar 综合征 I 型和 II 型
  新生儿黄疸
  母乳性黄疸
  药物抑制葡萄糖醛酸基转移酶活性（如氯霉素）
高结合胆红素血症
肝脏排泄受损
  家族性胆汁淤积（Dubin-Johnson 综合征、Rotor 综合征、良性复发性胆汁淤积、妊娠期胆汁淤积）
  肝细胞损伤（由浸润性疾病、血色病、α_1-抗胰蛋白酶缺乏症、淋巴瘤、结节病、恶性肿瘤广泛肝转移引起）
  肝硬化
  肝炎
  药物诱导的胆汁淤积（氯丙嗪、红霉素、异烟肼、氟烷等多种药物）
  原发性胆汁性肝硬化
  充血性心力衰竭
  感染中毒症

肝后性病因
肝外胆管梗阻
  胆结石引起胆总管梗阻
  胰腺良恶性肿瘤
  胆管癌和壶腹癌
  胆道狭窄（术后、胆结石相关、原发性硬化性胆管炎）
  先天性疾病（胆道闭锁、囊性纤维化）
  感染性胆管病变
  慢性胰腺炎（胰头纤维化）

减少。这些疾病通常不伴有严重肝脏疾病。

高胆红素血症的病因

多种原因可引起高胆红素血症，表 11.1 列出了主要原因。根据对胆红素生成、代谢和排泄机制的影响对这些病因进行分类，有助于更好地理解高胆红素血症。胆红素生成过多的典型病因是溶血，而胆红素摄取和代谢障碍的常见原因包括肝硬化及其他肝脏疾病，如病毒性肝炎、药物或毒物性肝损伤、肝缺血等。梗阻性黄疸最常见的原因是由癌症（多见于胆管癌或胰头癌）、胆石症或胆管狭窄引起的胆道梗阻。由于黄疸的发生涉及多种机制，其评估比较复杂。

肝前性黄疸

肝前性黄疸通常与胆红素生成过多相关（图 11.1），主要原因包括溶血（血管内或血管外溶血）、大血肿吸收消散或红细胞机械损伤（如弥散性血管内凝血）。某些遗传性疾病可导致红细胞破坏增多，进而引起溶血性黄疸。镰状细胞贫血是典型的病因，其他可能的病因还包括葡萄糖-6-磷酸脱氢酶缺乏症和遗传性球形红细胞增多症。此外，感染性疾病也可能直接（如疟疾）或间接（如通过自身免疫性损伤）导致溶血。溶血引起的黄疸通常较轻，在没有其他肝脏疾病的情况下，血清胆红素水平很少超过 5 mg/dl。巨幼红细胞贫血患者的无效造血显著增加，可能引起轻度黄疸。

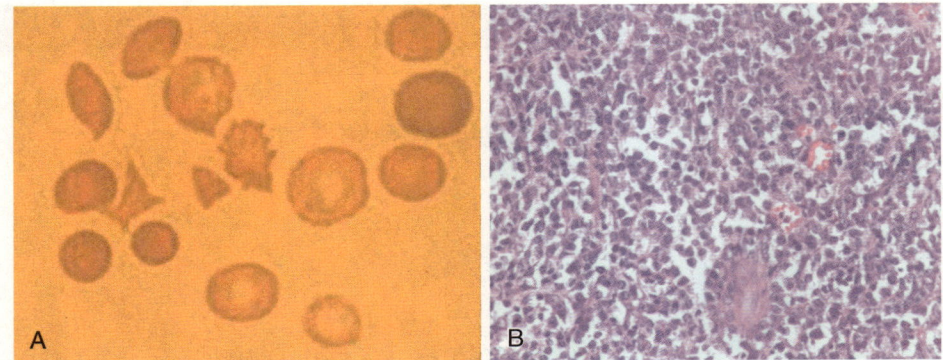

Fig. 11.1 Hemolytic anemia associated with lymphoma. (A) Blood smear shows the destroyed red blood cells. (B) Lymphoma.

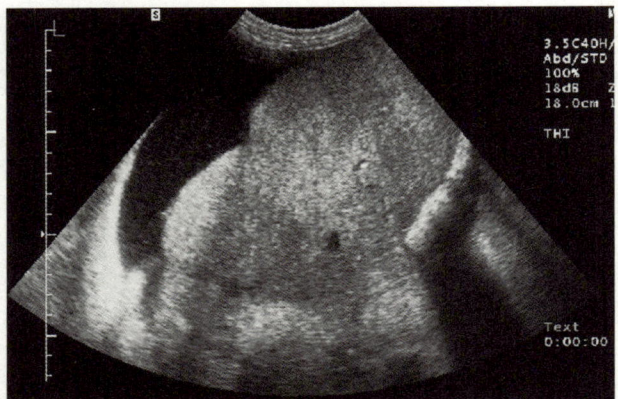

Fig. 11.2 Ultrasound image shows a cirrhotic liver with atrophy, irregular contours, and ascites.

Hemolysis should be considered in the evaluation of unconjugated hyperbilirubinemia and evaluated by examination of the peripheral blood smear (and, in some cases, the bone marrow smear and biopsy) as well as measurements of the reticulocyte count, haptoglobin, lactate dehydrogenase (LDH), erythrocyte fragility, and Coombs testing as indicated.

Hepatic or Hepatocellular Jaundice

Typically, considerable reserve exists within the liver, so jaundice of hepatocellular origin can be indicative of significant injury or dysfunction. The differential diagnosis is broad because the liver is susceptible to many different forms of injury (Fig. 11.2). The most common categories are viral hepatitis, exposure to toxins (e.g., alcohol, carbon tetrachloride, amanita, and increasingly herbs and supplements), medications (INH, antibiotics), autoimmune disorders (e.g., autoimmune hepatitis, primary biliary cholangitis [PBC], primary sclerosing cholangitis [PSC]), and liver tumors (primary or metastatic). Impaired hepatic uptake of bilirubin can be a cause of unconjugated hyperbilirubinemia. When present, it is typically caused by competition for bilirubin uptake by drugs such as rifampin. Removal of the competing agent usually leads to resolution of the jaundice.

Impaired Conjugation

Another common cause of unconjugated hyperbilirubinemia is Gilbert syndrome, a benign disorder that affects up to 7% of the population. This represents a normal variant that is not associated with intrinsic liver disease. Rather, it typically manifests during the second or third decade of life as mild unconjugated hyperbilirubinemia that is exacerbated by fasting or physical stress. Most of those affected have a total bilirubin level of less than 3 mg/dL, mostly of the unconjugated (indirect) fraction. The underlying genetic variant responsible is a homozygous abnormality in the TATAA element of the promoter region of the UDP-GT gene that results in lower enzymatic levels. The diagnosis is strongly suggested by unconjugated hyperbilirubinemia in the setting of normal hepatic enzyme levels, no known liver disease, and no evidence of hemolysis. Liver biopsy usually is not indicated, and therapy is not warranted. However, the bilirubin level does decrease significantly with phenobarbital administration. It is important to be aware of this common cause of unconjugated hyperbilirubinemia so that the patient can be reassured and more costly or invasive tests can be avoided. Although Gilbert syndrome has generally been thought to have a benign course, sometimes people with this condition might be at an increased risk of developing gallstones. On the other hand, patients with Gilbert syndrome might be at a lower risk to develop cardiovascular disease, because unconjugated bilirubin has antioxidant properties that may offer some protective effect and mitigate progression of atherosclerosis.

Crigler-Najjar syndrome is another cause of unconjugated hyperbilirubinemia in which the bilirubin levels may be much higher due to a genetically determined decrease or absence of UDP-GT activity. Conjugation may also be impaired by mild, acquired defects of UDP-GT induced by drugs such as chloramphenicol.

NEONATAL JAUNDICE

About 50% of term and 80% of preterm babies develop jaundice, which usually appears 2 to 4 days after birth and resolves spontaneously after 1 to 2 weeks. Most jaundice in newborn infants occurs for two main reasons. First, the enzymatic and transport pathways responsible for bilirubin metabolism are relatively immature and are unable to conjugate bilirubin as efficiently or as quickly as in adults. Second, bilirubin production is increased. Of those two mechanisms, the major defect is in bilirubin conjugation, which may cause mild to moderate unconjugated hyperbilirubinemia between the second and fifth days of life lasting until day 8 in normal births or about day 14 in premature births. This neonatal jaundice is usually harmless, and no specific therapy is required other than close observation.

More severe pathologic unconjugated hyperbilirubinemia can occur in neonates and usually is caused by a combination of hemolysis secondary to blood group incompatibility and defective conjugation. This neonatal jaundice is a serious condition that requires immediate

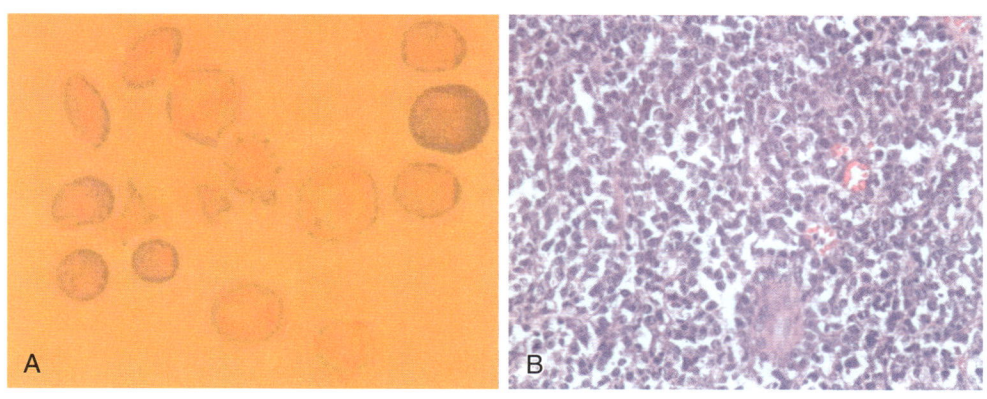

图 11.1 淋巴瘤相关的溶血性贫血。A. 血涂片显示被破坏的红细胞。B. 淋巴瘤

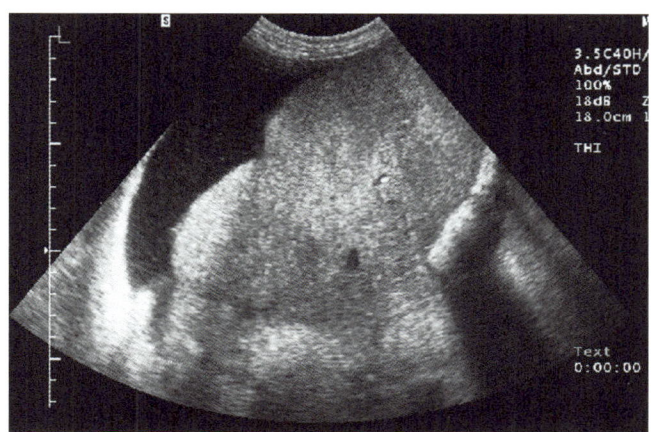

图 11.2 超声图像显示肝硬化，伴有肝脏萎缩、轮廓不规则和腹腔积液

在高非结合胆红素血症时，应考虑溶血的可能性，并进行外周血涂片（某些情况还应行骨髓涂片和活检）、网织红细胞计数、结合珠蛋白、乳酸脱氢酶（LDH）、红细胞脆性及 Coombs 试验等检测。

肝细胞性黄疸

肝脏有较强的储备能力，因此肝细胞性黄疸通常预示严重肝损伤或功能失调。多种原因可引起肝损伤（图 11.2），需仔细鉴别诊断。最常见的原因包括病毒性肝炎，毒物（如酒精、四氯化碳、鹅膏菌，以及部分草药和膳食补充剂），药物（如异烟肼、抗生素），自身免疫病［如自身免疫性肝炎、原发性胆汁性胆管炎（PBC）、原发性硬化性胆管炎（PSC）］和肝脏肿瘤（原发性或转移性）。肝脏对胆红素摄取受损可能是高非结合胆红素血症的原因之一，多见于某些药物（如利福平）与胆红素发生竞争性摄取。停用这些竞争性药物后，黄疸通常可消退。

胆红素结合受损

吉尔伯特综合征（Gilbert 综合征）是高非结合胆红素血症的另一个常见原因，人群中的发病率高达 7%，它是一种良性疾病，与肝脏疾病无关，属于正常的生理变异。通常在青少年或成年早期表现为轻度高非结合胆红素血症，在禁食或应激时加重。大多数患者总胆红素 < 3 mg/dl，以非结合胆红素升高为主。Gilbert 综合征主要是由于 *UDP-GT* 基因启动子区域 TATAA 元件的纯合突变，导致 UDP-GT 活性降低。在肝酶水平正常、无已知肝脏疾病或溶血的情况下，高非结合胆红素血症强烈提示 Gilbert 综合征。患者通常不需要肝活检和特殊治疗。当应用苯巴比妥后，患者胆红素水平会显著下降。了解 Gilbert 综合征的特点非常重要，因为这可避免患者不必要的担忧，并避免侵入性检查和更多费用。虽然 Gilbert 综合征总体上是一种良性疾病，但部分患者患胆石症的风险增加。另一方面，由于非结合胆红素具有抗氧化特性，有一定的保护作用，可减缓动脉粥样硬化的进展，Gilbert 综合征患者罹患心血管疾病的风险可能较低。

克-纳综合征（Crigler-Najjar 综合征）是另一种可导致高非结合胆红素血症的疾病，它是由于基因突变导致 UDP-GT 活性降低或完全缺失，患者的胆红素水平可能显著升高。此外，某些药物（如氯霉素）可引起 UDP-GT 获得性缺陷，影响胆红素结合。

新生儿黄疸

约 50% 的足月儿和 80% 的早产儿在出生后会出现黄疸，通常见于出生后 2～4 天内，黄疸于 1～2 周内可自行消退。大多数新生儿黄疸由两个主要原因引起。第一，参与新生儿胆红素代谢的酶和转运功能尚未完全成熟，不能高效、迅速地结合胆红素；第二，新生儿胆红素生成增加。两种机制中，胆红素结合能力不足更为关键，可导致轻中度高非结合胆红素血症（见于出生后第 2～5 天，足月儿可持续至第 8 天，早产儿可能持续至第 14 天）。新生儿黄疸通常为良性，除密切观察黄疸的程度外，不需要特殊治疗。

需要注意的是，新生儿期可能发生严重的病理性高非结合胆红素血症，通常是由血型不合引起溶血及胆红素结合缺陷所致。这种新生儿黄疸为临床急症，

attention because severe hyperbilirubinemia can lead to permanent neurologic damage (kernicterus). Phototherapy provided by conventional lighting or a fiberoptic light is the treatment of choice; it reduces neonatal jaundice (as assessed by serum bilirubin levels) compared with no treatment. Low-threshold compared with high-threshold phototherapy reduces neurodevelopmental impairment and hearing loss and reduces serum bilirubin on day 5 in infants with extremely low birth weight. However, it increases the duration of phototherapy, and it has no effect on mortality or on the rate of exchange transfusion. Close phototherapy, compared with distant light-source phototherapy, reduces the duration of phototherapy in infants with hyperbilirubinemia. If jaundice does not improve with phototherapy, other causes of neonatal jaundice should be assessed.

CONJUGATED HYPERBILIRUBINEMIA

Conjugated hyperbilirubinemia is associated with impaired formation or excretion of *all components* of bile, a situation termed *cholestasis*. The two major mechanisms of conjugated hyperbilirubinemia are defective excretion of bilirubin from hepatocytes into bile (intrahepatic cholestasis) and mechanical obstruction to the flow of bile through the bile ducts.

Impaired Hepatic Excretion (Intrahepatic Cholestasis)

Intrahepatic cholestasis can result from a wide range of conditions, including those that impair canalicular transport (e.g., certain drugs, circulating inflammatory cytokines during sepsis) and those that cause destruction of the small intrahepatic bile ducts. PBC, for example, is a chronic, progressive liver disease that occurs primarily in women and is characterized by the indolent destruction and subsequent disappearance over time of small lobular bile ducts. The gradual decrease in the number of bile ducts leads to progressive cholestasis, portal inflammation, fibrosis, and eventually cirrhosis. A similar loss of intrahepatic ducts can occur as a result of chronic rejection after liver transplantation.

Drug-induced cholestasis is increasingly common, and immune-mediated or idiosyncratic mechanisms can be the underlying cause. In some cases, there is associated hepatitis with significant cell injury (this can lead to hepatocellular damage and elevations in alanine aminotransferase [ALT] and aspartate aminotransferase [AST]). Representative drugs include, but are not limited to, nitrofurantoin, oral contraceptives, anabolic steroids, erythromycin, cimetidine, gold salts, chlorpromazine, prochlorperazine, imipramine, sulindac, tolbutamide, ampicillin, and other penicillin-based antibiotics. Given the broad access to drugs in Western societies and the unpredictable nature of the adverse liver effects, a high index of suspicion for drug-induced cholestasis is required. Drug-induced liver injury is generally considered a diagnosis of exclusion, after a thorough evaluation has ruled out other viral, autoimmune, and metabolic etiologies.

Intrahepatic cholestasis of pregnancy (ICP), also known as idiopathic jaundice of pregnancy, is a cholestatic disorder that is characterized by pruritus in the absence of a skin rash and elevation of aminotransferases (often up to 100 IU/L), alkaline phosphatase, 5-nucleotidase, and total and direct bilirubin concentrations. Total levels of bilirubin rarely exceed 6 mg/dL. The levels of γ-glutamyl transpeptidase are normal or only modestly elevated. ICP occurs in the second or third trimester of pregnancy and usually resolves spontaneously within 2 to 3 weeks after delivery. The diagnosis is suggested by the combination of pruritus and abnormal liver function tests with exclusion of other causes such as gallstones or intrinsic liver disease. ICP is associated with a higher risk for adverse perinatal outcome, including preterm birth, meconium passage, and fetal death.

The cause of ICP is not fully defined, but genetic, hormonal, and environmental factors are all likely to be involved. There is a high incidence of ICP in Chile and some other areas, and studies of potential genetic contributors are underway. Because adverse outcomes appear to occur predominantly after 37 weeks gestation, management by an experienced obstetrics team and consideration of early delivery are warranted. Ursodeoxycholic acid may be effective in ameliorating maternal pruritus and improving liver function test results; however, no medication has yet been shown to reduce the risk to the fetus.

The hemophagocytic syndrome, also known as hemophagocytic lymphohistiocytosis (HLH), is an uncommon hyperinflammatory disorder caused by severe hypercytokinemia. It manifests as fever, splenomegaly, and jaundice, with hemophagocytosis in the bone marrow and other tissues pathologically. Primary or familial HLH, also called familial erythrophagocytic lymphohistiocytosis, is a heterogeneous autosomal recessive disorder that has been found to be more prevalent with parental consanguinity. Secondary HLH is associated with malignancy, immunodeficiency, and infection, especially viral infection. In HLH, there is an inherent defect of natural killer cells and cytotoxic T cells, so they are unable to cope effectively with the infectious agent or antigen. Liver biopsies in HLH reveal sinusoidal dilation with hemophagocytic histiocytosis.

Postoperative jaundice typically occurs 1 to 10 days after surgery and has an incidence of approximately 15% after heart surgery and 1% after elective abdominal surgery. It is multifactorial in origin, with increased bilirubin load from bleeding and blood transfusions as well as impaired bilirubin conjugation and secretion caused by inflammatory cytokines. It typically resolves fully over time.

In hepatocellular disease, all three steps of hepatic bilirubin metabolism are impaired. Excretion, the rate-limiting step, is usually most affected, leading to predominantly conjugated hyperbilirubinemia.

Jaundice can be profound in acute hepatitis (see Chapter 12) without adverse prognostic implications. In chronic liver disease, however, persistent jaundice usually implies irreversible decrease in hepatic function and a poor prognosis.

Posthepatic Jaundice

Posthepatic jaundice, also called obstructive jaundice, results from a complete or partial obstruction of intrahepatic or extrahepatic bile ducts (Fig. 11.3). The most common causes are gallstones in the common bile duct and tumors of the pancreatic head. Not infrequently, the first sign of pancreatic cancer is jaundice. Other causes include strictures of the common bile duct resulting from prior surgery or passage of gallstones. Primary sclerosing cholangitis should be considered in the setting of jaundice and biliary strictures that may be seen on imaging studies (magnetic resonance cholangiopancreatography [MRCP] or endoscopic retrograde pancreatography [ERCP]). Less common causes include congenital biliary atresia, pancreatitis, pancreatic pseudocysts, and parasites such as liver flukes (e.g., *Clonorchis sinensis*, *Dicrocoelium dendriticum*, *Opisthorchis viverrini*).

Mirizzi syndrome is an uncommon cause of posthepatic jaundice observed in 0.7% to 1.4% of patients after cholecystectomy. This syndrome is caused by extrinsic compression from an impacted stone in the cystic duct that impinges on and obstructs the common bile duct (see Table 11.1). Portal hypertensive biliopathy (or vascular biliopathy) is characterized by anatomic and functional abnormalities of the intrahepatic, extrahepatic, and pancreatic ducts in patients with portal hypertension associated with extrahepatic portal vein obstruction or, less frequently, cirrhosis. These morphologic changes, consisting of dilatation and stenosis of the biliary tree, are caused by extensive venous collaterals that develop in an attempt to decompress the portal

需要立即治疗，因为严重的高胆红素血症会导致永久性神经损伤，即核黄疸。新生儿黄疸的首选治疗是使用传统照明灯或光纤灯进行光疗；光疗已被证明可降低血清胆红素水平，从而减轻新生儿黄疸的严重程度。与高阈值光疗相比，低阈值光疗可减轻极低体重儿的神经发育障碍和听力损失，同时降低出生后第5天的血清胆红素水平。但是，低阈值光疗可能会增加光疗的持续时间，且对死亡率或血浆置换需求没有显著影响。与使用远距离光源的光疗相比，近距离光疗能够缩短高胆红素血症婴儿的光疗时间。如果经光疗后黄疸状况没有改善，应进一步评估导致新生儿黄疸的其他可能原因。

高结合胆红素血症

高结合胆红素血症与所有胆汁成分的形成或排泄障碍有关，即胆汁淤积。导致高结合胆红素血症的两个主要机制包括：胆红素从肝细胞排泄到胆汁的过程障碍（肝内胆汁淤积）；胆汁在胆管中受到机械性阻塞。

肝排泄受损（肝内胆汁淤积）

肝内胆汁淤积可由多种因素引起，包括毛细胆管转运功能障碍（如特定药物、感染中毒症期间循环中的炎性细胞因子）和肝内小胆管破坏。例如，PBC是一种多见于女性的慢性进行性肝病，其特点是小叶内胆管的进行性破坏和消失。随着胆管数量的减少，会出现进行性肝内胆汁淤积、汇管区炎症、纤维化，最终发展为肝硬化。肝移植后的慢性排异反应也可引起类似的肝内胆管破坏消失。

药物诱导的胆汁淤积越来越常见，可能与免疫介导或特异质机制有关。部分患者伴有肝炎和明显的肝细胞损伤（ALT和AST水平升高）。代表性药物包括但不限于呋喃妥因、口服避孕药、合成类固醇、红霉素、西咪替丁、金盐、氯丙嗪、丙氯拉嗪、丙咪嗪、舒林酸、甲苯磺丁脲、氨苄西林和其他青霉素类抗生素等。由于药物的应用广泛，其引起的肝损伤不可预测，因此，应高度警惕药物诱导的胆汁淤积。药物诱导的肝损伤通常可通过排除法进行诊断，需要全面评估并排除病毒性、自身免疫性和代谢性病因等。

妊娠期肝内胆汁淤积（ICP）又称妊娠期特发性黄疸，是一种胆汁淤积性疾病，主要表现为无皮疹的瘙痒，以及转氨酶（通常不超过100 IU/L）、碱性磷酸酶、5-核苷酸酶、总胆红素和结合胆红素水平升高。总胆红素水平很少超过6 mg/dl，而γ-谷氨酰转移酶（GGT）水平通常正常或仅轻度升高。ICP多发生在妊娠中晚期，多于分娩后2～3周内自行消退。ICP的诊断需结合瘙痒症状和肝功能检查结果，同时排除其他原因，如胆石症或原发性肝脏疾病。ICP可导致发生围产期不良事件（如早产、羊水胎粪污染和死胎）的风险增加。

ICP的确切病因尚未完全明确，可能与遗传因素、激素水平和环境因素有关。在智利等地区，ICP的发病率相对较高，研究者正在探索可能涉及的遗传因素。ICP相关的不良事件主要发生于妊娠第37周之后，必须由产科专业团队进行诊疗，并评估是否需要提前终止妊娠。熊去氧胆酸已被证实能有效缓解ICP的瘙痒症状，改善肝功能指标，但目前尚无药物能够降低ICP相关胎儿不良事件的风险。

噬血细胞综合征（HLH）又称噬血细胞性淋巴组织细胞增生症，是一种少见的由大量炎性细胞因子引起的过度炎症反应综合征。HLH的临床表现包括发热、脾大和黄疸，以及在骨髓和其他组织中出现噬血现象。原发性或家族性HLH是一种杂合性常染色体隐性遗传病，在父母近亲结婚的子女中更常见。继发性HLH与恶性肿瘤、免疫缺陷和感染（尤其是病毒感染）有关。在HLH患者中，自然杀伤（NK）细胞和细胞毒性T细胞的功能缺陷，无法有效识别病原体或抗原。肝活检可显示肝窦扩张和噬血细胞浸润。

术后黄疸通常发生于外科手术后1～10天，心脏手术和择期腹部手术后的黄疸发病率分别约为15%和1%。术后黄疸的发生可能与多种因素有关，包括出血和输血导致的胆红素负荷增加，以及炎性细胞因子对胆红素结合和分泌的影响等。术后黄疸通常随时间而逐渐完全恢复。

在肝细胞性疾病中，胆红素代谢的各个步骤都可能受损。胆红素排泄过程（限速步骤）通常受影响最大，主要表现为高结合胆红素血症。

急性肝炎时黄疸可能较严重（见第12章），但通常不会导致预后不良。但是，慢性肝病出现持续性黄疸通常预示着肝功能不可逆性损伤和预后不良。

肝后性黄疸

肝后性黄疸（即梗阻性黄疸）通常由肝内或肝外胆管完全或部分梗阻所致（图11.3）。最常见的原因包括胆总管结石和胰头肿瘤。胰腺癌以黄疸为首发症状的情况并不少见。外科术后胆总管狭窄及胆道结石也是引起梗阻性黄疸的常见原因。出现黄疸伴胆道狭窄时应考虑原发性硬化性胆管炎，可通过影像学检查[如磁共振胰胆管成像（MRCP）或内镜逆行胰胆管造影（ERCP）]观察到胆道狭窄。少见原因包括先天性胆道闭锁、胰腺炎、胰腺假性囊肿，以及寄生虫感染（如华支睾吸虫、分支双腔吸虫、麝后睾吸虫）。

Mirizzi综合征是引起肝后性黄疸的少见原因，胆囊切除术后患者的发生率为0.7%～1.4%。主要原因是结石嵌顿于胆囊管从而对胆总管造成外压和梗阻（表11.1）。门静脉高压性胆病（又称血管性胆病）是因肝外门静脉阻塞或肝硬化（较少见）等引起门静脉高压，导致肝内、肝外血管及胰管出现解剖结构和功能异常。门静脉高压可导致广泛静脉侧支形成，继而导致胆道形态

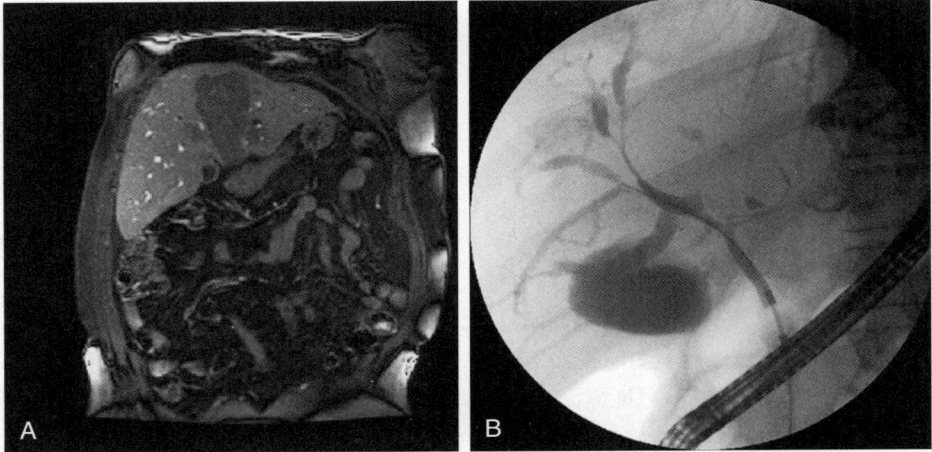

Fig. 11.3 Hepatocellular carcinoma compressing the bile ducts. (A) Sagittal view of computed abdominal tomography scan. (B) Endoscopic retrograde cholangiopancreatography demonstrates multiple strictures of the bile ducts.

venous blockage. The condition is usually asymptomatic until it has progressed to a more advanced stage such as biliary cirrhosis.

Immunoglobulin G4 (IgG4)–related sclerosing disease has recently been recognized as a distinct disease entity that can affect the bile ducts, gallbladder, pancreas, and other sites. Most cases of IgG4-related pancreatobiliary disease are associated with elevated serum IgG4 levels, extensive IgG4-positive plasma cells, and infiltration of lymphocytes into various organs, which leads to fibrosis. Several established systems are used to diagnose IgG4 disease; they rely on a combination of imaging findings of the pancreas, bile duct, and other organs; serologic findings; pancreatic histologic findings; and response to corticosteroid therapy.

CLINICAL APPROACH TO THE EVALUATION OF JAUNDICE

The differential diagnosis of jaundice is broad, thus a thorough history and physical examination along with judicious use of laboratory and imaging studies are necessary to define its underlying etiology. Jaundice appears as yellowing of the skin and sclera. Other conditions may mimic this presentation (e.g., carotenemia, Addison's disease, quinacrine ingestion), but scleral and mucosal discolorations are absent in these conditions. In hypercarotenemia, for example, the yellowish-orange coloration typically involves only the palms of the hands and soles of the feet.

An elevated serum bilirubin level, usually higher than 3 mg/dL, confirms the clinical impression of jaundice. The most important initial step is to define whether the jaundice is predominantly caused by an elevation of unconjugated or conjugated bilirubin. If jaundice is primarily the result of unconjugated bilirubin, evaluation for hemolysis and other conditions with shortened red blood cell survival is required. In patients with elevated conjugated bilirubin, the clinical challenge lies in determining whether biliary obstruction or impaired hepatic excretion is responsible (see Chapter 10).

In cholestatic jaundice caused by biliary obstruction, the alkaline phosphatase level is typically increased to more than three times normal, whereas serum transaminases are usually elevated less than 5-fold to 10-fold (see Chapter 10). Patients with cholestasis may also develop pruritus and malabsorption of fat and fat-soluble vitamins (vitamins A, D, E, and K). More specific causes of biliary obstruction are suggested by recurrent abdominal pain and nausea (gallstones) or epigastric pain radiating to the back with weight loss and gallbladder distention (carcinoma of the pancreatic head). In complete biliary obstruction, conjugated hyperbilirubinemia is prominent and usually peaks at about 30 mg/dL in the absence of renal failure. Eosinophilia may accompany drug-induced jaundice. Inquiring about the use of drugs known to cause cholestasis, serologic testing for antimitochondrial antibody in suspected PBC, and ERCP or MRCP to evaluate PSC may be helpful.

In jaundice produced by hepatocellular disease (see Chapters 10 and 12), serum transaminases are characteristically elevated more than 10-fold and alkaline phosphatase levels are less than three times normal. Evidence of hepatocellular damage is commonly associated and includes a prolonged prothrombin time, hypoalbuminemia, and clinical features of hepatic dysfunction (palmar erythema, spider angiomas, gynecomastia, and ascites). A careful evaluation includes inquiry about the use of drugs known to cause hepatocellular injury, alcohol, risk factors for viral hepatitis, and preexisting liver disease. More selected laboratory studies, such as serologic testing for hepatitis, are usually required (see Chapter 12).

If extrahepatic obstruction is suspected, noninvasive studies such as ultrasound or computed tomography should be used to determine whether bile ducts are dilated. If dilated ducts are found on noninvasive imaging, then direct cholangiography (either endoscopic or radiologic) provides the most reliable approach to management and potential treatment of cholestatic jaundice. If intrahepatic cholestasis is suggested clinically and extrahepatic obstruction is excluded by noninvasive means or by direct cholangiography, then the emphasis is placed on further laboratory testing to define the specific cause. Liver biopsy is sometimes required to define a specific histologic diagnosis, rule out other causes of disease, and assess the degree of injury and fibrosis.

For a deeper discussion on this topic, please see Chapter 138, "Approach to the Patient with Jaundice or Abnormal Liver Tests," in *Goldman-Cecil Medicine*, 26th Edition.

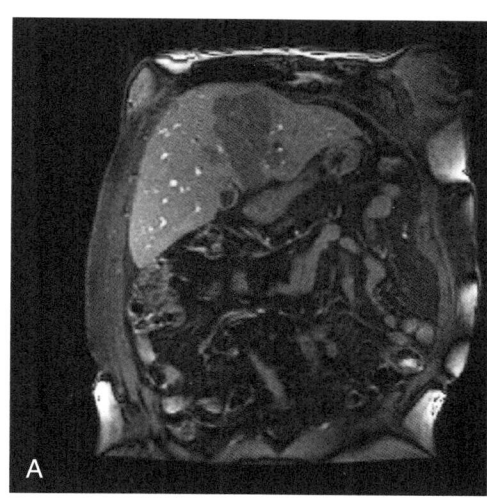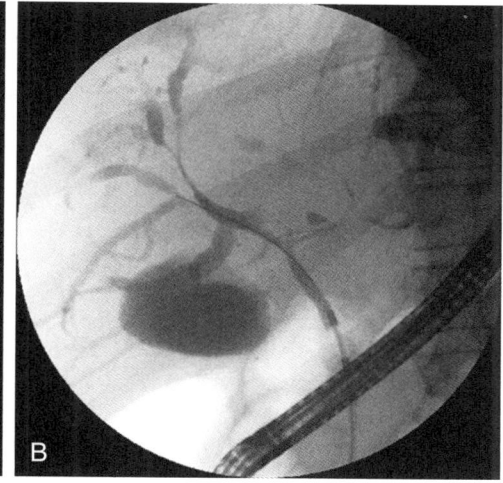

图 11.3　肝细胞癌压迫胆管。**A**. 腹部 CT 矢状位图。**B**. ERCP 显示胆管多处狭窄

学改变，如胆管及其分支扩张和狭窄。早期门静脉高压性胆病通常无症状，晚期可形成胆汁性肝硬化。

免疫球蛋白 G4（IgG4）相关性硬化性疾病被认为是一种可累及胆管、胆囊、胰腺等多个器官的疾病。大多数 IgG4 相关性胰胆管疾病可出现血清 IgG4 水平升高、大量 IgG4 阳性浆细胞及淋巴细胞浸润，这些病理学变化可导致器官纤维化。目前已有多种 IgG4 相关性疾病的诊断系统，需要结合影像学检查（胰腺、胆管和其他器官）、血清学检测、胰腺组织学结果和对皮质类固醇的治疗反应而做出诊断。

黄疸的临床评估方法

多种病因可导致黄疸，需仔细进行鉴别诊断，详尽的病史采集、体格检查，以及合理的实验室检查和影像学检查至关重要。皮肤和巩膜黄染是黄疸的特征性表现。胡萝卜素血症、艾迪生病（Addison 病）、使用奎宁等情况也可能引起皮肤黄染，但通常仅限于手掌和足底，而无巩膜和黏膜的黄染。

当血清胆红素 > 3 mg/dl 时，提示临床显性黄疸。首先应判断黄疸是以非结合胆红素水平升高为主还是以结合胆红素水平升高为主。以非结合胆红素水平升高为主时，需要评估溶血或其他导致红细胞寿命缩短的因素。以结合胆红素水平升高为主时，需鉴别胆道梗阻和肝排泄受损（见第 10 章）。

在由胆道梗阻引起的胆汁淤积性黄疸中，碱性磷酸酶水平通常会升至正常值上限的 3 倍以上，而血清转氨酶通常不超过正常值上限的 5～10 倍（见第 10 章）。胆汁淤积可能合并皮肤瘙痒、脂肪和脂溶性维生素（维生素 A、D、E 和 K）吸收不良。提示梗阻性黄疸特定病因的临床表现包括反复腹痛和恶心（可能由胆石症引起）或上腹痛向背部放射、体重减轻和胆管扩张（可能由胰头癌引起）。完全性胆道梗阻主要表现为结合胆红素水平显著升高，可高达约 30 mg/dl（无肾衰竭时）。药物诱导的黄疸可伴有嗜酸性粒细胞增多。询问用药史（是否使用过可能导致胆汁淤积的药物）、检测血清抗线粒体抗体以排查 PBC、行 ERCP 或 MRCP 评估 PSC，均有助于鉴别诊断。

当黄疸由肝细胞性疾病（见第 10 章和第 12 章）引起时，通常表现为血清转氨酶水平升高超过正常值上限的 10 倍，而碱性磷酸酶水平低于正常值上限的 3 倍。肝细胞损伤通常可导致凝血酶原时间（PT）延长、低白蛋白血症和肝功能障碍的临床表现（如肝掌、蜘蛛痣、男性乳房发育和腹腔积液）。应详细询问病史，包括可能导致肝损伤的用药史、饮酒史、病毒性肝炎的危险因素和既往肝病史。还需要进行相关实验室检查，如肝炎血清标志物检测等（见第 12 章）。

若怀疑存在肝外胆道梗阻，应首先行超声或 CT 等非侵入性检查确定是否有胆管扩张。如果非侵入性检查发现胆管扩张，直接胆道造影（通过内镜或放射介入）不仅是诊断胆汁淤积性黄疸的可靠方法，也是肝外胆道梗阻的治疗手段。如果临床提示肝内胆汁淤积，通过非侵入性检查或直接胆道造影排除肝外胆道梗阻后，应进一步行实验室检查以确定具体原因，必要时行肝穿刺组织学检查，以排除其他病因、评估肝损伤和纤维化的程度。

有关此专题的深入讨论，请参阅 *Goldman-Cecil Medicine* 第 26 版第 138 章"黄疸或肝功能试验异常患者的接诊"。

SUGGESTED READINGS

Berk PD: Approach to the patient with jaundice or abnormal liver tests. In Goldman L, Ausiello D, editors: Cecil textbook of medicine, ed 22, Philadelphia, 2004, Saunders, pp 897–905.

Pathak B, Sheibani L, Lee RH: Cholestasis of pregnancy, Obstet Gynecol Clin North Am 37:269–282, 2010.

Suárez V, Puerta A, Santos LF, et al.: Portal hypertensive biliopathy: a single center experience and literature review, World J Hepatol 5:137–144, 2013.

Trauner M, Wagner M, Fickert P, et al.: Molecular regulation of hepatobiliary transport systems: clinical implications for understanding and treating cholestasis, J Clin Gastroenterol 39(4 Suppl 2):S111–S124, 2005.

Vlachou PA, Khalili K, Jang HJ, et al.: IgG4-related sclerosing disease: autoimmune pancreatitis and extrapancreatic manifestations, Radiographics 31:1379–1402, 2011.

Woodgate P, Jardine LA: Neonatal jaundice, Clin Evid (Online) Epub Sep 15, 2011. Available at: http://www.ncbi.nlm.nih.gov/pubmed/21920055. Accessed September 19, 2014.

推荐阅读

Berk PD: Approach to the patient with jaundice or abnormal liver tests. In Goldman L, Ausiello D, editors: Cecil textbook of medicine, ed 22, Philadelphia, 2004, Saunders, pp 897–905.

Pathak B, Sheibani L, Lee RH: Cholestasis of pregnancy, Obstet Gynecol Clin North Am 37:269–282, 2010.

Suárez V, Puerta A, Santos LF, et al.: Portal hypertensive biliopathy: a single center experience and literature review, World J Hepatol 5:137–144, 2013.

Trauner M, Wagner M, Fickert P, et al.: Molecular regulation of hepatobiliary transport systems: clinical implications for understanding and treating cholestasis, J Clin Gastroenterol 39(4 Suppl 2):S111–S124, 2005.

Vlachou PA, Khalili K, Jang HJ, et al.: IgG4-related sclerosing disease: autoimmune pancreatitis and extrapancreatic manifestations, Radiographics 31:1379–1402, 2011.

Woodgate P, Jardine LA: Neonatal jaundice, Clin Evid (Online) Epub Sep 15, 2011. Available at: http://www.ncbi.nlm.nih.gov/pubmed/21920055. Accessed September 19, 2014.

12

Acute and Chronic Hepatitis

Nayan M. Patel, Jen Jung Pan, Michael B. Fallon

INTRODUCTION

The term *hepatitis* denotes inflammation of the liver. It is applied to a broad category of clinicopathologic conditions that result from the damage produced by viral, toxic, metabolic, pharmacologic, or immune-mediated injury to the liver.

ACUTE HEPATITIS

Acute hepatitis implies a recent-onset inflammatory condition lasting less than 6 months. It can culminate either in complete resolution of the liver damage with return to normal function and structure or rapid progression of the acute injury toward extensive necrosis and a fatal outcome. Depending on the etiology, some may also progress to develop a chronic hepatitis. The most common causes of acute hepatitis are viral hepatitis (hepatitis A through E) and nonviral causes such as drug-induced liver injury, alcohol, toxins, autoimmune hepatitis, and Wilson's disease.

Acute Viral Hepatitis

Five hepatotropic viruses cause classic acute viral hepatitis (Table 12.1), but other viruses, including cytomegalovirus, herpesviruses, and Epstein-Barr virus can also cause liver injury. All of the hepatotropic viruses are ribonucleic acid (RNA) viruses except hepatitis B virus (HBV), which has a deoxyribonucleic acid (DNA) genome.

Hepatitis A virus (HAV) is a nonenveloped, single-stranded RNA virus classified in the Picornaviridae family and in the *Hepatovirus* genus. It is stable at moderate temperature and low pH, allowing the virus to survive in the environment and be transmitted by the fecal-oral route. The course is generally self-limited and does not lead to chronic infection.

Hepatitis E virus (HEV) belongs to the genus *Hepevirus* in the Hepeviridae family and has four genotypes. HEV1 and HEV2 are restricted to human beings and are transmitted via contaminated water in developing countries. HEV1 occurs mainly in Asia, whereas HEV2 occurs in Africa and Mexico. HEV3 and HEV4 infect human beings, pigs, and other mammalian species and are responsible for sporadic cases of autochthonous hepatitis E in both developing and developed countries. HEV3 has a worldwide distribution. HEV4 mostly occurs in Southeast Asia. While typically self-limited, acute liver failure and hepatic decompensation can occur in patients who are pregnant, malnourished, or have preexisting liver disease. Additionally, patients with solid organ transplants can develop a chronic HEV infection.

HBV is a small DNA virus that belongs to the Hepadnaviridae family. Approximately 250 million persons are carriers of HBV worldwide; of these, 75% reside in Asia and the Western Pacific. Both acute and chronic HBV infection can occur. Chronic hepatitis B infection is a major cause of hepatocellular carcinoma worldwide and can occur without cirrhosis because of integration of HBV DNA into hepatocytes.

Hepatitis C virus (HCV) is a single-stranded positive-sense RNA virus that belongs to the Flaviviridae family and has been classified as the sole member of the genus *Hepacivirus*. Approximately 74 million people are infected with HCV worldwide and 2.4 million in the United States. HBV has eight genotypes (labeled A through H), and HCV has six genotypes (1 through 6). Both HBV and HCV viruses are transmitted parenterally. HBV is present in virtually all body fluids and excreta of carriers. Transmission occurs most commonly through blood and blood products, contaminated needles, and sexual contact. Historically, HCV was the main cause of post-transfusion hepatitis before 1992. It is currently the most common cause of hepatitis among intravenous drug users. The Centers for Disease Control and Prevention now recommends one-time screening of persons born between 1945 and 1965 for hepatitis C because of the high prevalence of the disease in this birth cohort.

Hepatitis D virus (HDV) is classified in a separate genus of the Deltaviridae family. It is a small, defective RNA virus that can propagate only in an individual who has coexistent HBV infection, either after simultaneous transmission of the two viruses or via superinfection of an established HBV carrier. HDV has at least eight genotypes, four of which (genotypes 5 through 8) seem to be of exclusively African origin. Of the 250 million chronic carriers of HBV worldwide, more than 15 million have serologic evidence of exposure to HDV. Like HBV, HDV is transmitted via the parenteral route through exposure to infected blood or body fluids. Because there is evidence for sexual transmission, people with high-risk sexual activity are at increased risk for infection.

Clinical and Laboratory Manifestations

Acute viral hepatitis typically involves an asymptomatic incubation period from exposure to the first appearance of symptoms. This can be weeks to months depending on the type of viral hepatitis. Next a prodromal phase lasting several days that is characterized by constitutional and gastrointestinal symptoms including malaise, fatigue, anorexia, nausea, vomiting, myalgia, and headache occurs. A mild fever may be present (Fig. 12.1). Clinical manifestations of hepatitis A depend on the age of the host: fewer than 30% of infected young children showed symptomatic hepatitis, whereas about 80% of infected adults had severe acute hepatitis with remarkably elevated serum aminotransferases (Fig. 12.2). Arthritis and urticaria resembling serum sickness, attributed to immune complex deposition, are present in 5% to 10% of cases of acute hepatitis B and C. Taste and smell alterations may also occur. Jaundice soon appears, with bilirubinuria and acholic (pale) stools, which are often accompanied by an improvement in the patient's sense of well-being. The liver is usually tender and enlarged; splenomegaly is found in about one fifth of patients. Notably, many patients with acute viral hepatitis are asymptomatic or have symptoms without jaundice (anicteric hepatitis). In such instances, medical attention often is not sought.

急性和慢性肝炎

李淑香　王倩怡　译　段维佳　赵新颜　审校　贾继东　通审

引言

"肝炎"一词是指肝脏的炎症。它可被用于描述由病毒、毒物、代谢、药物或免疫介导的肝损伤所致的一系列临床病理学改变。

急性肝炎

急性肝炎是指近期发生的、持续时间<6个月的肝脏炎症。急性肝炎的结局既可能是肝损伤完全消退，肝功能和结构恢复正常，也可能是迅速进展为广泛肝坏死而导致死亡。根据不同病因，部分患者也可能发展为慢性肝炎。病毒性肝炎（甲型、乙型、丙型、丁型和戊型肝炎）和非病毒性肝炎（如药物诱导的肝损伤、酒精性肝炎、毒物引起的肝炎、自身免疫性肝炎、肝豆状核变性）是急性肝炎最常见的类型。

急性病毒性肝炎

5种嗜肝病毒感染可引起经典的急性病毒性肝炎（表12.1），但其他病毒（包括巨细胞病毒、疱疹病毒和EB病毒）感染也可引起急性肝损伤。除乙型肝炎病毒（HBV）是脱氧核糖核酸（DNA）病毒外，其他嗜肝病毒均为核糖核酸（RNA）病毒。

甲型肝炎病毒（HAV）是一种无包膜单链RNA病毒，属于微小RNA病毒科嗜肝病毒属。该病毒在适当温度和低pH值环境中可稳定存活，能够通过粪-口途径传播。HAV感染的病程通常呈自限性，不会导致慢性感染。

戊型肝炎病毒（HEV）属于肝炎病毒科嗜肝病毒属，有4个基因型。HEV1和HEV2仅见于人类，在发展中国家通过受污染的水传播。HEV1主要分布在亚洲，而HEV2主要分布在非洲和墨西哥。HEV3和HEV4可感染人、猪和其他哺乳动物，在发展中国家和发达国家均可引起散发性本土戊型肝炎病例。HEV3呈全球性分布。HEV4主要分布在东南亚。尽管戊型肝炎大多为自限性疾病，但妊娠、营养不良或有基础肝病的患者感染HEV后可造成急性肝衰竭和肝脏失代偿。此外，接受实体器官移植的患者感染后可发展为慢性HEV感染。

HBV是一种小DNA病毒，属于肝炎病毒科。全球约有2.5亿HBV携带者；其中75%的患者分布在亚洲和西太平洋地区。急性和慢性HBV感染均可发生。慢性HBV感染是全球肝细胞癌的主要原因；由于HBV DNA可以整合到宿主的肝细胞内，因此肝细胞癌可以发生在无肝硬化的慢性乙型肝炎患者中。

丙型肝炎病毒（HCV）是一种单股正链RNA病毒，属于黄病毒科，是被归类为肝炎病毒属的唯一成员。全球约有7400万人感染HCV，美国有240万人感染。HBV有8种基因型（标记为A～H），HCV有6种基因型（标记为1～6）。HBV和HCV均通过肠外方式传播。HBV几乎存在于携带者的所有体液和排泄物中，最常见的传播途径是暴露于血液、血制品、受污染的针头和性接触。历史上，HCV感染在1992年以前是输血后肝炎的主要原因。目前，HCV感染是静脉吸毒者最常见的肝炎原因。美国疾病预防控制中心（CDC）推荐对1945—1965年出生的人群进行一次性丙型肝炎筛查，因为该队列人群的患病率较高。

丁型肝炎病毒（HDV）属于δ病毒科。它是一种有缺陷的小RNA病毒，只能在HBV感染的个体中繁殖，两种病毒可同时感染，也可在HBV携带者中发生重叠感染。HDV至少有8种基因型，其中4种（基因型5～8）似乎仅存在于非洲。全球约有2.5亿慢性HBV携带者，其中超过1500万人有HDV暴露的血清学证据。与HBV类似，HDV通过暴露于感染者血液或体液的肠外途径传播。由于有证据表明HDV可通过性传播，因此高风险性行为者感染的风险增加。

临床表现和实验室检查

急性病毒性肝炎从暴露于病毒到首次出现症状之间通常存在无症状潜伏期。根据病毒性肝炎的不同类型，潜伏期可能为数周至数月。随后进入持续数天的前驱期，主要表现为全身症状和胃肠道症状，包括全身不适、疲劳、食欲减退、恶心、呕吐、肌痛和头痛，还可能出现低热（图12.1）。甲型肝炎的临床表现取决于感染者的年龄：在幼儿患者中，症状性肝炎的比例不足30%，而成人患者约80%会出现血清转氨酶水平显著升高的严重急性肝炎（图12.2）。5%～10%的急性乙型肝炎和丙型肝炎患者会出现类似血清病的关节炎和荨麻疹，这归因于免疫复合物沉积。患者还可能出现味觉和嗅觉改变。随后很快出现黄疸，伴胆红素尿和白陶土样便，此时患者通常自觉病情改善。体格检查常可见肝大和肝区触痛，1/5的患者可有脾大。值得注意的是，许多急性病毒性肝炎患者通常无症状或无黄疸表现（无黄疸性肝炎）。在这种情况下，患者往往不会寻求医疗帮助。

TABLE 12.1 Characteristics of Acute Viral Hepatitides

	Hepatitis A	Hepatitis B	Hepatitis C	Hepatitis D	Hepatitis E
Causative agent	27–28 nm RNA virus Nonenveloped	42 nm DNA virus Enveloped	55–65 nm RNA virus Enveloped	36–43 nm RNA virus Enveloped	27–34 nm RNA virus Nonenveloped
Transmission	Fecal-oral	Blood-borne, sexual, percutaneous, perinatal	Similar to HBV; vertical and sexual route uncommon	Similar to HBV	Similar to HAV; transfusion; vertical transmission
Incubation period (days)	15–50	30–180	14–180	Similar to HBV	15–60
Onset	Acute	Acute, insidious	Insidious	Acute, insidious	Acute, insidious
Fulminant disease (%)	0.01–0.5	1	<0.1	5–20	1–2
Chronic hepatitis	No	Yes	Yes	Yes/No	Yes/No
Treatment	Supportive	Nucleos(t)ide analogues; IFN-α	DAA ± ribavirin	IFN-α	Supportive; ribavirin
Prophylaxis	Hygiene; immune globulin, vaccine	Similar to HAV	Hygiene	Hygiene, HBV vaccine	Hygiene, vaccine

DAA, Direct-acting antiviral; *HAV*, hepatitis A virus; *HBV*, hepatitis B virus; *IFN-α*, interferon-α.

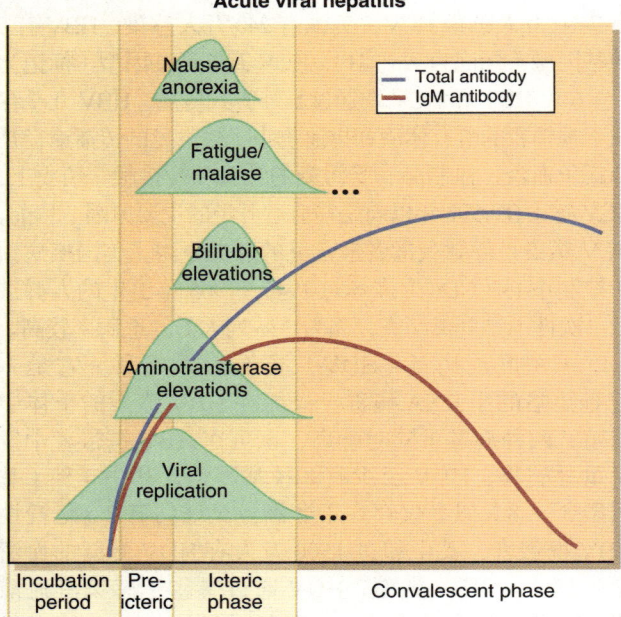

Fig. 12.1 Typical clinical, laboratory, and serological course in acute self-resolving viral hepatitis. *IgM*, Immunoglobulin M.

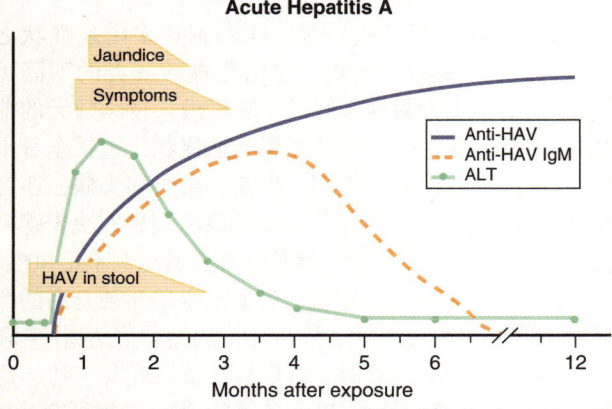

Fig. 12.2 Serologic course of acute hepatitis A. *ALT*, Alanine aminotransferase; *HAV*, hepatitis A virus; *IgM*, immunoglobulin M.

Alanine aminotransferase (ALT) and aspartate aminotransferase (AST) are released from acutely damaged hepatocytes, and serum levels can rise to 20-fold or more above normal. An elevated serum bilirubin level (>2.5 to 3 mg/dL) results in jaundice and is defined as icteric hepatitis. Values higher than 20 mg/dL are uncommon and correlate in a general way with the severity of disease. Elevations in serum alkaline phosphatase (ALP) are usually limited to three times normal levels except in cases of cholestatic hepatitis. A complete blood cell count most commonly shows mild leukopenia with atypical lymphocytes. Anemia and thrombocytopenia may also be present. The icteric phase of acute viral hepatitis may last days to weeks and is followed by gradual resolution of symptoms and laboratory values.

Diagnosis

Acute viral hepatitis can be diagnosed either directly, by detecting the nucleic acids of the infecting virus, or indirectly, by demonstrating an immune response in the host (Tables 12.2 and 12.3). Epstein-Barr virus and cytomegalovirus hepatitis are part of the differential diagnosis and also may be diagnosed by the appearance of specific antibodies of the immunoglobulin M (IgM) class.

In acute hepatitis B, hepatitis B surface antigen (HBsAg) and e antigen (HBeAg) are present in serum. Both are usually cleared within 3 months in acute self-limited infection, but HBsAg may persist in some patients with uncomplicated disease for 6 months to 1 year. Clearance of HBsAg is followed after a variable period by the emergence of antibodies against hepatitis B surface antigen (anti-HBs), which confers long-term immunity. Antibodies against hepatitis B core antigen (anti-HBc) and e antigen (anti-HBe) appear in the acute phase of the illness, but neither provides immunity. During the serologic window period, anti-HBc IgM, a marker of active viral replication suggesting recent infection, may be the only evidence of HBV infection (Fig. 12.3).

Every patient who is HBsAg positive should be tested for antibodies against HDV (anti-HDV IgG), which persist even after the patient has cleared HDV infection. Active HDV infection is now confirmed by the detection of serum HDV RNA with sensitive real-time polymerase chain reaction (PCR) assays. However, because of the variability of the genome sequence, assays of HDV RNA can produce false-negative results. Testing of anti-HDV IgM antibodies still has a role in patients who test negative for HDV RNA but have clinical features of HDV-related liver disease. While there is no diagnostic feature, suspicion for active HDV co-infection should be higher in acute liver failure from acute HBV infection.

Acute hepatitis C can be detected within 2 weeks after exposure with the use of a sensitive PCR assay for HCV RNA. Serum antibodies

表 12.1	急性病毒性肝炎特征				
	甲型肝炎	乙型肝炎	丙型肝炎	丁型肝炎	戊型肝炎
病原体	27～28 nm RNA 病毒 无包膜	42 nm DNA 病毒 有包膜	55～65 nm RNA 病毒 有包膜	36～43 nm RNA 病毒 有包膜	27～34 nm RNA 病毒 无包膜
传播途径	粪-口传播	血液传播、性传播、经皮传播、围产期传播	同 HBV；少数经垂直传播和性传播	同 HBV	同 HAV；输血传播；垂直传播
潜伏期（天）	15～50	30～180	14～180	同 HBV	15～60
起病形式	急性	急性，隐匿	隐匿	急性，隐匿	急性，隐匿
暴发性肝炎占比（%）	0.01～0.5	1	＜0.1	5～20	1～2
慢性肝炎	无	有	有	有/无	有/无
治疗	支持治疗	核苷(酸)类似物；IFN-α	DAA±利巴韦林	IFN-α	支持治疗；利巴韦林
预防	卫生措施；免疫球蛋白、疫苗	同 HAV	卫生措施	卫生措施、HBV 疫苗	卫生措施、疫苗

DAA，直接抗病毒药物；HAV，甲型肝炎病毒；HBV，乙型肝炎病毒；IFN-α，干扰素 α。

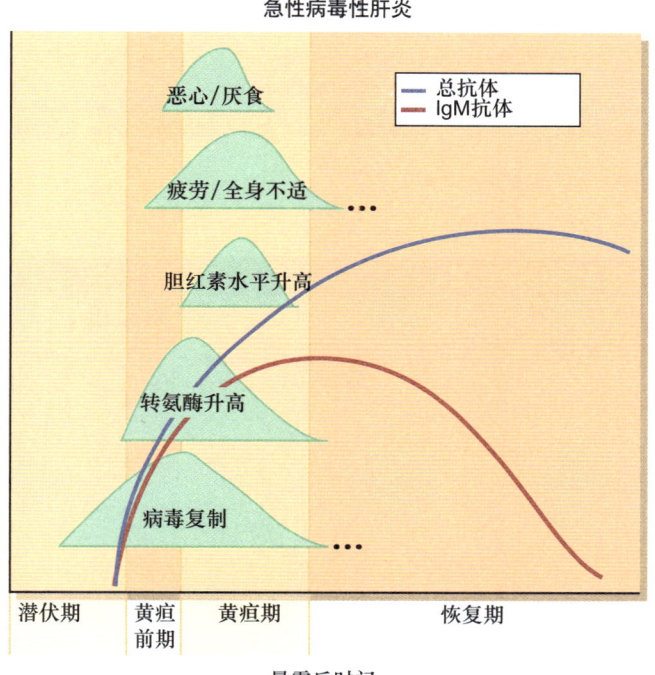

图 12.1 急性自愈性病毒性肝炎的典型临床表现、实验室检查和血清学演变过程。IgM，免疫球蛋白 M

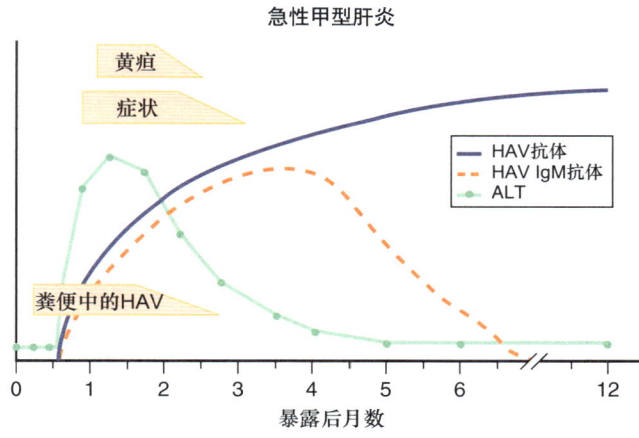

图 12.2 急性甲型肝炎的血清学演变过程。ALT，丙氨酸转氨酶；HAV，甲型肝炎病毒；IgM，免疫球蛋白 M

丙氨酸转氨酶（ALT）和天冬氨酸转氨酶（AST）从急性损伤的肝细胞中释放出来，使其血清水平可升至正常值上限的 20 倍或更高。血清胆红素水平升高（＞2.5～3 mg/dl）可导致黄疸，被定义为黄疸性肝炎。胆红素＞20 mg/dl 的情况不常见，通常与疾病的严重程度相关。出现胆汁淤积性肝炎时，血清碱性磷酸酶（ALP）水平升高通常不超过正常值上限的 3 倍。全血细胞计数最常见的改变是白细胞轻度减少伴有非典型淋巴细胞，也可能出现贫血和血小板计数减少。急性病毒性肝炎的黄疸期可持续数天至数周，随后患者的临床症状和实验室指标逐渐恢复。

诊断

急性病毒性肝炎可通过检测病毒核酸来直接诊断，也可通过证实存在宿主免疫应答来间接诊断（表 12.2 和表 12.3）。EB 病毒感染和巨细胞病毒性肝炎是鉴别诊断的一部分，可通过检测特异性免疫球蛋白 M（IgM）抗体来诊断。

急性乙型肝炎患者的血清中存在乙型肝炎表面抗原（HBsAg）和 e 抗原（HBeAg）。在急性自限性感染中，HBsAg 和 HBeAg 通常在 3 个月内清除，但在无并发症的患者中，HBsAg 可能持续存在 6 个月至 1 年。HBsAg 清除后一段时间会出现乙型肝炎表面抗体（HBsAb），从而产生长期免疫。乙型肝炎核心抗体（HBcAb）和 e 抗体（HBeAb）出现在疾病的急性期，但两者均不能提供保护性免疫。在血清学窗口期，抗 HBc IgM 抗体是病毒复制活跃的标志，提示近期感染，这可能是 HBV 感染的唯一证据（图 12.3）。

HBsAg 阳性的患者均应检测 HDV 抗体（抗 HDV IgG 抗体），即使在 HDV 感染清除后，这种抗体也会持续存在。目前，可通过实时聚合酶链反应（PCR）检测血清 HDV RNA，以确认活动性 HDV 感染。但是，由于基因组序列的变异性，HDV RNA 检测可能出现假阴性结果。对于 HDV RNA 检测阴性但有 HDV 相关肝病临床特征的患者，抗 HDV IgM 抗体检测仍有用。虽然没有特征性诊断标志物，但在急性 HBV 感染所致的急性肝衰竭患者中，应高度怀疑活动性 HDV 共感染的可能。

急性丙型肝炎可在暴露后 2 周内通过 PCR 检测到 HCV RNA。在暴露后 12 周内或发现生化指标异常后

TABLE 12.2 Serologic Markers of Viral Hepatitis

Agent	Marker	Definition	Significance
HAV	Anti-HAV IgM	IgM antibody to HAV	Marker of acute or recent infection
	Anti-HAV IgG	IgG antibody to HAV	Marker of acute or previous infection; post vaccination; confers protective immunity
HBV	HBsAg	Hepatitis B surface antigen	The presence of HBsAg indicates that the person is infectious
	HBeAg	Hepatitis B e antigen	Transiently positive in acute infection; may persist in chronic infection; reflection of active viral replication and high infectivity
	Anti-HBs	Antibody to surface antigen	Marker of acute self-limited infection; post vaccination; confers protective immunity
	Anti-HBe	Antibody to e antigen	Transiently positive in convalescence; positive in chronic infection before seroconversion; usually a reflection of low infectivity
	Anti-HBc IgM	IgM antibody to core antigen	Marker of acute or exacerbation of chronic infection
	Anti-HBc IgG	IgG antibody to core antigen	Appears at the onset of symptoms in acute infection and persists for life; not seen in vaccinees without prior infection
HCV	Anti-HCV	Antibody to HCV	Marker of acute and chronic infection; does not provide immunity
HDV	Anti-HDV IgM	IgM antibody to HDV	Positive in acute infection, negative in past infection but persists in a large proportion of patients with chronic infection
	Anti-HDV IgG	IgG antibody to HDV	Positive in all individuals exposed to HDV, and persists long-term, even after viral clearance
HEV	Anti-HEV IgM	IgM antibody to HEV	Marker of acute or recent infection[a]
	Anti-HEV IgG	IgG antibody to HEV	Marker of chronic or previous infection[a]

HAV, Hepatitis A virus; *HBV*, hepatitis B virus; *HCV*, hepatitis C virus; *HDV*, hepatitis D virus; *HEV*, hepatitis E virus; *IgG*, immunoglobulin G; *IgM*, immunoglobulin M.
[a]Serologic testing is unreliable, and seroconversion might never occur in immunosuppressed persons.

TABLE 12.3 Interpretation of Diagnostic Markers in Hepatitis B

	HBsAg	HBeAg	Anti-HBc IgM	Anti-HBc IgG	Anti-HBs	Anti-HBe	Blood HBV DNA
Acute infection	+	+	+	+	−	+/−	High
Acute self-limited infection	−	−	+	+	+	+/−	−
Vaccinated	−	−	−	−	+	−	−
Chronic infection							
HBeAg positive	+	+	−	+	−	−	High
HBeAg negative	+	−	−	+	−	+	Low
Immune escape	+	−	−	+	−	+	High
Occult infection	−	−	−	+	−	+/−	Very low
Reactivation of chronic infection	+	+	+/−	+	−	+/−	High

anti-HBc IgG, Immunoglobulin G antibody against hepatitis B core antigen; *anti-HBc IgM*, immunoglobulin M antibody against hepatitis B core antigen; *anti-HBe*, antibody against hepatitis B e antigen; *anti-HBs*, antibody against hepatitis B surface antigen; *HBeAg*, hepatitis B e antigen; *HBsAg*, hepatitis B surface antigen; *HBV DNA*, hepatitis B virus deoxyribonucleic acid.

to HCV develop within 12 weeks after exposure, or within 4 to 5 weeks after biochemical abnormalities are discovered. Importantly, these are not neutralizing antibodies and do not confer immunity (Fig. 12.4). At onset of symptoms, 30% of patients will be missed if checked by serum enzyme immunoassay (EIA) for HCV antibody alone.

Commercial EIAs for hepatitis E to detect both IgM and IgG class antibodies are also available but may lack sensitivity and specificity. Diagnosis of HEV infection should be established by PCR assays in immunosuppressed patients, because serologic testing is unreliable, and seroconversion might never occur.

Complications

Cholestatic hepatitis. In some patients, most commonly during HAV infection, a prolonged but self-limited period of cholestasis (total bilirubin >10 mg/dL) occurs that is characterized by marked conjugated hyperbilirubinemia, elevation of ALP, and pruritus. Further investigation may be required to rule out biliary obstruction (see Chapters 10, 11, and 15).

Relapsing hepatitis. For unknown reasons, up to 10% of patients can experience a relapse of HAV infection after an initial resolution. This is characterized by biochemical relapse, but often milder clinical symptoms, and will typically resolve spontaneously.

表 12.2　病毒性肝炎的血清学标志物

病毒类型	标志物	定义	临床意义
HAV	Anti-HAV IgM	抗 HAV IgM 抗体	急性或近期感染的标志物
	Anti-HAV IgG	抗 HAV IgG 抗体	急性或既往感染的标志物；疫苗接种后；可提供保护性免疫
HBV	HBsAg	乙型肝炎表面抗原	存在 HBsAg 提示患者具有传染性
	HBeAg	乙型肝炎 e 抗原	急性感染时呈短暂阳性；慢性感染时可能持续阳性；反映病毒复制活跃和传染性强
	HBsAb	乙型肝炎表面抗体	急性自限性感染的标志物；疫苗接种后；可提供保护性免疫
	HBeAb	乙型肝炎 e 抗体	恢复期呈短暂阳性；慢性感染血清阳转前呈阳性；反映传染性弱
	Anti-HBc IgM	抗乙型肝炎核心抗原 IgM 抗体	急性感染或慢性感染加重的标志物
	Anti-HBc IgG	抗乙型肝炎核心抗原 IgG 抗体	在急性感染症状开始时出现，并终生存在；无既往感染的疫苗接种者不会出现
HCV	Anti-HCV	抗 HCV 抗体	急性或慢性感染的标志物；不能提供保护性免疫
HDV	Anti-HDV IgM	抗 HDV IgM 抗体	急性感染呈阳性，既往感染呈阴性，但在大部分慢性感染者中持续存在
	Anti-HDV IgG	抗 HDV IgG 抗体	所有暴露 HDV 者均呈阳性，病毒清除后仍可长期存在
HEV	Anti-HEV IgM	抗 HEV IgM 抗体	急性或近期感染的标志物[a]
	Anti-HEV IgG	抗 HEV IgG 抗体	慢性或既往感染的标志物[a]

HAV，甲型肝炎病毒；HBV，乙型肝炎病毒；HCV，丙型肝炎病毒；HDV，丁型肝炎病毒；HEV，戊型肝炎病毒；IgG，免疫球蛋白 G；IgM，免疫球蛋白 M。
[a] 血清学检测不可靠，免疫抑制患者可能永远不会发生血清阳转。

表 12.3　乙型肝炎诊断性标志物的解读

	HBsAg	HBeAg	anti-HBc IgM	anti-HBc IgG	HBsAb	HBeAb	血液 HBV DNA
急性感染	+	+	+	+	−	+/−	高
急性自限性感染	−	−	+	+	+	+/−	−
疫苗接种	−	−	−	−	+	−	−
慢性感染							
HBeAg 阳性	+	+	−	+	−	−	高
HBeAg 阴性	+	−	−	+	−	+	低
免疫逃逸	+	−	−	+	−	+	高
隐匿性感染	−	−	−	+	+/−	+/−	极低
慢性感染再激活	+	+	+/−	+	−	+/−	高

anti-HBc IgG，抗乙型肝炎核心抗原 IgG 抗体；anti-HBc IgM，抗乙型肝炎核心抗原 IgM 抗体；HBeAb，乙型肝炎 e 抗体；HBsAb，乙型肝炎表面抗体；HBeAg，乙型肝炎 e 抗原；HBsAg，乙型肝炎表面抗原；HBV DNA，乙型肝炎病毒脱氧核糖核酸。

4～5周内，血清中会出现 HCV 抗体。重要的是，该抗体并非中和抗体，不会产生保护性免疫（图 12.4）。在症状出现时，如果只通过血清酶免疫分析（EIA）检测 HCV 抗体，30% 患者可能会被漏诊。

市售的戊型肝炎 EIA 试剂盒可同时检测 IgG 和 IgM 抗体，但可能缺乏敏感性和特异性。免疫抑制患者可通过 PCR 检测确诊 HEV 感染，因为血清学检测对于这些患者并不可靠，且血清阳转可能永远不会发生。

并发症

胆汁淤积性肝炎　部分患者可出现持续时间较长但呈自限性的胆汁淤积（总胆红素＞10 mg/dl），最常见于 HAV 感染期间，主要表现为明显的高结合胆红素血症、ALP 水平升高和瘙痒。需要进一步检查以排除胆道梗阻（见第 10 章、第 11 章和第 15 章）。

复发性肝炎　多达 10% 的患者在初次感染恢复后可能会经历 HAV 感染的复发，但原因尚不清楚。这种复发以生化指标反复为特征，但临床症状通常较轻，并且会自行缓解。

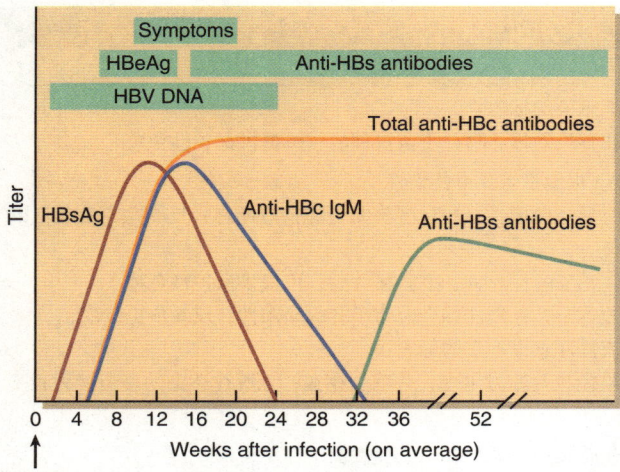

Fig. 12.3 Kinetics of hepatitis B virus (HBV) markers during acute self-resolving hepatitis B. The *arrow* indicates infection. *HBc,* Hepatitis B core; *HBeAg,* hepatitis B e antigen; *HBs,* hepatitis B surface; *HBsAg,* hepatitis B surface antigen; *IgM,* immunoglobulin M.

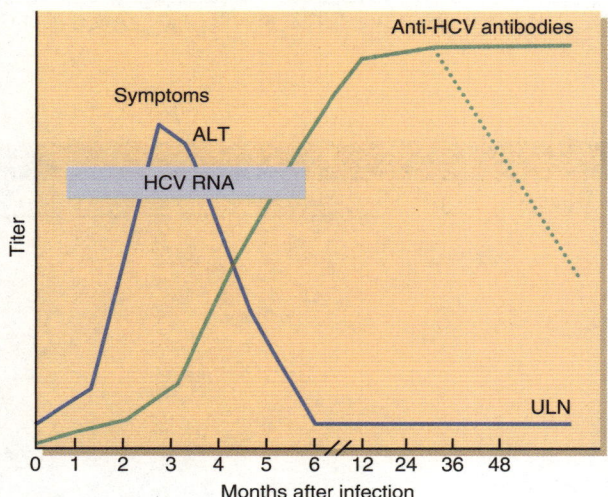

Fig. 12.4 Kinetics of hepatitis C virus markers during acute self-resolving hepatitis C. *ALT,* Alanine aminotransferase; *ULN,* upper limit of normal.

Fulminant hepatitis. Massive hepatic necrosis occurs in fewer than 1% of patients with acute viral hepatitis; it leads to a devastating and often fatal condition called acute liver failure. This condition is discussed in detail in Chapter 13.

Chronic hepatitis. Hepatitis A does not progress to chronic liver disease, although occasionally it has a relapsing course. Persistence of elevated levels of ALT and AST, viral antigens, or nucleic acids beyond 6 months in patients with hepatitis B or C suggests evolution to chronic hepatitis, although slowly resolving acute hepatitis may occasionally exhibit such test abnormalities for up to 12 months with eventual complete resolution. About 60% of organ transplant recipients infected with HEV fail to clear the virus and go on to develop chronic hepatitis. Chronic hepatitis is considered in detail later in this chapter.

Rare complications. Acute viral hepatitis may rarely be followed by aplastic anemia, which tends to affect mostly male patients and results in a mortality rate greater than 80%. Pancreatitis, myocarditis, pericarditis, pleural effusion, and neurologic complications including Guillain-Barré syndrome, aseptic meningitis, and encephalitis have also been reported. Extrahepatic manifestations such as cryoglobulinemia and glomerulonephritis are associated with hepatitis B and C, and polyarteritis nodosa is associated with hepatitis B. These manifestations are more common in patients who fail to clear acute HBV or HCV and develop chronic hepatitis.

Management

Unless complicated by fulminant hepatitis, cases of acute hepatitis A, B, and E are usually self-limited and are managed by supportive care including rest, maintenance of adequate hydration and dietary intake, and avoidance of alcohol use. Hospitalization may be needed for patients who cannot tolerate oral intake and for those with evidence of deteriorated liver function, such as hepatic encephalopathy or coagulopathy.

In general, hepatitis A and E may be regarded as noninfectious after 3 weeks, whereas hepatitis B is potentially infectious to sexual contacts throughout its course, although the risk is low once HBsAg has been cleared. Studies of antiviral therapy in acute hepatitis B have not shown clear benefit, although some experts advocate the use of nucleos(t)ide analogues, specifically in the setting of acute liver failure due to hepatitis B. Treatment of acute hepatitis C is not always needed because 20% to 50% of patients will spontaneous clear the virus. This typically occurs within 6 months of the time of infection. If a decision is made to initiate treatment, current guidelines suggest monitoring HCV RNA for 12 to 16 weeks before starting treatment to allow for possible spontaneous clearance. Because of the safety and efficacy of direct acting antivirals (DAAs), the same regimen of medication for chronic hepatitis C is recommended for acute HCV.

Prevention

In patients with hepatitis A or E, both feces and blood contain virus during the prodromal and early icteric phases. General hygiene measures should include handwashing by contacts and careful handling, disposal, and sterilization of excreta, contaminated clothing, and utensils. HAV vaccination is appropriate for children older than 12 months of age, travelers to endemic areas, individuals with immunodeficiency or chronic liver disease, and those with high-risk behaviors or occupations. HAV vaccination is preferred over immunoglobulin for postexposure prophylaxis, based on results from randomized trials. With the availability of two candidate vaccines, one of which is already licensed for use in China, HEV prevention through vaccination is now a realistic possibility.

HBV is rarely transmitted by body fluids other than blood; however, it is highly infectious, and strict adherence to universal precautions is mandatory. Efforts at preventing hepatitis B have involved the use of hepatitis B immunoglobulin (HBIG) and recombinant HBV vaccines. Prophylaxis with HBIG after blood or mucosal exposure should be given within 7 days along with HBV vaccine. Preventive vaccination is currently recommended for high-risk individuals—health care professionals, patients undergoing hemodialysis, patients with chronic liver disease, residents and staff of custodial care institutions, and sexually active homosexual men—and is advocated universally for children. In the United States, the first hepatitis B vaccination is recommended to be given within 12 to 24 hours of birth.

No accepted prevention strategies other than universal precautions are available for HCV, and serum immunoglobulin is not useful for postexposure prophylaxis. The advent of widespread blood product screening for hepatitis C has made such infection after transfusion a rarity.

Alcoholic Liver Disease

Alcohol abuse continues to be a major cause of liver disease in the Western world. The three major pathologic findings resulting from

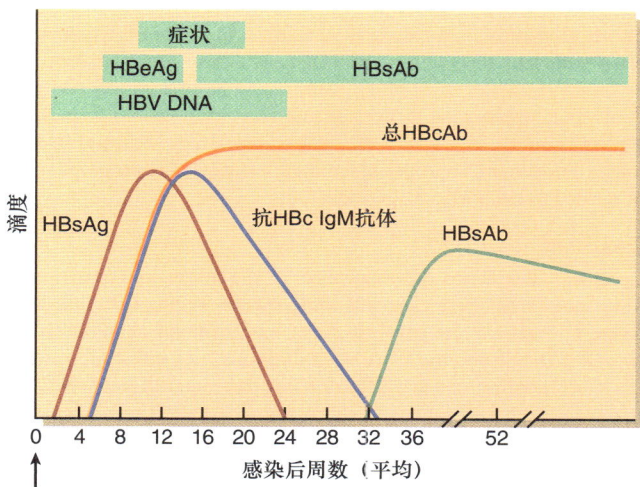

图 12.3 急性自愈性乙型肝炎期间 HBV 标志物的动态变化。箭头表示感染。HBcAb, 乙型肝炎核心抗体; HBeAg, 乙型肝炎 e 抗原; HBsAb, 乙型肝炎表面抗体; HBsAg, 乙型肝炎表面抗原; IgM, 免疫球蛋白 M

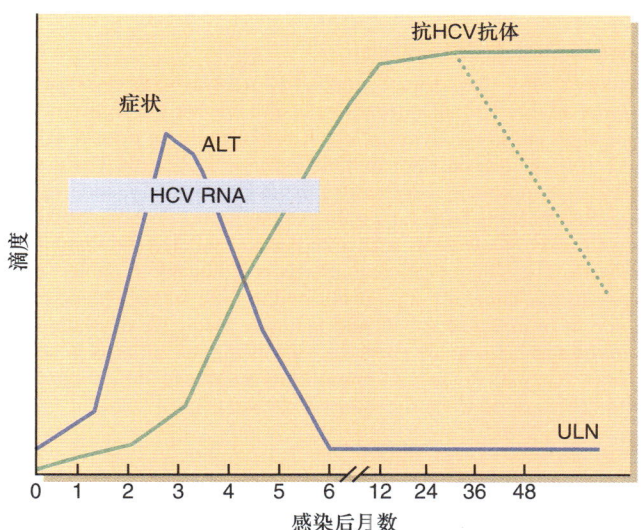

图 12.4 急性自愈性丙型肝炎期间 HCV 标志物的动态变化。ALT, 丙氨酸转氨酶; ULN, 正常值上限

暴发性肝炎 在急性病毒性肝炎患者中, 大量肝坏死的发生率 < 1%; 暴发性肝炎可导致毁灭性且危及生命的急性肝衰竭 (见第 13 章)。

慢性肝炎 甲型肝炎偶尔会复发, 但不会进展为慢性肝病。在乙型和丙型肝炎患者中, 若 ALT 和 AST、病毒抗原或核酸持续升高超过 6 个月, 则提示疾病演变为慢性肝炎, 但少数急性患者会表现为缓慢恢复, 其实验室指标异常长达 12 个月, 但最终可完全恢复。约 60% 的器官移植受者感染 HEV 后因无法清除病毒而发展为慢性肝炎。慢性肝炎的内容详见下文。

罕见并发症 极少数情况下, 急性病毒性肝炎可继发再生障碍性贫血, 主要见于男性患者, 且死亡率超过 80%。此外, 胰腺炎、心肌炎、心包炎、胸腔积液和神经系统并发症 (包括吉兰-巴雷综合征、无菌性脑膜炎和脑炎) 也有报道。冷球蛋白血症和肾小球肾炎等肝外表现与乙型和丙型肝炎有关, 结节性多动脉炎与乙型肝炎有关。这些表现更常见于急性感染 HBV 或 HCV 未能清除而发展为慢性肝炎的患者。

管理

除非并发暴发性肝炎, 急性甲型、乙型和戊型肝炎通常呈自限性, 可采用支持治疗, 包括休息、维持充足的水分和饮食摄入、避免饮酒。对于不能进食和有肝功能恶化征象 (如肝性脑病或凝血功能障碍) 的患者, 可能需要住院治疗。

一般来说, 急性甲型和戊型肝炎在 3 周后可视为无传染性, 而急性乙型肝炎在整个病程中都可能存在性传播风险, 尽管 HBsAg 被清除后其传染风险很低。急性乙型肝炎的抗病毒治疗研究尚未显示出明确的疗效, 但一些专家主张使用核苷 (酸) 类似物, 特别是在乙型肝炎导致急性肝衰竭的情况下。急性丙型肝炎通常不需要治疗, 因为 20% ~ 50% 的患者在感染后 6 个月内会自发清除病毒。如果需要治疗, 目前的指南建议在治疗开始前先监测 HCV RNA 12 ~ 16 周, 以评估实现病毒自发清除的可能性。由于直接抗病毒药物 (DAA) 的安全性和有效性, 建议对急性丙型肝炎采取与慢性丙型肝炎相同的治疗方案。

预防

在甲型或戊型肝炎患者中, 前驱期和黄疸早期时粪便和血液中均含有病毒。一般卫生措施应包括接触后洗手, 对排泄物、受污染的衣物和用具进行仔细处理、处置和消毒。HAV 疫苗接种适用于 12 个月以上儿童、前往甲型肝炎流行地区的旅行者、免疫缺陷或慢性肝病患者, 以及有高风险行为或职业的个体。随机试验证实, 对于 HAV 暴露后的预防, 接种 HAV 疫苗优于免疫球蛋白。随着两种候选疫苗的问世 (其中一种已在中国获得使用许可), 通过接种疫苗预防 HEV 感染已成为现实。

HBV 很少通过除血液以外的体液传播; 但它具有高度传染性, 必须严格遵守标准预防措施。预防乙型肝炎的方法包括使用乙型肝炎免疫球蛋白 (HBIG) 和重组 HBV 疫苗。血液或黏膜暴露后应立即注射 HBIG 预防, 同时 7 天内接种 HBV 疫苗。目前建议高危人群预防性接种乙型肝炎疫苗, 如医护人员、接受血液透析的患者、慢性肝病患者、托管机构的托管人员和工作人员, 以及性活跃的男男性关系者, 且提倡儿童普遍接种。在美国, 建议在出生后 12 ~ 24 h 内进行第一次乙型肝炎疫苗接种。

除普遍预防措施外, 目前尚无其他公认的针对 HCV 感染的预防策略, 血清免疫球蛋白对暴露后预防无效。随着血液制品 HCV 筛查工作的广泛开展, 输血后感染的情况已变得罕见。

酒精性肝病

酒精滥用仍然是西方国家肝脏疾病的主要原因。酒精滥用导致的 3 种主要病变包括脂肪肝、酒精性肝炎和肝硬

alcohol abuse are fatty liver, alcoholic hepatitis, and cirrhosis. These findings are not mutually exclusive and may all be present in the same patient. The first two conditions are potentially reversible. Alcoholic cirrhosis is discussed in Chapter 14.

Mechanism of Injury

The mechanisms of liver injury caused by alcohol are complex. Ethanol and its metabolites, acetaldehyde and nicotinamide adenine dinucleotide phosphate, are directly hepatotoxic and cause a large number of metabolic derangements. Induction of cytochrome P-450 (i.e., CYP2E1) stimulates reactive oxidant species and cytokine pathways, particularly tumor necrosis factor-α (TNF-α). These are critical in initiating and perpetuating hepatic injury, as well as causing fibrosis through stellate cell activation. Excess alcohol leads to increased intestinal permeability, and the resultant endotoxemia from bacterial lipopolysaccharide leads to hepatic inflammation from upregulation of TNF-α.

Hepatotoxic effects from alcohol vary considerably among individuals based on dose, duration, drinking patterns, sex, ethnicity, genetic factors, and comorbidities that may affect the liver. The amount of alcohol ingested is the most important risk factor for the development of alcoholic liver disease. Women have a lower threshold of injury than men and have decreased amounts of gastric alcohol dehydrogenase as compared to men. The risk of cirrhosis is increased in men who drink greater than 60 to 80 grams of alcohol daily and women who drink more than 20 grams of alcohol daily. Malnutrition and other forms of chronic liver disease may potentiate the toxic effects of alcohol on the liver.

Clinical and Pathologic Features

Alcoholic fatty liver may manifest as incidentally discovered hepatomegaly or elevated aminotransferase levels on screening blood tests. Vague discomfort in the right upper quadrant of the abdomen may be the only symptom. Jaundice is rare, and aminotransferases are only mildly elevated (<5 times normal). Liver biopsy shows either diffuse or centrilobular fat occupying most of the hepatocytes.

Alcoholic hepatitis is a distinct entity characterized by acute hepatic inflammation that carries a high morbidity and mortality in its most severe form. It is characterized on liver biopsy by the histologic triad of Mallory bodies, infiltration by polymorphonuclear leukocytes, and a network of interlobular connective tissue surrounding hepatocytes and central veins (pericellular, perivenular, and perisinusoidal fibrosis). Patients with alcoholic hepatitis may be asymptomatic, or they may be extremely ill with hepatic failure. Other common symptoms are anorexia, nausea, vomiting, weight loss, and abdominal pain. For those with fever, infection needs to be ruled out. Rapid onset of jaundice is commonly present and may be pronounced, with cholestatic features that require differentiation from biliary tract disease (see Chapters 10, 11, and 15). Physical examination may reveal cutaneous signs of chronic liver disease, including spider angiomas and palmar erythema. In addition, gynecomastia, parotid enlargement, testicular atrophy, and loss of body hair may be found. The presence of ascites and hepatic encephalopathy can occur. Aminotransferases are only moderately increased (200 to 400 U/L) in alcoholic hepatitis compared with other forms of acute hepatitis. The ratio of AST to ALT almost always exceeds 2:1, in contrast to viral hepatitis, in which the aminotransferases are usually increased in parallel. The white blood cell count may be strikingly increased.

Diagnosis

A history of excessive and prolonged alcohol intake is frequently difficult to obtain from patients with alcoholic liver disease. However, historical, clinical, and biochemical features of alcoholic hepatitis are often sufficient to establish the diagnosis. Many patients suspected or found to imbibe alcohol excessively may have causes in addition to alcohol contributing to liver disease (e.g., chronic viral hepatitis). Therefore, when other causes of liver disease are suggested, and alcohol intake is uncertain, appropriate serologic testing and a liver biopsy may be needed to establish a diagnosis.

Treatment

Complete abstinence from alcohol is the most important step. Meticulous supportive care, including enteral feeding for those with severe anorexia, is the cornerstone of treatment for acute alcoholic hepatitis. In the absence of contraindications (i.e., infection, gastrointestinal bleeding, or renal failure), some patients with alcoholic hepatitis may benefit from treatment with corticosteroids. A calculated discriminant function (DF) value greater than 32 (where DF = 4.6 × [prothrombin time (in seconds) − control (in seconds)] + total bilirubin [in mg/dL]) may identify a subgroup of patients who are more likely to benefit from the use of corticosteroids, but these patients have advanced liver disease and a high mortality rate. Similarly, a Model for End-stage Liver Disease (MELD) score greater than 21 predicts a 90-day mortality of 20%. Pentoxifylline, an oral TNF-α antagonist, was shown to reduce the risk of renal failure but not mortality in a single randomized trial but has not shown benefit in other trials.

Complication and Prognosis

Alcoholic fatty liver disease completely resolves with cessation of alcohol intake. Alcoholic hepatitis can also resolve, but it commonly progresses either to cirrhosis, which may already be present at the time of initial diagnosis, or to hepatic failure and death. The development of encephalopathy, ascites, acute kidney injury, and gastrointestinal bleeding from varices often complicates alcoholic hepatitis (see Chapter 14). Patients with a DF greater than 32 have a high risk of death. The Lille model combines six reproducible variables (age, renal insufficiency, albumin, prothrombin time, bilirubin, and evolution of bilirubin at day 7) and is highly predictive of death at 6 months and helps guide corticosteroid therapy if initiated. A score greater than 0.45 predicts a 6-month survival rate of 25%, compared with 85% survival when the score is less than 0.45.

Drug-Induced Liver Injury

Drug-induced liver injury (DILI) refers to liver injury caused by drugs or other chemical agents and represents a special type of adverse drug reaction. More than 1000 medications and supplements are known to cause hepatotoxicity. Antibiotics remain the drugs most commonly responsible for DILI in the United States and Europe; the annual incidence of antibiotic-associated DILI is 1 in 10,000 to 100,000 individuals.

DILI may be classified by the pattern of liver injury observed. *Acute hepatocellular injury* is characterized by elevated levels of serum ALT and minimal elevations of serum ALP. *Cholestatic injury* is characterized by a disproportionately elevated level of ALP, which is synthesized and released by injured bile ducts. Liver injury that has both hepatocellular and cholestatic features is called *mixed liver injury*. DILI can also be classified into two broad categories, predictable and unpredictable, depending on the hepatotoxins involved. Predictable hepatotoxins, such as acetaminophen and carbon tetrachloride, cause dose-dependent liver injury. Acetaminophen is now the leading cause of life-threatening acute liver failure in the United States and Europe. Unpredictable hepatotoxins cause DILI in a so-called idiosyncratic fashion. Idiosyncratic reactions are difficult to predict and are not dose dependent. They generally tend to occur within the first 3 months of

化。这些病变可同时存在于同一患者。其中，前两种病变可能是可逆的。酒精性肝硬化将在第 14 章中讨论。

发病机制

酒精引起的肝损伤机制较为复杂。乙醇及其代谢产物（乙醛和烟酰胺腺嘌呤二核苷酸磷酸）对肝脏有直接毒性，可导致多种代谢紊乱。细胞色素 P450（即 CYP2E1）的诱导可激活活性氧类和细胞因子通路，特别是肿瘤坏死因子-α（TNF-α）。这在肝损伤的启动和维持、星状细胞激活导致肝纤维化等方面至关重要。此外，过量饮酒可导致肠道通透性增加，从而产生由细菌脂多糖引起的内毒素血症，进而引起 TNF-α 上调，导致肝脏炎症。

酒精的肝毒性作用在不同个体之间差异很大，这取决于酒精摄入量、饮酒时间、饮酒模式、性别、种族、遗传因素及可能累及肝脏的合并症。其中，酒精摄入量是影响酒精性肝病进展最重要的危险因素。与男性相比，女性的损伤阈值更低，且胃内酒精脱氢酶的含量更少。当男性每日酒精摄入量 > 60 ~ 80 g、女性 > 20 g 时，肝硬化的发生风险增加。营养不良和其他类型的慢性肝病可能增强酒精的肝毒性作用。

临床表现和病理学特征

酒精性脂肪肝可表现为偶然发现的肝大或血液筛查化验发现转氨酶水平升高。右上腹隐痛可能是唯一的症状。转氨酶多表现为轻度升高（< 正常值上限的 5 倍），很少合并黄疸。肝活检可表现为弥漫性或小叶中心性肝细胞脂肪变性。

酒精性肝炎是一种以急性肝脏炎症为特征的独立疾病，危重患者的并发症发生率和死亡率很高。肝活检可表现为三联征：马洛里小体（Mallory 小体）、多形核白细胞浸润，以及围绕肝细胞和中心静脉的纤维组织增生（肝细胞周围、中心静脉周围和窦周纤维化）。酒精性肝炎患者可无症状，病情危重时可伴有肝衰竭。其他常见症状包括食欲减退、恶心、呕吐、体重减轻和腹痛。对于发热患者，需排除感染。黄疸急性发作较常见，且可能非常明显，具有胆汁淤积的特征，需要与胆道疾病鉴别（见第 10 章、第 11 章和第 15 章）。体格检查可见慢性肝病的皮肤改变，如蜘蛛痣和肝掌。此外，还可见男性乳房发育、腮腺肿大、睾丸萎缩和体毛丧失。患者可发生腹腔积液和肝性脑病。与其他病因导致的急性肝炎相比，酒精性肝炎患者的转氨酶水平仅中度升高（200 ~ 400 U/L），通常 AST/ALT 比值 > 2∶1，这可与病毒性肝炎相鉴别。此外，白细胞计数可显著增加。

诊断

通常很难从酒精性肝病患者处获取长期过量饮酒的病史。然而，通过病史、临床和生化特征，通常足以确定酒精性肝炎的诊断。许多有过量饮酒史的患者可能同时合并除酒精以外的其他病因（如慢性病毒性肝炎）。因此，当提示存在其他引起肝病的病因且饮酒史不明确时，可能需要进行适当的血清学检查甚至肝活检来明确诊断。

治疗

完全戒酒是酒精性肝病最重要的治疗措施。细致全面的支持性措施（包括对严重厌食症患者进行肠内营养）是急性酒精性肝炎治疗的基石。在没有禁忌证（即感染、消化道出血或肾衰竭）的情况下，部分酒精性肝炎患者可能从皮质类固醇治疗中获益。可根据计算出的判别函数（DF）值 > 32 {其中 DF = 4.6 × [凝血酶原时间（s）- 对照（s）] + 总胆红素（mg/dl)} 来识别出皮质类固醇治疗的目标患者，但这些患者均为进展期肝病且病死率高。同样，终末期肝病模型（MELD）评分 > 21 分可预测 90 天内死亡率达 20%。一项随机试验显示，己酮可可碱（一种口服 TNF-α 拮抗剂）可降低肾衰竭的风险，但并未降低死亡率，其疗效在其他试验中未被证实。

并发症和预后

酒精性脂肪肝在戒酒后可获得痊愈。酒精性肝炎在戒酒后也可得到改善，但多数会进展为肝硬化（初诊时可能已经存在），甚至肝衰竭和死亡。出现肝性脑病、腹腔积液、急性肾损伤和食管静脉曲张破裂出血等并发症会使酒精性肝炎的病情更加复杂（见第 14 章）。DF 值 > 32 的患者死亡风险更高。Lille 模型结合了 6 个可重复的变量（年龄、肾功能不全、白蛋白、凝血酶原时间、胆红素和第 7 天时的胆红素变化），可预测 6 个月内的死亡风险，并有助于指导皮质类固醇治疗。Lille 模型得分 > 0.45 分和 < 0.45 分预测的 6 个月生存率分别为 25% 和 85%。

药物性肝损伤

药物性肝损伤（DILI）是由药物或其他化学制剂引起的肝损伤，它是药物不良反应的一种特殊类型。已知超过 1000 种药物和膳食补充剂能够引起肝毒性。在美国和欧洲，抗生素是最常见的导致 DILI 的药物；抗生素相关 DILI 的年发病率为（1 ~ 10）/100 000。

根据肝损伤模式可对 DILI 进行分类。急性肝细胞损伤的特点是血清 ALT 水平升高，而血清 ALP 水平仅有轻微升高。胆汁淤积性损伤的特点是 ALP 水平不成比例地异常升高，因为受损的胆管合成并释放 ALP。同时具有肝细胞损伤和胆汁淤积性损伤特征的肝损伤被称为混合性肝损伤。此外，根据涉及的肝毒素，可将 DILI 分为两大类：可预测和不可预测。可预测的肝毒素（如对乙酰氨基酚和四氯化碳）会导致剂量依赖性肝损伤。对乙酰氨基酚目前是美国和欧洲危及生命的急性肝衰竭的主要原因。不可预测的肝毒素以特异质的形式引起 DILI。特异质反应难以预测，且不依赖于剂量，通常在开始用药后的前 3 个月内发生，其发

initiating a medication. They occur relatively rarely in individuals with unique genetic and environmental characteristics.

Clinical and Laboratory Manifestations

DILI symptoms are similar to those associated with viral hepatitis and include malaise, anorexia, nausea and vomiting, right upper quadrant abdominal pain, jaundice, acholic stools, and dark (tea-colored) urine. Patients with cholestatic DILI may also have pruritus. Fever and rash, hallmarks of hypersensitivity, may be present with DILI caused by certain drugs such as anticonvulsants and sulfamethoxazole-trimethoprim. Cholestatic or mixed hepatitis related to amoxicillin-clavulanic acid (Augmentin) may develop shortly after the drug has been stopped, usually within 2 to 3 weeks. Nitrofurantoin (Macrobid) characteristically causes a chronic hepatitis after many weeks, months, or even years of therapy and is often associated with the presence of serum antinuclear antibodies (ANA).

Diagnosis

The diagnosis of DILI is challenging because of the lack of specific or uniform clinical features or laboratory tests in the majority of cases. A high level of suspicion for DILI is essential for diagnosis, as is the exclusion of other possible causes of liver injury. Generally, DILI occurs within the first 3 months of initiation of a medication but can occur after longer periods. The Russel-Uclaf Causality Assessment Method (RUCAM) provides objective and consistent assessment but can be cumbersome for routine clinical use. Moreover, a study conducted by Grant and Rockey suggested that expert opinion outperforms RUCAM in making a diagnosis of DILI. There is definitely a need for a simple, accurate, and reproducible method for diagnosing DILI.

Hepatitis E appears to be a small but important alternative diagnosis for suspected DILI. Of 318 patients in the multicenter U.S. Drug-Induced Liver Injury Network (DILIN) with suspected drug hepatotoxicity, 9 (3%) were found to be positive for HEV IgM.

Treatment

The mainstay of management of DILI is withdrawal of the offending agent and supportive care, which is usually sufficient in cases of mild to moderate DILI. Rechallenge of the implicated drug should be avoided. Specific therapies are available for some types of DILI. Timely administration of N-acetylcysteine (NAC) for acetaminophen overdose can be lifesaving. NAC may also improve outcomes of patients with early acute liver failure from etiologies other than acetaminophen. Corticosteroids are probably ineffective for DILI from most drugs; however, a short course of steroids is sometimes used for treatment of immune-mediated DILI with the manifestations of rash, fever, and eosinophilia. Ursodeoxycholic acid is safe and may possibly hasten the resolution of jaundice and pruritus.

Complication and Prognosis

With supportive care and discontinuation of the offending drug, mild to moderate DILI usually resolves rapidly. Cholestatic liver injury may take many weeks and even months to completely resolve. Occasionally, cholestatic DILI can progress to permanent bile duct injury with so-called vanishing bile duct syndrome. Patients may develop progressive liver injury or develop acute liver failure manifesting with encephalopathy and coagulopathy, and may need liver transplantation.

CHRONIC HEPATITIS

Chronic hepatitis is defined as a sustained inflammatory process in the liver lasting longer than 6 months. On initial presentation, chronic hepatitis can be difficult to differentiate from acute hepatitis on clinical or histologic criteria alone. Except for hepatitis A, acute viral hepatitis, especially that caused by HBV or HCV, can ultimately lead to chronic hepatitis. Nonalcoholic steatohepatitis (NASH) is now the most frequent cause of chronic hepatitis in the United States and Western Europe. Several drugs can cause chronic hepatitis including methyldopa, isoniazid, minocycline, propylthiouracil, and hydralazine. In contrast to acute hepatitis, an etiologic agent is sometimes difficult to identify in cases of chronic hepatitis. The pathogenesis of these idiopathic forms may represent quiescent autoimmune disease, undetected past DILI or NASH, antibody-negative viral infection, or misdiagnosed cholestatic liver injury (e.g., primary biliary cirrhosis [PBC], primary sclerosing cholangitis [PSC]).

Chronic Viral Hepatitis

In Western countries, acute HBV infection usually occurs in adults; 5% to 10% of patients fail to clear the virus and develop chronic hepatitis. In other areas, vertical transmission and childhood acquisition is common. Children who are infected within 2 years of birth have a much higher rate of chronic hepatitis B. HBV infection without evidence of any liver damage may persist, resulting in asymptomatic hepatitis B carriers. In Asia and Africa, many such carriers appear to have acquired the virus from infected mothers during infancy (vertical transmission).

Patients who are HBsAg and HBeAg positive and have high blood HBV DNA (>20,000 IU/mL), coupled with elevated serum aminotransferases, are in a high replicative phase (see Table 12.3). In contrast, patients in a low replicative phase are HBsAg and anti-HBe positive, have low blood HBV DNA (<20,000 IU/mL), and have near-normal or normal aminotransferase levels. These patients likely have HBV with precore and/or core promoter mutation. Patients infected with HBV in a high replicative phase are at high risk for cirrhosis and hepatocellular carcinoma. Such patients, and those who have already progressed to early cirrhosis, are the primary candidates for antiviral therapy.

Currently, eight drugs are approved for the treatment of adults with chronic hepatitis B in the United States, including interferon-α and its pegylated form and six nucleos(t)ide analogues (lamivudine, telbivudine, adefovir dipivoxil, tenofovir disoproxil, entecavir, and tenofovir alafenamide). The primary aim of therapy is to eliminate or permanently suppress HBV and thus reduce the activity of hepatitis and slow or limit the progression of liver disease. It is important to start therapy with a nucleos(t)ide analogue that has a high genetic barrier to resistance, such as entecavir or tenofovir, as first-line therapy. Long-term follow-up studies have shown interferon-based therapy increases HBsAg seroclearance over time. HBsAg seroclearance is less common in patients who are treated with nucleos(t)ide analogues rather than interferon-based therapy. All patients with chronic HBV are at risk for hepatocellular carcinoma and should undergo screening based on age, sex, and ethnicity. The risk of hepatocellular carcinoma decreases with decreasing viral load.

In patients with HBV and HDV coinfection, the fate of HDV is determined by the host response to HBV, which in more than 95% of adults results in viral clearance. By contrast, HDV superinfection of an individual with chronic hepatitis B usually results in chronic HDV infection. Treatment with nucleos(t)ide analogues is not effective in reducing HDV replication. The accepted practice for treatment of chronic HDV infection is weekly pegylated interferon for at least 48 weeks. In patients with a high concentration of HBV DNA, the addition of a potent nucleos(t)ide analogue to inhibit HBV replication is logical, but long-term effectiveness has yet to be defined.

Chronic hepatitis C develops in up to 75% of individuals who are acutely exposed to HCV (Fig. 12.5). Approximately 1.6% of the United States population (4.1 million people) are positive for antibodies to HCV (anti-HCV), and 2.4 million of them have chronic infection. Up

生率较低且主要见于具有特定遗传和环境特征的个体。

临床表现和实验室检查

DILI的症状与病毒性肝炎相似,包括全身不适、食欲减退、恶心和呕吐、右上腹疼痛、黄疸、白陶土样便和深色(茶色)尿液。患有胆汁淤积性DILI的患者可能会出现皮肤瘙痒。发热和皮疹(超敏反应的标志)可见于由特定药物(如抗惊厥药和磺胺甲噁唑-甲氧苄啶)引起的DILI。阿莫西林-克拉维酸相关胆汁淤积性或混合性肝损伤可在停药后短时间内(2~3周)出现。呋喃妥因相关DILI的特点是可在治疗数周、数月甚至数年后引起慢性肝炎,且常伴有血清抗核抗体(ANA)阳性。

诊断

因缺乏特异的临床特征或实验室检查标志物,DILI的诊断具有挑战性。最重要的是临床高度怀疑DILI并排除其他可能导致肝损伤的原因。一般情况下,DILI发生在开始用药后的3个月内,但也可能在较长时间后才发生。Russel-Uclaf因果关系评估方法(RUCAM)可提供客观且一致的评估,但在临床工作中使用较为繁琐。此外,Grant和Rockey的研究表明,专家意见在DILI诊断方面优于RUCAM。临床上亟需一种简便、准确和可重复的DILI诊断方法。

对于疑诊DILI的患者,戊型肝炎是一个少见但重要的鉴别诊断。在多中心美国药物性肝损伤协作网(DILIN)的318例疑似DILI的患者中,9例(3%)被发现HEV IgM阳性。

治疗

及时停用可疑药物及对症支持治疗是最主要的措施,这对于轻中度DILI患者通常已经足够。应避免再次使用可疑药物。特殊类型的DILI有其特定的治疗方法。及时给予N-乙酰半胱氨酸(NAC)可挽救对乙酰氨基酚过量患者的生命。NAC也可能改善由非对乙酰氨基酚引起的早期急性肝衰竭患者的预后。皮质类固醇对大多数药物引起的DILI可能无效;然而,在伴有皮疹、发热和嗜酸性粒细胞增多的免疫介导性DILI患者中,可考虑短期应用。对于胆汁淤积型DILI,熊去氧胆酸是安全的,并可能加速改善黄疸和瘙痒症状。

并发症和预后

在停用可疑肝损伤药物及对症支持治疗的情况下,轻中度DILI患者通常可迅速缓解。胆汁淤积型DILI可能需要数周甚至数月才能完全恢复,少数患者可能会进展为慢性胆管损伤,即胆管消失综合征。少数患者可能出现进行性肝损伤,或发展为以肝性脑病和凝血功能障碍为表现的急性肝衰竭,并可能需要肝移植。

慢性肝炎

慢性肝炎被定义为持续超过6个月的肝脏炎症。在初次就诊时,仅凭临床表现或组织学特点可能很难将慢性肝炎与急性肝炎区分开来。除甲型肝炎外,急性病毒性肝炎(特别是乙型肝炎或丙型肝炎)最终可能导致慢性肝炎。非酒精性脂肪性肝炎(NASH)目前是美国和西欧地区慢性肝炎最常见的原因。此外,多种药物(包括甲基多巴、异烟肼、米诺环素、丙硫氧嘧啶和肼屈嗪)也可引起慢性肝炎。与急性肝炎不同,在慢性肝炎患者中,有时很难明确致病因子。这些特发性慢性肝炎的发生机制可能包括自身免疫性肝病的静止期、既往未被发现的DILI或NASH、抗体阴性的病毒感染,或被误诊的胆汁淤积性肝损伤[如原发性胆汁性胆管炎(PBC)、原发性硬化性胆管炎(PSC)]。

慢性病毒性肝炎

在西方国家,急性HBV感染常见于成人;5%~10%的患者不能清除病毒而发展为慢性肝炎。在其他地区,垂直传播和儿童期感染较为常见。在出生后2年内感染HBV的儿童更易发展为慢性乙型肝炎。HBV感染可能会持续存在但没有肝脏损伤的证据,即无症状HBV携带者。在亚洲和非洲,多数HBV携带者可能是在婴儿期通过受感染的母亲而感染病毒(垂直传播)。

HBsAg和HBeAg阳性、血液中HBV DNA水平高(> 20 000 IU/ml)且伴有血清转氨酶水平升高的患者,提示处于高复制期(表12.3)。相比之下,处于低复制期的患者HBsAg和HBeAb阳性,但血液中HBV DNA水平低(< 20 000 IU/ml),且转氨酶水平接近正常或正常。这些患者可能携带具有前核心和(或)核心启动子突变的HBV。处于高复制期的HBV感染者发展为肝硬化和肝细胞癌的风险更高。这些患者和已经发展至早期肝硬化的患者是抗病毒治疗的主要目标人群。

目前,美国批准了8种药物用于治疗成人慢性乙型肝炎,包括干扰素-α及其聚乙二醇化形式和6种核苷(酸)类似物(拉米夫定、替比夫定、阿德福韦酯、替诺福韦酯、恩替卡韦和丙酚替诺福韦)。治疗的主要目标是消除或长期抑制HBV复制,从而减少肝炎活动并减缓或限制肝脏疾病的进展。选择具有高耐药屏障的核苷(酸)类似物作为起始治疗非常重要,如恩替卡韦或替诺福韦酯。长期随访研究表明,基于干扰素的治疗会随时间而提高HBsAg的血清清除率。与接受核苷(酸)类似物治疗的患者相比,接受干扰素治疗的患者HBsAg的血清清除率更高。所有慢性乙型肝炎患者均有进展为肝细胞癌的风险,因此应根据年龄、性别和种族进行定期筛查。肝细胞癌的风险会随病毒载量的降低而减小。

在HBV和HDV共感染的患者中,HDV感染的转归取决于宿主对HBV的反应,超过95%的成人感染者可完全清除病毒。相比之下,慢性乙型肝炎患者重叠感染HDV通常会导致慢性HDV感染。核苷(酸)类似物治疗在减少HDV复制方面无效。治疗慢性HDV感染的公认方法是每周使用聚乙二醇干扰素,至少48周。在血清HBV DNA水平高的患者中,应加用1种强效核苷(酸)类似物,以抑制HBV复制,但其长期效果尚不明确。

高达75%的急性HCV感染者会发展为慢性丙型肝炎(图12.5)。约1.6%的美国人口(约410万人)

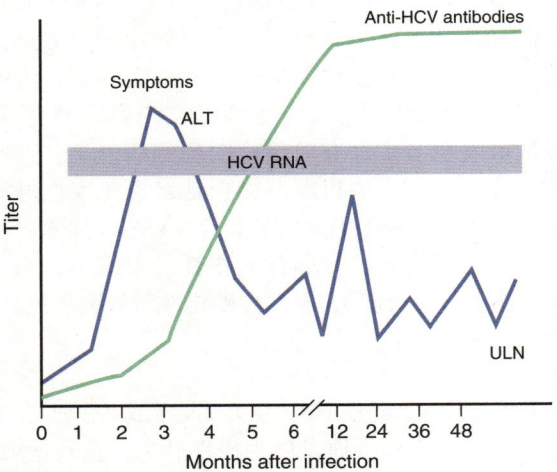

Fig. 12.5 Kinetics of hepatitis C virus (HCV) markers during acute hepatitis C that evolves toward chronic infection. *ALT,* Alanine aminotransferase; *ULN,* upper limit of normal.

to 20% of HCV cases progress to cirrhosis, usually within 20 to 30 years after infection. HCV has six major genotypes, of which genotype 1 is the most common in the United States, followed by genotypes 2 and 3. The genotype helps determine the treatment regimen and duration of therapy. The goal of antiviral therapy is to achieve a sustained virologic response (SVR12) or cure, defined as an undetectable HCV RNA level 12 weeks after treatment discontinuation. The current medications for hepatitis C are very effective and achieve cure in 98% to 99% of treatment naïve patients. These newer second-generation direct-acting antivirals target HCV replication, and have dramatically increased cure rates, shortened treatment duration, and minimized side effects. These medications work via novel mechanisms of action that target HCV enzymes needed for replication such as NS5B polymerase, NS3/4 protease, and the HCV protein NS5A. Pegylated interferon-α and ribavirin are now historical medications for treatment of chronic hepatitis C, where patients were treated for 24 or 48 weeks with SVR rates of 50% and a high incidence of side effects.

Among organ transplant recipients, the consumption of game meat, pork products, or mussels may result in HEV infection, which is most commonly asymptomatic without jaundice. About 60% of such infections become chronic, and up to 10% of patients progress to cirrhosis. Treatment includes careful reduction in immunosuppression, which results in viral clearance in 30% of patients on ribavirin monotherapy.

Autoimmune Hepatitis

Autoimmune hepatitis (AIH) has several clinical forms that share typical histologic findings including significant hepatic inflammation with a preponderance of plasma cells and fibrosis. Type 1, or classic, AIH is characterized by the presence of hypergammaglobulinemia, as well as the autoantibodies ANA or anti–smooth muscle antibodies (ASMA) in up to 80% of cases. Type 2 AIH is characterized by the presence of anti–liver/kidney microsomal antibodies (anti-LKM1) and the absence of ANA and ASMA. The type 1 variant can affect people of any age or gender, whereas the less common type 2 variant primarily affects girls and young women. A third type of AIH with antibodies to soluble liver antigen or liver-pancreas antigen (anti-SLA/LP) is no longer considered a unique entity because these antibodies may be found in type 1 and 2 variants as well. There are also uncommon overlap variants of AIH that have features of both AIH and other liver diseases such as PBC or PSC.

There are no pathognomonic features of AIH, and the diagnosis is made by a combination of factors. A simplified diagnostic algorithm that includes the presence of autoantibodies, hypergammaglobulinemia, typical liver histology, and absence of viral hepatitis has proved useful in identifying patients with AIH. Extrahepatic manifestations such as amenorrhea, rashes, acne, vasculitis, thyroiditis, and Sjögren's syndrome are common. Evidence of hepatic failure and the presence of chronic disease on liver biopsy are often discernable at the time of diagnosis. Indications for treatment include abnormal liver function tests and significant hepatic inflammation on biopsy.

Corticosteroids are the mainstay of treatment, typically in combination with azathioprine as a steroid-sparing agent. This regimen is efficacious in most patients (>80%) and in many instances prolongs survival.

Nonalcoholic Fatty Liver Disease

Nonalcoholic fatty liver disease (NAFLD) has a spectrum of presentations from simple steatosis, which usually does not progress to advanced liver disease, to NASH, which may exhibit or lead to cirrhosis. It is the most common cause of abnormal liver function tests among adults in the United States and Western Europe. NAFLD is commonly seen in people with central obesity, hypertension, diabetes, and hyperlipidemia, although it can be observed in persons with normal weight as well. Insulin resistance plays a central role in the pathophysiology of NAFLD. Estimates indicate that about 80 to 100 million Americans have NAFLD; of these, 18 million have NASH and almost 20% have signs of advanced disease (i.e., bridging fibrosis, cirrhosis) on histologic examination.

Liver biopsy is the "gold standard" for diagnosis of NASH. The NAFLD Activity Score has been developed and represents the sum of scores for steatosis, lobular inflammation, and hepatocyte ballooning that are typically seen on liver biopsy. It ranges from 0 to 8, with a score of 5 or higher considered diagnostic of NASH. Liver biopsy is invasive, costly, and can cause complications including a small mortality risk (0.01% to 0.1%). The use of liver biopsy has declined with newer noninvasive assessments of liver fibrosis and steatosis. Liver biopsy predominantly is used when there is diagnostic uncertainty to the etiology of disease. Radiologic imaging studies based on ultrasound and MRI can determine fibrosis by measuring liver stiffness with transient elastography technology and can also estimate the degree of steatosis.

Currently, this is no FDA-approved treatment available for NASH. Clinical trials of agents that therapeutically target the development of hepatic steatosis and fibrosis are underway and have shown beneficial effects on hepatic fibrosis. However, weight reduction with a goal of 5% to 7% of body weight loss and regular exercise are associated with biochemical and histologic improvement and are important components of therapy. Vitamin E and pioglitazone have been shown to improve hepatic inflammation in nondiabetic patients with NASH, but they are not routinely recommended because of questions regarding long-term safety and side effects.

Genetic and Metabolic Hepatitis

Hemochromatosis is an autosomal recessive genetic disorder that causes low levels of the iron regulatory hormone hepcidin causing defective sensing of iron stores and leads to excessive absorption of iron from the digestive tract. In the United States, about 1 of every 250 Caucasians have the condition; however, clinical expression is variable. Elevated ferritin and transferrin saturation values are typically used to screen patients with evidence of chronic liver disease and guide the need for further genetic testing. Most patients with hemochromatosis are homozygous for the C282Y mutation in the *HFE* gene, and a subset of

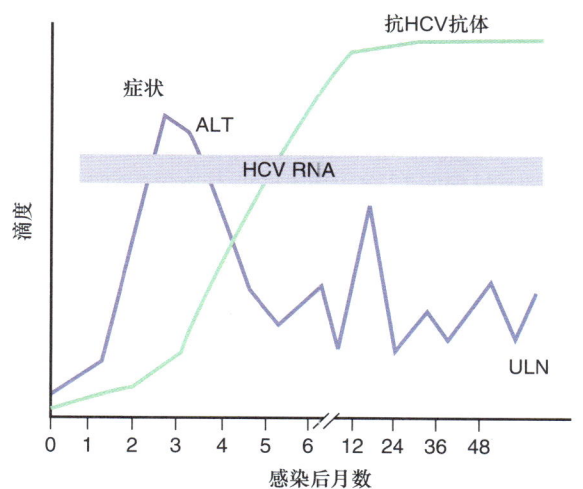

图 12.5 急性丙型肝炎向慢性感染演变期间 HCV 标志物的动态变化。ALT，丙氨酸转氨酶；ULN，正常值上限

抗 HCV 抗体呈阳性，其中约 240 万人患有慢性丙型肝炎。约 20% 的 HCV 感染者进展为肝硬化，通常见于感染后 20～30 年内。HCV 有 6 种基因型，其中基因 1 型在美国最常见，其次是基因 2 型和 3 型。基因分型有助于确定治疗方案和治疗持续时间。抗病毒治疗的目标是实现持续的病毒学应答（SVR12）或治愈，其定义为治疗停止后 12 周 HCV RNA 水平仍无法测出。目前治疗丙型肝炎的药物非常有效，98%～99% 的初治患者可实现治愈。这些新型第二代 DAA 针对 HCV 复制，显著提高了治愈率，缩短了治疗持续时间，并大大减少了副作用。这些药物通过针对 HCV 复制所需的酶来发挥作用，如 NS5B 聚合酶、NS3/4 蛋白酶和 HCV 蛋白 NS5A。聚乙二醇干扰素-α 和利巴韦林作为治疗慢性丙型肝炎的首选药物已成为历史，因为患者接受 24 周或 48 周治疗后的 SVR 率仅为 50%，且副作用发生率较高。

器官移植受者在食用野生动物肉类、猪肉制品或贝类时，可能会感染 HEV。此类感染通常无症状，不伴有黄疸。器官移植受者在感染 HEV 后，约 60% 会发生慢性化，且高达 10% 的患者会进展为肝硬化。其治疗方案包括谨慎地降低免疫抑制剂的剂量，这可使 30% 的利巴韦林单药治疗患者获得病毒清除。

自身免疫性肝炎

自身免疫性肝炎（AIH）有多种临床表现形式，但组织学上均以显著的肝脏炎症、浆细胞浸润和肝纤维化为典型特征。1 型（经典型）AIH 的特征是高丙种球蛋白血症、抗核抗体（ANA）或抗平滑肌抗体（ASMA）阳性（见于 80% 的病例）。2 型 AIH 的特征是抗肝肾微粒体抗体（抗 LKM1）阳性。1 型 AIH 可见于任何年龄或性别人群，而 2 型 AIH 主要见于女童和年轻女性。由于见于 3 型的可溶性肝抗原或肝-胰抗原（抗 SLA/LP）抗体阳性也可见于 1 型和 2 型 AIH，因此 3 型不再作为一种特殊类型。此外，还有较少见的 AIH 重叠变异型，即同时具有 AIH 和其他肝病（如 PBC 或 PSC）的特征。

AIH 没有特异性临床特征，诊断主要通过综合多种因素来确定。一项简化诊断流程（包括自身抗体阳性、高丙种球蛋白血症、典型的肝组织学特征及缺乏病毒性肝炎证据）已被证明可较好地用于 AIH 的诊断。AIH 常见的肝外表现包括闭经、皮疹、痤疮、血管炎、甲状腺炎和干燥综合征。诊断时通常可发现肝衰竭的证据及肝活检提示存在慢性肝病。治疗指征包括肝功能异常及组织学明显的肝脏炎症。

皮质类固醇是治疗的首选方案，通常与硫唑嘌呤联合使用，以减少皮质类固醇的用量。该方案在大多数患者（＞80%）中有明显疗效，且能够延长生存期。

非酒精性脂肪性肝病

非酒精性脂肪性肝病（NAFLD）的疾病谱可从单纯性脂肪肝（通常不会发展为严重肝脏疾病）到 NASH（可表现为或导致肝硬化）。NAFLD 是美国和西欧地区成人肝功能异常的最常见原因。NAFLD 通常见于向心性肥胖、高血压、糖尿病和高脂血症人群，但在正常体重人群中也可观察到。胰岛素抵抗在 NAFLD 的发病机制中发挥核心作用。据估计，美国有 8000 万到 1 亿人患有 NAFLD；其中，1800 万人患有 NASH，近 20% 的 NAFLD 患者有进展期肝病的组织学表现（如桥接纤维化、肝硬化）。

肝活检是诊断 NASH 的"金标准"。NAFLD 活动度评分（NAS）为肝细胞脂肪变性、气球样变性和小叶性炎症的评分之和，范围为 0～8 分，≥5 分考虑为 NASH。肝活检为有创性检查，价格较为昂贵，且可能导致并发症，包括死亡风险（0.01%～0.1%）。随着新型评估肝纤维化和脂肪变性的无创性方法的出现，肝活检的应用已有所减少，目前主要用于病因不明确的病例。基于超声和 MRI 的影像学技术可通过瞬时弹性成像技术测量肝硬度来评估纤维化，并能估计脂肪肝的程度。

目前，美国食品药品监督管理局（FDA）尚未批准治疗 NASH 的方法。针对肝脏脂肪变性和纤维化进展的新药临床试验正在进行中，并已显示出一定治疗效果。然而，减重 5%～7% 和定期运动可使生化和组织学改善，目前仍是重要的治疗手段。维生素 E 和吡格列酮已被证明可改善非糖尿病性 NASH 患者的肝脏炎症，但由于长期安全性和副作用问题，不推荐常规应用。

遗传性和代谢性肝炎

血色病是一种常染色体隐性遗传病，可引起铁调素（调节铁平衡的激素）水平降低，从而使机体对铁储备的感应缺陷，导致从消化道吸收过量的铁。在美国，白人的发病率约为 1/250；然而，临床表现可能多种多样。对于慢性肝病患者，通常选择血清铁蛋白和转铁蛋白饱和度来进行初步筛查，并指导是否需要进一步行基因检测。大多数血色病患者为 HFE 基因 C282Y 纯合突变，部分同时携带 C282Y 和 H63D 复合杂合突变的个体也可出现铁过载。在 H63D 纯合突变

individuals who are heterozygous for both C282Y and the H63D mutation may also develop iron overload. Iron overload is very uncommon among those who are homozygous for the H63D mutation. Genetic mutations in a number of other proteins involved in iron sensing have also been associated with iron overload but are not routinely tested in clinical practice.

Hemochromatosis is a systemic disease that causes iron deposition in parenchymal cells in various organs including the liver, heart, pancreas, and pituitary glands. Patients may develop liver cirrhosis and cancer, heart failure, diabetes mellitus, hypogonadism, and arthralgias. A high index of suspicion is required to detect the disorder in early stages. The standard treatment for hemochromatosis is therapeutic phlebotomy. For patients who cannot undergo phlebotomy, chelation therapy may be offered.

Wilson's disease is an autosomal recessive genetic disorder that results from mutations in the *ATP7B* gene located on chromosome 13. These mutations result in excessive accumulation of copper in a number of organs, most notably the liver, cornea, and brain. The prevalence of the disease is approximately 1 in 30,000 live births in most populations. Wilson's disease can occur at any age. Measurement of the 24-hour urine copper excretion, slit lamp examination of corneas for Kayser-Fleischer rings, and direct measurement of hepatic copper confirm the diagnosis. Patients should receive lifelong chelation treatment with either penicillamine or trientine. Zinc may be used to maintain stable copper levels in the body.

α_1-*Antitrypsin deficiency* (AAT) is an autosomal recessive genetic disorder of chromosome 14 that causes retention of AAT in the liver, resulting in liver damage. AAT is a protease inhibitor of the proteolytic enzyme elastase. The normal gene product is designated as PiM, and the deficiency variants are PiS (50% to 60%) and PiZ (10% to 20%). The most common carrier phenotypes are PiMS and PiMZ, and the disease phenotypes are PiZZ, PiSS, and PiSZ. Low serum AAT and diastase-positive staining of hepatocellular AAT inclusions on liver biopsy support the diagnosis. Phenotypic testing in the serum has been the traditional gold standard for the diagnosis. However, genotypic testing is now available and widely used. Lung disease results from a loss of protective effects in patients with low levels of circulating AAT. AAT replacement therapy is an option for those with lung disease but is not useful for patients with liver disease.

For a deeper discussion on this topic, please see Chapters 139, "Acute Viral Hepatitis," and 140, "Chronic Viral and Autoimmune Hepatitis," in *Goldman-Cecil Medicine*, 26th Edition.

SUGGESTED READINGS

Asselah T, Marcellin P: Interferon free therapy with direct acting antivirals for HCV, Liver Int 33(Suppl 1):93–104, 2013.

Feldman M, Friedman LS, Brandt LJ: Sleisenger and Fordtran's gastrointestinal and liver disease-2 Volume Set, ed 10, 2015, Chapters 78-82.

Grant LM, Rockey DC: Drug-induced liver injury, Curr Opin Gastrointesterol 28:198–202, 2012.

Hughes SA, Wedemeyer H, Harrison PM: Hepatitis delta virus, Lancet 378:73–85, 2011.

Jeong SH, Lee HS: Hepatitis A: clinical manifestations and management, Intervirology 53:15–19, 2010.

Kamar N, Bendall R, Legrand-Abravanel F, et al: Hepatitis E, Lancet 379:2477-2488, 2012.

Liaw YF: Impact of therapy on the outcome of chronic hepatitis B, Liver Int 33(Suppl 1):111–115, 2013.

中,铁过载非常罕见。除 *HFE* 外,还有一些基因突变与铁过载有关,这些基因编码的蛋白质参与了铁的感应和调节过程,但在临床实践中并不常规检测。

血色病是一种系统性疾病,可导致多种器官的实质细胞中出现铁沉积,主要包括肝、心脏、胰腺和腺垂体。患者可能会进展为肝硬化和肝细胞癌、心力衰竭、糖尿病、性腺功能减退和关节痛。该病的早期症状可能不明显,因此需要保持高度警惕,以便及早进行诊断和治疗。血色病的标准治疗是放血疗法。对于不能进行静脉放血的患者,可考虑使用铁螯合剂进行驱铁治疗。

肝豆状核变性是一种常染色体隐性遗传病,由位于 13 号染色体上的 *ATP7B* 基因突变引起,导致铜在多个器官(特别是肝、角膜和脑)中过度沉积。该病在大多数人群中的患病率约为 1/30 000。肝豆状核变性可发生于任何年龄。通过 24 h 尿铜排泄量、角膜裂隙灯检查[有无凯-弗环(K-F 环)]及直接测量肝脏铜含量,可以确定诊断。患者应终身接受驱铜治疗,包括青霉胺或曲恩汀。锌可用于维持体内铜含量的稳定。

α_1-抗胰蛋白酶(AAT)缺乏症是一种常染色体隐性遗传病,致病基因位于 14 号染色体,可导致 AAT 在肝细胞内聚积,引起肝损伤。AAT 是弹性蛋白酶(蛋白水解酶)抑制剂。正常基因产物为 PiM,而缺陷变异产物为 PiS(50%~60%)和 PiZ(10%~20%)。最常见的携带者表型为 PiMS 和 PiMZ,致病表型为 PiZZ、PiSS 和 PiSZ。血清 AAT 水平降低和肝活检中肝细胞内有淀粉酶染色阳性的 AAT 包涵体支持该病的诊断。血清表型分析是诊断 AAT 缺乏症的传统金标准。然而,基因检测现已被广泛应用。由于患者血清 AAT 水平显著下降,丧失了对肺泡壁的保护作用,可导致肺部疾病。AAT 替代治疗对肺部疾病有效,但对肝脏受累无明显效果。

有关此专题的深入讨论,请参阅 *Goldman-Cecil Medicine* 第 26 版第 139 章 "急性病毒性肝炎" 和第 140 章 "慢性病毒性肝炎和自身免疫性肝炎"。

推荐阅读

Asselah T, Marcellin P: Interferon free therapy with direct acting antivirals for HCV, Liver Int 33(Suppl 1):93–104, 2013.

Feldman M, Friedman LS, Brandt LJ: Sleisenger and Fordtran's gastrointestinal and liver disease-2 Volume Set,ed 10, 2015, Chapters 78-82.

Grant LM, Rockey DC: Drug-induced liver injury, Curr Opin Gastrointesterol 28:198–202, 2012.

Hughes SA, Wedemeyer H, Harrison PM: Hepatitis delta virus, Lancet 378:73–85, 2011.

Jeong SH, Lee HS: Hepatitis A: clinical manifestations and management, Intervirology 53:15–19, 2010.

Kamar N, Bendall R, Legrand-Abravanel F, et al: Hepatitis E, Lancet 379:2477-2488, 2012.

Liaw YF: Impact of therapy on the outcome of chronic hepatitis B, Liver Int 33(Suppl 1):111–115, 2013.

Acute Liver Failure

Anil Seetharam, Michael B. Fallon

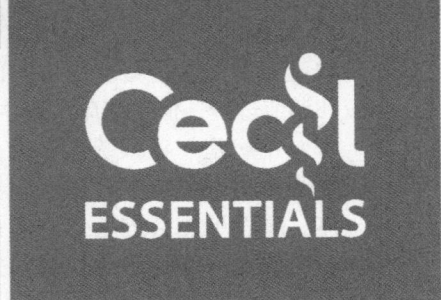

DEFINITIONS

Acute liver failure (ALF) is an infrequent condition characterized by rapid deterioration of liver function resulting in altered mentation and coagulopathy in individuals without preexisting liver disease. A widely accepted working definition includes International Normalized Ratio (INR) greater than 1.5 and any degree of altered mentation (encephalopathy) in a subject without preexisting cirrhosis and illness of less than 26 weeks' duration. Associated multisystem organ dysfunction and encephalopathy with chance for brainstem herniation mandate prompt recognition and transfer to an intensive care unit (ICU). Though etiologic specific treatment and supportive measures can be employed, liver transplantation remains the only chance for cure in those who do not spontaneously recover.

PATHOGENESIS

ALF develops as a result of severe, unrelenting inflammation with hepatocyte necrosis and collapse of the liver's architectural framework. This feature contrasts with the changes of cirrhosis and complications of portal hypertension that dominate chronic liver disease (see Chapter 14). ALF may result from infection with hepatotropic viruses A, B, C, D, or E (see Chapter 12) or from herpes simplex virus (HSV). Additionally, dose-dependent or idiosyncratic exposure to hepatotoxins such as acetaminophen, isoniazid, halothane, valproic acid, or mushroom toxins *(Amanita phalloides)* can produce ALF. Reye's syndrome, a disease that predominantly affects children, and acute fatty liver of pregnancy often resemble ALF; and are characterized by microvesicular fatty infiltration and little hepatocellular necrosis. Rare causes of ALF include: Wilson's disease, hepatic ischemia, autoimmune hepatitis, and malignancy.

CLINICAL PRESENTATION

The clinical presentation includes progressive jaundice and hepatic encephalopathy without clinical evidence of underlying chronic liver disease. Other common but nonspecific symptoms include nausea, vomiting, loss of appetite, right upper abdominal pain from hepatomegaly, fever, fatigue, dark urine, and clay-colored stools. Typically, the features of impaired hepatic synthetic and metabolic function predominate, with portal hypertension much less common compared to patients with established cirrhosis.

DIAGNOSIS

The clinical presentation of ALF can be dramatic, with jaundice and advanced systemic manifestations as the first indication of a severe and potentially life-threatening illness. A thorough medical history is essential and focused on potential exposure to viruses and hepatotoxins, pregnancy, an event associated with hypotension, and clues to suggest autoimmune causes.

Early laboratory testing should focus on assessing the severity of hepatic dysfunction and on detection of possible acetaminophen exposure, for which specific antidote treatment must be promptly initiated. Further specialized laboratory testing is designed to identify specific viral causes—with tests for anti–hepatitis A immunoglobulin M (IgM), hepatitis B surface antigen (HBsAg), anti–hepatitis B core antigen (anti-HBc) IgM, hepatitis D antigen, anti–hepatitis C antibody and/or hepatitis C virus RNA, anti–hepatitis E IgM, anti-varicella IgM, and herpes simplex IgM—or other causes (e.g., ceruloplasmin level or autoimmune markers). Acute fatty liver of pregnancy may progress to ALF in the peripartum period; however, a pregnancy test should be performed in all females of childbearing age because viral illnesses (HSV, hepatitis E) may have a more severe course in pregnancy.

A negative serum acetaminophen level does not exclude acetaminophen overdose because the drug is rapidly cleared from the blood. Importantly, acetaminophen overdose accounts for approximately 50% of all cases of ALF and 20% of all cases of presumed indeterminant causes in Western countries. Small quantities of acetaminophen (or acetaminophen-containing compounds) may precipitate ALF in the context of consistent alcohol use due to constitutive activation (by ethanol) of cytochrome pathways creating toxic acetaminophen metabolites.

Imaging of the liver including ultrasound with Doppler may be utilized to assess liver architecture and blood flow into/out of the liver. Though not obligatory, a liver biopsy may be considered to assess for etiology; biopsy is often performed via the transjugular route secondary to coagulopathy and acuity of illness.

TREATMENT

Treatment of ALF is largely supportive, because specific treatment for the underlying cause of liver failure is often not available. However, many processes that result in widespread liver cell necrosis and ALF are transient events, and liver cell regeneration with recovery of liver function often occurs if patients survive the initial insult. Acetaminophen toxicity and hypotension causing hepatic necrosis are representative. In contrast, ALF resulting from viral hepatitis or idiosyncratic drug-induced liver injury (DILI) typically has a longer time course and an uncertain prognosis. In either case, meticulous supportive treatment in an intensive care unit setting has been shown to improve survival. Patients with ALF should be treated in centers with experience with this disease and with a liver transplantation program. Numerous systemic complications can result from ALF, and each must be thoroughly identified and treated (Table 13.1). As liver failure progresses,

急性肝衰竭

王艳 译 赵新颜 段维佳 审校 贾继东 通审

定义

急性肝衰竭（ALF）是指在没有基础肝病的患者中出现肝功能迅速恶化并导致肝性脑病和凝血功能障碍的少见综合征。目前公认的定义是：无肝硬化及基础肝病的患者在 26 周内出现国际标准化比值（INR）＞1.5 和任何程度的肝性脑病。急性肝衰竭并发多系统器官功能障碍和可能出现脑疝的肝性脑病时，需要迅速识别并转至重症监护病房（ICU）治疗。尽管可以采取对因治疗和支持性治疗，但对于经上述治疗未自发恢复的患者，肝移植仍然是唯一的治愈机会。

发病机制

ALF 是严重的持续性炎症反应引起肝细胞坏死和肝脏正常架构塌陷的后果。这一特征不同于慢性肝病（主要表现为肝硬化和门静脉高压相关并发症；见第 14 章）。ALF 可由嗜肝病毒 HAV、HBV、HCV、HDV 或 HEV 感染引起（见第 12 章），或由单纯疱疹病毒（HSV）引起。此外，剂量依赖性或特异质型肝毒物[如对乙酰氨基酚、异烟肼、氟烷、丙戊酸或蘑菇毒素（如毒伞蕈）]也能引起 ALF。瑞氏综合征（Reye 综合征；一种主要见于儿童的疾病）和妊娠期急性脂肪肝的表现与 ALF 类似，其特征是肝细胞微泡性脂肪变，但很少有肝细胞坏死。ALF 的罕见原因包括肝豆状核变性、缺血性肝病、自身免疫性肝炎和肝癌。

临床表现

临床表现为逐渐加重的黄疸和肝性脑病，且没有慢性肝病的临床证据。其他常见但非特异性的症状包括恶心、呕吐、食欲减退、肝大引起右上腹痛、发热、疲劳、尿色加深、白陶土样便。与肝硬化不同的是，ALF 患者肝脏合成和代谢功能受损的表现突出，而门静脉高压少见。

诊断

ALF 的临床表现可能非常明显，黄疸和进展性多系统受累是病情严重甚至危及生命的第一征象。全面采集病史非常重要，需要重点关注是否有病毒感染、接触肝毒性药物、妊娠、低血压及自身免疫性肝炎等因素。

针对 ALF 患者的初始实验室检查应集中在评估肝功能受损的严重程度，以及检测是否服用对乙酰氨基酚，并对服用者立即启动特定的解毒治疗。进一步实验室检查应筛查特定的病毒学指标，如抗 HAV IgM 抗体、HBsAg、抗 HBc IgM 抗体、HDV 抗原、抗 HCV 抗体和（或）HCV RNA、抗 HEV IgM 抗体、抗水痘病毒 IgM 抗体及抗 HSV IgM 抗体，同时需要筛查其他原因，如血清铜蓝蛋白和自身免疫标志物。妊娠期急性脂肪肝可能在围产期进展为 ALF；所有育龄期女性均应进行妊娠试验，因为病毒感染性疾病（如 HSV、HEV）可能在妊娠期加重。

由于对乙酰氨基酚会迅速从血液中清除，因此血清检测阴性并不能排除对乙酰氨基酚过量的可能性。在西方国家，对乙酰氨基酚过量约占所有 ALF 病例的 50%，占不明原因 ALF 病例的 20%。长期饮酒患者即使服用少量的对乙酰氨基酚（或含对乙酰氨基酚的复方制剂）也可能引发 ALF，这是因为乙醇可通过激活细胞色素途径而产生毒性对乙酰氨基酚代谢产物。

影像学检查（包括多普勒超声）有助于评估肝脏结构和血流进出肝脏的变化。尽管肝脏活检不是必须的，但可考虑用于病因评估。由于凝血功能障碍和病情快速进展，通常选择经颈静脉肝穿刺活检。

治疗

ALF 的治疗主要是支持性治疗，因为通常缺乏针对病因的特异性治疗。然而，许多导致广泛肝细胞坏死和 ALF 的过程是一过性事件，如果患者能渡过最初的打击，通常会出现肝细胞再生和肝功能恢复。对乙酰氨基酚中毒和低血压导致的肝坏死就是典型的例子。相比之下，由病毒性肝炎或特异质药物性肝损伤（DILI）引起的 ALF 通常病程更长、预后不确定。研究表明，无论是上述何种情况，在 ICU 进行细致的支持性治疗可以提高生存率。ALF 患者应在经验丰富且能进行肝脏移植的中心接受治疗。ALF 可能导致许多系统性并发症，需要全面评估和治疗（表 13.1）。随着

TABLE 13.1 Management of Selected Problems in Fulminant Hepatic Failure

Organ System	Pathogenesis	Supportive Measures
Hepatic encephalopathy	Diminished hepatocyte function	Identification of treatable causes (e.g., hypoglycemia, drugs used for sedation, sepsis, gastrointestinal bleeding, electrolyte imbalance, decreased Po_2, increased Pco_2)
		Lactulose and rifaximin
Cerebral edema	Systemic and local inflammation and circulating neurotoxins, including arterial ammonia	Elevate head of bed 20–30 degrees
		Hyperventilate (Pco_2 reduction)
		ICP monitor placement
		Mannitol
Renal	Prerenal kidney injury from diminished effective circulating volume, acute tubular necrosis, or functional leading to acid/base/electrolyte imbalance	Continuous renal replacement therapy
Cardiovascular	Low systemic vascular resistance	Intravenous resuscitation with normal saline and changed to half-normal saline containing 75 mEq/L sodium bicarbonate if acidotic
	Diminished central vascular tone compromises peripheral tissue oxygenation	Vasopressor support to maintain a mean arterial pressure of at least 75 mm Hg or a cerebral perfusion pressure of 60–80 mm Hg
Hematologic	Concomitant reduction in levels of both procoagulant and natural anticoagulant proteins, in conjunction with elevation of factor VIII (FVIII) and Von Willebrand factor, resulting in reduced thrombin generation capacity	Vitamin K 10 mg IV × 1
		Fresh-frozen plasma, platelets, and rFVIII generally reserved for active bleeding or need for invasive procedure
		Acid suppression to prevent luminal GI tract bleeding
Infectious	Immune dysfunction	Surveillance cultures of blood, urine, and tracheal aspirate when applicable
		Low threshold to initiate broad-spectrum antibiotic and antifungal therapy

a syndrome of multisystem organ failure can result; this can include encephalopathy, coagulopathy, infection, and renal failure.

Hepatic encephalopathy is often the first and most dramatic sign of liver failure. The precise pathogenesis of hepatic encephalopathy in ALF remains unclear and is likely multifactorial; however, it differs from that associated with chronic liver disease or portal hypertension in two important aspects. First, it often responds to therapy only when liver function improves, and second, it is frequently associated with hypoglycemia or cerebral edema, two other potentially treatable causes of coma. Therapy for hepatic encephalopathy in ALF differs slightly from the principles outlined in Chapter 14. Use of lactulose may be considered (orally or through a nasogastric tube) but should be discontinued if there is no significant improvement in mentation. Rifaximin, a nonabsorbable antibiotic, can be given as an adjunct orally or per tube. Intubation is often necessary to protect the airway from aspiration and to allow ventilation in patients with advanced encephalopathy.

Cerebral edema, the pathogenesis of which is unknown, is a leading cause of death in ALF. Differentiation between cerebral edema and hepatic encephalopathy can be difficult, and computed tomography of the head is often unreliable as observable architectural changes of edema may lag behind clinical progression. Measurement of intracranial pressure (ICP) can be considered, although it is associated with complications including bleeding. The goal is to maintain an ICP of less than 20 mm Hg while maintaining a cerebral perfusion pressure (calculated as mean arterial pressure minus ICP) greater than 60 mm Hg. Supportive measures to limit ICP elevation include: control of agitation, head elevation of 20 to 30 degrees, hyperventilation, systemic vasopressors to maintain mean arterial pressure, administration of mannitol, barbiturate-induced coma, and urgent liver transplantation.

As hepatic synthetic function deteriorates, *hypoglycemia* can occur as a result of impaired hepatic gluconeogenesis and insulin degradation. All patients at risk should receive 10% glucose IV infusions with frequent monitoring of blood glucose levels. Other metabolic abnormalities commonly occur, including hyponatremia, hypokalemia, respiratory alkalosis, and metabolic acidosis. Therefore, frequent monitoring of blood electrolytes and pH is indicated. Renal replacement therapy may be employed to regulate acid/base/electrolyte balance, with continuous modes preferred over intermittent hemodialysis.

Bleeding occurs frequently and is commonly caused by gastric erosions in the setting of impaired synthesis of clotting factors and prolonged prothrombin times. All patients should receive vitamin K and prophylactic gastric acid suppression. Fresh-frozen plasma administration is reserved for when clinically significant bleeding occurs or if major procedures, including ICP monitoring and central line placement, are performed. Studies in ALF have found a concomitant and proportional reduction in plasma levels of both procoagulants and natural anticoagulant proteins, in conjunction with a significant elevation in plasma levels of factors-VIII (FVIII) and Von Willebrand factor, resulting in an overall efficient, albeit reduced, thrombin generation capacity in comparison with healthy controls. Global hemostasis as assessed with thromboelastography (TEG) may be normal by several compensatory mechanisms, even in patients with markedly elevated INR.

Up to 80% of patients with ALF develop infection at some point in their illness; both bacterial (≈80% of infections) and fungal (≈20% of infections) have been implicated. Patients are at higher risk for infection as a result of impaired immunity resulting from liver failure and the need for invasive monitoring. Severe infection may occur without fever or leukocytosis. Therefore, frequent cultures are recommended and warranted with abrupt changes in status, and there should be a low threshold for beginning antibiotic therapy.

Although often employed to guide evaluation, no single prognostic model discriminates those who will spontaneously recover and those who will require transplant. The United States Acute Liver Failure Group (ALFSG) prospectively enrolled over 1900 subjects with ALF managed with and without transplantation and aimed to develop a model for ALF to predict transplant-free survival at 21 days. Clinical demographics and laboratory parameters were collected at enrollment and recorded serially up to 1 week. Variables of prognostic value adopted in the predictive model included: admission coma grade, liver

表 13.1	暴发性肝衰竭并发症的管理	
受累系统	发病机制	治疗措施
肝病脑病	肝细胞功能减退	积极寻找可治疗的病因（如低血糖、镇静药、感染中毒症、消化道出血、电解质紊乱、氧分压降低、二氧化碳分压升高） 乳果糖和利福昔明
脑水肿	全身性和局部炎症反应，神经毒素（包括血氨）进入循环系统	床头抬高 20°～30° 过度通气（降低二氧化碳分压） 监测颅内压 甘露醇
肾	有效循环血容量减少导致肾前性肾损伤、急性肾小管坏死、酸碱失衡及电解质紊乱	连续性肾脏替代治疗
心血管系统	全身血管阻力降低 中心血管张力降低导致周围组织的氧气供应减少	生理盐水静脉补液；酸中毒时更换为含 75 mmol/L 碳酸氢钠的半生理盐水补液 使用血管升压药，以维持平均动脉压≥75 mmHg 或脑灌注压 60～80 mmHg
血液系统	促凝血因子和天然抗凝血因子水平降低，凝血因子Ⅷ（FⅧ）和血管性血友病因子（vWF）水平升高，导致凝血酶生成减少	单次静脉注射 10 mg 维生素 K 活动性出血或需要进行侵入性操作的患者，输注新鲜冰冻血浆、血小板和重组凝血因子Ⅷ 抑酸治疗，以预防消化道出血
感染	免疫功能紊乱	尽可能监测血液、尿液和气管抽吸物病原学培养 放宽广谱抗生素和抗真菌治疗的指征

肝衰竭的进展，可能出现多器官功能障碍综合征，包括肝性脑病、凝血功能障碍、感染和肾衰竭。

肝性脑病通常是肝衰竭最显著的首发症状。ALF 患者发生肝性脑病的确切发病机制尚不明确，很可能由多因素共同作用引起。然而，ALF 与慢性肝病或门静脉高压相关的肝性脑病在两个重要方面有所不同。首先，只有在肝功能改善时，ALF 才对治疗有应答；其次，ALF 常伴有低血糖或脑水肿，这两种情况都是会导致昏迷但可被及时纠正的病因。ALF 相关肝性脑病的治疗与第 14 章中介绍的治疗原则略有不同：可考虑使用乳果糖（口服或经鼻胃管给药），如果患者的意识状况没有显著改善，则应停止使用；可口服或经鼻胃管给予利福昔明（一种不经肠道吸收的抗生素）辅助治疗；严重肝性脑病患者需要气管插管，以保护气道免受吸入性损伤并保证通气。

脑水肿是 ALF 致死的主要原因，其发病机制尚不明确。鉴别脑水肿和肝性脑病有一定难度，因水肿造成的脑结构改变往往滞后于临床表现，故头颅 CT 常不可靠；测量颅内压（ICP）可能有助于鉴别，但应注意该操作可能导致并发症（如出血）。治疗目标是维持 ICP < 20 mmHg 和脑灌注压（平均动脉压－ICP）> 60 mmHg。有助于抑制 ICP 升高的支持治疗包括：避免情绪激动、头部抬高 20°～30°、过度通气、使用全身血管升压药维持平均动脉压、给予甘露醇、巴比妥类药物诱导昏迷、紧急肝移植。

随着肝脏合成功能的恶化，由于肝脏糖异生和胰岛素降解受损，患者可能出现低血糖。所有存在低血糖风险的患者均应接受 10% 葡萄糖静脉注射，并密切监测血糖水平。其他常见的代谢异常包括低钠血症、低钾血症、呼吸性碱中毒和代谢性酸中毒。因此，建议密切监测血清电解质及 pH 值。肾脏替代治疗可用于调节酸碱及电解质平衡，连续性血液透析优于间歇性血液透析。

出血是 ALF 的常见并发症。由于凝血因子合成受损和凝血酶原时间延长，胃黏膜糜烂通常会导致消化道出血。因此，所有患者均应使用维生素 K 和预防性使用抑酸药物。当发生临床显著的出血事件或需要进行侵入性操作时（如 ICP 监测和中心静脉置管），应输注新鲜冰冻血浆。研究发现，ALF 患者血液中的促凝血因子和天然抗凝血因子水平成比例降低，而凝血因子Ⅷ（FⅧ）和血管性血友病因子的水平显著升高，与健康对照组相比，尽管凝血功能减低，但总体上仍保留有效的凝血能力。此外，由于机体存在一定代偿机制，通过血栓弹力图（TEG）评估全身出凝血功能时可能显示正常结果，即使是 INR 明显升高的患者。

高达 80% 的 ALF 患者在病程中会发生感染，包括细菌感染（约占 80%）和真菌感染（约占 20%）。肝衰竭导致的免疫功能受损和侵入性监测是 ALF 患者感染风险高的主要原因。即使发生严重感染，也可能没有发热或白细胞增多，因此，建议反复采集标本进行病原学培养，尤其是在病情突然变化时，同时应放宽抗生素治疗指征。

尽管常被用于评估病情，但尚无单一预测模型能够准确区分自发恢复和需要移植的患者。美国急性肝衰竭小组（ALFSG）前瞻性入组了 1900 多例接受和未接受肝移植的 ALF 患者，旨在开发一种能预测 21 天无肝移植生存率的 AFL 模型。该研究收集了基线人口学和实验室指标，并连续记录 1 周。该预测模型包含以下指标：入院时昏迷程度分级、肝衰竭病因、是否

failure etiology and vasopressor requirement, as well as admission INR and bilirubin values. The model correctly predicted outcome in 66.3% of subjects, slightly outperforming historic King's College Criteria and the Model for End-stage Liver Disease (MELD) score.

Liver transplantation (see Chapter 14) has been performed with success in patients with ALF and is the treatment of choice for patients who appear unlikely to recover spontaneously. Because of high risk of abrupt clinical deterioration, the optimal approach is for potential candidates to be transferred to transplantation centers before significant complications develop (e.g., coma, cerebral edema, hemorrhage, infection). ALF subjects who meet transplant program criteria for listing in the United Sates are granted status 1A, placing them at the highest priority on the waiting list.

PROGNOSIS

Etiology of ALF and the degree of hepatic encephalopathy are key determinants of prognosis. Patients with ALF resulting from acetaminophen overdose or viral hepatitis A or B have a better survival rate than do patients with Wilson's disease or those with indeterminate etiology. The short-term survival rate for patients with ALF in coma is 20% without liver transplantation.

Currently, ALF accounts for approximately 8% of all liver transplants, as per data from the Scientific Registry of Transplant Recipients (SRTR) with 1-year survival rates of 84% in the United States. Patients who survive without transplantation also have an excellent prognosis because liver tissue usually regenerates normally regardless of the cause of ALF.

SUGGESTED READINGS

Bernal W, Wendon J: Acute liver failure, N Engl J Med 369(26): 2525–3, 2013.

Koch DG, Tillman H, Durkalski V, Lee WM, Reuben A: Development of a model to predict transplant-free survival of patients with acute liver failure, Clin Gastroenterol Hepatol 14(8):1199–1206, 2016.

Lee WM, Larson AM, Stravitz RT: AASLD position paper: the management of acute liver failure—update 2011. Available at: http://www.aasld.org/practiceguidelines/Documents/AcuteLiverFailureUpdate2011.pdf.

需要使用血管升压药、入院时 INR 和胆红素水平。该模型可准确预测 66.3% 的受试者的临床结局，略优于 King's College 标准和终末期肝病模型（MELD）。

肝移植（见第 14 章）是救治 ALF 患者的有效手段，也是不能自发恢复患者的首选治疗方法。由于 ALF 患者病情突然恶化的风险极高，建议在出现严重并发症（如昏迷、脑水肿、出血、感染等）前，将可能需要肝移植的患者转诊至移植中心。在美国，符合移植等待名单标准的 ALF 患者将获得 1A 评级，使他们在等待名单上享有最高优先级。

预后

ALF 的病因和肝性脑病的严重程度是决定预后的关键因素。对乙酰氨基酚过量或 HAV 和 HBV 导致的 ALF 患者生存率高于肝豆状核变性或不明病因引起的 ALF。若未行肝移植，发生昏迷的 ALF 患者的短期生存率为 20%。

根据美国移植受者科学登记数据库（SRTR），在美国，ALF 约占肝移植总例数的 8%，移植后 1 年生存率为 84%。未行肝移植的存活患者预后也很好，这是因为无论何种病因导致的 ALF，肝组织通常都能再生。

推荐阅读

Bernal W, Wendon J: Acute liver failure, N Engl J Med 369(26): 2525–3, 2013.

Koch DG, Tillman H, Durkalski V, Lee WM, Reuben A: Development of a model to predict transplant-free survival of patients with acute liver failure, Clin Gastroenterol Hepatol 14(8):1199–1206, 2016.

Lee WM, Larson AM, Stravitz RT: AASLD position paper: the management of acute liver failure—update 2011. Available at: http://www.aasld.org/practiceguidelines/Documents/AcuteLiverFailureUpdate2011.pdf.

Cirrhosis of the Liver and Its Complications

Shivang Mehta, Michael B. Fallon

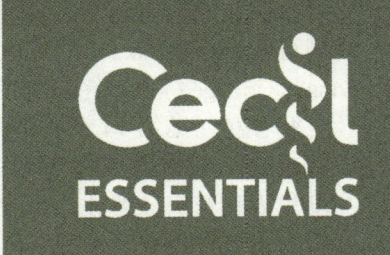

LIVER CIRRHOSIS

Definition
Cirrhosis is a slowly progressive disease that is characterized by formation in the liver of fibrous and scar tissue that eventually replaces normal hepatocytes and impairs portal blood flow. Fibrosis can be a self-perpetuating result of many initial processes, including infectious, inflammatory, toxic, metabolic, genetic, and vascular insults that lead to liver damage. Most of the clinical features of cirrhosis develop as a result of portal hypertension, hepatocellular dysfunction, or altered cellular differentiation.

Etiology
Alcoholic liver disease, nonalcoholic steatohepatitis (NASH), and hepatitis C virus infection are the most common causes of cirrhosis in industrialized nations; hepatitis B virus is the major cause in Asia and in most of Africa. There are many other significant causes of cirrhosis, including biliary cirrhosis (primary and secondary), autoimmune hepatitis, inherited diseases (e.g., α_1-antitrypsin deficiency), and drug-induced injury, that require specific evaluation. However, a significant number of patients with cirrhosis at presentation have no readily identifiable cause. These cases are referred to as idiopathic or cryptogenic in origin, and it remains a diagnosis of exclusion. Common and uncommon conditions that may lead to cirrhosis are listed in Table 14.1. Chronic active hepatitis, nonalcoholic fatty liver disease (NAFLD)/NASH, and α_1-antitrypsin deficiency are discussed in Chapter 12.

Pathology
The typical sequence of events that leads to development of cirrhosis involves significant hepatocyte injury followed by ineffective repair that results in hepatic fibrosis. The injury can be acute or chronic in nature, depending on the mechanism. The fibrotic response to injury leads to development of nodules surrounded by fibrous tissue that consist of foci of regenerating hepatocytes, formation of fibrovascular membranes, rearrangement of blood vessels, and finally cirrhosis. This disruption of the normal hepatic lobular architecture distorts the vascular bed and contributes to development of portal hypertension and intrahepatic shunting. On gross morphology, cirrhosis can be referred to as macronodular (>3 mm regenerating nodules), commonly seen as a result of chronic active hepatitis, or micronodular (<3 mm regenerating nodules) a typical feature of alcoholic cirrhosis or cirrhosis of mixed origin.

Clinical Presentation
Symptoms of liver cirrhosis are often nonspecific in the early stages and include fatigue, malaise, weakness, weight change, anorexia, and nausea. With progression of portal hypertension or loss of hepatocytes, increased abdominal girth, sexual dysfunction, altered mental status, and gastrointestinal bleeding may be noted. Physical findings depend on the stage at presentation. Table 14.2 highlights the pathogenic mechanisms underlying these diverse signs and symptoms.

Diagnosis
Owing to significant reserves of liver function, patients with cirrhosis are often asymptomatic and the diagnosis is established incidentally at the time of physical examination or laboratory testing. Alternatively, patients abruptly experience specific life-threatening complications of cirrhosis, most notably variceal bleeding, ascites, spontaneous bacterial peritonitis, and hepatic encephalopathy (HE). If cirrhosis is suspected on clinical grounds, the diagnosis can be made reliably by a combination of clinical, laboratory, and radiologic findings in most cases. Although liver biopsy is still considered the "gold standard" for accurate diagnosis, new noninvasive modalities to estimate fibrosis have come to the forefront. The predominant modalities utilized to assess fibrosis non-invasively are FibroSure, FibroScan (ultrasound with shear wave elastography), and magnetic resonance elastography (MRE). With these advances, biopsy is now done more often to assess the stage and severity of disease, assign prognosis, and monitor the response to treatment.

Laboratory Findings
Hepatocellular dysfunction leads to impaired protein synthesis (hypoalbuminemia), hyperbilirubinemia, low levels of blood urea nitrogen (BUN), and elevated serum ammonia levels. Portal hypertension causes hypersplenism, which results in anemia, thrombocytopenia, and leukopenia. Patients with ascites often develop dilutional hyponatremia as a result of avid renal retention of sodium (Na^+) and water. The liver enzymes alanine aminotransferase (ALT) and aspartate aminotransferase (AST) are good markers of active hepatocyte necrosis, whereas elevations of alkaline phosphatase and bilirubin out of proportion to ALT and AST suggest intrahepatic or extrahepatic biliary obstruction. FibroSure is a laboratory test that consists of a panel comprising total bilirubin, GGT, α_2-macroglobulin, haptoglobin, and apolipoprotein A1 corrected for age and sex to provide a surrogate for advanced fibrosis validated in populations with hepatitis B and C.

Radiology
Various radiologic modalities including ultrasound (with and without Doppler imaging of the portal and hepatic venous vasculature), computed tomography, and magnetic resonance imaging have complementary profiles in the evaluation of suspected cirrhosis. Findings supportive of the diagnosis of cirrhosis include relative enlargement of the left hepatic and caudate lobes as a result of right lobe atrophy, surface nodularity, and features of portal hypertension such as ascites, intra-abdominal varices, and splenomegaly.

肝硬化及其并发症

孙亚朦　王冰琼　译　尤红　审校　贾继东　通审

肝硬化

定义

肝硬化是一种慢性进行性疾病，其特征是肝脏纤维瘢痕组织形成，最终取代正常肝细胞并影响门静脉血流。纤维化可以是多种初始过程（包括感染、炎症、毒性、代谢因素、遗传因素和血管损伤引起的肝损伤）引起的自我持续性损伤修复的结果。肝硬化的大多数临床特征由门静脉高压、肝细胞功能障碍或细胞分化异常引起。

病因

酒精性肝病、非酒精性脂肪性肝炎（NASH）和丙型肝炎病毒（HCV）感染是工业化国家最常见的肝硬化病因；乙型肝炎病毒（HBV）感染是亚洲和非洲大部分地区的主要病因。肝硬化的其他重要病因包括胆汁性肝硬化（原发性和继发性）、自身免疫性肝炎、遗传病（如 α_1-抗胰蛋白酶缺乏症）和药物性肝损伤，因此需要进行有针对性的评估检查。然而，许多肝硬化患者在就诊时并没有明确的病因，即特发性或隐源性肝硬化，属于排除性诊断。表 14.1 中列出了肝硬化的常见或少见病因。慢性活动性肝炎、非酒精性脂肪性肝病（NAFLD）/NASH 和 α_1-抗胰蛋白酶缺乏症见第 12 章。

病理学

导致肝硬化形成的典型过程包括肝细胞严重损伤修复无效，进而导致肝纤维化。根据其机制不同，损伤可分为急性或慢性。损伤引起的纤维增生反应形成纤维组织包绕的、内含再生肝细胞灶的结节，并形成纤维血管膜及重新排列的血管结构，最终导致肝硬化。正常肝小叶结构遭到破坏会导致血管床扭曲，引起门静脉高压和肝内分流。从大体形态上看，肝硬化可分为大结节性（再生结节直径＞3 mm）和小结节性（再生结节直径＜3 mm），前者常见于慢性活动性肝炎，后者是酒精性肝硬化或混合型肝硬化的典型特征。

临床表现

在肝硬化早期阶段，症状通常无特异性，包括疲劳、全身不适、乏力、体重变化、食欲减退和恶心。随着门静脉高压或肝细胞破坏的加剧，可能出现腹围增大、性功能障碍、精神状态改变和消化道出血等症状。体格检查取决于肝硬化的病程阶段。表 14.2 总结了不同症状和体征的发生机制。

诊断

由于肝脏具有很强的储备功能，肝硬化患者通常没有明显症状，仅在体格检查或实验室检查中偶然被诊断。但是，患者也可能会突然出现危及生命的肝硬化并发症，主要包括静脉曲张出血、腹腔积液、自发性细菌性腹膜炎和肝性脑病。对于临床怀疑肝硬化的患者，多数情况下可通过综合分析临床表现、实验室检查和影像学检查结果做出可靠的诊断。虽然肝活检仍被认为是确诊肝硬化的"金标准"，但新型非侵入性纤维化评估技术已崭露头角。用于无创性评估肝纤维化的主要技术包括 FibroSure、FibroScan（一种带有剪切波弹性成像的超声技术）和磁共振弹性成像（MRE）。随着这些技术的进步，肝活检现在被更多地用于评估疾病分期和严重程度、判断预后和监测治疗应答。

实验室检查

肝细胞功能障碍会导致蛋白质合成障碍（低白蛋白血症）、高胆红素血症、血尿素氮（BUN）水平下降和血氨水平升高。门静脉高压会引起脾功能亢进，从而导致贫血、血小板减少和白细胞减少。腹腔积液患者通常会因过度水钠潴留而出现稀释性低钠血症。肝酶中 ALT 和 AST 是活动性肝细胞坏死的标志物，而当碱性磷酸酶和胆红素水平升高与 ALT 和 AST 升高不成比例时，则提示肝内或肝外胆道梗阻。FibroSure 是一种由总胆红素、GGT、α_2-巨球蛋白、血红蛋白和载脂蛋白 AI 组成的实验室检测方法，并根据年龄和性别进行校正，是诊断进展期肝纤维化的替代指标，并已在乙型肝炎和丙型肝炎患者中得到验证。

影像学检查

超声（伴或不伴门静脉和肝静脉血管多普勒成像）、CT 和 MRI 等影像学检查对疑似肝硬化的诊断具有辅助作用。支持肝硬化诊断的征象包括：因肝右叶萎缩导致的左肝和尾状叶相对增大、肝表面呈结节状和门静脉高压的特征（如腹腔积液、腹腔内静脉曲张和脾大）。

TABLE 14.1 Common Causes of Cirrhosis

Alcohol abuse
Nonalcoholic steatohepatitis
Viral hepatitis (chronic hepatitis B, C, and D)
Cardiac cirrhosis
Chronic right-sided heart failure
Constrictive pericarditis
Drug-induced liver injury (DILI)
Autoimmune hepatitis
Primary biliary cirrhosis
Hemochromatosis (primary and secondary)
Wilson's disease
α_1-Antitrypsin deficiency

TABLE 14.2 Clinical Features and Pathogenesis of Cirrhosis

Signs and Symptoms	Pathogenesis
Constitutional	
Fatigue, anorexia, malaise, weakness, weight loss	Liver synthetic or metabolic dysfunction
Cutaneous	
Spider angiomas, palmar erythema	Altered estrogen and androgen metabolism
Jaundice	Decreased bilirubin excretion
Caput medusae	Portosystemic shunting due to portal hypertension
Endocrine	
Gynecomastia, testicular atrophy, decreased body hair in men	Altered estrogen and androgen metabolism
Decreased libido, virilization, and menstrual irregularities in women	
Gastrointestinal	
Abdominal pain	Hepatomegaly, hepatocellular carcinoma
Abdominal swelling	Ascites due to portal hypertension
Gastrointestinal bleeding	Variceal hemorrhage due to portal hypertension
Hematologic	
Anemia, leukopenia, thrombocytopenia	Hypersplenism secondary to portal hypertension
Ecchymosis	Decreased synthesis of coagulation factors
Neurologic	
Altered sleep pattern, somnolence, confusion, asterixis	Hepatocellular dysfunction: inability to metabolize ammonia to urea

Transient elastography (FibroScan) is a newer noninvasive modality that provides an indirect measure of liver fibrosis and cirrhosis by calculating liver stiffness. Abnormal liver stiffness suggests underlying fibrosis; in the presence of clinical and laboratory features of cirrhosis, this finding may obviate the need for diagnostic liver biopsy in some patients. Other modalities include ultrasound with shear wave velocity (50 Hz), which uses velocity within the liver to determine stiffness. MRE is an addition to imaging provided by MR that incorporates acoustic vibrations across the entire liver to determine liver stiffness. It is currently the most accurate noninvasive modality but is limited by availability and cost. Biopsy is more invasive and is usually reserved for situations in which the results of noninvasive studies are indeterminate or the cause of the liver disease is in doubt.

COMPLICATIONS OF CIRRHOSIS

The major sequelae of cirrhosis are illustrated diagrammatically in Fig. 14.1 and can be categorized broadly into features of hepatocellular dysfunction and portal hypertension. The pathophysiologic interrelationships among these complications are described in the following sections.

Hepatocellular Dysfunction

The loss of hepatocyte mass that occurs in cirrhosis results in impaired synthesis of many important proteins, which in turn leads to hypoalbuminemia, deficient production of vitamin K–dependent coagulation factors, and diminished capacity for hepatic detoxification (see Chapters 10 to 13 for details). In addition, there is a decline in the capacity for conjugation and excretion of bilirubin.

Portal Hypertension

Under normal circumstances, the portal circulation is a low-pressure system with only small changes in pressure as blood flows from the portal vein, through the liver, and into the inferior vena cava. The hepatic venous pressure gradient (HVPG), which reflects sinusoidal pressure, is the gradient between the wedged hepatic venous pressure and the free hepatic venous pressure measured by direct catheterization. Normal HVPG values range between 3 and 5 mm Hg. In cirrhosis, the distortion of hepatic architecture by fibrous tissue and regenerative nodules, along with an increased intrahepatic vascular tone, leads to increased resistance to portal venous flow and resultant portal hypertension. Portal hypertension is defined as an HPVG greater than 5 mm Hg, and clinically significant complications typically develop at values greater than 10 mm Hg.

Although cirrhosis is the most important cause of portal hypertension, any process that increases resistance to portal blood flow through the presinusoidal, sinusoidal, or hepatic venous outflow tracts may result in portal hypertension (Table 14.3). In addition, cirrhosis is associated with increased cardiac output, which leads to greater splanchnic blood flow, further aggravating portal hypertension. It is important to recognize that the HVPG is reliably increased only in sinusoidal portal hypertension.

With sustained portal hypertension, portosystemic collaterals are formed that have the benefit of decreasing portal pressures at the expense of bypassing the liver. Major sites of collateral formation include the gastroesophageal junction, retroperitoneum, rectum, and falciform ligament of liver (abdominal and periumbilical collaterals). Clinically, the most important collaterals are those connecting the portal to the azygos vein through the dilated and tortuous vessels (varices) in the submucosa of the gastric fundus and esophagus.

VARICEAL HEMORRHAGE

Definition and Pathology

Varices are abnormally large veins that are most commonly recognized near the gastroesophageal junction or the stomach wall. Gastroesophageal varices usually develop when the portal pressure

表 14.1　肝硬化的常见病因

酒精滥用
非酒精性脂肪性肝炎
病毒性肝炎（慢性乙型肝炎、慢性丙型肝炎和慢性丁型肝炎）
心源性肝硬化
慢性右心衰竭
缩窄性心包炎
药物性肝损伤（DILI）
自身免疫性肝炎
原发性胆汁性肝硬化
血色病（原发性和继发性）
肝豆状核变性（Wilson 病）
α_1-抗胰蛋白酶缺乏症

表 14.2　肝硬化的临床特征和发病机制

症状和体征	发病机制
全身症状	
疲劳、食欲减退、全身不适、乏力、体重下降	肝脏合成或代谢功能障碍
皮肤表现	
蜘蛛痣、肝掌	雌激素和雄激素代谢改变
黄疸	胆红素排泄减少
脐周静脉曲张	门静脉高压导致门体分流
内分泌系统症状	
男性乳房发育、睾丸萎缩、男性体毛减少	雌激素和雄激素代谢异常
性欲减退、女性男性化、女性月经失调	
消化道症状	
腹痛	肝大、肝细胞癌
腹胀	门静脉高压引起腹腔积液
消化道出血	门静脉高压引起静脉曲张破裂出血
血液系统症状	
贫血、白细胞减少、血小板减少	门静脉高压引起脾功能亢进
瘀斑	凝血因子合成减少
神经系统症状	
睡眠模式改变、嗜睡、意识错乱、扑翼样震颤	肝细胞功能障碍：无法将氨代谢为尿素

瞬时弹性成像（FibroScan）是一种较新的无创性方法，它是通过计算肝脏硬度来间接评估肝纤维化和肝硬化。肝脏硬度异常提示可能存在肝纤维化，结合肝硬化的临床表现和实验室检查异常结果，可避免部分患者进行诊断性肝活检。其他方法还包括超声剪切波弹性成像（50 Hz），它是利用剪切波在肝内的传播速度来测量肝脏硬度。MRE 是磁共振成像技术的补充，通过整个肝脏的声波振动来测量肝脏硬度，是目前最准确的无创性检查，但其应用受到可及性和成本的限制。肝组织活检为有创性检查，通常用于无创性检查结果不确定或病因存疑的情况。

肝硬化的并发症

如图 14.1 所示，肝硬化的主要并发症可大致分为肝细胞功能障碍和门静脉高压。下文将介绍这些并发症之间的病理生理学联系。

肝细胞功能障碍

肝硬化时肝细胞大量损伤，导致许多重要蛋白质合成障碍，进而导致低白蛋白血症、维生素 K 依赖性凝血因子生成不足和肝脏解毒能力下降（见第 10 章至第 13 章）。此外，肝脏对胆红素的结合和排泄能力下降。

门静脉高压

正常情况下，门静脉循环是一个低压力系统，血液从门静脉经肝脏进入下腔静脉的过程仅有微小的压力变化。肝静脉压力梯度（HVPG）反映了肝窦压力，是通过直接导管测量的肝静脉楔压与肝静脉自由压之间的差值。HVPG 的正常值范围为 3～5 mmHg。肝硬化时，肝纤维化和再生结节使肝脏结构变形，同时肝内血管张力增加，导致门静脉血流阻力增加，最终引起门静脉高压。门静脉高压的定义为 HPVG > 5 mmHg；HPVG > 10 mmHg 时常出现临床显著的并发症。

虽然肝硬化是导致门静脉高压的最重要原因，但任何增加门静脉窦前、窦内或肝静脉流出道血流阻力的过程都可能导致门静脉高压（表 14.3）。此外，肝硬化可引起心输出量增加，导致内脏血流量增加，从而进一步加重门静脉高压。需要强调的是，只有在窦性门静脉高压时，HVPG 的升高才有意义。

在持续门静脉高压的情况下，会形成门体静脉侧支循环，以降低门静脉的压力，但代价是血液绕过了肝脏。侧支循环形成的主要部位包括胃食管交界处、腹膜后、直肠和肝镰状韧带（腹部和脐周侧支循环）。在临床上，最重要的侧支是通过胃底和食管黏膜下层扩张和迂曲的血管（静脉曲张）连接门静脉和奇静脉的侧支循环。

静脉曲张破裂出血

定义和病理学

静脉曲张是一种异常扩张的大静脉，最常发生于胃食管交界处或胃壁。胃食管静脉曲张通常在 HVPG

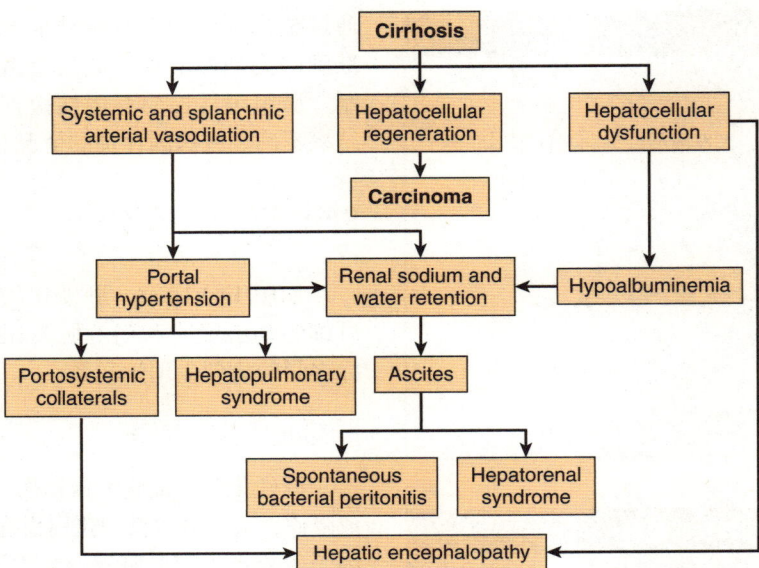

Fig. 14.1 Interrelationships among the complications of cirrhosis.

TABLE 14.3 Causes of Portal Hypertension

Increased Resistance to Flow
Presinusoidal
Extrahepatic
  Portal or splenic vein occlusion
Intrahepatic
  Schistosomiasis
  Congenital hepatic fibrosis
  Sarcoidosis
Sinusoidal
Cirrhosis (many causes)
Alcoholic hepatitis
Postsinusoidal
Extrahepatic
  Budd-Chiari syndrome
  Cardiac causes: constrictive pericarditis
Intrahepatic
  Veno-occlusive disease

Increased Portal Blood Flow
Splenomegaly not caused by liver disease
Arterioportal fistula

gradient (HVPG) exceeds 10 mm Hg, and the risk for variceal rupture increases when the gradient is higher than 12 mm Hg. Bleeding occurs most commonly from large varices in the esophagus when high tension in the walls of these vessels leads to rupture. Among gastric varices, fundal varices have the highest rate of bleeding and may bleed with portal pressure gradients of less than 12 mm Hg.

Clinical Presentation

Variceal bleeding usually manifests as painless hematemesis, melena, or hematochezia, which typically leads to hemodynamic compromise due to higher portal pressures. Bleeding is further aggravated by impaired hepatic synthesis of coagulation factors and thrombocytopenia from hypersplenism.

Treatment

The management of gastroesophageal varices includes prevention of initial bleeding (primary prophylaxis), treatment of acute variceal hemorrhage, and prevention of rebleeding (secondary prophylaxis) (Fig. 14.2). If varices are large, primary prophylaxis is commonly undertaken with nonselective β-adrenergic receptor blocking (NSBB) agents such as propranolol and nadolol. Surveillance for varices using esophagogastroduodenoscopy (EGD) is advocated only if endoscopic band ligation (EBL) is the initial treatment modality. EGD is recommended every 2 to 8 weeks until obliteration of varices, then in 3 to 6 months, after which surveillance can be done every 6 to 12 months. Periodic EBL is also effective if the patient has contraindications or intolerance to β-blockers. Isosorbide mononitrate therapy should not be used for prophylaxis because it has been shown to increase adverse events. EBL and NSBB should not be used in combination to prevent first variceal bleed.

When varices are present, 5% to 15% of patients experience an initial episode of bleeding annually, and this episode carries a significant mortality risk of 7% to 15% at 6 weeks. Management includes stabilization (airway, breathing, and circulation) and blood transfusions to maintain a hemoglobin level of 7 to 8 g/dL. Combined pharmacologic and endoscopic therapy is the current standard for control of bleeding and is superior to either therapy alone. Prophylactic intravenous antibiotics should be administered early because they reduce the risk for infection, rebleeding, and death.

Current pharmacologic therapy consists of octreotide, a somatostatin analogue, which is widely used because of a good safety profile. This agent is best instituted before endoscopic examination. Endoscopic therapy includes EBL or sclerotherapy or both. EBL is the preferred modality given the lower incidence of adverse effects and complications. In patients with gastric variceal hemorrhage, endoscopic variceal ablation with cyanoacrylate glue is superior to EBL, although this therapy is not approved in the United States. Balloon tamponade (Sengstaken-Blakemore tube, Linton tube, or Minnesota tube) or esophageal stenting have been used as temporary measures reserved only for cases in which endoscopic therapy has failed in the setting of massive hemorrhage. A recent meta-analysis in limited studies for esophageal stenting versus

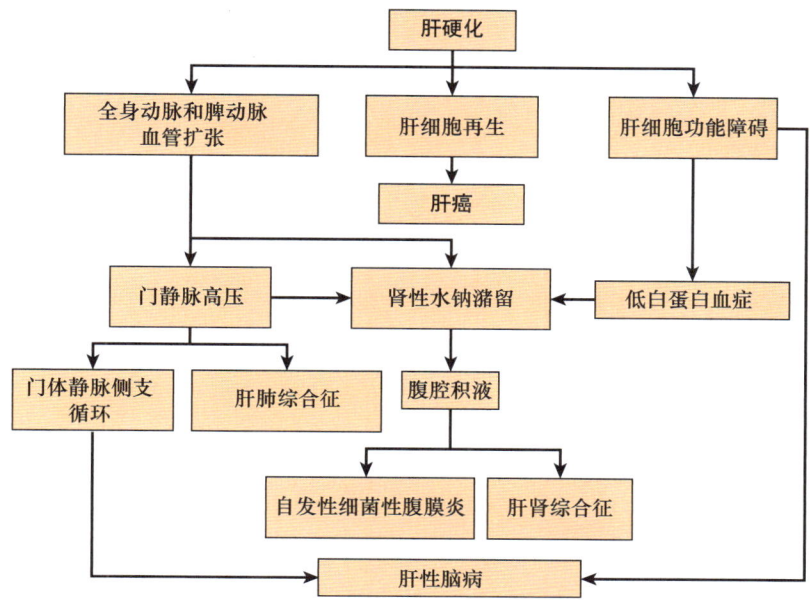

图 14.1　肝硬化并发症之间的相互联系

表 14.3　门静脉高压的原因

血流阻力增加
窦前性
肝外原因
　门静脉或脾静脉阻塞
肝内原因
　血吸虫病
　先天性肝纤维化
　结节病

窦性
肝硬化（多种原因）
酒精性肝炎

窦后性
肝外原因
　布-加综合征
　心脏原因：缩窄性心包炎
肝内原因
　肝小静脉闭塞性疾病

门静脉血流量增加
非肝脏疾病引起的脾大
动脉门静脉瘘

> 10 mmHg 时形成，而当 HVPG > 12 mmHg 时，胃食管静脉曲张破裂的风险会增加。最常见的出血来自大的食管静脉曲张，因为这些血管壁的高张力会导致破裂。在胃静脉曲张中，胃底静脉曲张的出血发生率最高，且可发生于 HVPG < 12 mmHg 时。

临床表现

静脉曲张破裂出血通常表现为无痛性呕血、黑便或鲜血便，并通常因门静脉压力升高而导致血流动力学异常。此外，肝脏合成凝血因子的能力受损和脾功能亢进引起的血小板数量减少也会加重肝硬化患者的出血。

治疗

胃食管静脉曲张的治疗包括预防首次出血（一级预防）、治疗急性静脉曲张破裂出血和预防再出血（二级预防）（图 14.2）。对于较大的静脉曲张，一级预防通常使用非选择性 β 受体阻滞剂（NSBB），如普萘洛尔和纳多洛尔。仅当选择内镜套扎术（EBL）作为初始预防治疗时，才推荐行食管胃十二指肠镜（EGD）监测胃食管静脉曲张变化。建议每 2～8 周进行 1 次 EGD，直至静脉曲张消失；然后每 3～6 个月进行 1 次 EGD；此后可每 6～12 个月进行 1 次 EGD。如果患者有 NSBB 禁忌证或不耐受，定期进行 EBL 也有效。单硝酸异山梨酯已被证明会增加不良反应，因此不应将其用于预防性治疗。不推荐 EBL 和 NSBB 联合用于预防首次静脉曲张出血。

一旦形成静脉曲张，每年有 5%～15% 的患者会出现首次出血，出血发生后 6 周内的死亡率为 7%～15%。治疗包括维持生命体征稳定（气道、呼吸和循环支持）和输血，输血的目标是维持患者的血红蛋白水平为 7～8 g/dl。药物和内镜联合治疗是目前控制出血的标准治疗方案，其效果优于单一治疗。预防性使用抗生素可显著降低感染、再出血和死亡的风险，应尽早使用。

目前的治疗药物包括奥曲肽（一种生长抑素类似物），其安全性良好且已被广泛使用。该药最好在内镜检查前使用。内镜治疗包括 EBL 和（或）硬化剂注射。由于不良反应和并发症的发生率较低，EBL 是首选方式。对于胃静脉曲张破裂出血患者，内镜下注射氰基丙烯酸酯胶比 EBL 更有效，但这种治疗在美国尚未获得批准。气囊填塞（Sengstaken-Blakemore 管、Linton 管或 Minnesota 管）或食管支架置入术可作为临时措施，仅用于内镜治疗失败的大出血病例。近期一项纳入关于食管支架置入术与气囊填塞研究的荟萃分析显示，食管支架置入术可有效控制出血，尽管存在支架移位的问题。此

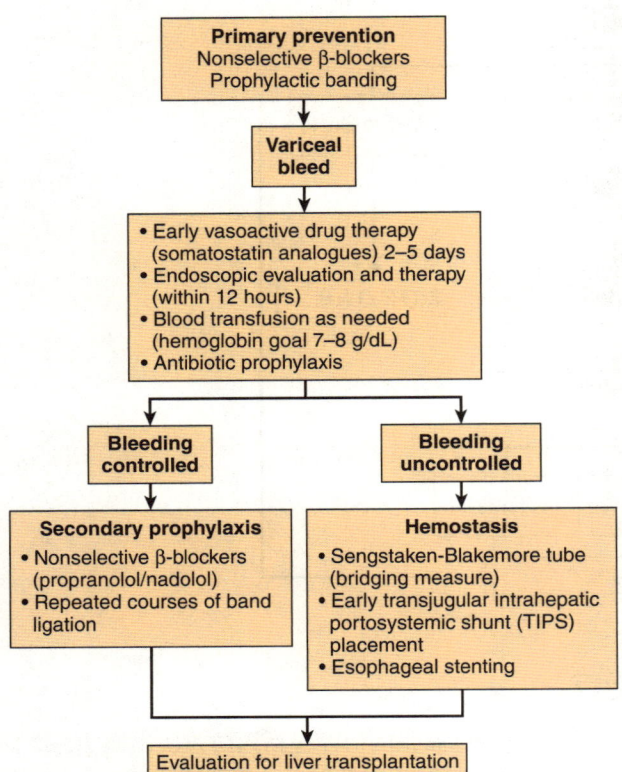

Fig. 14.2 Prevention and treatment of variceal bleeding.

TABLE 14.4	Classification of Ascites
SAAG High (>1.1 g/dL)	**SAAG Low (<1.1 g/dL)**
Cirrhosis	Peritoneal carcinomatosis
Alcoholic hepatitis	Peritoneal tuberculosis
Chronic hepatic congestion	Pancreatic and biliary disease
Right ventricular heart failure	Nephrotic syndrome
Budd-Chiari syndrome	
Constrictive pericarditis	
Massive liver metastases	
Myxedema	
Mixed ascites	

SAAG, Serum-ascites albumin gradient.

balloon tamponade revealed esophageal stenting to have improvement in bleeding control despite issues with stent migration. Also, there is evidence that early (within 72 hours of admission) placement of a transjugular intrahepatic portosystemic shunt (TIPS) in a subset of patients with advanced liver disease improves survival after bleeding. The most common side effect of the TIPS is postprocedural encephalopathy.

Recommendations for secondary prophylaxis to prevent rebleeding include a combination of nonselective β-blockers (propranolol and nadolol) and variceal obliteration through repeated courses of EBL. In patients who undergo TIPS, the patency must be assessed using Doppler ultrasound on a regular basis.

Prognosis

Overall, the frequency and mortality rates from variceal bleeding appear to be decreasing in the United States over the past 2 decades. However, variceal hemorrhage is life-threatening, and after an initial episode the risk of rebleeding approaches 60% with a mortality rate of approximately 33% if secondary prophylaxis is not instituted.

ASCITES

Definition and Pathology

Ascites represents the accumulation of excess fluid in the peritoneal cavity. Although cirrhosis is the most common cause of ascites, there are also other important causes (Table 14.4). The precise sequence of events leading to the development of cirrhotic ascites remains debated.

Diagnosis

Physical examination is relatively insensitive for detection of small volumes of ascites, but bulging flanks, shifting dullness, and evidence of portal hypertension (e.g., distended veins over the abdominal wall and caput medusae) become evident with increasing amounts of fluid. Abdominal ultrasound is both sensitive and specific and is widely used in screening. When fluid is present, abdominal paracentesis is the quickest and most direct approach for confirmation of the presence of fluid in the abdominal cavity and initial characterization of the cause. In addition to standard measures such as cell count, the serum-ascites albumin gradient (SAAG), which is proportional to the sinusoidal portal pressure, is calculated as follows:

$$SAAG = \text{(Serum albumin concentration)} - \text{(Ascitic fluid albumin concentration)}$$

An elevated SAAG (>1.1 g/dL) correlates well with portal hypertension as the likely cause of fluid accumulation (see Table 14.4).

Clinical Presentation

Patients usually report increasing abdominal girth, fullness of the flanks, and weight gain with or without peripheral edema. Ascites becomes clinically detectable with fluid accumulation greater than about 500 mL. Shifting dullness to percussion is the most sensitive clinical sign of ascites, but about 1500 mL of fluid must be present for reliable detection.

Treatment

Management of cirrhotic ascites depends on the cause. Patients with high SAAG (>1.1 g/mL), which is used as a surrogate measure for elevated portal pressures, usually respond to salt restriction (<2 g/day) and diuretics to stimulate renal Na^+ loss. The administration of spironolactone, an aldosterone antagonist, supplemented with a loop diuretic (e.g., furosemide), is effective in about 90% of patients. Diuresis should be monitored closely because aggressive diuretic therapy may result in electrolyte disturbances (e.g., hyponatremia, hypokalemia) and hypovolemia, leading to impaired renal function and potentially precipitating HE. Water restriction is implemented when the serum sodium concentration is less than 120 to 125 mEq/L.

Prognosis

Refractory ascites occurs in up to 10% of patients with cirrhosis and is defined as the persistence of tense ascites despite maximal diuretic therapy (spironolactone, 400 mg/day, and furosemide, 160 mg/day) or the development of azotemia or electrolyte disturbances at submaximal doses of diuretics. Treatment includes repeated large-volume paracentesis and colloid volume expansion with albumin (6 to 8 g/L of fluid removed), TIPS placement in appropriate candidates, and eventually liver transplantation (Fig. 14.3). Peritoneovenous shunts are rarely used and are reserved for patients who are not candidates for paracentesis, TIPS, or transplantation.

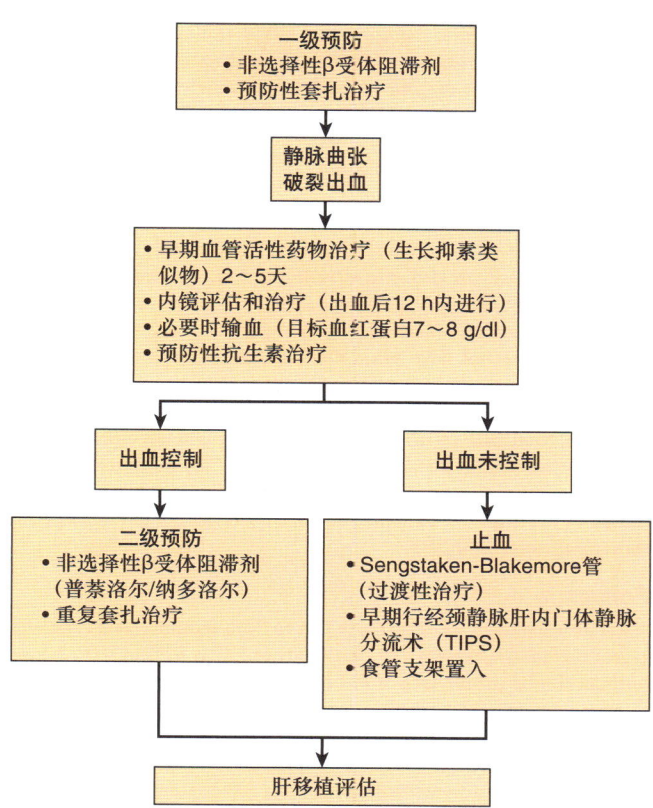

图 14.2 胃食管静脉曲张破裂出血的预防和治疗

表 14.4 腹腔积液的分类	
SAAG 高（> 1.1 g/dl）	SAAG 低（< 1.1 g/dl）
肝硬化	腹膜癌
酒精性肝炎	结核性腹膜炎
慢性肝淤血	胰腺和胆道疾病
右心室衰竭	肾病综合征
布-加综合征	
晚期肝转移	
黏液性水肿	
混合性腹腔积液	

SAAG，血清-腹水白蛋白梯度。

外，研究表明，对部分进展期肝病患者早期（入院72 h内）进行经颈静脉肝内门体静脉分流术（TIPS）可提高患者出血后的生存率。TIPS最常见的副作用是术后肝性脑病。

预防再出血的二级预防建议包括联合使用 NSBB（普萘洛尔和纳多洛尔）和多次 EBL 消除胃食管静脉曲张。对于接受 TIPS 的患者，必须定期进行多普勒超声检查，以评估支架的通畅性。

预后

总体上，美国在过去20年中静脉曲张破裂出血的发生率和死亡率呈下降趋势。但是，静脉曲张破裂出血会危及生命，如果不采取二级预防措施，首次出血后再出血的风险接近60%，发生再出血时死亡率约为33%。

腹腔积液

定义和病理学

腹腔积液是指腹腔内液体的过量积聚。肝硬化是腹腔积液最常见的原因，但一些其他的重要因素也可导致腹腔积液（表 14.4）。关于肝硬化导致腹腔积液的具体病理生理学机制，目前仍存在争议。

诊断

腹腔积液量较小时，体格检查相对不敏感，但随着腹腔积液量的增加，腹部膨隆、移动性浊音和门静脉高压的证据（如腹壁静脉曲张和海蛇头征）是诊断肝硬化腹腔积液的重要依据。腹部超声的敏感性和特异性较高，已被广泛用于腹腔积液的筛查。出现腹腔积液时，腹腔穿刺术是确认腹腔积液和初步明确病因最快速、最直接的方法。除了进行细胞计数等标准方法外，血清-腹水白蛋白梯度（SAAG）也是重要的诊断工具，SAAG与窦性门静脉压力成正比。SAAG 的计算公式如下：

$$SAAG = 血清白蛋白浓度 - 腹腔积液白蛋白浓度$$

SAAG > 1.1 g/dl 时，提示患者可能是门静脉高压所致的腹腔积液（表 14.4）。

临床表现

患者通常表现为腹围增加、腹部饱满、体重增加，伴或不伴外周水肿。当腹腔积液超过约 500 ml 时，临床上即可发现。叩诊移动性浊音阳性是腹腔积液最敏感的临床体征，但需要腹腔积液量达到约 1500 ml 时才能可靠地检测到这一体征。

治疗

肝硬化腹腔积液的治疗取决于病因。高 SAAG（> 1.1 g/dl）患者通常对限盐（< 2 g/d）和利尿剂（促进肾排泄 Na^+）治疗有应答。服用螺内酯（醛固酮拮抗剂）辅以袢利尿剂（如呋塞米）对约 90% 的患者有效。应密切监测利尿情况，因为激进的利尿治疗可能会导致电解质紊乱（如低钠血症、低钾血症）和低血容量，进而导致肾功能受损，并有可能诱发肝性脑病。当血清 Na^+ < 120～125 mmol/L 时，应限制饮水。

预后

难治性腹腔积液在肝硬化患者中的发生率高达 10%，其定义为接受最大剂量利尿剂治疗（螺内酯 400 mg/d，呋塞米 160 mg/d）后仍持续存在大量腹腔积液，或在尚未达到最大剂量利尿剂治疗的情况下即出现氮质血症或电解质紊乱。治疗方法包括反复进行大容量腹腔穿刺引流联合白蛋白胶体扩容（每移除 1 L 腹腔积液需补充 6～8 g 白蛋白）、在合适的患者中行 TIPS，以及肝移植（图 14.3）。腹腔静脉分流术很少使用，仅用于不适合进行腹腔穿刺术、TIPS 或肝移植的患者。

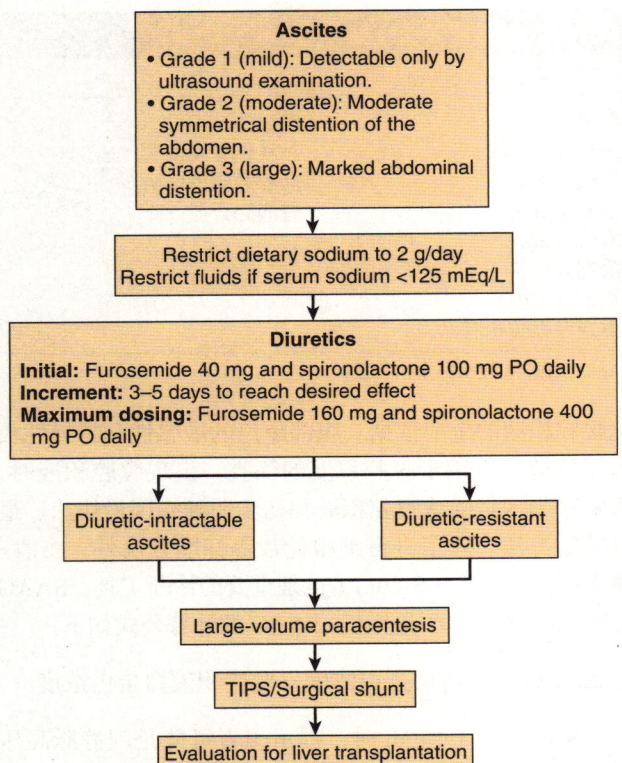

Fig. 14.3 Management of ascites in cirrhosis. *TIPS,* Transjugular intrahepatic portosystemic shunt.

SPONTANEOUS BACTERIAL PERITONITIS

Definition and Pathology

Cirrhotic patients may develop infection of ascitic fluid in the absence of an obvious source of contamination or surgically treatable source, a condition known as acute spontaneous bacterial peritonitis (SBP). The exact mechanism of contamination of the ascitic fluid is unclear. Factors such as bacterial overgrowth, altered motility, and increased intestinal permeability causing transient translocation of bacteria into the bloodstream and eventual seeding of the peritoneal fluid may contribute. The microbiology of SBP includes most commonly *Escherichia coli* and Enterobacteriaceae *(Klebsiella)*. Gram-positive organisms such as *Streptococcus (viridans)*, *Enterococcus*, and *Pneumococcus* species may also be found. With the use of prophylactic antibiotics for SBP there has been a shift to gram-positive organisms being isolated. Anaerobes are uncommon, and a single organism is isolated on culture in most cases; the presence of multiple organisms suggests bowel perforation or other causes of peritonitis.

Clinical Presentation

Clinical features may include fever, abdominal pain, and signs of peritoneal irritation, particularly in advanced cases. Often, early infection is clinically silent or manifests with worsening of HE, diarrhea, ileus, or renal insufficiency.

Diagnosis

Diagnostic paracentesis should be considered in any patient with cirrhotic ascites who deteriorates clinically. The diagnosis of SBP is highly likely if a high concentration (>250 cells/mm^3) of polymorphonuclear leukocytes (PMNs) is present in the ascitic fluid, and this finding should prompt empiric therapy while blood and ascitic fluid culture results are pending. The use of rapid bedside diagnostic methods such as leukocyte esterase reagent strips is not routinely recommended in view of their low sensitivity. However, inoculation of both aerobic and anaerobic blood culture bottles with the first samples of peritoneal fluid retrieved at bedside significantly increases the yield of capturing potential pathogens.

Treatment

Patients are usually treated with intravenous third-generation cephalosporin (e.g., ceftriaxone, 2 g every 24 hours); quinolones, in particular ciprofloxacin, are routinely used in the United States, provided that the patient does not have prior exposure and is not in overt shock. Response to treatment is usually seen within 72 hours; therapy is continued for a minimum of 5 days and can extend up to 14 days. Repeat peritoneal fluid analysis may be done if recovery is delayed or to ensure that the ascitic fluid is sterile after treatment. The administration of intravenous albumin on day 1 (1.5 g/kg) and day 3 (1 g/kg) has been shown to decrease the incidence of renal dysfunction and to improve short-term survival in SBP.

Prognosis

There is a high rate of recurrence, up to 70% within 1 year, and the 1-year mortality rate with a prior episode of SBP is 50% to 70%. Long-term antibiotic prophylaxis is indicated to reduce the recurrence rate to approximately 20%. Short-term prophylaxis should be considered for patients with cirrhosis and ascites who are hospitalized with upper gastrointestinal bleeding. Common prophylactic regimens for SBP include fluoroquinolones (ciprofloxacin, 500 mg/daily; norfloxacin, 400 mg/day) and trimethoprim-sulfamethoxazole (1 double-strength tablet daily). Long-term antibiotic prophylaxis can lead to infection with resistant extended-spectrum β-lactamase (ESBL)-producing organisms or methicillin-resistant *Staphylococcus aureus* (MRSA).

HEPATORENAL SYNDROME

Definition and Pathology

Hepatorenal syndrome (HRS) is a form of functional renal failure that occurs in the presence of significant hepatic synthetic dysfunction and ascites. Three mechanisms of kidney dysfunction have been proposed: splanchnic arterial vasodilation, renal arterial vasoconstriction, and cardiac dysfunction.

Clinical Presentation and Diagnosis

Patients with HRS typically have advanced ascites and other manifestations of cirrhosis but are not otherwise symptomatic. However, some patients may notice decreased urine output or signs of encephalopathy. There is no single laboratory or imaging study that can be used alone to diagnose HRS. However, the 5-year probability of developing HRS in patients with cirrhosis and ascites is 40%, and HRS develops in approximately 30% of cirrhotic patients who are admitted with SBP. Therefore, a high clinical suspicion is warranted along with a systematic approach to diagnosis based on fulfillment of certain criteria.

The International Club of Ascites (ICA) developed updated diagnostic criteria incorporating new definitions of acute kidney injury (AKI) in 2015:

1. Cirrhosis with ascites
2. Diagnosis of AKI according to ICA-AKI criteria: 50% increase in the serum creatinine level from baseline which is known or presumed to have occurred within the 7 days prior OR Rise of 0.3 mg/dL (26.4 µmol/L) in the serum creatinine level in less than 48 hours

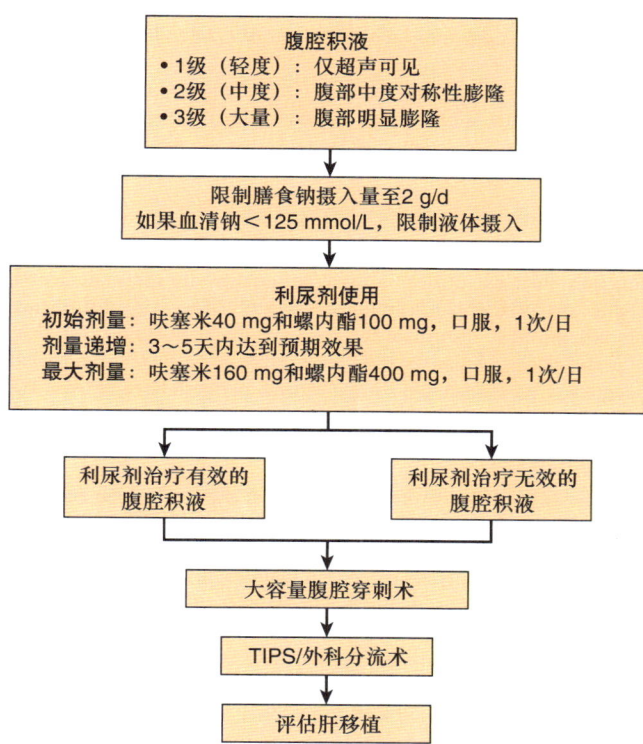

图 14.3 肝硬化腹腔积液的管理。TIPS，经颈静脉肝内门体静脉分流术

自发性细菌性腹膜炎

定义和病理学

肝硬化患者可能会在没有明确污染源或外科可清除病灶的情况下发生腹腔积液感染，这种情况被称为急性自发性细菌性腹膜炎（SBP）。腹腔积液感染的确切机制尚不清楚。细菌过度生长、肠道动力改变、肠道黏膜通透性增加等因素均会导致细菌短暂入血，最终在腹腔内播种，导致腹腔积液感染。引起SBP最常见的病原体是大肠埃希菌和肠杆菌科细菌（克雷伯菌）。革兰氏阳性菌［如链球菌（草绿色链球菌）、肠球菌和肺炎球菌］也可引起SBP。随着预防性抗生素在SBP患者中的应用，分离出的革兰氏阳性菌有所增多，但厌氧菌并不常见。大多数情况下，培养分离出的是单一菌种，若培养结果显示存在多种微生物，提示存在肠穿孔或其他引起腹膜炎的原因。

临床表现

临床表现可包括发热、腹痛和腹膜刺激症状，晚期患者上述症状更为明显。早期感染往往无临床症状，或表现为肝性脑病症状加重、腹泻、肠梗阻或肾功能不全。

诊断

任何临床病情恶化的肝硬化腹腔积液患者均应考虑进行诊断性腹腔穿刺。如果腹腔积液中多形核白细胞（PMN）计数 > 250 个 / 立方毫米，则极有可能是SBP。在等待血培养和腹腔积液培养结果期间，应及时进行经验性抗感染治疗。由于白细胞酯酶测定试纸等床旁快速诊断性方法的敏感性较低，不建议常规使用。但是，将床旁获得的腹腔积液样本立即接种到需氧和厌氧血培养瓶中，可显著提高潜在病原体的检出率。

治疗

推荐选用静脉注射第三代头孢菌素（如头孢曲松 2 g/24h）；喹诺酮类药物，尤其是环丙沙星（在美国常规使用），但用药的前提是患者既往未使用过类似药物，且没有明显的休克症状。治疗反应通常在用药 72 h 内出现，治疗时间应至少持续 5 天，最长可达 14 天。若患者的病情恢复未达到预期，或需要确认是否成功消除腹腔积液感染，可重复进行腹腔积液分析。治疗第 1 天和第 3 天分别给予静脉注射白蛋白 1.5 g/kg 和 1.0 g/kg 已被证明可降低 SBP 患者发生肾功能不全的风险，并改善患者的短期生存率。

预后

SBP 患者的复发率很高，1 年内复发率高达 70%，对于曾经发生过 SBP 的患者，1 年死亡率为 50% ～ 70%。长期使用抗生素预防可将复发率降至约 20%。对于因上消化道出血住院的肝硬化腹腔积液患者，应考虑短期预防性使用抗生素。常见的 SBP 预防方案包括氟喹诺酮类药物（环丙沙星 500 mg/d，诺氟沙星 400 mg/d）和甲氧苄啶-磺胺甲噁唑（1 片 / 日）。长期预防性使用抗生素可导致耐药菌感染，特别是超广谱 β-内酰胺酶（ESBL）细菌或耐甲氧西林金黄色葡萄球菌（MRSA）。

肝肾综合征

定义和病理学

肝肾综合征（HRS）是功能性肾衰竭的一种形式，出现于严重肝脏合成功能障碍和腹腔积液的情况下。目前提出了 3 种肾衰竭的可能机制：内脏动脉扩张、肾动脉收缩和心功能不全。

临床表现和诊断

HRS 患者通常有严重腹腔积液和肝硬化的其他表现，但除此之外没有其他症状。部分患者可能出现尿量减少或脑病征象。目前尚无任何实验室检查或影像学检查可单独用于诊断 HRS。肝硬化腹腔积液患者 5 年内发生 HRS 的概率为 40%，约 30% 因 SBP 入院的肝硬化患者会出现 HRS。因此，临床上需要高度警惕，并基于特定标准进行系统性诊断。

2015 年，国际腹腔积液俱乐部（ICA）结合急性肾损伤（AKI）的新定义，制定了最新的诊断标准：

1. 肝硬化伴腹腔积液
2. 根据 ICA-AKI 标准被诊断为 AKI：7 天内血清肌酐水平较已知或推断的基线值升高 ≥ 50%，或在入院 48 h 内血清肌酐水平升高 ≥ 0.3 mg/dl（26.4 μmol/L）

3. Lack of response after at least 2 days of diuretic withdrawal and volume expansion with albumin (1 g/kg of body weight/day, to a maximum of 100 g/day)
4. Absence of shock
5. Lack of current or recent treatment with nephrotoxic drugs
6. Absence of parenchymal kidney disease as indicated by proteinuria of more than 500 mg/day, microhematuria (>50 red blood cells/high-power field), or abnormal renal US findings

HRS has two types, HRS-AKI type 1 and HRS-CKD (chronic kidney disease) type 2. HRS-AKI is characterized as an increase in serum creatinine 0.3 mg/dL or greater within 48 hrs or 50% or greater from baseline value according to ICA consensus document *and/or* urinary output 0.5 mL/kg body weight or less for longer than 6 hours. HRS-CKD is defined as eGFR less than 60 mL/min per 1.73 m^2 for 3 months or greater in the absence of other (structural) causes.

Typically, the kidneys are histologically normal and can regain normal function in the event of recovery of liver function (e.g., after liver transplantation). Severe cortical vasoconstriction has been demonstrated angiographically, and such vasoconstriction reverses when these kidneys are transplanted into patients who do not have cirrhosis.

Treatment and Prognosis

The mortality rate is high in HRS, and so prevention is important. In all patients with cirrhosis, precipitating factors (e.g., diuretics, lactulose, nonsteroidal anti-inflammatory drugs, angiotensin-converting enzyme inhibitors) should be avoided if possible. Patients should be promptly diagnosed and treated for any signs of SBP, and colloid (albumin) should be administered if rising creatinine levels are observed. Prevention of variceal bleeding should also be optimized by primary and secondary prophylaxis.

Studies have shown an increased mortality rate with AKI among hospitalized cirrhotic patients. Several medical therapies are currently under review, including use of terlipressin, a vasopressin V_1 receptor analogue, in combination with albumin for type 1 HRS. Other studies have evaluated the combination of octreotide and midodrine (an α-adrenergic agonist) and intravenous albumin. Placement of TIPS has also been reported to stabilize or even improve renal function, mainly in patients with HRS-CKD. However, a significant limitation of TIPS is the possibility of worsening hepatic function in decompensated cirrhosis. Liver transplantation has become the accepted treatment for HRS because it is the only known therapeutic intervention that reverses the process. It is limited by rapid progression of HRS and lack of available organs.

HEPATIC ENCEPHALOPATHY

Definition

HE is a complex, reversible neuropsychiatric syndrome that occurs in patients with chronic liver disease, portal hypertension, or portosystemic shunting. HE is also seen in patients with acute liver failure. HE develops in about 30% to 45% of cirrhotic patients, and when it is present, the survival probability is approximately 23% at 3 years.

Pathophysiology

The pathogenesis of HE in the setting of cirrhosis is thought to be multifactorial and may differ in acute and chronic liver disease. Contributors include the inadequate hepatic removal of potential endogenous neurotoxins, altered permeability of the blood-brain barrier, and abnormal neurotransmission. Elevation of blood ammonia levels, derived from both amino acid deamination and bacterial hydrolysis of nitrogenous compounds in the gut, has been the best studied factor, but its specific role in the pathogenesis of HE remains uncertain. Many other potential contributors to HE have been investigated, including increased tone of the inhibitory GABAA/benzodiazepine neurotransmitter system, activation of the astrocytic 18-kDa translocator protein (PTBR), production of endogenous benzodiazepine-like compounds, altered cerebral metabolism, zinc deficiency, increase in serotonin levels, upregulation of H1 receptors, altered melatonin production, and deposition of manganese in the basal ganglia.

Clinical Presentation

The clinical features of HE include disturbances of higher neurologic function such as intellectual and personality disorders, dementia, inability to copy simple diagrams (constructional apraxia), disturbance of consciousness, disturbances of neuromuscular function (asterixis, hyperreflexia, myoclonus), and, rarely, a Parkinson-like syndrome and progressive paraplegia. One of the earliest manifestations of overt HE is alteration of the normal sleep-wake cycle.

Diagnosis

There is no laboratory or imaging study that allows a specific diagnosis of HE. Rather, it is a clinical syndrome. Blood levels of ammonia are commonly measured, but elevated levels are neither sensitive nor specific for HE. Neuropsychometric and neurocognitive tests such as the Portosystemic Encephalopathy Syndrome Test (PSET) and the earlier Stroop Color-Word Test evaluate the patient's attention, concentration, fine motor skills, and orientation and have been shown to be highly specific for the diagnosis of HE, but they are reasonably labor intensive. Therefore, a smartphone-based application known as EncephalApp was created incorporating the Stroop test that is validated for use in detection of covert/minimal HE. It is imperative that reversible causes of neurologic dysfunction, such as hypoglycemia, subdural hematoma, meningitis, and drug overdose, be considered and excluded early in the differential diagnosis of altered mental status in patients with cirrhosis.

Classification of Hepatic Encephalopathy

There are three major types of HE: type A (Acute), which is associated with acute liver failure; type B (Bypass), which is associated with portosystemic shunts in the absence of liver disease; and type C (Cirrhosis), which is associated with liver cirrhosis and is subdivided into episodic, persistent, and minimal types.

HE has been further graded based on the West Haven Criteria from 0 to 4. A new nomenclature, termed the Spectrum of Neurocognitive Impairment in Cirrhosis (SONIC) classification, has been proposed to improve recognition of earlier forms of HE that require specialized testing for detection and to facilitate research studies. Patients are divided into those who are unimpaired, those with covert HE, and those with overt HE (Table 14.5).

Treatment

Treatment of HE starts with identifying and addressing any precipitating factors (Table 14.6), reducing and eliminating substrates for the generation of nitrogenous compounds, and preventing ammonia absorption from the bowel. Protein restriction was considered to be important in preventing excess ammonia production in the past; however, studies have demonstrated that dietary restriction of protein is not of significant benefit. Short-term protein restriction may be considered for patients with severe encephalopathy, but long-term restriction is associated with worsening malnutrition. Treatment with formulas rich in branched-chain amino acids has shown no benefit in improving encephalopathy or mortality.

Nonabsorbable disaccharides (e.g., lactulose) are the mainstay treatment of HE. These agents are fermented to organic acids by colonic bacteria, processes that lower stool pH and trap NH_4^+ in the colon, thereby decreasing absorption. In addition, the cathartic effect

3. 停用利尿剂并给予白蛋白［1 g/（kg·d），最大剂量为 100 g/d］扩充血容量治疗 2 天后仍无应答

4. 无休克

5. 目前或近期未使用肾毒性药物

6. 无肾实质性疾病，即无如下表现：尿蛋白＞500 mg/d、镜下血尿（红细胞＞50 个 / 高倍视野）、肾脏超声检查异常

HRS 分为两种类型：1 型［即 HRS-AKI（急性肾损伤型）］和 2 型［即 HRS-CKD（慢性肾脏病型）］。根据 ICA 共识文件，HRS-AKI 的特征是 48 h 内血清肌酐水平升高＞0.3 mg/dl 或升高≥基线值的 50%，和（或）尿量≤0.5 ml/kg，持续 6 h 以上。HRS-CKD 的定义为估算的肾小球滤过率（eGFR）在 3 个月或更长时间内＜60 ml/（min·1.73 m^2），且无其他（结构性）原因。

通常情况下，患者的肾脏组织学正常，且在肝功能恢复（如肝移植后）的情况下肾功能也可以恢复至正常。血管造影显示 HRS 患者存在严重的肾皮质血管收缩，如果将这些肾脏移植到没有肝硬化的患者体内，这种血管收缩会逆转。

治疗和预后

一旦发生 HRS，则死亡率很高，因此预防 HRS 非常重要。对于所有肝硬化患者，应尽可能避免诱发因素（如利尿剂、乳果糖、非甾体抗炎药、血管紧张素转换酶抑制剂等）。如果患者出现任何 SBP 征象，应及时进行诊断和治疗。若观察到血清肌酐水平升高，则应给予胶体输注（白蛋白）。此外，应对静脉曲张破裂出血进行一级和二级预防。

研究显示，合并 AKI 的肝硬化住院患者的死亡率升高。目前正在对几种药物治疗进行研究，其中包括特利加压素（一种血管升压素 V$_1$ 受体类似物）与白蛋白联合治疗 1 型 HRS，其他研究评估了奥曲肽和米多君（一种 α 受体激动剂）与静脉输注白蛋白联合治疗的效果。研究表明，TIPS 可稳定甚至改善肾功能，主要在 HRS-CKD 患者中。然而，TIPS 的一个重要局限性是可能导致失代偿期肝硬化患者的肝功能恶化。肝移植是目前已知的唯一能逆转 HRS 的治疗方法，但其应用受到 HRS 疾病进展迅速和器官短缺的限制。

肝性脑病

定义

肝性脑病（HE）是一种复杂、可逆的神经精神综合征，多发于慢性肝病、门静脉高压或门体静脉分流的患者。急性肝衰竭患者也会出现 HE。30%～45% 的肝硬化患者会出现 HE，一旦出现 HE，患者的 3 年生存率仅约 23%。

病理生理学

多种机制可导致肝硬化患者发生 HE，且在急性和慢性肝病中可能有所区别。主要机制包括肝脏对潜在的内源性神经毒素清除不足、血脑屏障通透性改变和神经传递异常。其中研究最透彻的因素是氨基酸脱氨和细菌水解肠道中的含氮化合物引起的血氨水平升高，但其在 HE 发病机制中的具体作用仍不明确。研究还发现了许多可能导致 HE 的因素，包括抑制性神经递质 γ-氨基丁酸（GABA）系统 / 苯二氮䓬受体系统上调、星形胶质细胞 18-kDa 转运蛋白（PTBR）激活、内源性苯二氮䓬类化合物的产生、大脑代谢改变、锌缺乏、5-羟色胺水平升高、H$_1$ 受体上调、褪黑素分泌改变及基底节区锰沉积。

临床表现

HE 的临床特征包括高级神经功能紊乱［如智力和人格障碍、痴呆、无法复制简单的图表（结构性失用）］，意识障碍，神经肌肉功能紊乱（扑翼样震颤、反射亢进、肌阵挛），以及罕见的帕金森样综合征和进行性截瘫。显性 HE 最早的表现之一是的睡眠-觉醒周期异常。

诊断

HE 是一种临床综合征，目前尚缺乏特异性实验室或影像学检查可以明确诊断。通常进行血氨测定，但血氨水平升高对诊断 HE 既不敏感也不特异。神经心理测试和神经认知测试［如门体静脉分流脑病综合征测试（PSET）和早期 Stroop Color-Word 测试］可评估患者的注意力、专注力、精细动作技能和定向力，这些测试对 HE 诊断具有高度特异性。但是，这些测试需要大量人力。因此，为了检测隐性 / 轻度 HE，开发了一款名为 EncephalApp 的智能手机应用程序，它包含了经过验证的 Stroop 测试。应注意，对于肝硬化患者出现的精神状态改变，在鉴别诊断过程中必须及早考虑并排除可逆性原因，如低血糖、硬膜下血肿、脑膜炎和药物过量。

HE 的分类

HE 有 3 种主要类型：A 型（急性），与急性肝衰竭有关；B 型（分流型），与门体静脉分流有关，无基础肝脏疾病；C 型（肝硬化型），与肝硬化有关，可进一步分为发作型、持续型和轻微型。

根据 West-Haven 标准，HE 可进一步分为 0～4 级。肝硬化神经认知功能变化谱（SONIC）分类法是一种新的命名法，旨在更好地识别需要专门检测才能发现的早期 HE，以及便于研究。患者可分为未受损、隐匿性 HE 和显性 HE（表 14.5）。

治疗

治疗 HE 首先要明确并去除诱发因素（表 14.6），减少和消除产生含氮化合物的底物，并阻止肠道吸收氨。既往认为，限制蛋白质摄入对防止氨的过量产生非常重要；但研究表明，限制蛋白质摄入并无明显益处。对于严重脑病患者，可考虑短期限制蛋白质摄入，但长期限制蛋白质摄入会加重营养不良。使用富含支链氨基酸的配方奶粉治疗既不能改善脑病，也不能降低死亡率。

非吸收性双糖（如乳果糖）是治疗 HE 的主要方

TABLE 14.5 Clinical Stages of Hepatic Encephalopathy as Defined by the West Haven Criteria and the Proposed Sonic Classification

	WEST HAVEN CRITERIA		SONIC			
Grade	Intellectual Function	Neuromuscular Function	Classification	Mental Status	Special Tests	Asterixis
0	Normal	Normal	Unimpaired	Not impaired	Normal	Absent
Minimal	Normal examination findings. Subtle changes in work or driving	Minor abnormalities of visual perception or on psychometric or number tests	Covert HE	Not impaired	Abnormal	Absent
1	Personality changes, attention deficits, irritability, depressed state	Tremor and incoordination				
2	Changes in sleep-wake cycle, lethargy, mood and behavioral changes, cognitive dysfunction	Asterixis, ataxic gait, speech abnormalities (slow and slurred)	Overt HE	Impaired	Abnormal	Present (absent in coma)
3	Altered level of consciousness (somnolence), confusion, disorientation, and amnesia	Muscular rigidity, nystagmus, clonus, Babinski sign, hyporeflexia				
4	Stupor and coma	Oculocephalic reflex, unresponsiveness to noxious stimuli				

SONIC, Spectrum of Neuro-Cognitive Impairment in Cirrhosis.
Modified from Nevah MI, Fallon MB: Hepatic encephalopathy, hepatorenal syndrome, hepatopulmonary syndrome, and systemic complications of liver disease. In Feldman M, Friedman LS, Brandt LJ, editors: Sleisenger and Fordtran's gastrointestinal and liver disease, ed 9, Philadelphia, 2010, Saunders.

TABLE 14.6 Hepatic Encephalopathy: Precipitating Factors

Gastrointestinal bleeding
Increased dietary protein
Constipation
Infection
Central nervous system depressant drugs (benzodiazepines, opiates, tricyclic antidepressants)
Deterioration in hepatic function
Hypokalemia: most often induced by diuretics
Azotemia: most often induced by diuretics
Alkalosis: most often induced by diuretics
Hypovolemia: most often induced by diuretics

of lactulose eliminates ammonia and other nitrogenous compounds. Patients are usually directed to achieve two to three soft stools per day as the goal of lactulose therapy. Reduction and elimination of nitrogenous compound substrates can also be achieved by administering enemas and using nonabsorbable antibiotics such as rifaximin in patients who do not tolerate or respond to lactulose. Rifaximin (Xifaxan), 550 mg PO twice daily, is approved by the US Food and Drug Administration for the treatment of HE and has a favorable side effect profile; however, cost is the limiting factor. Other agents that affect intestinal motility and ammonia generation are being evaluated, including acarbose and probiotics.

HEPATOPULMONARY SYNDROME AND PORTOPULMONARY HYPERTENSION

The effects of cirrhosis and portal hypertension on the pulmonary circulation manifest as two distinct disorders, hepatopulmonary syndrome (HPS) and portopulmonary hypertension (PoPH).

Hepatopulmonary Syndrome

HPS occurs in 5% to 30% of patients with cirrhosis and is a progressive disease. It is characterized by gas exchange abnormalities (increased alveolar-arterial gradient and hypoxemia) resulting from intrapulmonary vascular dilation. The vascular dilation leads to vascular remodeling and angiogenesis, resulting in impaired oxygen transfer from the alveoli to the central stream of red blood cells within capillaries. Usually, this functional intrapulmonary right-to-left shunt significantly improves with the administration of 100% oxygen. HPS also has been reported in cases of hepatic venous outflow obstruction without cirrhosis.

Diagnosis

HPS is diagnosed based on high clinical suspicion and measurement of a widened alveolar-arterial oxygen gradient on room air in the presence or absence of hypoxemia. The gradient is calculated by analyzing arterial blood gases. HPS is graded from mild, in which the arterial partial pressure of oxygen (Pao_2) is greater than 80 mm Hg) to very severe (Pao_2 <50 mm Hg). Intrapulmonary shunting is demonstrated by contrast echocardiography, in which agitated saline is injected into a peripheral vein during the performance of two-dimensional echocardiography. Delayed appearance of microbubbles in the left cardiac chambers (more than three to six cardiac cycles after injection) indicates intrapulmonary vasodilation. Early visualization of microbubbles in the left cardiac chambers indicates intracardiac shunting. Other tests, including chest radiography, computed tomography, and pulmonary function tests, are performed to exclude intrinsic cardiopulmonary disorders.

Clinical Presentation

Clinical features range from subclinical abnormalities in gas exchange to profound hypoxemia causing significant dyspnea. Classically in HPS, the dyspnea is worse on standing and improves when the patient

表 14.5　由 West-Haven 标准和 SONIC 分类定义的肝性脑病临床分期

West-Haven 标准			SONIC			
分级	智力功能	神经肌肉功能	分类	精神状态	特殊检查	扑翼样震颤
0	正常	正常	未受损	未受损	正常	无
轻微	检查结果正常 工作或驾驶时有细微改变	视知觉或心理测验或数字测试显示轻微异常	隐匿性 HE	未受损	异常	无
1	性格改变、注意力缺陷、易怒、抑郁状态	震颤和协调运动障碍	显性 HE	受损	异常	有 （昏迷中无）
2	睡眠-觉醒周期改变、嗜睡、情绪和行为改变、认知功能障碍	扑翼样震颤、共济失调步态、言语异常（语速变慢和说话含糊不清）				
3	意识水平改变（嗜睡）、意识模糊、定向障碍和失忆	肌肉僵硬、眼球震颤、阵挛、巴宾斯基征、反射减弱				
4	木僵、昏迷	眼脑反射、对有害刺激反应迟钝				

SONIC，肝硬化神经认知功能变化谱。
改编自 Nevah MI，Fallon MB：Hepatic encephalopathy, hepatorenal syndrome, hepatopulmonary syndrome, and systemic complications of liver disease. In Feldman M，Friedman LS，Brandt LJ，editors：Sleisenger and Fordtran's gastrointestinal and liver disease, ed 9，Philadelphia，2010，Saunders.

表 14.6　肝性脑病：诱发因素

消化道出血
饮食摄入蛋白质增加
便秘
感染
中枢神经系统抑制药物（苯二氮䓬类药物、阿片类药物、三环类抗抑郁药）
肝功能恶化
低钾血症：通常由利尿剂引起
氮质血症：通常由利尿剂引起
碱中毒：通常由利尿剂引起
低血容量：通常由利尿剂引起

法。这些药物在结肠中被肠道细菌发酵为有机酸，从而降低粪便的 pH 值。这一过程有助于将氨（NH_3）转化为不可吸收的离子形式（NH_4^+），并使其在结肠中滞留，减少了氨的吸收。此外，乳果糖的导泻作用还能促进氨和其他含氮化合物的排泄，治疗目标通常是促使患者每天排 2～3 次软便。对于不能耐受乳果糖或乳果糖治疗无效的患者，也可通过灌肠和使用非吸收性抗生素（如利福昔明）来减少和消除氮化合物底物。FDA 已批准利福昔明用于治疗 HE，剂量为口服 550 mg，2 次/日。虽然利福昔明的副作用较少，但其治疗费用较高。目前正在对其他影响肠道蠕动和氨生成的药物进行评估，包括阿卡波糖和益生菌。

肝肺综合征和门静脉高压性肺动脉高压

肝硬化和门静脉高压对肺循环的影响可表现为两种异常，即肝肺综合征（HPS）和门静脉高压性肺动脉高压（PoPH）。

肝肺综合征

5%～30% 的肝硬化患者会出现 HPS。HPS 是一种进行性疾病，其特点是肺内血管扩张导致气体交换异常（肺泡-动脉血氧梯度升高和低氧血症）。血管扩张会引起血管重塑和血管新生，导致红细胞从肺泡运输氧气到毛细血管的功能受损。这种功能性肺内右向左分流通常在吸入 100% 氧气后可明显改善。HPS 在无肝硬化的肝静脉流出道阻塞病例中也有报道。

诊断

HPS 的诊断基于临床高度怀疑，并在患者吸入室内空气的情况下检测到肺泡-动脉血氧梯度升高，无论是否存在低氧血症。肺泡-动脉血氧梯度可通过动脉血气分析计算得出。HPS 可分为轻度［动脉血氧分压（PaO_2）> 80 mmHg］和重度（PaO_2 < 50 mmHg）。肺内分流可通过造影超声心动图显示，即在进行二维超声心动图检查时将震荡的生理盐水注入外周静脉。左心室延迟出现微气泡（注射后超过 3～6 个心动周期）则提示肺内血管扩张。左心室早期出现微气泡表明存在心内分流。其他检查（包括胸部 X 线检查、CT 和肺功能检查）可排除固有的心肺疾病。

临床表现

临床特征包括从亚临床气体交换异常，到导致明显呼吸困难的严重低氧血症。HPS 的典型表现为站立时呼吸困难加重，躺下时呼吸困难减轻（分别为直立型低氧血症和平卧呼吸）。患者还可能出现明显的夜间低氧血症。

lies down (orthodeoxia and platypnea, respectively). Patients may also have marked nocturnal hypoxemia.

Screening and Treatment
Screening by pulse oximetry typically targets patients with values lower than 96% at rest on room air for further evaluation; however, recent data suggest that this may not be an appropriate screening tool. Currently, there is no established medical therapy for HPS. Recent evaluation of newer agents such as sorafenib showed no significant improvement. Liver transplantation remains the only option and reverses HPS in most patients. The use of TIPS to treat HPS is not established.

Prognosis
HPS carries a mortality rate of up to 40% in 2.5 years.

Portopulmonary Hypertension
PoPH is defined as the presence of pulmonary arterial hypertension in the setting of portal hypertension.

Diagnosis and Pathology
The diagnosis of PoPH is based entirely on results of right heart catheterization. The diagnostic values include a mean pulmonary arterial pressure greater than 25 mm Hg at rest or 30 mm Hg with exercise, a pulmonary capillary wedge pressure lower than 15 mm Hg, and a pulmonary vascular resistance greater than 240 dynes, all in the presence of portal hypertension or liver disease or both. PoPH is graded according to the mean pulmonary artery pressure, from mild (>25 to 35 mm Hg) to moderate (35 to 50 mm Hg) to severe (>50 mm Hg). Patients with mild PoPH do not appear to have increased operative risk. Moderate PoPH carries a high intraoperative risk and should be medically managed before transplantation. Severe PoPH is generally considered a contraindication to surgery. The exact mechanisms of PoPH are poorly understood. Histologically, it has characteristics similar to those of pulmonary hypertension.

Clinical Presentation
The most common symptom of PoPH is dyspnea on exertion, but many cirrhotic patients with PoPH are asymptomatic.

Treatment
In addition to symptomatic treatment (oxygen for dyspnea and diuretics for volume overload), the medical management of PoPH is similar to that for pulmonary arterial hypertension. The drugs most commonly used in treatment for PoPH are prostacyclins (intravenous, inhaled or subcutaneous), oral treatments including phosphodiesterase inhibitors, and endothelin receptor antagonist.

If moderate PoPH responds to therapy, liver transplantation may be considered. However, it has not been established whether successful liver transplantation reliably reverses PoPH. Liver transplantation is contraindicated in severe PoPH because of high transplant-related morbidity and mortality. However, there were no dedicated randomized clinical trials of these therapies until the PORTICO trial. The PORTICO trial was a double-blind, placebo-controlled, multicenter study of macitentan, an endothelin receptor antagonist. Macitentan showed improved pulmonary vascular resistance without hepatotoxicity. More novel agents are being studied.

Prognosis
Untreated PoPH carries high rates of morbidity and mortality; the mean survival time from diagnosis is 15 months. A study on the U.S.-based Registry to Evaluate Early and Long-term Pulmonary Arterial Hypertension Disease Management (REVEAL) showed a 5-year survival rate of 40% from the time of diagnosis in patients with PoPH.

HEPATOCELLULAR CARCINOMA

Epidemiology
Liver cancer is the fifth most common cancer in men and the seventh most common in women worldwide; HCC is the most common type of liver cancer. In the United States, approximately 90% of liver cancers are HCC, and cholangiocarcinomas account for most of the rest. In other areas of the world, including sub-Saharan Africa, China, Japan, and Southeast Asia, HCC is one of the most frequent malignancies and is an important cause of mortality, particularly among middle-aged men.

Etiology
HCC often arises from a cirrhotic liver, and it is closely associated with chronic viral hepatitis. Hepatitis B virus DNA has been shown to integrate into the host cell genome, where it may disrupt tumor suppressor genes and activate oncogenes. In areas of high prevalence, vaccination to prevent infection with hepatitis B virus has reduced the incidence of HCC. The exact pathophysiologic mechanisms leading to tumor genesis in patients with other causes of cirrhosis (e.g., hemochromatosis, alcohol, hepatitis C viral infection) remain poorly understood. Risk factors for the development of HCC and its clinical manifestations are listed in (Table 14.7).

Diagnosis
Table 14.8 lists currently used imaging techniques for detection of HCC and the most common findings. A tissue specimen may be necessary to confirm the diagnosis in some cases, but it is not needed if characteristic clinical and radiologic features are present, especially if they are accompanied by a rise in serum α-fetoprotein levels. The Hepatic Carcinoma Early Detection Screening (HES) algorithm for early detection of HCC was developed and has been validated in the Veterans affairs (VA) cohort. The algorithm includes patient's age, ALT level, platelet count, and current and rate of change to AFP level. It has shown an improvement in early detection in patients with cirrhosis in comparison to AFP alone.

Staging
Although many staging systems for HCC are in use, the Barcelona Clinic Liver Cancer (BCLC) system is most commonly used.

Treatment
Patients with well-compensated cirrhosis may undergo surgical resection or liver transplantation, with a 5-year survival rate of up to 70%. Nonsurgical options include percutaneous ethanol injection, transarterial chemoembolization (TACE), and radiofrequency ablation. The first-line treatment for many years was Sorafenib (a receptor tyrosine kinase angiogenesis inhibitor) for use in patients with unresectable HCC. However, recently another agent was approved, lenvatinib, which works by the same mechanism, and both have been shown to prolong survival of these patients. Second-line agents have also been approved, which include regorafenib, cabozantinib, and nivolumab.

Prognosis
In patients with widespread, multifocal disease and in those with vascular invasion, the prognosis is poor, with a 5-year survival rate of 5% to 6%. Accordingly, emphasis is placed on prevention of viral hepatitis and other causes of liver disease and on screening by ultrasound of those who are at higher risk, including patients with known cirrhosis.

筛查和治疗

使用脉搏血氧仪进行筛查时，对于在吸入室内空气的情况下静息手指脉氧饱和度 < 96% 的患者，通常会进行进一步评估；但近期数据表明，这可能不是一种合适的筛查工具。目前，HPS 尚无公认的药物治疗。近期对索拉非尼等新药的评估未显示出明显的病情改善。肝移植可逆转大多数患者的 HPS，是治疗的唯一选择。能否使用 TIPS 治疗 HPS 尚无定论。

预后

HPS 患者在 2.5 年内的死亡率高达 40%。

门静脉高压性肺动脉高压

PoPH 的定义为在门静脉高压的情况下出现肺动脉高压。

诊断和病理学

PoPH 的诊断完全基于右心导管检查。诊断标准包括：在门静脉高压和（或）肝脏疾病的情况下，静息时平均肺动脉压 > 25 mmHg 或运动时 > 30 mmHg，肺毛细血管楔压 < 15 mmHg，肺血管阻力 > 240 达因。根据平均肺动脉压，可将 PoPH 分为轻度（> 25 ~ 35 mmHg）、中度（35 ~ 50 mmHg）和重度（> 50 mmHg）。轻度 PoPH 患者似乎不会增加手术风险；中度 PoPH 患者的术中风险较高，移植前应进行药物治疗；重度 PoPH 通常被视为手术禁忌证。PoPH 的确切机制尚不明确，其组织学特征与肺动脉高压相似。

临床表现

PoPH 最常见的症状是运动时呼吸困难，但许多伴有 PoPH 的肝硬化患者并无症状。

治疗

除了对症治疗（呼吸困难时吸氧、容量超负荷时使用利尿剂）外，PoPH 的药物治疗与肺动脉高压相似。治疗 PoPH 最常用的药物是前列环素（静脉注射、吸入或皮下注射）和口服治疗药物（包括磷酸二酯酶抑制剂和内皮素受体拮抗剂）。

如果 PoPH 为中度且上述治疗有效，可考虑进行肝移植。然而，尚未确定成功的肝移植手术能否可靠地逆转 PoPH。重度 PoPH 是肝移植的禁忌证，因为此时移植相关并发症的发病率和死亡率都很高。在 PORTICO 试验之前，没有针对这些治疗方法的随机临床试验。PORTICO 试验是一项关于内皮素受体拮抗剂马昔腾坦的多中心双盲安慰剂对照试验。结果显示，马昔腾坦可改善肺血管阻力，且无肝毒性。目前多种新药正在研究中。

预后

未经治疗的 PoPH 患者死亡率很高，确诊后平均生存期为 15 个月。美国肺动脉高压疾病早期和长期管理评估登记处（REVEAL）的一项研究显示，PoPH 患者确诊后的 5 年生存率为 40%。

肝细胞癌

流行病学

肝癌是全球男性的第五大癌症，是女性的第七大癌症；肝细胞癌（HCC）是最常见的肝癌类型。在美国，约 90% 的肝癌为 HCC，其余大部分为胆管癌。在世界其他地区，包括撒哈拉以南非洲地区、中国、日本和东南亚地区，HCC 是最常见的恶性肿瘤之一，也是导致死亡的重要原因，尤其是在中年男性中。

病因

HCC 常源于肝硬化，与慢性病毒性肝炎密切相关。研究表明，HBV DNA 可整合到宿主细胞基因组，破坏抑癌基因并激活癌基因。在乙型肝炎高发地区，接种疫苗预防 HBV 感染可降低 HCC 的发生率。对于其他病因（如血色病、酒精性肝病、HCV 感染）所致的肝硬化患者发生 HCC 的确切病理生理学机制，目前仍知之甚少。发生 HCC 的危险因素及其临床表现见表 14.7。

诊断

表 14.8 总结了目前可用于诊断 HCC 的影像学技术及其最常见的表现。部分患者可能需要进行组织活检以确诊，但如果存在特征性的临床和影像学表现，尤其是伴有血清甲胎蛋白（AFP）水平升高时，则不需要组织标本。肝癌早期检测筛查（HES）算法可用于早期识别肝癌，该算法已在美国退伍军人事务部的队列中得到验证。该算法包括患者的年龄、ALT 水平、血小板计数、AFP 水平的当前值及其变化率。与 AFP 单一指标相比，该算法提高了肝硬化患者中肝癌的早期检出率。

分期

尽管目前有多种 HCC 分期系统，但最常用的是巴塞罗那临床肝癌（BCLC）分期系统。

治疗

肝功能代偿良好的肝硬化患者可接受手术切除或肝移植，5 年生存率可达 70%。非手术治疗方案包括经皮乙醇注射、经导管动脉化疗栓塞（TACE）和射频消融。多年来，索拉非尼（一种酪氨酸激酶血管生成抑制剂）是不可切除的 HCC 患者的一线治疗药物。近期又批准了仑伐替尼（作用机制与索拉非尼相同），两种药物均可延长患者的生存期。二线药物也已获得批准，包括瑞戈非尼、卡博替尼和纳武利尤单抗。

预后

病灶广泛、多发和有血管侵犯的患者预后较差，5 年生存率仅为 5% ~ 6%。因此，重点在于预防病毒性肝炎和其他病因导致的肝脏疾病，并通过超声筛查高危人群，如肝硬化患者。

TABLE 14.7 Hepatocellular Carcinoma
Associations
Chronic hepatitis B infection
Chronic hepatitis C infection
Hemochromatosis (with cirrhosis)
Cirrhosis (alcoholic, cryptogenic)
Aflatoxin ingestion, Thorotrast exposure
α_1-Antitrypsin deficiency
Androgen administration
Common Clinical Presentations
Abdominal pain
Abdominal mass
Weight loss
Deterioration of liver function
Unusual Manifestations
Bloody ascites
Tumor emboli (lung)
Jaundice
Hepatic or portal vein obstruction
Metabolic effects
Erythrocytosis
Hypercalcemia
Hypercholesterolemia
Hypoglycemia
Gynecomastia
Feminization
Acquired porphyria
Clinical and Laboratory Findings
Hepatic bruit or friction rub
Serum α-fetoprotein >400 ng/mL

TABLE 14.8 Imaging Characteristics of Hepatocellular Carcinoma
Ultrasonography
Mass lesion with varying echogenicity but usually hypoechoic
Dynamic Computed Tomography
Arterial phase: tumor enhances quickly
Venous phase: quick de-enhancement of tumor relative to parenchyma
Magnetic Resonance Imaging
T1-weighted images: hypointense
T2-weighted images: hyperintense
After gadolinium administration, tumor increases in intensity

VASCULAR DISEASE OF THE LIVER

Disorders of the hepatic vasculature are uncommon and include portal vein thrombosis (PVT), hepatic vein thrombosis (Budd-Chiari syndrome), and veno-occlusive disease. Affected patients usually have portal hypertension with or without associated liver dysfunction, which may mimic the presentation of cirrhosis.

Portal Vein Thrombosis
Definition and Etiology
Thrombosis of the portal vein may develop after blunt abdominal trauma, umbilical vein infection, neonatal sepsis, intra-abdominal inflammatory diseases (e.g., pancreatitis), or hypercoagulable states, and in association with cirrhosis. Myeloproliferative diseases (including polycythemia vera, essential thrombocytosis, and myelofibrosis) are now being recognized as possible causes of PVT. One study observed that as many as 25% to 65% of patients with splanchnic vein thrombosis in the absence of cirrhosis had a myeloproliferative disease. The Janus kinase 2 (JAK2) mutation is a marker for myeloproliferative disease and is often checked in patients with PVT. The disease produces the manifestations of portal hypertension, but the liver histology is usually normal.

Diagnosis
The diagnosis is established by angiography, but noninvasive imaging modalities such as Doppler ultrasonography, computed tomography, and magnetic resonance imaging may reveal thrombus, collateral circulation near the porta hepatis, and splenomegaly. In long-standing PVT, tortuous venous channels develop within the organized clot, leading to cavernous transformation.

Treatment
In acute PVT, thrombolysis may be attempted, but anticoagulation with warfarin remains the mainstay of therapy. In most patients, recanalization of the thrombus occurs within 6 months after initiation of anticoagulation. Recommendations for duration of anticoagulation after an acute event vary and are usually 3 to 6 months. Long-term anticoagulation may be used in cases of chronic thrombosis, especially when associated with hypercoagulable states.

Concern exists that anticoagulation may precipitate hemorrhage from varices that arise as a consequence of portal hypertension; however, studies have not shown an increased risk for variceal bleeding in anticoagulated patients with chronic PVT. In fact, studies suggest a role for prophylactic anticoagulation (enoxaparin) for prevention of PVT and hepatic decompensation in cirrhosis. If variceal hemorrhage occurs, it is best managed with endoscopic obliteration. Prophylaxis with β-blockers to prevent variceal bleeding may decrease the portal pressure, potentially propagating thrombus, and therefore is not usually recommended. If endoscopic treatment fails, surgical management with portosystemic shunting may be attempted, but this approach is often difficult because of the absence of suitable patent vessels. The use of TIPS has also been studied in nonocclusive PVT and may be beneficial in establishing patency of the portal vein for future interventions such as liver transplantation in lieu of anticoagulation only.

Budd-Chiari Syndrome
Definition and Etiology
Occlusion of the major hepatic veins or the inferior vena cava, especially in the intrahepatic and suprahepatic segments, causes Budd-Chiari syndrome. Most cases are associated with hematologic disease (e.g., polycythemia vera, paroxysmal nocturnal hemoglobinuria, essential thrombocytosis, other myeloproliferative disorders), pregnancy, oral contraceptive use, tumors (especially HCC), or other causes of a hypercoagulable state (e.g., factor V Leiden mutation, protein C and S deficiency). Abdominal trauma and congenital webs of the vena cava are also related to Budd-Chiari syndrome. About 20% of cases are idiopathic, but many of these patients prove to have early, subclinical myeloproliferative disease or genetic mutations associated with a hypercoagulable state.

Clinical Presentation
Budd-Chiari syndrome can manifest acutely, possibly in association with acute liver failure, or it can manifest as a subacute or chronic illness. Acute disease produces right upper quadrant abdominal pain, hepatomegaly, ascites, and jaundice, whereas the subacute or chronic form produces primarily portal hypertension. Elevation of serum

表 14.7　肝细胞癌
相关因素 慢性乙型肝炎病毒感染 慢性丙型肝炎病毒感染 血色病（伴肝硬化） 肝硬化（酒精性、隐源性） 接触黄曲霉毒素、使用钍造影剂 α_1-抗胰蛋白酶缺乏症 服用雄激素
常见临床表现 腹痛 腹部肿块 体重减轻 肝功能恶化
少见临床表现 血性腹腔积液 癌栓（肺部） 黄疸 肝静脉或门静脉阻塞 代谢紊乱 红细胞增多症 高钙血症 高胆固醇血症 低血糖 男性乳房发育 男性女性化 获得性卟啉病
临床和实验室检查发现 肝动脉杂音或摩擦音 血清甲胎蛋白 > 400 ng/ml

表 14.8　肝细胞癌的影像学特征
超声 占位性病变，有不同的回声改变，但通常为低回声
动态 CT 动脉期：肿瘤快速强化 静脉期：相对于肝实质，肿瘤强化快速消退
MRI T1 加权像：低信号 T2 加权像：高信号 注射钆造影剂后，肿瘤信号增强

肝血管疾病

肝血管疾病并不常见，包括门静脉血栓形成（PVT）、肝静脉血栓形成（布-加综合征）和肝小静脉闭塞病。受累患者通常有门静脉高压，伴或不伴肝功能异常，可能与肝硬化的表现相似。

门静脉血栓形成

定义和病因

腹部钝性外伤、脐静脉感染、新生儿感染中毒症、腹腔内炎症性疾病（如胰腺炎）、高凝状态及肝硬化均可导致 PVT。骨髓增生性疾病（包括真性红细胞增多症、原发性血小板增多症和骨髓纤维化）也被认为是 PVT 的可能病因。一项研究发现，在没有肝硬化的脾静脉血栓患者中，25%～65% 的患者患有骨髓增生性疾病。*JAK2* 突变是骨髓增生性疾病的标志物，PVT 患者通常需进行检查。PVT 会导致门静脉高压相关表现，但肝组织学通常正常。

诊断

血管造影可确诊 PVT，但多普勒超声检查、CT 和 MRI 等非侵入性成像方法可显示血栓、肝门附近的侧支循环和脾大。PVT 长期存在时，血栓内会形成迂曲的静脉通道，导致门静脉海绵样变。

治疗

急性 PVT 可尝试溶栓治疗，但使用华法林进行抗凝治疗仍然是主要的治疗方法。大多数患者的血栓会在开始抗凝治疗后 6 个月内再通。对急性血栓形成后的抗凝疗程建议各不相同，通常为 3～6 个月。对于慢性血栓，尤其是伴有高凝状态时，可采用长期抗凝治疗。

抗凝治疗可能引发人们对门静脉高压引起的静脉曲张出血的担忧；但研究并未显示接受抗凝治疗的慢性 PVT 患者静脉曲张出血的风险增加。事实上，研究表明，预防性抗凝治疗（依诺肝素）在预防肝硬化患者 PVT 和失代偿方面均有一定作用。如果发生静脉曲张出血，首选内镜治疗。使用 β 受体阻滞剂预防静脉曲张出血可降低门静脉压，但可能会引起血栓扩展，因此通常不建议使用。如果内镜治疗失败，可尝试门体静脉分流术，但由于缺乏合适的通畅血管，该方法难度较大。研究显示，使用 TIPS 治疗非闭塞性 PVT 可能有利于门静脉通畅，以便后续的干预措施（如肝移植），从而取代单纯的抗凝治疗。

布-加综合征

定义和病因

肝主要静脉或下腔静脉闭塞（尤其是肝内段和肝上段闭塞）可导致布-加综合征。大多数病例与血液病（如真性红细胞增多症、阵发性睡眠性血红蛋白尿症、原发性血小板增多症、其他骨髓增生性疾病），妊娠，口服避孕药，肿瘤（尤其是 HCC）或其他导致高凝状态的原因（如因子 V Leiden 突变、蛋白 C 和 S 缺乏）有关。腹部创伤和先天性腔静脉隔膜形成也与布-加综合征有关。约 20% 的布-加综合征为特发性，但其中许多患者被证明存在早期亚临床骨髓增生性疾病或与高凝状态相关的基因突变。

临床表现

布-加综合征可呈急性起病，可能伴有急性肝衰竭，也可表现为亚急性或慢性。急性起病表现为右上腹疼痛、肝大、腹腔积液和黄疸，而亚急性或慢性以门静脉高压为主要表现。患者的血清胆红素和转氨酶

bilirubin and transaminase levels may be mild, but liver function is often poor, with profound hypoalbuminemia and coagulopathy.

Diagnosis

The diagnosis can be established noninvasively with Doppler ultrasonography, which shows decreased or absent hepatic vein blood flow, and computed tomography, which shows delayed or absent contrast filling of the hepatic veins and hypertrophy of the caudate lobe. Magnetic resonance angiography may also demonstrate these findings. Hepatic venography is especially useful if the results of noninvasive imaging are inconclusive. Venography often shows an inability to catheterize and visualize the hepatic veins; the characteristic spider-web pattern of collateral vessels may also be demonstrated, and the inferior vena cava may appear compressed owing to hepatomegaly or an enlarged caudate lobe. On liver biopsy, centrilobular congestion, hemorrhage, and necrosis (nutmeg liver) are seen, with cirrhosis developing in patients with chronic obstruction.

Treatment

Treatment should be individualized and is dependent on the mode and severity of presentation and the potential cause of the disease. Supportive therapy to relieve ascites and edema (e.g., dietary sodium restriction, diuretics) and chronic anticoagulation may be considered for patients with chronic Budd-Chiari syndrome in whom methods to decompress congestion are not feasible. Thrombolysis followed by anticoagulation is most useful in patients with acute forms of the disease. In selected patients (such as those with venous webs or strictures or single-vessel thrombosis), angioplasty with or without stent placement may be used. Decompressive modalities are most useful before the development of cirrhosis and include transjugular intrahepatic portacaval and side-to-side portacaval shunts. In patients with cirrhosis, liver transplantation followed by continued anticoagulation is often considered the best option.

Veno-Occlusive Disease

Definition and Etiology

Hepatic veno-occlusive disease, also called sinusoidal obstruction syndrome, often occurs after cytoreductive therapy and before bone marrow transplantation but may also follow exposure to other drugs or herbal preparations (e.g., azathioprine, pyrrolizidine alkaloids). Endothelial cell injury leads to obstruction at the level of the hepatic venules and the sinusoids.

Clinical Presentation

The disease is characterized by jaundice, painful hepatomegaly, and fluid retention. Clinical manifestations can be rapidly progressive and lead to multiorgan dysfunction and death in 20% to 25% of patients.

Diagnosis

The diagnosis is clinically suspected when weight gain, epigastric or right upper quadrant abdominal pain, and jaundice develop within the first 3 to 4 weeks after bone marrow transplantation. Laboratory abnormalities include hyperbilirubinemia, elevated transaminases, and, in severe cases, profound synthetic dysfunction. Doppler abdominal ultrasonography may reveal ascites, reversal of portal vein flow, and an elevated hepatic artery resistance index. Liver biopsy is diagnostic and is usually obtained with use of the transjugular approach. The advantages of this approach compared with the percutaneous route include the ability to measure the hepatic venous pressure gradient (which is typically elevated in veno-occlusive disease) and a lower incidence of bleeding.

Treatment

Mild forms of the disease may favorably respond to supportive therapy alone. In moderate to severe disease, treatment has been attempted with tissue plasminogen activator and heparin, antithrombin III, prostaglandin E_1, and glutamine plus vitamin E, although the efficacies of these treatments have not been clearly established. Defibrotide (a mixture of porcine-derived single-stranded phosphodiester oligonucleotides) has been evaluated as a potential treatment option for severe veno-occlusive disease; however, evidence for efficacy has been mixed.

LIVER TRANSPLANTATION

MELD Score

The Model for End-stage Liver Disease (MELD) score was originally calculated based on the serum creatinine concentration, prothrombin time (International Normalized Ratio), and bilirubin level and has been used to predict short-term mortality in cirrhosis and to prioritize patients awaiting liver transplantation. However, in 2016 an adjustment was made to the MELD score to include the serum sodium, now commonly referred to as the MELD-Na. The MELD-Na score ranges from 6 to 40. Higher scores are associated with more advanced disease and increased predicted mortality. Patients are typically considered for liver transplantation when the MELD-Na score reaches 15.

Prognosis

Liver transplantation is a highly successful procedure in patients with progressive, advanced, and otherwise untreatable liver disease. Advances in surgical techniques and supportive care, the use of cyclosporine and tacrolimus for immunosuppression, and careful selection of patients have all contributed to the excellent results of liver transplantation. Between 70% and 80% of patients undergoing liver transplantation survive at least 5 years, usually with good quality of life. The most common indication for liver transplantation in the United States is chronic liver disease resulting from alcohol. Other liver diseases for which transplantation is commonly performed include cirrhosis from NAFLD, hepatitis C virus, autoimmune hepatitis, primary biliary cirrhosis, and primary sclerosing cholangitis. Patients with hepatitis B are candidates for liver transplantation if they can be given hepatitis B immunoglobulin or nucleoside analogues to help prevent recurrence. Excellent results have also been obtained in selected patients with acute liver failure (see Chapter 13). Liver transplantation for malignant hepatobiliary disease has been less successful because of recurrent disease in the transplanted liver.

For a deeper discussion on this topic, please see Chapter 144, "Cirrhosis and Its Sequelae," in *Goldman-Cecil Medicine*, 26th Edition.

SUGGESTED READINGS

Angeli Paolo, Garcia-Tsao G, Nadim MK, Parikh CR. News in pathophysiology, definition and classification of hepatorenal syndrome: a step beyond the international Club of ascites (ICA) consensus document, J Hepatol 71(4):811–822, 2019.

Garcia–Tsao G, Abraldes JG, Berzigotti A, Bosch J. Portal hypertensive bleeding in cirrhosis: Risk stratification, diagnosis, and management: 2016 practice guidance by the American Association for the study of liver diseases, Hepatology 65(1):310–335, 2017.

Kamath PS, Kim W: The model for end-stage liver disease (MELD), Hepatology 45:797–805, 2007.

水平轻度升高，但肝功能储备通常较差，多伴有严重低白蛋白血症和凝血功能障碍。

诊断

多普勒超声检查和 CT 可以确诊，前者可显示肝静脉血流减少或消失，后者可显示肝静脉显影延迟或缺失、尾状叶肥大。磁共振血管成像也可显示上述表现。如果上述无创性影像学检查无法确定诊断，肝静脉造影尤其有用。静脉造影通常表现为导管无法通过肝静脉，从而无法观察到肝静脉；也可能显示侧支血管形成所致的特征性蜘蛛网状模式，下腔静脉可能因肝大或尾状叶增大而有受压的征象。肝活检可见小叶中心充血、出血和坏死（槟榔肝），慢性静脉阻塞患者会发展为肝硬化。

治疗

治疗应个体化，取决于发病方式、严重程度和潜在病因。对于不能进行减压治疗缓解肝脏充血的慢性布-加综合征患者，可采用缓解腹腔积液和水肿的支持性治疗（如限盐、使用利尿剂）和长期抗凝治疗。溶栓后再进行抗凝治疗对急性布-加综合征患者最有效。对于特定患者（如存在静脉网状结构或狭窄、单支血管血栓形成），可使用伴或不伴支架置入的血管成形术。减压治疗在肝硬化发生之前最有效，包括 TIPS 和侧-侧门腔静脉分流术。对于肝硬化患者，肝移植后继续进行抗凝治疗通常被认为是最佳选择。

肝小静脉闭塞病

定义和病因

肝小静脉闭塞病又称肝窦阻塞综合征，常发生在减细胞治疗后和骨髓移植前，也可能发生在接触其他药物或草药制剂（如硫唑嘌呤、吡咯烷生物碱）后。内皮细胞损伤可引起肝小静脉和肝窦水平的阻塞。

临床表现

该病以黄疸、痛性肝大和体液潴留为特征。临床表现可迅速进展，且在 20%～25% 的患者中导致多器官功能障碍和死亡。

诊断

若患者在骨髓移植后 3～4 周内出现体重增加、上腹痛或右上腹痛和黄疸，临床应怀疑该病。实验室指标异常包括胆红素水平和转氨酶水平升高，严重者会出现严重的合成功能障碍。腹部多普勒超声检查可发现腹腔积液、门静脉血流逆行和肝动脉阻力指数升高。肝活检具有诊断意义，通常采用经颈静脉肝穿刺获取组织样本。与经皮肝穿刺相比，这种方法的优势在于能够测量肝静脉压力梯度（肝小静脉闭塞时通常会升高），且出血发生率较低。

治疗

轻症患者对单纯支持治疗的反应良好。对于中重度患者，可尝试使用组织型纤溶酶原激活物和肝素、抗凝血酶Ⅲ、前列腺素 E_1、谷氨酰胺联用维生素 E 进行治疗，但这些药物的疗效尚未明确。去纤苷（一种猪源性单链磷酸二酯寡核苷酸混合物）被作为治疗重度肝小静脉闭塞病的潜在方案进行了评估，但其疗效证据参差不齐。

肝移植

MELD 评分

终末期肝病模型（MELD）评分最初是由血清肌酐浓度、凝血酶原时间（国际标准化比值）和胆红素水平计算得出，用于预测肝硬化患者的短期死亡率，并对等待肝移植的患者进行优先排序。然而，在 2016 年对 MELD 评分进行了调整，纳入了血清钠，目前常被称为 MELD-Na。MELD-Na 评分的范围为 6～40 分。分数越高提示疾病越晚期，预测死亡率越高。当 MELD-Na 评分达到 15 分时，通常考虑对患者进行肝移植。

预后

对于进展性、晚期和无法用其他方法治疗的肝脏疾病患者，肝移植是非常成功的治疗方法。外科技术和支持性治疗的进步、免疫抑制剂（如环孢素和他克莫司）的使用，以及谨慎的患者选择，都是肝移植取得良好效果的原因。70%～80% 接受肝移植的患者至少能存活 5 年，通常生活质量良好。在美国，肝移植最常见的适应证是酒精导致的慢性肝病。其他常见的肝脏疾病包括 NAFLD、丙型肝炎、自身免疫性肝炎、原发性胆汁性肝硬化和原发性硬化性胆管炎导致的肝硬化。乙型肝炎患者如果能通过接受乙型肝炎免疫球蛋白或核苷类似物来预防复发，即可作为肝移植候选人。经过筛选的急性肝衰竭患者接受肝移植后也可获得很好的治疗效果（见第 13 章）。肝移植治疗肝胆恶性疾病的成功率较低，因为这些疾病会在移植肝内复发。

有关此专题的深入讨论，请参阅 *Goldman-Cecil Medicine* 第 26 版第 144 章"肝硬化及其并发症"。

推荐阅读

Angeli Paolo, Garcia-Tsao G, Nadim MK, Parikh CR. News in pathophysiology, definition and classification of hepatorenal syndrome: a step beyond the international Club of ascites (ICA) consensus document, J Hepatol 71(4):811–822, 2019.

Garcia–Tsao G, Abraldes JG, Berzigotti A, Bosch J. Portal hypertensive bleeding in cirrhosis: Risk stratification, diagnosis, and management: 2016 practice guidance by the American Association for the study of liver diseases, Hepatology 65(1):310–335, 2017.

Kamath PS, Kim W: The model for end-stage liver disease (MELD), Hepatology 45:797–805, 2007.

Kim WR, Biggins SW, Kremers WK, et al: Hyponatremia and mortality among patients on the liver-transplant waiting list, N Engl J Med 359(10):1018–1026, 2008.

Krowka MJ, Miller DP, Barst RJ, et al: Portopulmonary hypertension: a report from the US-based REVEAL registry, Chest 141:906–915, 2012.

Runyon BA: Management of adult patients with ascites due to cirrhosis: update 2012, AASLD Practice Guideline, AASLD 3(1):5–8, 2012.

Valla DC: Thrombosis and anticoagulation in liver disease, Hepatology 47:1384–1393, 2008.

Villa E, Cammà C, Marietta M, et al: Enoxaparin prevents portal vein thrombosis and liver decompensation in patients with advanced cirrhosis, Gastroenterology 143:1253–1260, 2012.

Kim WR, Biggins SW, Kremers WK, et al: Hyponatremia and mortality among patients on the liver-transplant waiting list, N Engl J Med 359(10):1018–1026, 2008.

Krowka MJ, Miller DP, Barst RJ, et al: Portopulmonary hypertension: a report from the US-based REVEAL registry, Chest 141:906–915, 2012.

Runyon BA: Management of adult patients with ascites due to cirrhosis: update 2012, AASLD Practice Guideline, AASLD 3(1):5–8, 2012.

Valla DC: Thrombosis and anticoagulation in liver disease, Hepatology 47:1384–1393, 2008.

Villa E, Cammà C, Marietta M, et al: Enoxaparin prevents portal vein thrombosis and liver decompensation in patients with advanced cirrhosis, Gastroenterology 143:1253–1260, 2012.

15

Disorders of the Gallbladder and Biliary Tract

Stacie A. F. Vela, Michael B. Fallon

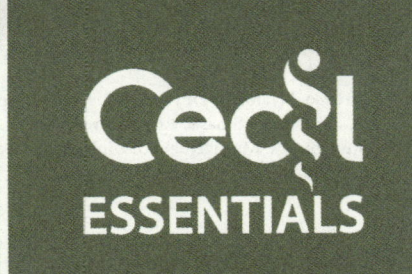

INTRODUCTION

The gallbladder and biliary tract transport bile from the liver into the intestines, a process central to digestion of fat and absorption of lipids and fat-soluble vitamins. Gallbladder and biliary tract diseases are among the most common and costly of all digestive disorders. This chapter examines the principal gallbladder and biliary tract disorders, focusing on cholelithiasis. The reader is referred to Chapter 11 for a detailed discussion of bilirubin metabolism and the diagnostic approach to jaundice and to Chapter 5 for a review of the various imaging techniques used to study the biliary tract.

NORMAL BILIARY ANATOMY AND PHYSIOLOGY

Fig. 15.1 outlines the basic anatomy of the liver and biliary tract. The liver produces 500 to 1500 mL of bile per day. The secretory product of individual hepatocytes contains bile acids, phospholipids, and cholesterol, which are transported across the apical membrane and into the canalicular space between cells. These canaliculi merge to form larger intrahepatic bile ducts and then the common hepatic duct. During fasting, tonic contractions of the sphincter of Oddi, located in the region of the ampulla of Vater, divert about one half of the bile through the cystic duct into the gallbladder, where it is stored and concentrated by water resorption. Cholecystokinin, which is released after food enters the small intestine, causes the sphincter of Oddi to relax, allowing delivery of a timed bolus of bile into the intestine. Bile acids are present in millimolar concentrations. They are detergent molecules that possess both fat-soluble and water-soluble moieties. Cholesterol is secreted by the liver to the intestine, where it undergoes fecal excretion. In the intestinal lumen, bile acids solubilize dietary fat and promote its digestion and absorption. Bile acids are, for the most part, efficiently reabsorbed by the small intestinal mucosa, particularly in the terminal ileum. They are then recycled to the liver for re-excretion, a process termed *enterohepatic circulation*.

GALLBLADDER DISORDERS

Gallstones (Cholelithiasis)

Gallstone formation constitutes a significant health problem, affecting 10% to 15% of the adult population. Complications from gallstones are a leading cause for hospital admissions related to gastrointestinal problems. In the United States, gallstone disease leads to more than 750,000 cholecystectomies annually, making this the most common elective abdominal surgery, with estimated costs of $6.5 billion per year. Gallstones are of two types: 75% are made of cholesterol, and 25% are pigmented stones (black or brown). The latter are composed of calcium bilirubinate and other calcium salts. The risk factors for cholelithiasis are shown in Table 15.1.

Pathogenesis of Cholelithiasis

The three main factors that lead to cholesterol gallstone formation are cholesterol supersaturation of bile, nucleation, and gallbladder hypomotility. These are influenced by both genetic background and intestinal factors (Fig. 15.2).

The liver is the most important organ in regulating total-body cholesterol stores. Once it is secreted, cholesterol, which is insoluble in water, is solubilized in bile through the formation of mixed micelles with bile acids and phospholipids. In most individuals, there is more cholesterol in bile than can be maintained in stable solution. This is even more pronounced in the setting of insulin resistance. As bile becomes supersaturated, microscopic cholesterol molecules aggregate into coalescent vesicles that crystallize, a process referred to as *nucleation*. The gradual deposition of additional layers of cholesterol leads to the appearance of macroscopic stones. Factors that influence nucleation include bile transit time, gallbladder contraction, bile composition (concentrations of cholesterol, phospholipids, and bile salts), and presence of bacteria, mucin, and glycoproteins, which can act as a nidus to initiate cholesterol crystal formation. The interplay between *pronucleating* and *antinucleating* factors in the gallbladder may determine whether cholesterol gallstones will form from supersaturated bile. Gallbladder sludge is a super-concentrated mixture of bile acids, bilirubin, cholesterol, mucus, and proteins that exhibits various degrees of fluidity and is prone to precipitate into a semisolid or solid form.

The pathophysiologic factors leading to pigment stone formation are less well understood; however, increased production of bilirubin conjugates (hemolytic states), increased biliary calcium (Ca^{2+}) and bicarbonate (HCO^-_3) levels, cirrhosis, and bacterial deconjugation of bilirubin to a less soluble form are all associated with pigment stone formation. Black pigment stones, which are composed primarily of calcium bilirubinate, are formed in sterile bile in the gallbladder and are common in chronic hemolytic states, in cases of cirrhosis, and in patients with ileal resection. Their brown pigment counterparts, composed primarily of calcium salts, are formed in the bile ducts and are seen in the setting of infection of the biliary tract.

Many of the recognized predisposing factors for cholelithiasis and gallbladder sludge can be understood in terms of the pathophysiologic scheme outlined previously:

1. Biliary cholesterol saturation is increased by insulin resistance, estrogens, multiparity, oral contraceptives, obesity, rapid weight loss, and terminal ileal disease, which decreases the bile acid pool.
2. Nucleation is enhanced by biliary parasites, recurrent bacterial infection of the biliary tract, altered intestinal microbiome, and antibiotics such as ceftriaxone, which has a proclivity to concentrate and crystallize with calcium in the biliary tree. Total parenteral nutrition and blood transfusions also promote bile pigment accumulation and *gelfaction* of sludge.

胆囊和胆道疾病

单姗　张冠华　译　王宇　尤红　审校　贾继东　通审

引言

胆囊和胆道将胆汁从肝脏输送到肠道，这一过程对脂肪的消化和脂类及脂溶性维生素的吸收至关重要。胆囊和胆道疾病是最常见、医疗费用最高的消化系统疾病之一。本章将介绍主要的胆囊和胆道疾病，重点关注胆石症。关于胆红素代谢和黄疸的诊断方法请见第11章；关于针对胆道的各种成像技术请见第5章。

正常解剖学和生理学

图15.1概括了肝脏和胆道的基本解剖结构。肝脏每天产生500～1500 ml胆汁。肝细胞分泌胆汁酸、磷脂和胆固醇，这些物质通过顶部细胞膜转运至细胞间的毛细胆管。毛细胆管汇合形成较大的肝内胆管，进一步汇合成肝总管。空腹时，位于肝胰壶腹的Oddi括约肌处于收缩状态，使得约1/2的胆汁通过胆囊管进入胆囊，并在其中储存和浓缩。当食物进入小肠后，胆囊收缩素被释放，引起Oddi括约肌松弛，从而定时将胆汁送入小肠。胆汁酸的浓度为毫摩尔级，它们是具有脂溶性和水溶性部分的去污分子。肝脏分泌的胆固醇进入肠道，随粪便排出。在肠道中，胆汁酸溶解食物中的脂肪，促进其消化和吸收。大部分胆汁酸被小肠黏膜（特别是末段回肠）重吸收，从而被运回肝脏，然后重新分泌至小肠，这一过程称为胆汁酸的肠肝循环。

胆囊疾病

胆石症（胆囊结石）

胆石症是一个重要的健康问题，可见于10%～15%的成人造。胆石症引起的并发症是因胃肠疾病住院的主要原因。在美国，每年有超过750 000名患者因胆石症而接受胆囊切除术，使该手术成为最常用的腹部择期手术，每年产生的医疗费用约65亿美元。胆石症有两种类型：75%为胆固醇结石，25%是胆色素结石（黑色或棕色）。后者由胆红素钙和其他钙盐组成。胆石症的危险因素见表15.1。

发病机制

胆固醇结石形成的3个主要因素为胆汁中胆固醇过度饱和、成核和胆囊排空障碍，这些因素同时受遗传背景和肠道因素的影响（图15.2）。

肝脏是调节全身胆固醇储存最重要的器官。不溶于水的胆固醇一旦被分泌，就会通过与胆汁酸和磷脂形成微粒而溶解于胆汁中。在大多数个体中，胆汁中的胆固醇含量高于血液中的含量，这种情况在合并胰岛素抵抗时尤为明显。当胆汁中的胆固醇过饱和时，胆固醇分子聚集成聚结囊泡并结晶，这一过程被称为成核。胆固醇逐渐沉积，形成肉眼可见的结石。影响成核的因素包括胆汁转运时间，胆囊收缩功能，胆汁成分（胆固醇、磷脂和胆盐的浓度），以及细菌、黏蛋白和糖蛋白，这些物质可作为促成核因子参与胆固醇晶体的形成。胆囊内促进成核和抑制成核的因素之间的相互作用可能决定了过饱和的胆汁是否会形成胆固醇结石。胆泥是由胆汁酸、胆红素、胆固醇、黏液和蛋白质组成的超浓缩混合物，具有不同程度的流动性，易沉淀为半固体或固体。

胆色素结石形成的病理生理学因素尚不完全清楚；但是，胆红素轭合物增加（溶血状态）、胆汁中钙离子（Ca^{2+}）和碳酸氢盐（HCO_3^-）浓度增加、肝硬化、细菌将胆红素分解为难溶解形式均与胆色素结石形成有关。黑色素结石（主要由胆红素钙组成）在胆囊中的无菌性胆汁中形成，常见于慢性溶血状态、肝硬化和回肠切除后的患者。棕色结石（主要由钙盐组成）常见于胆道感染。

许多已知的诱发因素可通过上述病理生理学机制促进胆石症和胆泥的形成：

1. 胰岛素抵抗、雌激素、经产、口服避孕药、肥胖症、快速减重和末端回肠疾病可使胆汁酸减少，从而使胆汁中胆固醇饱和度增加。

2. 胆道寄生虫、胆道反复细菌感染、肠道微生物群改变、抗生素（如头孢曲松，易在胆道系统浓缩并与钙形成结晶）均具有促进成核的作用。全肠外营养和输血也会促进胆色素和胆泥的沉积。

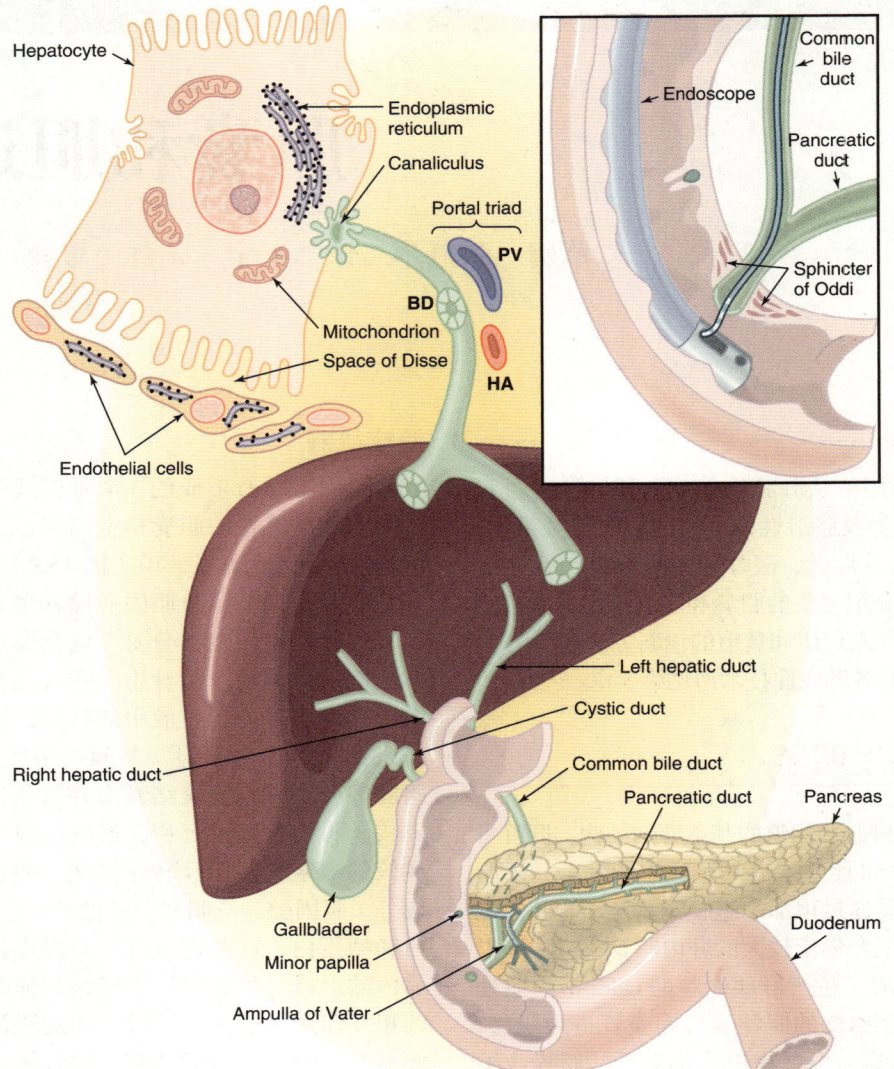

Fig. 15.1 Normal anatomy and histology of the liver and biliary tract. Materials destined for metabolism or excretion by the liver (such as unconjugated bilirubin) enter the sinusoidal bed and cross the endothelial barrier and the space of Disse. Unconjugated bilirubin is taken up by the hepatocyte, conjugated with glucuronide to become water soluble, and excreted into bile across the canalicular membrane of the hepatocyte. The canaliculi empty into bile ductules (BD), which lead to the interlobular (small), septal (medium), and large intrahepatic bile ducts and finally to the main branches of the common bile duct. The portal areas, or portal triads, are composed mainly of portal vein (PV), hepatic artery (HA), and BD branches. During fasting, tonic contraction of the sphincter of Oddi, located in the region of the ampulla of Vater, diverts about one half of the bile through the cystic duct into the gallbladder, where it is stored and concentrated to be released later during meal times. Disease at any level of the biliary tree can lead to cholestasis and obstructive jaundice. The *inset* shows an endoscopic retrograde cholangiopancreatography procedure. See Figs. 15.5, 15.6, and 15.7 for radiographic depictions in specific biliary tract disorders.

3. Bile stasis is caused by gallbladder hypomotility (resulting from pregnancy, somatostatin, or fasting), bile duct strictures, choledochal cysts, biliary parasites, and total parenteral nutrition.

Clinical Manifestations of Gallstones

Gallstones develop at some point in 10% to 20% of Americans. Between 50% and 60% of these individuals remain asymptomatic, but about one third develop biliary colic or chronic cholecystitis, and 15% develop acute complications. The natural history of gallstone disease is outlined in Fig. 15.3. Obstruction of the biliary tract at any level by stones or sludge is the underlying cause of the clinical manifestations of gallstone disease. Obstruction by gallstones can occur at the level of the cystic duct, common hepatic duct, common bile duct, or ampulla of Vater (see Figs. 15.1 and 15.3). Symptoms arise from contraction of the gallbladder during transient obstruction of the cystic duct by gallstones, and persistent obstruction of the cystic duct leads to superimposed inflammation or infection of the gallbladder (i.e., acute cholecystitis). Obstruction of the distal common bile duct may result

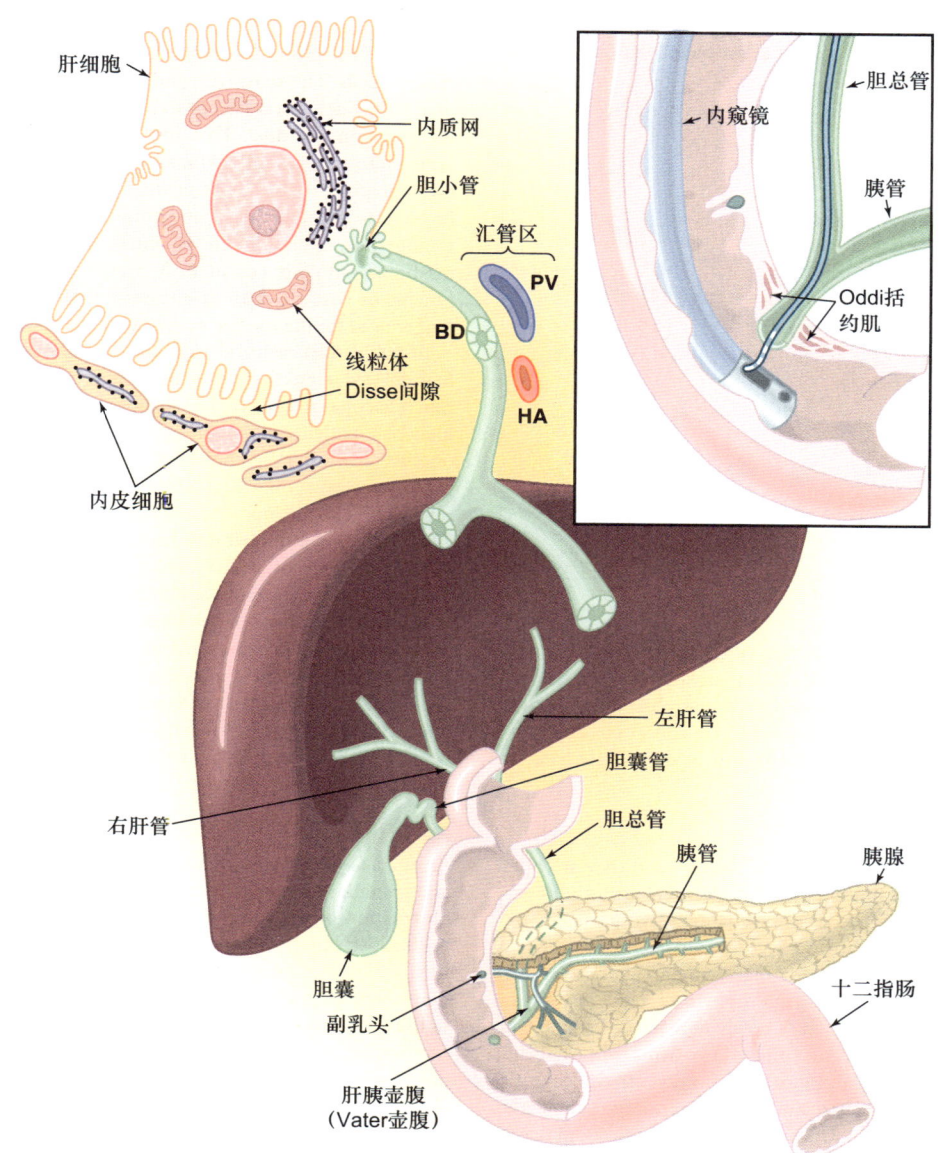

图 15.1　肝脏和胆道系统的正常解剖和组织学结构。肝脏代谢或分泌的物质（如非结合胆红素）进入肝窦间隙，穿过内皮屏障和 Disse 间隙。非结合胆红素被肝细胞摄取，与葡萄糖醛酸结合成水溶性物质，并通过肝细胞的胆小管膜分泌到胆汁中，进入小叶内胆管（BD）、小叶间胆管（小胆管）、隔胆管（中等胆管）和肝内大胆管，最后进入胆总管的大分支。门静脉区或汇管区主要由门静脉（PV）、肝动脉（HA）和胆管分支组成。在空腹期间，位于肝胰壶腹（Vater 壶腹）区的 Oddi 括约肌持续收缩，使得约 1/2 的胆汁通过胆囊管进入胆囊，胆囊储存并浓缩胆汁，并在进餐时分泌。胆道系统任何部位的疾病都可能导致胆汁淤积和梗阻性黄疸。右上角插图展示了内镜逆行胰胆管造影（ERCP）过程的示意图。胆道疾病的影像学图像请参见图 15.5、图 15.6 和图 15.7

3.胆汁淤积可由胆囊排空障碍（由妊娠、生长抑素或禁食导致），胆管狭窄，胆总管囊肿，胆道寄生虫和全肠外营养引起。

临床表现

10%～20% 的美国人患有胆石症，其中 50%～60% 的患者没有症状，约 1/3 的患者会出现胆绞痛或慢性胆囊炎，15% 会出现急性并发症。胆石症的自然病程见图 15.3。结石或胆泥引起的任何胆道水平的梗阻是导致胆石症临床表现的根本原因。结石可在胆囊管、肝总管、胆总管或肝胰壶腹（Vater 壶腹）处引发阻塞（图 15.1 和图 15.3）。当结石暂时阻塞胆囊管时，可因胆囊收缩而引发临床症状；当结石持续阻塞胆囊管时，可导致胆囊炎症或感染（即急性胆囊炎）。胆总管

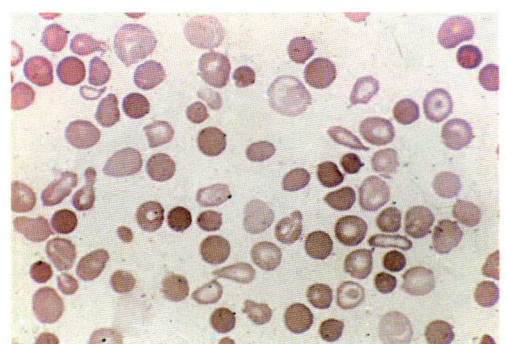
彩图 4-5　MDS—RA 血象

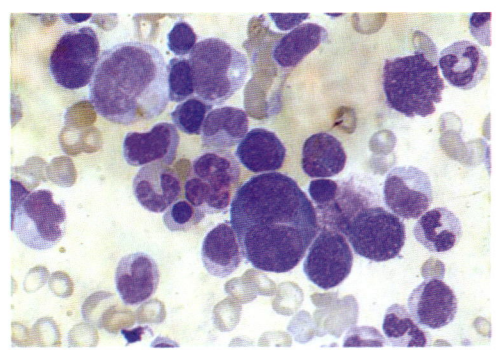
彩图 4-6　MDS—RAS 骨髓象

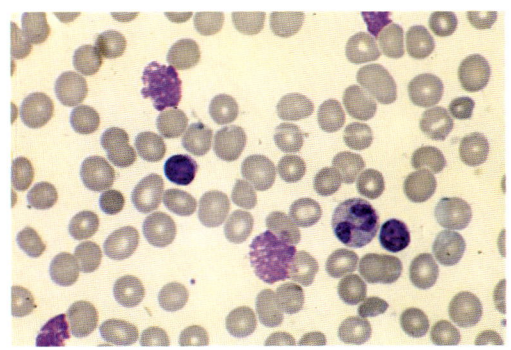
彩图 4-7　CLL 血象

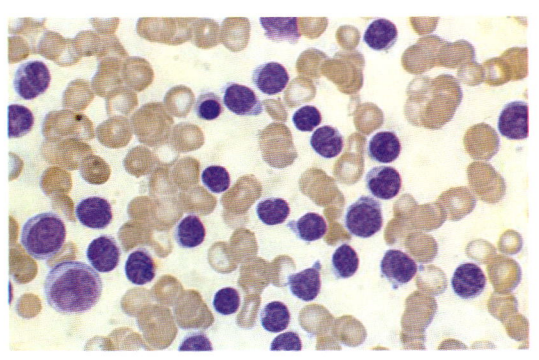
彩图 4-8　CLL 骨髓象

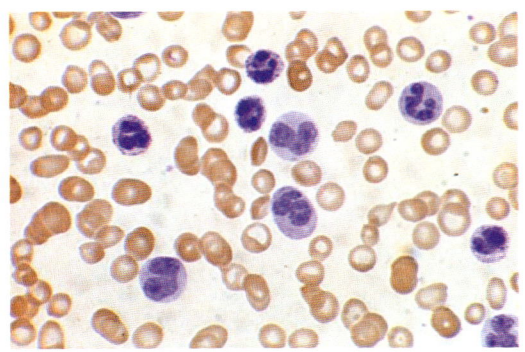
彩图 4-9　CML 血象

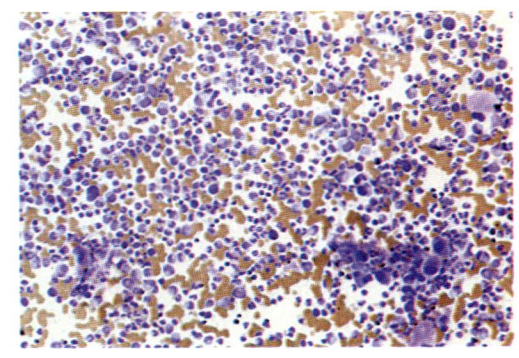
彩图 4-10　CML 骨髓象

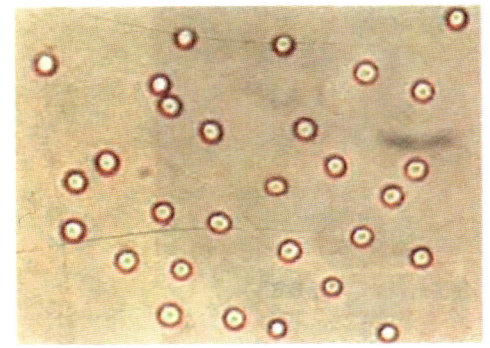
彩图 6-1　尿沉渣直接涂片（未染色，×400）：尿红细胞

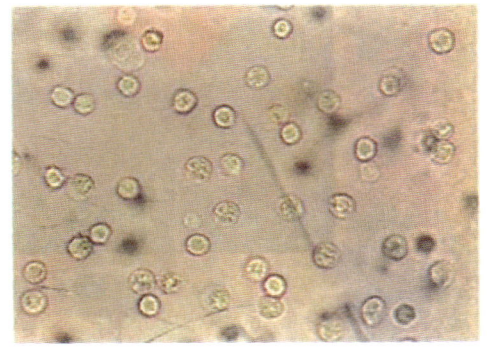
彩图 6-2　尿沉渣直接涂片（未染色，×400）：尿白细胞

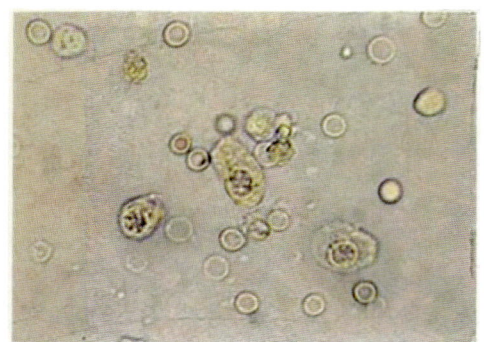

彩图 6-3　尿沉渣直接涂片（未染色，×400）：肾小管上皮细胞

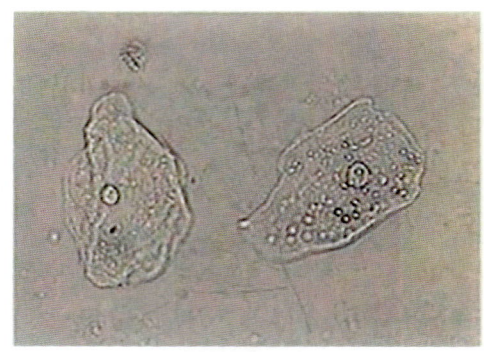

彩图 6-4　尿沉渣直接涂片（未染色，×400）：鳞状上皮细胞（扁平上皮细胞）

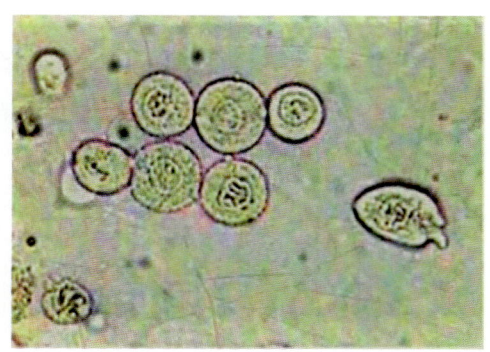

彩图 6-5　尿沉渣直接涂片（未染色，×400）：小圆形上皮细胞

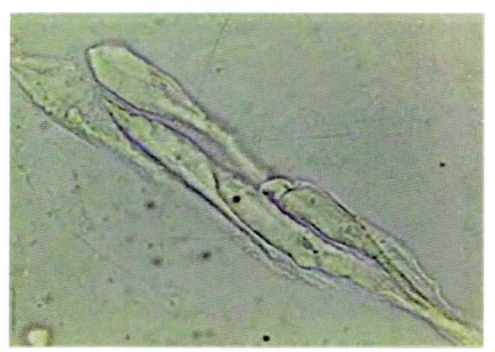

彩图 6-6　尿沉渣直接涂片（未染色，×400）：尾形上皮细胞

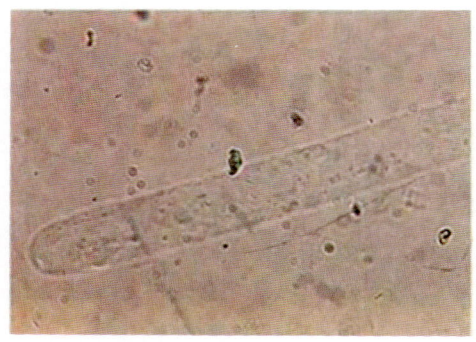

彩图 6-7　尿沉渣直接涂片（未染色，×400）：透明管型

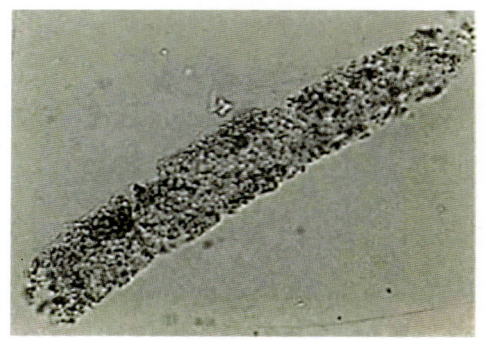

彩图 6-8　尿沉渣直接涂片（未染色，×400）：颗粒管型

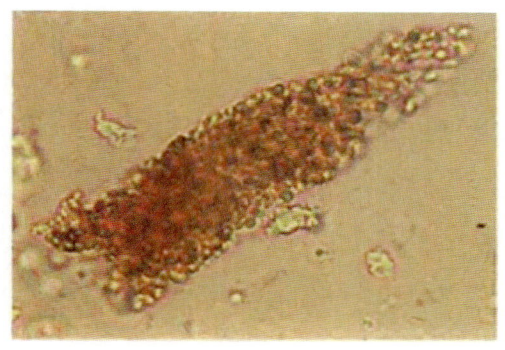

彩图 6-9　尿沉渣直接涂片（未染色，×400）：红细胞管型

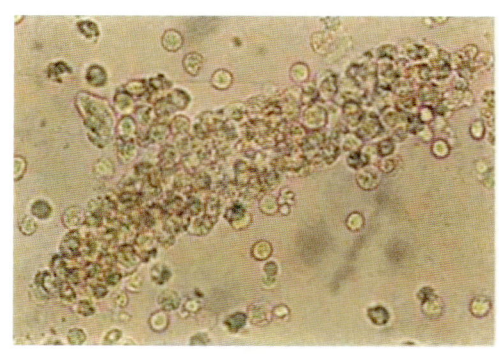

彩图 6-10　尿沉渣直接涂片（未染色，×400）：白细胞管型

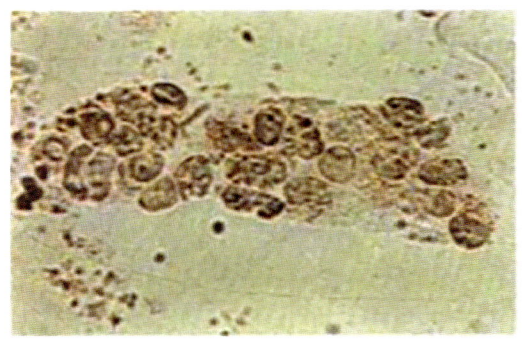

彩图 6-11　尿沉渣直接涂片（未染色，×400）：上皮细胞管型

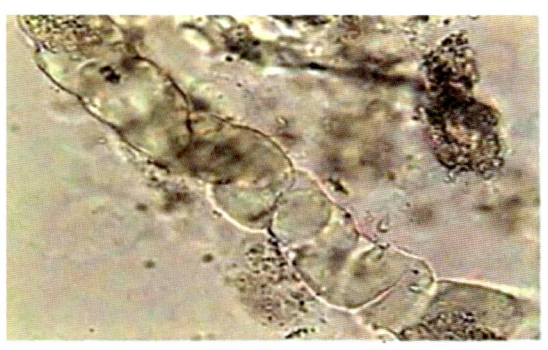

彩图 6-12　尿沉渣直接涂片（未染色，×400）：蜡样管型

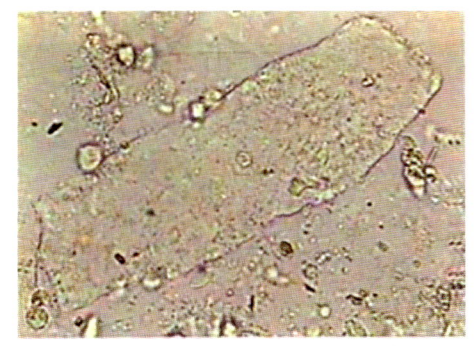

彩图 6-13　尿沉渣直接涂片（未染色，×400）：肾衰竭管型

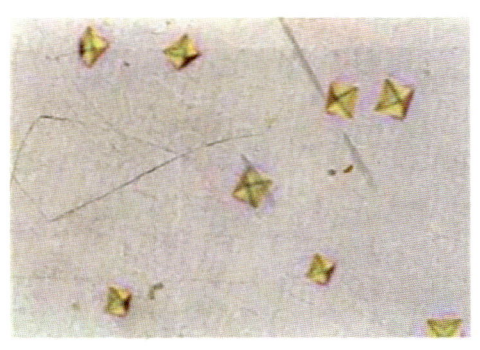

彩图 6-14　尿沉渣直接涂片（未染色，×400）：草酸钙结晶

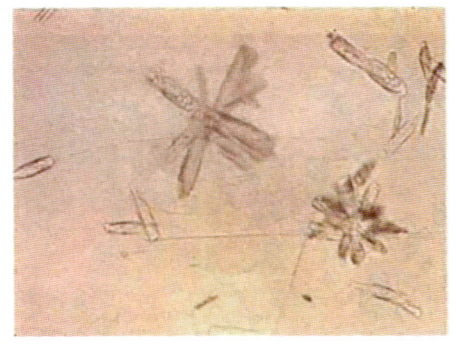

彩图 6-15　尿沉渣直接涂片（未染色，×400）：碳酸钙结晶

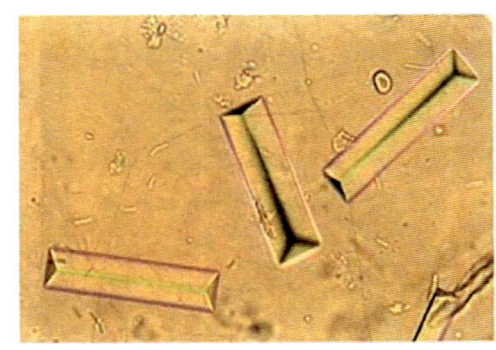

彩图 6-16　尿沉渣直接涂片（未染色，×400）：磷酸盐结晶

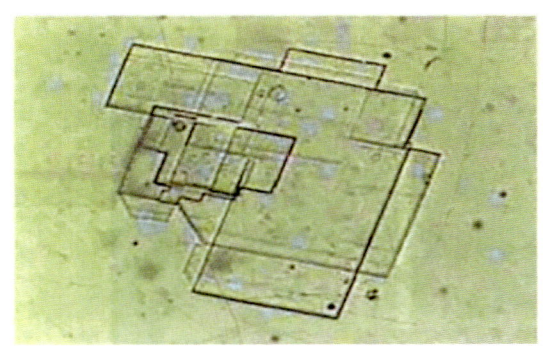

彩图 6-17　尿沉渣直接涂片（未染色，×400）：胆固醇结晶

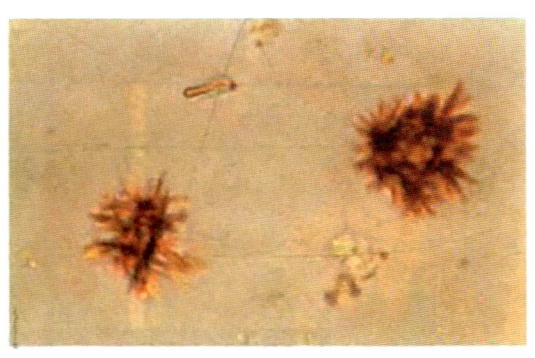

彩图 6-18　尿沉渣直接涂片（未染色，×400）：胆红素结晶

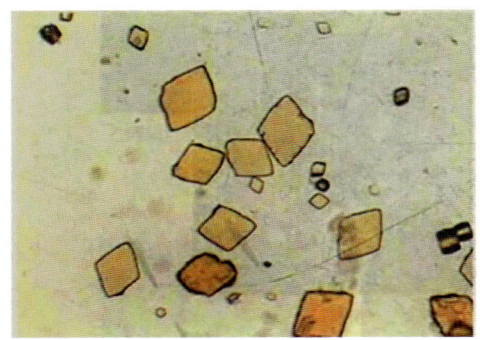
彩图 6-19 尿沉渣直接涂片（未染色，×400）：尿酸结晶

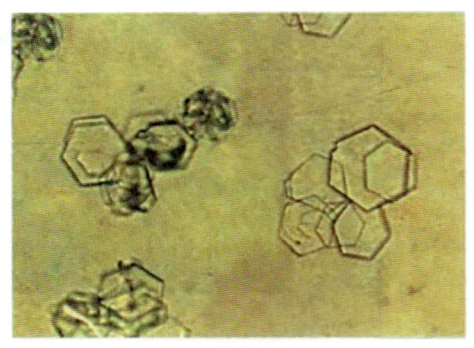
彩图 6-20 尿沉渣直接涂片（未染色，×400）：胱氨酸结晶

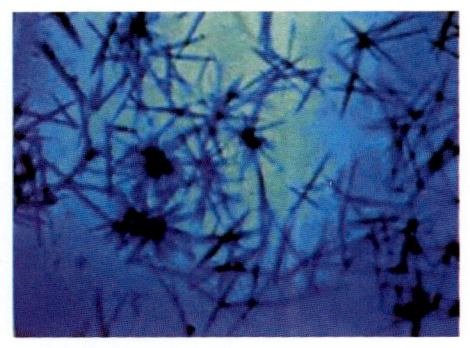
彩图 6-21 尿沉渣直接涂片（未染色，×400）：酪氨酸结晶

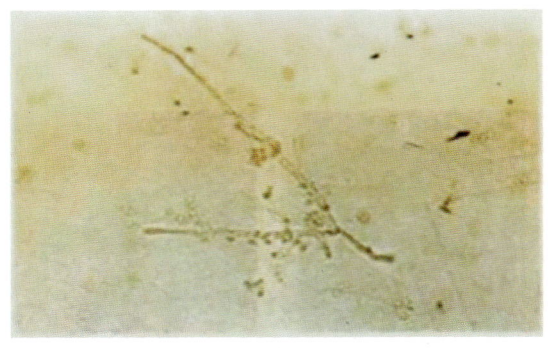
彩图 6-22 尿沉渣直接涂片（未染色，×400）：尿液中的真菌

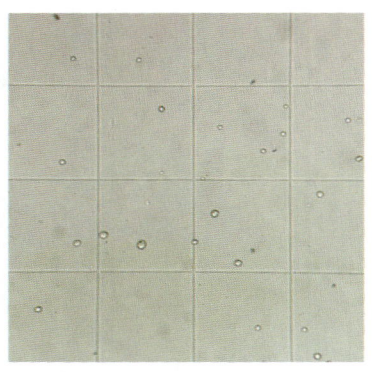
彩图 8-2 白细胞稀释计数

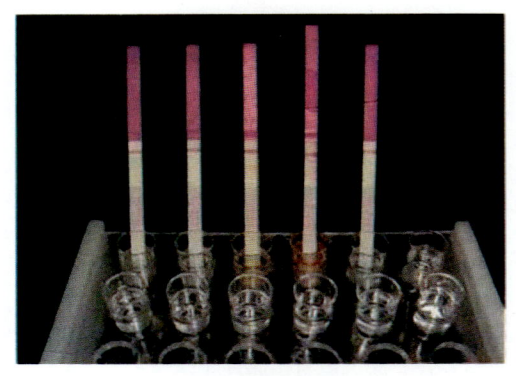
彩图 8-3 粪便隐血试验结果判断

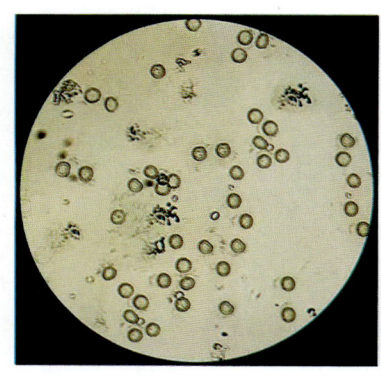
彩图 8-4 粪便中的红细胞

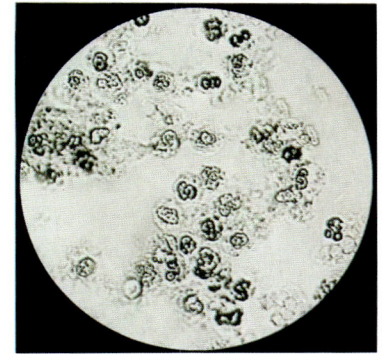 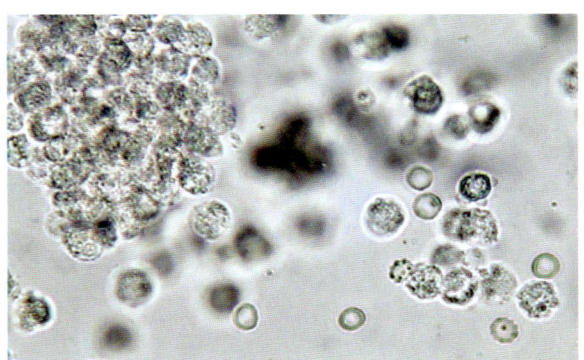

彩图 8-5　粪便中的白细胞

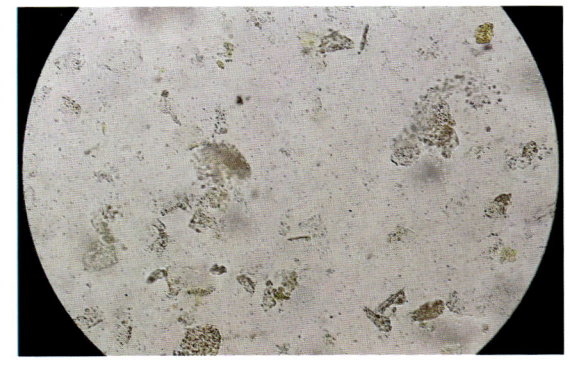 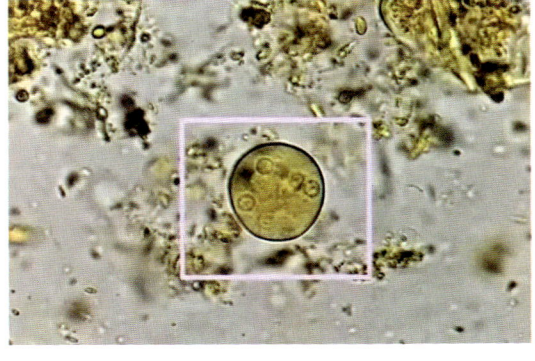

彩图 8-6　粪便中的上皮细胞　　　　　彩图 8-7　粪便中的巨噬细胞

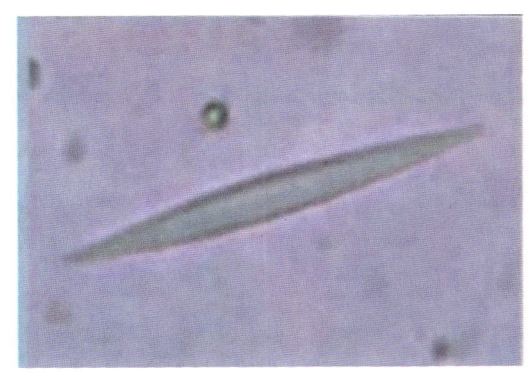 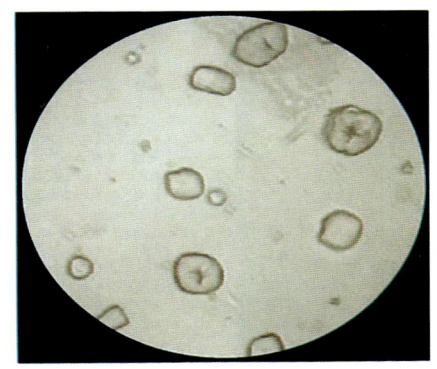

彩图 8-8　粪便中的夏科 - 莱登结晶　　　彩图 8-9　粪便中的淀粉颗粒

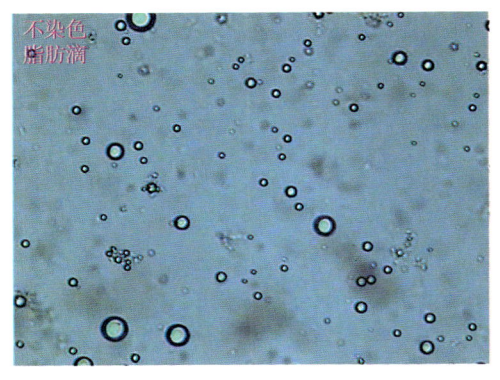 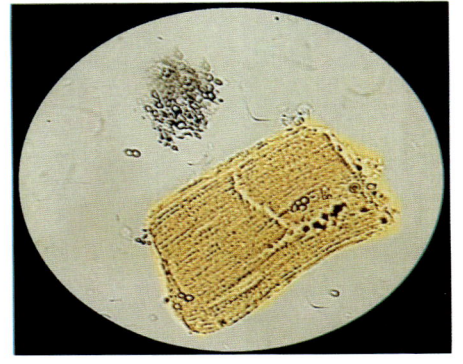

彩图 8-10　粪便中的脂肪小滴　　　　彩图 8-11　粪便中的肌肉纤维

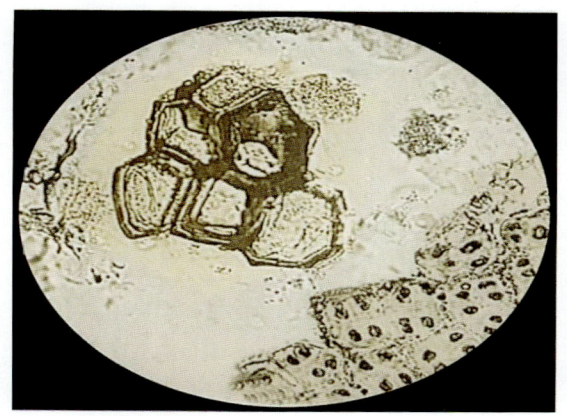
彩图 8-12 粪便中的植物细胞

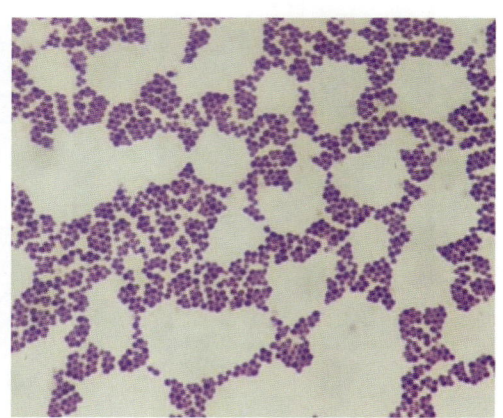
彩图 11-4 葡萄球菌

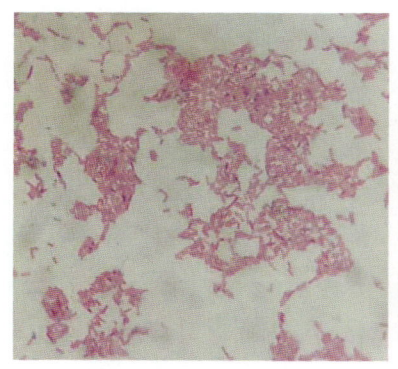
彩图 11-5 大肠埃希菌

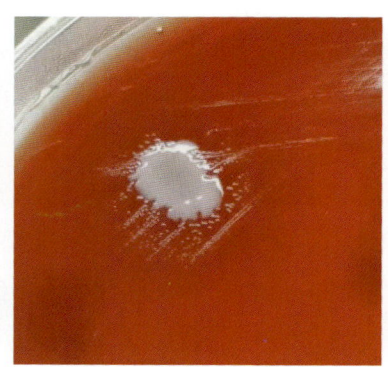
彩图 11-10 卫星现象（+）

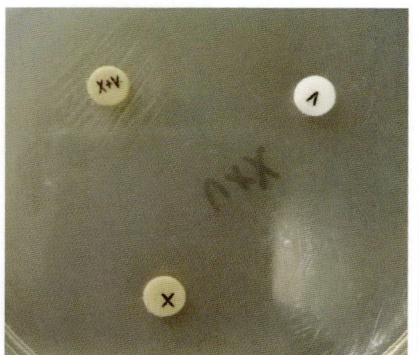
彩图 11-11 流感嗜血杆菌 V、X 因子试验

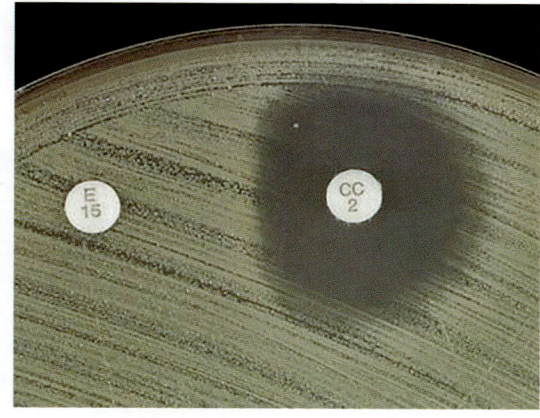
彩图 11-12 "D 试验"阳性结果

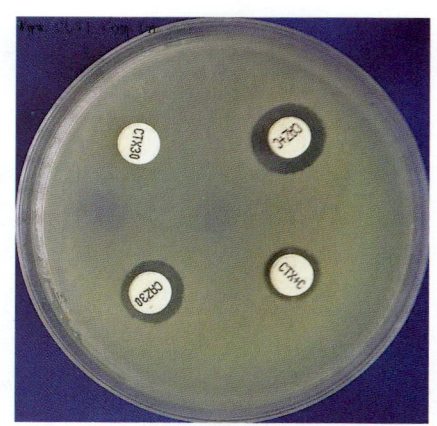
彩图 11-13 ESBLs（阳性菌株）CAZ+C 比 CAZ 环>5 mm

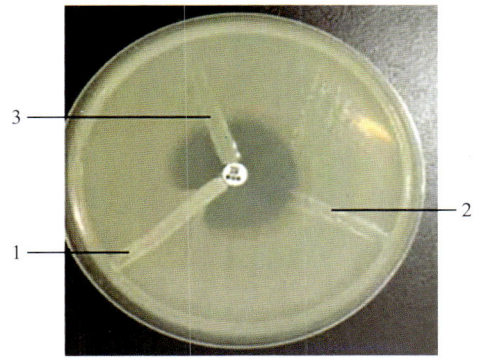

彩图 11-14　改良 Hodge 试验图

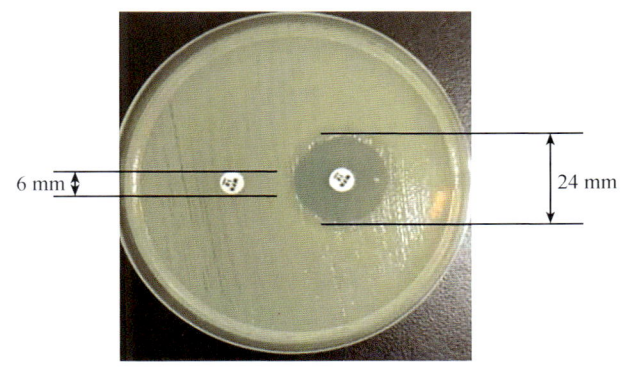

彩图 11-15　mCIM 和 eCIM 试验图

左：mCIM 试验（抑菌圈直径为 6 mm，箭头为两直线间的垂直距离）；右：eCIM 试验（抑菌圈直径 24 mm，箭头为两直线间的垂直距离）。实验结果：mCIM 试验阳性，eCIM 试验阳性，抑菌圈直径之差为 18 mm

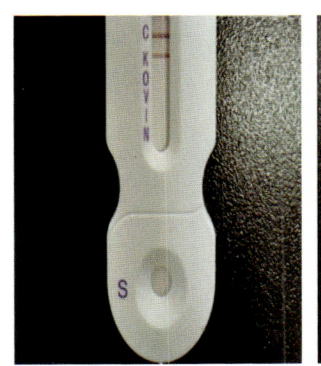
1. KPC 型

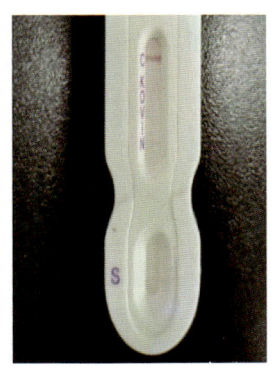
2. NDM 型

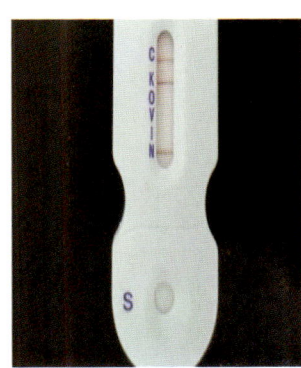
3. KPC+NDM 型

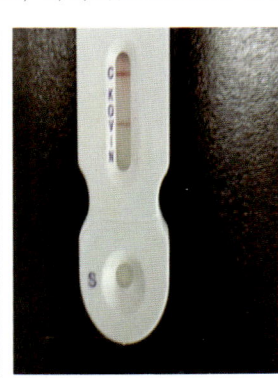
4. VIM 型

彩图 11-16　常见碳青霉烯酶基因型

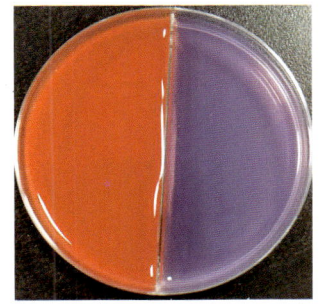

A. 血琼脂平板和中国蓝琼脂平板

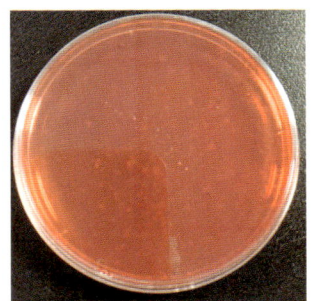

B. SS 琼脂平板

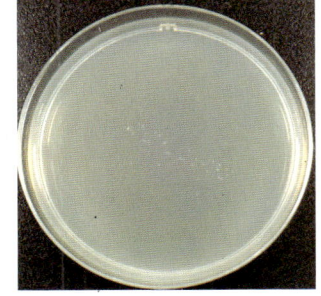

C. 水解酪蛋白（M-H）培养基

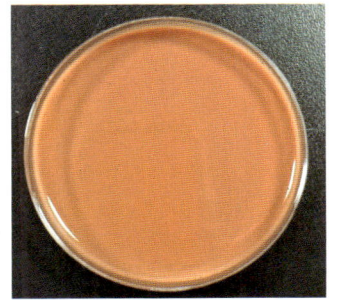

D. 巧克力培养基

彩图 11-17　细菌培养基

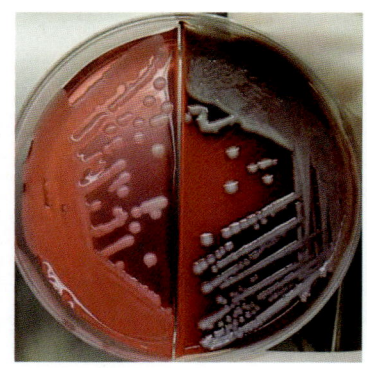
彩图 11-18　黏液型菌落

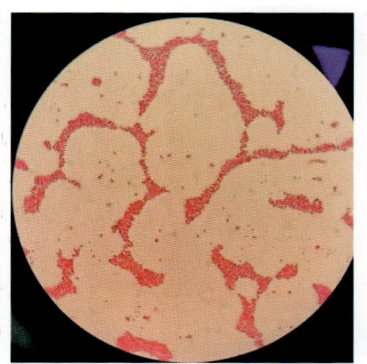
彩图 11-19　菌落涂片

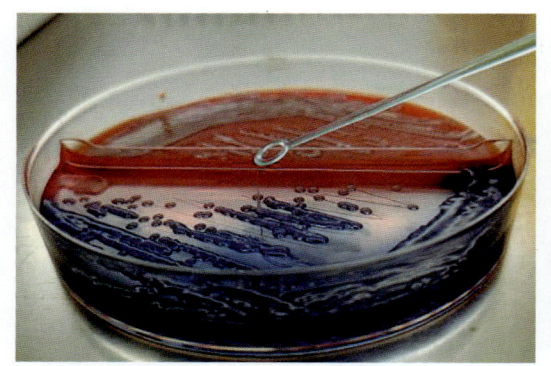
彩图 11-20　菌落黏液丝

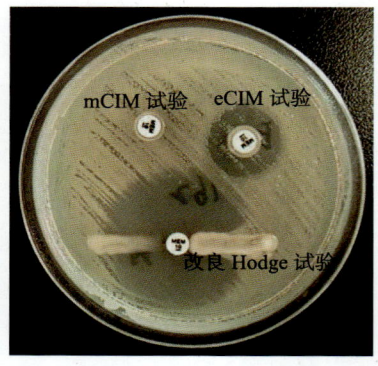
彩图 11-21　碳青霉烯酶检测结果

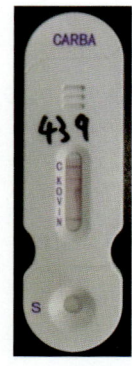
彩图 11-22　复检结果